THE REALITIES
OF AGING

CONTRIBUTING AUTHORS

Ruth E. Dunkle, Ph.D.
Associate Professor of Social Work
The University of Michigan

Eileen S. Metress, Ph.D.
Associate Professor of Health Promotion
The University of Toledo

Seamus P. Metress, Ph.D.
Professor of Anthropology
The University of Toledo

THE REALITIES OF AGING:
AN INTRODUCTION TO GERONTOLOGY

THIRD EDITION

Cary S. Kart
The University of Toledo

Allyn and Bacon
Boston · London · Sydney · Toronto

To the memory of my father

Library of Congress Cataloging-in-Publication Data

Kart, Cary S. (Cary Steven), 1946–
  The realities of aging.

  "Contributing authors: Ruth E. Dunkle, Eileen S.
Metress, Seamus P. Metress."
  Includes index.
  1. Gerontology. I. Dunkle, Ruth E. II. Metress,
Eileen S. III. Metress, Seamus P. IV. Title.
HQ1061.K36 1989 305.26   89-6980
ISBN 0-205-11893-3

Printed in the United States of America

10 9 8 7 6 5 4 3 2 1   95 94 93 92 91 90

Series editor: Karen Hanson
Editorial/production service: Editing, Design and Production, Inc.
Production administrator (in-house): Peter Petraitis
Text designer: Marie McAdam
Cover coordinator: Linda Dickinson
Manufacturing buyer: Tamara McCracken

Photo credits: page 11, H. Armstrong Roberts; page 34, H. Armstrong Roberts; page 47, H. Armstrong Roberts; page 76, H. Armstrong Roberts; page 102, H. Armstrong Roberts; page 119, H. Armstrong Roberts; page 143, © Frank Siteman 1980; page 169, H. Armstrong Roberts; page 198, © Elizabeth Crews/Icon/Stock, Boston, Inc. 1981; page 233, H. Armstrong Roberts; page 256, © Frank Siteman 1983; page 301, H. Armstrong Roberts; page 327, © Jeff Albertson/Stock, Boston, Inc. 1977; page 339, H. Armstrong Roberts; page 366, H. Armstrong Roberts; page 393, © Ulrike Welsch; page 428, H. Armstrong Roberts; page 458, © Frank Siteman 1984; page 473, © Michael Hayman/Stock, Boston, Inc. 1981; page 502, H. Armstrong Roberts.

CONTENTS

CHAPTER 19
DEATH AND DYING   470
Cary S. Kart and Eileen S. Metress

EPILOGUE
CAREERS IN THE AGING NETWORK   494

GLOSSARY   507

INDEX   519

PREFACE

Allyn and Bacon deserves a thank you for providing me with a second opportunity to make substantive and stylistic changes in *Realities*. The field of gerontology continues to grow rapidly, and my efforts in this edition have been aimed at trying to keep pace. This has been a more difficult task than in the past, because gerontology has strengthened its multidisciplinary identity.

A recent survey of gerontology programs carried out by the Association for Gerontology in Higher Education (AGHE) and the University of Southern California (USC) has identified four courses as most commonly offered in gerontological instruction programs in institutions of higher education in the United States. Some describe these four courses as representing a core curriculum in gerontology. The courses are Social Gerontology, Psychology of Aging, Biology and Physiology of Aging, and Sociology of Aging. From my biased perspective, this edition of *Realities* remains the text of choice for an introductory course in gerontology precisely because it has strengths in the sociology of aging, the biology and physiology of aging, and the psychology of aging.

The basic structure of the book has been retained with some alteration from the second edition. Again, Part I introduces the study of aging and consists of three chapters. Chapter 1 discusses ten myths about aging. Chapter 2 defines the field of gerontology, presents a history of aging, and includes updated material on methodological issues current in aging research. Chapter 3 presents the population dynamics and demographic characteristics of the aged, updated to include the most current data. Part II presents material on the biomedical aspects of aging. Chapters 4 and 5 are devoted to the biological aspects of aging. Chapter 6 describes the health status of the elderly population.

Part III places aging in psychological and sociological perspective. Separate chapters are devoted to the psychological aspects of aging (Chapter 7) and to sociological theories of aging (Chapter 9). A new chapter in this part is entitled "Social Aspects of Aging" (Chapter 8). Part IV considers the relationship between the aged and society. Chapter 10 presents material on the family life of older people; Chapters 11, 12, and 13 deal with the economics of aging, work, retirement and leisure, and the politics of aging, respectively. A new chapter in this part deals with the relationship between religion and aging (Chapter 14).

Part V identifies five special issues of concern for older people: the problems of racial and ethnic aging (Chapter 15); living environments (Chapter 16); long-term care (Chapter 17); health policy for the aged in the United States (Chapter 18); and death and dying (Chapter 19). The future of the field and career opportunities are discussed in an epilogue.

New as well as revised chapters from the second edition were read in various stages of development by Ruth Dunkle, Carol Engler, Daniel J. Klenow, William C. Lane, Chuck Longino, Eileen and Seamus Metress, Neil Palmer, and Jill Quadagno. Much of what is good here comes from their collective wisdom. Errors of fact and judgment can only be attributed to the author. Ruth Dunkle and Eileen and Seamus Metress deserve special thanks for the chapters they have contributed to this volume.

The University of Toledo continues to be a productive environment for me. Joyce Rothschild has relieved me of chairmanship duties and carries these out more ably than I ever did. The Department of Sociology, Anthropology, and Social Work has some new faces and a new spirit that make it a more exciting and rewarding place in which to work.

By the time this book appears Michelle will have put up with twenty years of this—and it has not been easy! Through it all she has remained a caring and loving partner in our "business," while at the same time pursuing her own career. I really have been lucky! In the preface to an earlier edition I wrote that Renee is old enough for me to start thinking about her using the third edition in a college course. That time has now come. Jeremy begins his high school career as well. I have reason to be a proud father!

I hope the publication of this book finds Grandma Eleanor in continued good health and spirits; Ina, Charlie, and the girls happy and prosperous; and Grandpa Max and Grandma Sylvia in good health. I am saddened by the recent deaths of my uncles Paul Ortner, Irving Feinstein, and Sam Herman. Each was a good man, devoted to family and friends. I am one among many enriched by their lives. In particular, Uncle Paul deserves special mention. He gave time, energy, and love to all his nieces and nephews; no doubt each felt a special bond with him. Our joys and successes were his, as was our grief. Finally, as with the first two editions of this text, the third edition is formally dedicated to the memory of my father.

PART I

INTRODUCTION TO THE STUDY OF AGING

CHAPTER 1

FIRST THE GOOD NEWS . . . THE MYTHS OF AGING

CHAPTER 2

THE STUDY OF AGING

CHAPTER 3

THE DEMOGRAPHY OF AGING

CHAPTER 1

FIRST THE GOOD NEWS . . . THE MYTHS OF AGING

According to Greek mythology (Hamilton 1942, 428), Aurora, the goddess of the Dawn, was in love with Tithonus, a Trojan. Aurora asked Zeus to make Tithonus immortal, and Zeus agreed, but Aurora did not think to ask Zeus to allow Tithonus to retain his youthfulness. For a while the lovers lived happily, but then the consequences of Aurora's error began to appear. Tithonus's hair turned gray, and soon he could move neither hand nor foot. He prayed for death, but there was no release for him. At last, in pity, Aurora left him alone in his room, locking the door behind her. As the story goes, Tithonus still lies in that room, babbling endlessly.[1]

The legend of Tithonus reflects a number of themes relevant to contemporary life in the United States, not the least of which is the prevalent fear of old age and its concomitant hardships and infirmities. Some see this fear of growing old as the root of a negative attitude toward old age and the tendency on the part of many Americans to avoid the word *old* and to substitute euphemisms such as "golden years." A recent nationwide opinion poll reported that only 2 percent of the public feel that the years between sixty and sixty-nine are "the best years of a person's life"; fewer than one-half of 1 percent feel that way about the seventies. Even among those in the poll who were sixty-five years of age or over themselves, only 8 percent considered the sixties and seventies to be optimal years (NCOA 1976).

Dr. Robert N. Butler, winner of the Pulitzer Prize for his book *Why Survive? Being Old in America*, coined the term *ageism* to describe this negative attitude

---

[1] There is another version of the story that says that Tithonus shrank in size until Aurora, with a feeling for the natural fitness of things, turned him into a skinny and noisy grasshopper (Hamilton 1942, 428).

3

toward aging and the aged. He equates ageism with racism and sexism and defines it as simply "not wanting to have all those ugly old people around" (Butler 1975). Just as racism has generated some unfortunate stereotypes of people in different racial groups, so too has ageism fostered some unfortunate myths about old people and the aging process. Moreover, like racism, ageism has roots in the early American experience.

According to the historian David Hackett Fischer (1977), colonial America was a place in which age, not youth, was exalted and venerated, honored, and obeyed. This respect for older people found expression in a variety of forms including the iconography of Puritanism, the distribution of honored seats in the meetinghouses of Massachusetts, and the patterns of officeholding in church and state. Fashions were also styled to flatter age, and census data suggest that people attempted to enhance their status by reporting themselves as older than they actually were.

This era of *gerontophilia* was succeeded by a period of transformation (1780–1820) during which attitudes toward old age began to change. In the nineteenth century, Fischer argues, there was truly a revolution in age relations in the United States, evidenced by new expressions of contempt for the aged (such as *fogey* and *geezer*), by the appearance of mandatory retirement policies, and by the development of a cult of youth in literature.

Fischer attributes the decline in the status of old people to two important factors. The first is demographic. Declines in both birth and death rates along with increases in life expectancy—long-term trends beginning in the colonial period—changed the age composition of the U.S. population. Old people increased in numbers as well as in the proportion of the population they constituted. Second, and perhaps more important for Fischer, is the radical expansion of the ideas of equality and liberty that occurred during the late eighteenth and early nineteenth centuries. These ideas altered forever the conception of the world upon which the old order had rested. Not only did the aged suffer the apparent misfortune of being identified with the old order, but they were also a constant reminder of what the new order hoped to avoid: dependence, disease, failure, and sin (Cole 1983).

Ageism is a cultural phenomenon whose acceptance is long-standing and crosscuts differences in age, region, and social class. It may be passed from generation to generation by means of socialization. Some theories of prejudice against racial and religious minorities also seem to help explain ageist attitudes in the United States. According to Levin and Levin (1980), persons who hold unfavorable attitudes toward the aged also dislike blacks, the mentally ill, and the physically disabled.

How is ageism perpetuated today? One way is through so-called commonsense observations. Everyday aphorisms, such as "You can't teach an old dog new tricks," reflect a common sense that is negative as well as inconsistent with scientific knowledge. Scientific knowledge can also reinforce negative stereotypes about old people. This was especially the case in the early post–World War II period as the study of aging began to develop (see Chapter 2).

As Steffl (1978) points out, "Early research described characteristics of . . . aged congregated in poor farms, nursing homes, and state mental hospitals leading to a general picture of impaired elderly." Add to this picture the testimony of physicians and social workers, whose elderly clients were (and are) often physically and socially dependent. Finally, as Clark Tibbitts (1979) suggests, the private agencies and public program bureaucracies helped perpetuate negative stereotypes by pleading with Congress for legislation on behalf of "the impaired, deprived, dependent elderly."

Myths and stereotypes of the elderly may also be transmitted through the mass media. Virtually all analyses of the content of television programming show an underrepresentation of older people in comparison with their numbers in the total population as well as a striking imbalance in the ratio of older males to females (Kubey 1980). For example, Aronoff (1974) found that elderly prime-time TV characters made up only about one-half their share in the general population. Northcott (1975) analyzed television characterizations, concentrating on role portrayals lasting two minutes or longer. Of the almost 500 such roles analyzed, only about 8 percent appeared to be sixty years of age or older, and over 90 percent of these were minor characters. Northcott concluded that television drama is dominated by mature adult males below the age of fifty-five who competently deal with various problems that in the real world more frequently affect the elderly, children, and women.

What of the quality of the image of older people in television? Aronoff (1974) found this image to be quite negative. Only about 40 percent of older male and 10 percent of older female characters could be described in positive terms such as "good," "happy," or "successful." Moreover, the number and proportion of males playing "bad guys" increased with age. This finding is supported by Signorelli and Gerbner (1977), who observe that a greater proportion of the elderly than of other age groups portray roles that are classified as bad or unsuccessful. Still, these authors also found that class status on the screen increased with age; the elderly had the greatest proportion of their numbers (18.6 percent) categorized as belonging to the upper class.

Harris and Feinberg (1977) examined the image of the elderly across various types of television programming and discovered a mixed bag. On the one hand, old TV characters could be described as one-dimensional with a narrow range of emotions. No romantic involvements whatsoever were shown among characters over sixty years of age; only one was counted among individuals aged fifty to sixty years. On the other hand, news and talk shows presented the greatest percentages of older people, and on these programs the older person's image was most positive. This was reflected in high ratings of "authority" and "esteem" given to older politicians, journalists, and business executives who appear on such programs. These authoritative old people are overwhelmingly male. Harris and Feinberg believe that these data highlight the disparity that exists between the real world as reported on the news and life as it is recreated on entertainment programs.

Television drama does not purport to be a one-to-one representation of reality, but is of necessity a selected view of life, chosen for its supposed dramatic appeal. The areas of business and politics are rarely selected as the stage for dramatic representations. Therefore, older people who are in true life eminently successful in these fields are not portrayed in such roles in the simulated world of television entertainment. (p. 466)

Nevertheless, Passuth and Cook (1985) offer a caution about exaggerating the relationship between television viewing and ageism. In response to the question, "Does heavy television viewing make a consistently negative contribution to the public's knowledge and attitudes about older persons?" they answer, "No." Only for adults under age thirty do Passuth and Cook report a modest relationship between heavy viewing and low knowledge levels about aging; for adults thirty years of age and older they report no such relationship. From their point of view, we must examine other socializing institutions and contexts to understand how knowledge and attitudes about aging and older people are developed.

Television is not the only mass medium in which stereotypes about old people have been found. Researchers have examined aging in literature (for example, Loughman 1977; Sohngen 1977), humor (Davies 1977; Palmore 1971; Smith 1979), letters to "Dear Abby" (Gaitz and Scott 1975), periodicals (Duncan 1963), advertising (Francher 1973; Smith 1976), poetry (Sohngen and Smith 1978), newspapers (Buchholz and Bynum 1982), and fairy tales (Chinen, 1987).

Some research does indicate a positive shift in attitudes toward older persons. Austin (1985) reports a sample of midwestern university students more accepting of close relationships with older people than of close relationships with disabled people. Included in the latter group were the blind, paraplegics, and the mentally retarded. Austin proposes that people have developed more positive attitudes toward old age in recent years as increasing numbers of older people have become visible in productive roles. This does not suggest that ageist attitudes have disappeared in the United States, only that, as compared with other groups, older people are seen as more productive and more conforming to societal values.

Holtzman and Akiyama (1985) compared the frequency and quality of the portrayal of older characters on Japanese and U.S. television programs most often watched by children. They found American television to portray older characters more frequently and more positively than did Japanese television. This was particularly surprising given commonly held beliefs about the cultural importance of older persons in non-Western cultures.

Still, ageism can be subtle as well as flexible. According to Robert Binstock (1983), former President of the Gerontological Society of America, new distortions of the reality of older people have appeared to provide the foundation for the emergence of the aged as scapegoat for a variety of economic and political frustrations in the United States. These distortions, identified by Binstock as classic examples of "tabloid thinking," include the belief that the aged are a potent self-interested political force, and that they pose an unsustainable burden on the U.S. economy. Binstock identifies three important consequences of this scapegoating of the aged for U.S. society. First, it diverts attention from other public policy issues, including unemployment and the deficit in the federal budget. Second, it produces conflict between generations as representatives of the young and the old battle for scarce resources. Third, it diverts attention from long-standing issues of equity and justice in public programs of support for older people.

One aim of this book is to refute negative stereotypes and present a more realistic view of aging in the United States, a view that is more positive than many students of aging have admitted. The following list of ten statements about old people and the aging process should be treated as a quiz. Read each item carefully and indicate whether you believe it to be true or false.

_____ **1.** Senility inevitably accompanies old age.
_____ **2.** Most old people are isolated from their families.
_____ **3.** The majority of old people are in poor health.
_____ **4.** Old people are more likely than younger people to be victimized by crime.
_____ **5.** The majority of old people live in poverty.
_____ **6.** The increasing growth of federal programs for the aged is the principal cause for the budget deficits of the 1980s.
_____ **7.** Older workers are less productive than younger ones.
_____ **8.** Old people who retire usually suffer a decline in health and an early death.
_____ **9.** Most old people have no interest in, or capacity for, sexual relations.
_____ **10.** Most old people end up in nursing homes and other long-term care institutions.

If you answered false to all ten statements you have a perfect score; true responses indicate misconceptions about old people and the aging process.

DEBUNKING THE MYTHS
MYTH: Senility Inevitably Accompanies Old Age

We have only to think of people like the Honorable Claude Pepper, Betty Friedan, Maggie Kuhn, and Vladimir Horowitz to debunk the myth that senility is inevitable. These are individuals whose quality of achievement has not been diminished by age.

This myth is part of the conventional view that aging brings with it a decline in intelligence, memory, and learning. Yet, empirical evidence shows that these relationships are quite complex and decline is anything but inevitable. Age-related changes in learning ability appear to be quite small, even after the keenness of the senses has begun to decline. Memory and learning are functions of the central nervous system. Thus, when there is impairment, it is often due to some disease (arteriosclerosis, for example) or an associated condition; we should not assume that some typical process of normal aging is at work.

MYTH: Most Old People Are Isolated from Their Families

Marvin Sussman (1965) has argued that the isolation of the nuclear family in the United States is a myth, and that there exists in modern urban-industrial societies an extended kin system made up of numerous nuclear families that exchange services and are partially dependent on each other. This service exchange includes the contributions made by family members in direct care-giving roles to their elderly relations. Instrumental tasks—managing money, for example—are more likely to be provided by sons; expressive tasks—providing personal care and social/emotional support—are more likely to be provided by daughters (Lopata 1973; Treas 1977).

More recently, Sussman (1976) has suggested that the proliferation of services for the elderly such as Medicare and nutrition programs has brought additional contact within families as kin act as mediators, advocates, protectors, and buffers between institutional bureaucracies and elderly relations. This indirect care has been defined as "care management," the most important care providing function that a family can fulfill on behalf of an elderly relative (Lowy 1983).

Brody and her colleagues (1983) have concluded that values regarding family care have not eroded in the United States despite demographic and socioeconomic changes over time. They studied the responses of elderly grandmothers, middle-generation daughters, and young adult granddaughters. A large majority from all three generations felt that adult children should adjust their family schedules in order to help a dependent parent. They also believed that financial help should be provided, especially by working children.

Still, most older people prefer to live near, but not in the same household with, their adult children. In addition, emphasis on care provided to dependent parents often causes us to forget that substantial assistance in the form of goods and services and financial aid also flows from elderly parents to their adult children (Troll 1971; Troll et al. 1979).

MYTH: The Majority of Old People Are in Poor Health

I recently asked a group of third-year medical students what proportion of older people did they believe are sick and institutionalized. The consensus was that more than half the older population are in ill health, and perhaps half of that population (25 percent of the total) are in institutions. *This is simply not the case.*

The majority of older people do *not* have the kinds of health problems that limit their ability to be employed or to manage their own households, and only about 5 percent of those sixty-five and over can be found in an old-age institution on a given day. According to The Special Committee on Aging of the United States Senate (1980), in a recent household-interview survey of the noninstitutionalized population, 69 percent of the older persons reported their health as "good" or "excellent" in comparison with "others of their own age." Only 9 percent reported themselves as being in poor health. Counting the approximately 5 percent of the elderly who live in institutional settings as being in poor health, a total of about 14 percent of all older people consider themselves in poor health.

More important is that, although 80 percent of the noninstitutionalized elderly population reported the presence of some chronic condition—most frequently, arthritis and hearing and vision impairments—less than 18 percent said that it limited their ability to work or do household chores.

MYTH: Old People Are More Likely Than Younger People to Be Victimized by Crime

Concerns about crimes against elderly Americans are quite high—especially among elderly Americans. Many surveys show that older persons are more fearful of crime than are younger persons. This concern appears to stem from the popular belief that elderly persons are victimized more often than others and suffer more serious consequences as a result. Nevertheless, no evidence supports this belief.

National and local surveys show that victimization rates are lower for the elderly than for other age groups, except for personal larceny with contact, which is equal to or slightly higher for the elderly than for some other age groups (Antunes et al. 1977; Alston 1986). Covey and Menard (1988) report that criminal victimization rates declined for all types of crime between 1973 and 1984 and the elderly have experienced greater declines over time than the general population. These authors speculate that changes in the demographic structure of the American population may contribute to these declines. Relatively smaller numbers of youth in the population may have lowered the crime rates, as youth and young adults commit a high percentage of crime.

Some have argued that because elderly victimization is relatively rare and fear of victimization is so widespread among the elderly, the fear of crime is the real problem and is more harmful than actual victimization (Braungart et al. 1980). Many older people tend to restrict their activity because of this fear (Dowd et al. 1981). A sense of helplessness against an intruder or attacker may make older persons more conscious of their need to protect themselves from crime, and may produce levels of fear that are incongruent with the statistics about their relative vulnerability to crime.

MYTH: The Majority of Old People Live in Poverty

It used to be easy to write about the economic problems of the old. If you did not know they were poor, you only had to ask one of them. Today's situation, though more complex, is much improved. Many private and public programs have been developed in the last decades to deal with the economic problems of old age. According to James H. Schulz (1988) of Brandeis University these programs include the following:

1. Substantial increases in social security old-age benefits in the last 15 years, a faster rate of climb than inflation in the same period.
2. The growth of private pension plans with increased benefit levels.
3. The creation of public health insurance and nutrition programs.
4. The legislation of property tax and other tax relief laws in virtually all states.
5. The Supplemental Security Income Program (SSI), which now covers more than twice as many low-income elderly as did the now abolished old-age assistance plan and raises benefit levels above previous levels of old-age assistance.

Part of the complexity in analyzing the economic situation of the aged stems from the fact that they receive money income from so many available sources. Wages and salaries, retirement benefits, veterans' benefits, unemployment insurance, workman's compensation, public assistance, dividends, interest, rents, royalties, private pensions, and annuities are only some of their sources of money income. In addition, approximately three out of four elderly Americans own homes, and most have substantial equity in these homes. Finally, the elderly receive indirect or in-kind income in the form of goods and services that they obtain free or at reduced cost. Medicare, food stamps, and housing subsidies are examples of programs providing in-kind benefits to older people.

MYTH: The Increasing Growth of Federal Programs for the Aged Is the Principal Cause for the Budget Deficits of the 1980s

Annual federal budget deficits in the range of $200 billion have not been unusual during the 1980s. Some have argued that this deficit results from the insatiable demands of older people for additional Social Security and health benefits. From this view, current generations of younger workers are taxed at a bur-

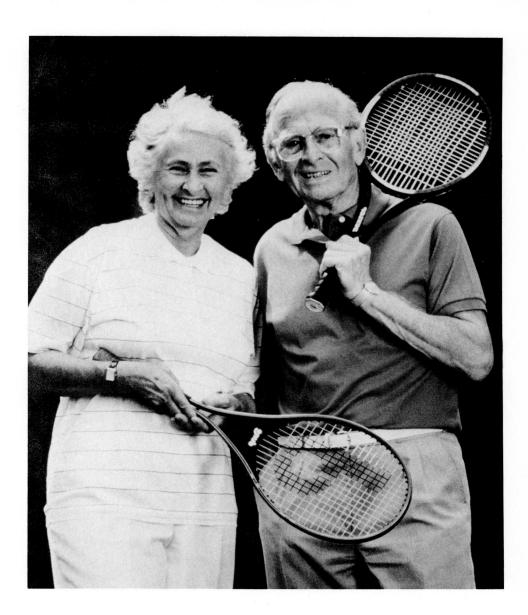

densome level in order to support social programs for the elderly. In addition, future generations are promised a diminished standard of living as a result of the vast amounts of federal debt to be serviced (Villers Foundation 1987).

The Social Security system has had financial problems in the past and may face such problems again in the future. Legislation passed by Congress in 1978 sought to correct these problems for fifty years into the future. With the severe economic downturn in the late 1970s and early 1980s, legislative relief was again required in 1983. New amendments to the Social Security Act, passed in 1983, have placed the system back on sound financial footing. Actuaries of the Social Security system itself, as well as those of the nonpartisan Congressional Budget Office and the House and Senate Budget Committees, agree that Social Security is currently helping to *reduce* the federal budget deficit because it is taking in more than it is spending. It is expected that Social Security will have a *surplus* of $142 billion across fiscal years 1987–1990 (Social Security Administration 1986). According to the Budget Committee of the U.S. House of Representatives (1986), were it not for Medicare and Social Security, the budget deficit would have been substantially greater in 1986. The Committee noted that Social Security and Medicare swung substantially out of deficit to balance during the 1980s, while the rest of the budget plunged deeply into deficit. Like many contemporary analysts, Martin Feldstein, former chairman of President Reagan's Council of Economic Advisors, has identified the major causes of the deficit increase since 1981 as including sustained increases in military spending and substantial federal tax decreases, not programs for the elderly (Blaustein 1983).

The increase in the elderly population has created demand for federal, state, and local programs to benefit the elderly. It is important to remember, though, that the biggest of these programs, Social Security, Medicare, and veterans' and civil service pensions, are not welfare programs. They are entitlements to which the elderly have contributed throughout their working years. Old people and the programs that benefit them cannot be held accountable for the massive federal budget deficits that have burdened the economy since 1981.

MYTH: Older Workers Are Less Productive Than Younger Ones

This myth, based on misconceptions about the aging process and the employment of older people, is often raised by proponents of mandatory retirement. This argument assumes that older persons as a group may be less well suited for work than are younger workers because older people do not learn new skills as well as younger persons do, older workers are more inflexible with respect to changes in work schedules and regimens, and declining physical and mental capacities are found in greater proportion among older persons.

These arguments are not based on fact. Many studies indicate that older workers produce a quality of work equal or superior to that of younger workers. In addition, as we have already indicated, there is no reason to expect a decline in intellectual capacities with age and every reason to assume that older workers in good health are capable of learning new skills when circumstances require it. Many workers can continue to work effectively beyond age sixty-five and may be better employees than younger workers because of greater experience and job commitment.

Finally, some proponents of age-based mandatory retirement policies argue that needed jobs would be opened for the young. Although this is an appealing argument (perhaps especially to the young), no study can be cited that demonstrates that the termination of older workers because of mandatory retirement was the direct cause of the hiring of young workers. Interestingly, the declining birth rate (discussed in Chapter 3) will mean a proportionately smaller labor force supporting a larger retiree population early in the next century. The potentially problematic economics of this situation could be alleviated by inducing older workers to *remain* in the labor force rather by forcing them out through mandatory retirement policies.

The field of child care, plagued by labor shortages, is already courting older workers. Kinder-Care Learning Centers, Inc., the largest U.S. day-care chain, has been actively recruiting older workers for the past three years. According to one official of the company, older workers are productive and motivated. In addition, the hiring of older workers has cut absenteeism and helped stabilize the Kinder-Care work force (Eastman 1988).

MYTH: Old People Who Retire Usually Suffer a Decline in Health and an Early Death

It is widely held that retirement has an adverse effect on health. Most of us have heard at least one story about a retiree who "went downhill fast." The story usually describes an individual who carefully plans for retirement, only to become sick and die within a brief period of time—the story is the same regardless of whether the retirement is mandatory or voluntary.

One problem with such stories is that the health status of the retiree before retirement is never made clear. Another problem is that most retirees themselves are older, and, although the majority of old people do not have major health problems, it is true that older people have a greater risk of illness than younger people do. In a well-known study, *Retirement in American Society*, Gordon Streib and Clement Schneider (1971) concluded that retired people are no more likely to be sick than are people of the same age who are still on the job. That is, *health declines appear to be associated with age, not with retirement!* In fact, as some researchers have pointed out, unskilled workers and others who work in harsh environments and in high-risk occupations may show *improvements* in health following retirement.

MYTH: Most Old People Have No Interest in, or Capacity for, Sexual Relations

Sexual interests, capacities, and functions change with age. Nevertheless, older men and women in reasonably good health can have an active and satisfying sex life.

Dr. Adrian Verwoerdt and his colleagues (1969a, 1969b) at Duke University studied 254 men and women ranging from sixty to ninety-four years of age. They found that the incidence of sexual interest does not show an age-related decline. In fact, interest may persist indefinitely. Most important, these researchers found that sexual behavior patterns of the later years correlate with those of the younger years. If there was interest and satisfying activity in the early years, there is likely to be interest and satisfying activity in the later years.

Some decline in sexual activity among the old is due to their acceptance of stereotypes about the sexless older years. Old people may feel shame and embarrassment about having sexual interests. Further, some older people relate normal changes in sexual functioning and impotence, and so they avoid sexual opportunities because they fear failure. Older people need not duplicate the sexual behavior of youth in order to enjoy their sexual experiences. Sex is qualitatively different in the later years. Sexual activity in later years may fulfill the human need for the warmth of physical closeness and the intimacy of companionship. Older people should be encouraged to seek this fulfillment.

MYTH: Most Old People End up in Nursing Homes and Other Long-Term Care Institutions

Most old people do *not* end up in nursing homes. The 1980 U.S. Census reports about 5 percent of the elderly population residing in old-age institutions of one kind or another. Still, this does not mean that the odds of being institutionalized are one in twenty. The Census only gives us a picture of the institutional population at one point in time.

In 1976 Erdman Palmore of Duke University reviewed the cases of 207 individuals from the Piedmont, North Carolina, area who were studied in the Duke First Longitudinal Study of Aging beginning in 1955 until their deaths prior to the spring of 1976. He observed that 54 of the 207 persons, or 26 percent, had been institutionalized in some type of extended-care facility one or more times before death. On the basis of this and other findings, he concluded that among normal-aged persons living in the community the chance of institutionalization before death would be about one in four. Other researchers, using different populations and different methods, have substantiated these findings. This suggests that three in four aged persons have no reason to view a nursing home stay as inevitable.

CONCLUSION

This brief chapter opened with a look at the legendary Tithonus, an unfortunate man who suffered the infirmities of old age endlessly. Actually, this myth appears in the middle of a Homeric hymn describing an adventure of Aphrodite, the goddess of love (Evelyn-White 1936). It seems that Aphrodite had considerable power over other gods and was often able to beguile them into mating with mere mortals, an act considered demeaning. In order to temper her arrogance, Zeus managed to infect her with desire for Anchises, a handsome Trojan.

Aphrodite arranged a rendezvous with Anchises, but after the lovemaking, Anchises, concerned about his ability to sustain a love affair with the goddess, begged Aphrodite to do something to preserve his good health. At first she seemed sympathetic to Anchises, but then she recounted to him the legend of Tithonus. She emphasized that she would not want Anchises to be deathless if he had to suffer the fate of Tithonus. Unwilling to grant him "youthful immortality," Aphrodite finally turned down Anchises's request with these words: "But as it is, harsh old age will soon enshroud you— ruthless old age which stands someday at the side of every man, deadly, wearying, dreaded even by the gods."

Although most people in our society *do* live to experience old age (almost 83 percent of females born today and about 70 percent of males are expected to reach age sixty-five), not many of us must expect to endure as Tithonus has. And although some in the United States do experience the "harsh" and "ruthless" old age that Aphrodite described for Anchises, *many do not*. Further, the debunking of prevalent myths about aging and the aged does not require that old people reflect the mirror opposite of ageism: Old people do not have to be intellectually gifted, happy, wealthy, and sexually active. Rather, the myths of aging discussed here simply suggest the diversity of aging experiences represented in our society. The rest of this book explores the biological, psychological, and social factors that contribute to this wide range in the experience of old age.

STUDY QUESTIONS

1. How is the myth of Tithonus relevant to aging in contemporary society?

2. Define the term *ageism*. What are its origins and how is it perpetuated today? What special role has television played in maintaining myths about the aged? Does television have a role in combatting these myths?

3. Why do gerontologists argue that senility is not an inevitable part of the aging process?

4. A common misconception is that most old people are lonely and isolated from their families. Can you present evidence to the contrary?

5. How sick are the elderly in the United States? Discuss this in terms of their ability to work and carry out other daily activities, their risks of being institutionalized, and their capacity for sexual relations.

6. Many elderly are in need of costly health and social services. What role does provision of these services play in the generation of the federal budget deficit?

BIBLIOGRAPHY

Alston, L.T. 1986. *Crime and older Americans*. Springfield, Ill.: Charles C Thomas.

Antunes, G.E., Cook, F., Cook, T., and Skogan, W. 1977. Patterns of personal crime against the elderly. *Gerontologist* 17:321–327.

Aronoff, C. 1974. Old age in prime time. *Journal of Communication* 24:86–87.

Austin, D.R. 1985. Attitudes toward old age: A hierarchical study. *Gerontologist* 25(4):431–434.

Binstock, R.H. 1983. The aged as scapegoat. *Gerontologist* 23(2):136–143.

Blaustein, P. 1983. Reagan economist blames deficit growth on arms outlays, lower taxes, debt costs. *Wall Street Journal,* November 20:3.

Braungart, M.M., Braungart, R.G., and Hoyer, W.J. 1980. Age, sex, and social factors in fear of crime. *Sociological Focus* 13:55–66.

Brody, E., Johnsen, P.T., Fulcomer, M.C., and Lang, A.M. 1983. Women's changing roles and help to elderly parents: Attitudes of three generations of women. *Journal of Gerontology* 18:597–607.

Buchholz, M., and Bynum, J.E. 1982. Newspaper presentation of America's aged: A content analysis of image and role. *Gerontologist,* 22(1):83–88.

Butler, R. 1975. *Why survive? Being old in America.* New York: Harper and Row.

Chinen, A.B. 1987. Fairy tales and psychological development in late life: A cross-cultural hermeneutic study. *Gerontologist* 27(3):340–352.

Cole, T.R. 1983. The 'enlightened' view of aging: Victorian morality in a new key. *Hastings Center Report* 13(3):34–40.

Covey, H.C., and Menard, S. 1988. Trends in elderly criminal victimization from 1973 to 1984. *Research on Aging* 10:329–341.

Davies, L.J. 1977. Attitudes toward old age and aging as shown by humor. *Gerontologist* 17:220–226.

Dowd, J., Sisson, R.P., and Kern, D.M. 1981. Socialization to violence among the aged. *Journal of Gerontology* 36:350–361.

Duncan, K.J. 1963. Modern society's attitude toward aging. *Geriatrics* 18:629–635.

Eastman, P. 1988. New role for older workers. *NRTA News Bulletin* 30(1):1, 12.

Evelyn-White, H.G. 1936. *Hesiod, the Homeric hymns and Homerica.* London: William Heinemann Ltd.

Fischer, D.H. 1977. *Growing old in America.* New York: Oxford University Press.

Francher, J.S. 1973. It's the Pepsi generation . . . : Accelerated aging and the television commercial. *International Journal of Aging and Human Development* 4:245–255.

Gaitz, C.M., and Scott, J. 1975. Analysis of letters to Dear Abby concerning old age. *Gerontologist* 15:47–50.

Hamilton, E. 1942. *Mythology.* Boston: Little, Brown and Co.

Harris, A.J., and Feinberg, J.F. 1977. Television and aging: Is what you see what you get? *Gerontologist* 17:464–468.

Holtzman, J.M., and Akiyama, H. 1985. What children see: The aged on television in Japan and the United States. *Gerontologist* 25(1):62–67.

Johnson, E., and Bursk, B. 1977. Relationships between the elderly and their adult children. *Gerontologist* 17(1):90–96.

Kubey, R. 1980. Television and aging: Past, present, and future. *Gerontologist* 20:16–35.

Levin, J., and Levin, W.C. 1980. *Prejudice and discrimination against the elderly.* Belmont, Calif.: Wadsworth Publishing Co.

Lopata, H. 1973. *Widowhood in an American city.* Cambridge, Mass.: Schenkman Publishing Co., Inc.

Loughman, C. 1977. Novels of senescence: A new naturalism. *Gerontologist* 17:79–84.

Lowy, L. 1983. The older generation: What is due, what is owed. *Social Casework* 64:371–376.

National Council on the Aging. 1976. *The myth and reality of aging in America.* Washington, D.C.: NCOA.

Northcott, H. 1975. Too young, too old—Age in the world of television. *Gerontologist* 15:184–186.

Palmore, E. 1971. Attitudes toward aging as shown by humor. *Gerontologist* 11:181–186.

———. 1976. Total chance of institutionalization among the aged. *Gerontologist* 16:504–507.

Passuth, P.M., and Cook, F.L. 1985. Effects of television viewing on knowledge and attitudes about older people: A critical reexamination. *Gerontologist* 25(1):69–77.

Schulz, J.H. 1988. *The economics of aging* (4th ed.). Dover, Mass.: Auburn House Publishing Co.

Signorelli, N., and Gerbner, G. 1977. *The image of the elderly in prime-time network television drama* (Report No. 12). Philadelphia: Institute for Applied Communication Studies, University of Pennsylvania.

Smith, M.C. 1976. Portrayal of elders in prescription drug advertising: A pilot study. *Gerontologist* 16:329–334.

Smith, M.D. 1979. The portrayal of elders in magazine cartoons. *Gerontologist* 19:408–412.

Social Security Administration, Office of the Actuary. 1986. *1986 Annual Report, Board of Trustees: Old age, survivors, disability insurance programs.* Washington, D.C.: Social Security Administration.

Sohngen, M. 1977. The experience of old age as depicted in contemporary novels. *Gerontologist* 17:70–78.

Sohngen, M., and Smith, R.J. 1978. Images of old age in poetry. *Gerontologist* 18:181–186.

Special Committee on Aging, United States Senate. 1980. *Every ninth American.* Washington, D.C.: Government Printing Office.

Steffl, B.M. 1978. Gerontology in professional and preprofessional curricula. In M. Seltzer, H. Sterns, and T. Hickey (eds.), *Gerontology in higher education: Perspectives and issues.* Belmont, Calif.: Wadsworth Publishing Co.

Streib, G., and Schneider, C. 1971. *Retirement in American society.* Ithaca, N.Y.: Cornell University Press.

Sussman, M. 1965. Relationships of adult children with their parents in the U.S. In E. Shanas and G. Streib (eds.), *Social structure and the family.* Englewood Cliffs, N.J.: Prentice-Hall, Inc.

————. 1976. The family life of old people. In R. Binstock and E. Shanas (eds.), *Handbook of aging and the social services*. New York: Van Nostrand Reinhold Co.

Tibbitts, C. 1979. Can we invalidate negative stereotypes of aging? *Gerontologist* 19(1):10–20.

Treas, J. 1977. Family support systems for the aged. *Gerontologist* 17:486–491.

Troll, L. 1971. The family of later life: A decade review. *Journal of Marriage and the Family* 33:263–290.

Troll, L., Miller, S., and Atchley, R. 1979. *Families in later life*. Belmont, Calif.: Wadsworth Publishing.

U.S. House of Representatives, Committee on the Budget. 1986. *President Reagan's fiscal year 1987 budget*. Washington, D.C.: U.S. Government Printing Office.

Verwoerdt, A., Pfeiffer, E., and Wang, H.S. 1969a. Sexual behavior in senescence. I. *J. Geriatric Psychiatry* 2:163–180.

————. 1969b. Sexual behavior in senescence. II. *Geriatrics* 24:137–154.

Villers Foundation. 1987. *On the other side of easy street: Myths and facts about the economics of old age*. Washington, D.C.: The Villers Foundation.

CHAPTER 2

THE STUDY OF AGING

Concerns about aging and death have been present in the written and oral records of societies dating back many thousands of years. Two of the most prominent themes contrast somewhat: One reflects the belief that extended life is neither possible nor desirable; the other refers to the desirability of attempting to lengthen life (Gruman 1966). Clearly, the latter has been the most prevalent throughout history. Three different themes represent the quest for the prolongation of life. The *antediluvian theme* involves the belief that in the past people lived much longer, best exemplified in the Book of Genesis, which records the life spans of ten Hebrew patriarchs who lived before the Flood. Noah lived for 950 years, Methuselah for 969 years, Adam for 930 years, and so on. The *hyperborean theme* develops the idea that in some remote part of the world there are people who enjoy a remarkably long life. According to the traditions of ancient Greece, a people live *hyper Boreas* (beyond the north wind): "Their hair crowned with golden bay-leaves they hold glad revelry; and neither sickness nor baneful eld mingleth among the chosen people; but, aloof from toil and conflict, they dwell afar" (Pindar in Gruman 1966, 22).

Finally, the *fountain theme* is based on the idea that there is some unusual substance that has the property of greatly increasing the length of life (Gruman 1966). The search for the "fountain of youth" in 1513 by Juan Ponce de Leon (who accidentally discovered Florida instead) is a good example of this rejuvenation theme. According to the earliest account of Ponce de Leon's adventure, published by a Spanish official in the New World in 1535, the explorer was "seeking that fountain of Biminie that the Indians had given to be understood would renovate or resprout and refresh the age and forces of he who drank or bathed himself in that fountain" (Lawson 1946, in Gruman 1966).

These themes remain current. Our fascination with reportedly long-lived peoples like the Abkhasians of the Georgian Republic of Russia (see Chapter 5) reflects a modern-day hyperborean theme. Similarly, any student of American billboard and television advertising will recognize the fountain theme. Skin creams, hair colorings, body soaps, foods, and vitamins are all depicted as unusual substances that we may use to remain eternally young.

The persistence of these themes suggests that throughout history and up to the present it has been difficult to distinguish between myth and history, between magic and science. The development of the systematic study of aging can be seen in this light, for it attempts to make clear distinctions between myth and history, magic and science.

WHY STUDY AGING?

Some will surely ask, "Why study aging?" At first the question may seem odd, but this is because we so rarely ask individuals to explain why they chose to work in a particular substantive area or why they chose one discipline over another (for example, gerontology instead of demography). The answer comes in five parts.

First, despite what has been written about the long history of aging, aging is a relatively new phenomenon: Never before have so many lived to be old. The historian Ronald Blythe (1979) suggests that if a Renaissance or Georgian man could return, he would be just as astonished by the sight of the increased numbers of aged people as he would be by a television set. This is because in his world it was the exception to go grey, to retire, to become old. Today, this process is ordinary, but because it is now ordinary does not make it any less novel. This is a real-life experiment of sorts. As Blythe points out, these "are the first generations of the full-timers and thus the first generations of old people for whom the state . . . is having to make special supportive conditions." The novelty, the experimentation, and the uncertainty all make gerontology an exciting field to be a part of today, and as a result have drawn many people to the study of aging.

Second, students of gerontology have come to view aging as a lifelong process in which we and all other living things participate. From this perspective, aging is seen as ongoing, starting at conception and ending with death. Thus, aging is not reserved for senior citizens or golden-age clubbers; it is shared by infants, children, teenagers, and young adults, as well as the more mature. It occupies the total life span, not merely the final stage of life. Without knowledge and understanding of the entire life span, it is difficult to understand the events of any one life phase. In this sense, we study the aged to learn not only about the final phase of life but also about youth and the middle years.

Third, as George Maddox (1979) has indicated, many sociologists and psychologists (and others) have begun to study aging because they see the later years as a strategic site for examining a wide range of scientific issues of fundamental importance in their disciplines. Examples of these issues are numerous and include status maintenance (Henratta and Campbell 1976), role loss and role transitions (Rosow 1976; Lowenthal 1977), and family structure and intergenerational relations (Sussman 1976).

Fourth, another reason to study aging has simply to do with the dramatic increase in interest in the problems of old people in the United States. Although it has been said sarcastically by many that people admire aging only in bottles, within the last decades, as more people have encountered old age, a large number of elaborate programs have been promoted and financed on behalf of our aged citizens. One reason behind the promotion of these governmental and nongovernmental programs is that the situation of the elderly has come to be defined by many as the responsibility of society as a whole. The burden of this responsibility is reason enough for studying the aged. Only by knowing more about the aged and the difficulties and changes they face can we really come to grips with their problems.

Finally, it is understood that different matters have intrinsic fascination for different scientists. This may explain, in part, why some choose gerontology. This author, like so many others, finds the study of aging to be intrisicially exciting and interesting. And so for his (and perhaps for many others) one answer to the question "Why study aging?" is "because the study of aging can become an end in itself."

DEFINING THE FIELD

Gerontology is the term used to describe the systematic study of the aging process. Though gerontology may include the study of aging in plants and animals below humans on the evolutionary scale, the term generally refers to the study of later adulthood among humans. Gerontology is an interdisciplinary study. Its major elements are drawn from the physical and social sciences, although the humanities and arts, business, and education are also represented in the content of gerontology. In 1954 Clark Tibbitts, a pioneer in the modern scientific era of gerontology, introduced the term *social gerontology* to describe the study of the impact of social and sociocultural factors on the aging process. Tibbitts and others recognized that aging does not occur in a vacuum. Rather, the aging process occurs in some social context—a social context that helps determine the meaning of aging as both an individual and a societal experience.

Gerontology is not only an academic discipline, it is also a field of practice that involves aspects of public policy and human service. In 1909 a Vienna-born physician, I. L. Nascher, coined the term *geriatrics* to describe one subfield of gerontological practice, the medical care of the aging.

The student of aging faces three main tasks: theoretical, methodological, and applied (Bromley 1974). The theoretical task involves confirming and extending the conceptual frameworks that explain the observed facts of aging. The methodological task involves developing suitable methods of research for examining the nature of aging. The applied task involves attempts to prevent or reduce the adverse effects of aging. Some gerontologists specialize in one or another task area: others find it difficult to separate theory, research, and practice. Gerontology is not a "disinterested science." Apparently, for many gerontologists, understanding the aging process is not enough. They must also address the practical and immediate problems of old people.

Gerontology is a complex field, encompassing a wide variety of substantive areas of study—health, family life, political economy, and retirement, among others. Yet there are no dominant paradigms in the broader field; and standardization of measurement, a common conceptualization of issues, and systematic testing of hypotheses derived from theory are for the most part lacking (Maddox and Wiley 1976). As Maddox and Wiley point out, applied, problem-oriented studies of the societal consequences of aging have dominated the field. This book reflects these facts. It attempts to introduce undergraduate and beginning graduate students to the major concepts and issues in the field of gerontology. But, in doing so, this volume recognizes the current state of affairs in gerontology. It recognizes, first, the importance of making the connection between basic and applied research without minimizing the role applied research has played in the development of gerontology or the need for additional research at a basic level and, second, the need to bring diverse disciplinary and interdisciplinary approaches to the study of aging.

THE HISTORY OF AGING

The study of aging is now considered to be scientific. Yet, as we have seen, particular nonscientific themes in concepts of human aging have persisted with some consistency through the prescientific and into the scientific era. This is especially clear when one looks at the imagery in discussions of the causes of aging. Bromley (1974) summarizes this imagery into three categories. In the first the body is a container full of some essential substance or spirit. This substance is gradually depleted or destroyed, leading to diminished capacities and increased vulnerability to disease and death. In the second image, aging represents a conflict within each person between positive and negative forces. Eventually, the negative forces of evil, disease, corruption, and so on prevail. Finally, aging is seen as symbolizing a process of renewal of life. Like the seed within the dry decaying shell, or the reptile that sheds its outer skin, aging represents the casting off of our "mortal coil" in preparation for life after death.

The astute reader of this brief history will recognize these images in the theories of aging from Greco-Roman medicine to modern times. The similarity of imagery employed by different theorists at different times reflects the enormous difficulty involved in conceptualizing human aging, for example, in distinguishing between aging as a cause and aging as an effect (Bromley 1974). The careful reader may also conclude that much of what passes for new knowledge in gerontology today is not new at all, but is rather the result of a systematizing and "scientizing" of ideas that have been in circulation for a long time.

Greece and Rome

In the Western world, the first full explicit theory of the causation of aging is found in Greco-Roman medicine and the Hippocratic theory (about fourth century B.C.) (Grant 1963). According to the Hippocratic theory, the essential factor in life is heat. At that time the common belief was that individuals have a fixed quantity of some life force. This material, characterized by Hippocrates as "innate heat," is used up during the course of a lifetime, although the rate of utilization varies with the individual. In general, old age was equated with a continuous diminishing of innate heat, and aging was seen as a consequence of a natural course of events. The latter point in itself constitutes a remarkable breakthrough of sorts, because many writers of the time confused the aging process with diseases in the old.

About a century after Hippocrates, Aristotle expanded on the "innate heat" theory of aging in his book *On Youth and Old Age, On Life and Death and On Respiration*. Aristotle likened the heat to a fire that had to be maintained and provided with fuel. Just as a fire could run out of fuel or be put out, innate heat could also be exhausted (as in the case of a natural death caused by aging) or extinguished (as in a death resulting from violence or disease). The contributions of Greek philosophers reached their peak with Galen (circa A.D. 130–200) who clearly differentiated between aging and dying and who was perhaps the first to characterize aging as a process beginning with conception (Grant 1963). To Aristotle's innate heat Galen added the elements of blood and semen. Blood and semen were sources of generation; drying in the form of heat produced the tissues (Grant 1963).

> By this means, then, the embryo is first formed and takes on a little firmness; and after this, drying more, acquires the outlines and faint patterns of each of its parts. Then, drying even more, it assumes not merely their outlines and patterns, but their exact appearance. And now, having been brought forth, it keeps growing larger and drier and stronger, until it reaches full development. Then all growth ceases, the bones elongating no more on account of their dryness, and every vessel increases in width, and thus all the parts become strong and attain their maximum power.
>
> But in ensuing time, as all the organs become even drier, not only are their functions performed less well but their vitality becomes more feeble and

restricted. And drying more, the creature becomes not only thinner but also wrinkled, and the limbs weak and unsteady in their movements. This condition is called old age. . . . This, then, is one innate destiny of destruction for every mortal creature. . . .

These processes, then, it is permitted no mortal body to escape; but others, which ensure, it is possible for the forethoughtful to avoid. Moreover, the source of these is from attempting to correct the aforesaid inevitable processes. (Galen, quoted in Grant, 1963. From Robert Green, *A Translation of Galen's Hygiene*, 1951:7. Courtesy of Charles C Thomas, Publisher, Springfield, Illinois.)

It is interesting that, for Galen, the very element that appears to bring life (drying) leads quite naturally (and unequivocally) to its end.

The attitude of the Greeks expressed their ambivalence toward aging. They emphasized family love and the wisdom of age, but also recognized the weaknesses and eccentricities of the aged (Bromley 1974). Aristotle condemned old age, and presented youth and old age as opposites. He characterized youth as a time of excess and later life as a time of conservativeness and small-mindedness (Hendricks and Hendricks 1977). Plato had a somewhat positive view of old age. In *The Republic* he refers to two important features of late life: the persistence of characteristics from earlier life and the relief of having outgrown some of life's difficulties (including frustrated ambition and unfulfilled sexual desire).

Cicero (106–43 B.C.) in his *De Senectute* has become a favorite source for contemporary writers on aging. Nevertheless, as Bromley points out, he is typical of his day. Although Cicero recognized that advanced age brought biological degeneration, he emphasized the relationship between aging and development, including the continuing capacity for psychological growth, and placed great value on experience accumulated over time. In fact, he recommended intellectual activity as part of a regimen to resist premature aging.

The Greek influence persisted. Freeman (1965), a noted historian of aging, has written of the physician, Villanova, and the Franciscan friar, Roger Bacon, thirteenth-century experts on aging, who essentially "followed the Galenic thought that aging was due to the loss of innate heat." Bacon, however, was in many respects a precursor of the scientific era to come. He argued that three factors tended to hasten the diminution of heat: infection, negligence, and ignorance of matters related to health. He proposed a method of hygiene that would allow men and women to achieve their rightful term of years in good health.

The Early Scientific Era

The scientific method, born during the sixteenth and seventeenth centuries, involved a radical break from earlier modes of thought. Magic, faith, and speculation no longer sufficed; observation, experimentation, and verification were the order of the day. One of the chief proponents of this new way of thinking, Francis Bacon, also wrote on aging. He attempted to dispel prior theories of aging because he believed them "corrupt with false opinion." Bacon wrote that "for both these things, which the vulgar physicians talk[e], of radical moisture, and natural heat, are but meer fictions." Unfortunately, Bacon himself was unable to escape completely the old ways of thinking. He simply replaced the Greek notion of innate heat with that of "spirit" or "pneuma" and argued that every body part (bones, blood, and so on) has such a spirit enclosed within it. With use, these spirits were consumed or dissolved—hence, old age. Bacon was, as might be expected, unable to verify this idea; yet he believed that with the proper method the "secrets of nature" could be discovered (Grant 1963).

Despite the new scientific approach, many people's basic ambivalence toward old age did not change. Bacon reflects this ambivalence in his discussion of the qualities intrinsic to youth and age: "[M]en of age object too much, consult too long, adventure too little, repent too soon, and seldom drive business home to the full period, but content themselves with a mediocrity of success . . . [yet] age doth profit rather in the powers of understanding, than in the virtues of the will and affections" (quoted in Hendricks and Hendricks 1977). A more positive sixteenth-century view was put forth by Paleotti who, in terms reminiscent of Cicero sixteen centuries before, concluded that "wisdom, maturity, and a cooling down of certain emotional currents give old age its peculiar form of creativeness unobtainable at other life periods" (quoted in Hendricks and Hendricks 1977).

In Europe and America, many books were written on, and advances made in, physiology, anatomy, pathology, and chemistry during the seventeenth and eighteenth centuries, although pre-Enlightenment ideas were still around in abundance. One of the first Americans to write about aging was Cotton Mather (1663–1728). His orientation was theological: Illness was conceived as punishment for original sin and only through temperance could longevity be achieved. Longevity was also the issue in what, perhaps, was the first complete American work on aging. William Barton, in his *Observations on the Progress of Population and the Probabilities of the Duration of Human Life, in the United States of America* (1791), attempted to show that the people of the United States lived longer and were healthier than people in Europe. He deduced that the likelihood of a person living past eighty was greater in America than abroad (Achenbaum 1978).

The first American work in geriatrics, *Account of the State of the Body and Mind in Old Age*, was published in 1793 by the physician Benjamin Rush. Perhaps more accurately than had anyone before him, Rush described the changes in the body and the mind that accompany old age. A historian of aging describes Rush as striking one of the last blows at the idea that old age is itself a disease: "Few persons appear to die of old age. Some of the diseases which have been mentioned generally cuts [*sic*] the last thread of life" (Rush, quoted in Grant 1963). Rush and his contemporaries—Hufeland in Germany and Bichat in

France, for example—represent the beginning of a more modern period. Science flowered, and writers of the time believed the principles of life would be discovered by scientific observation and experimentation.

In the nineteenth century we see an increased capacity for scientific research and some outstanding technological innovations, including advances in microscopy and thermometry. Lister, Pasteur, and Metchnikoff revolutionized public health by their discoveries of methods to control epidemic diseases and infection. Medical specialization was increasing, and one could begin to envision the outlines of a fledgling branch dealing with old age. The French physician Charcot attended particularly to the clinical aspects of old age; he believed the management of diseases of aging and the aged should be based on an established clinical regimen. According to Freeman (1965), Charcot is responsible for dividing the study of aging into two permanent lines of inquiry. One investigates the facts of aging and involves describing its effects and measuring its changes in capacities. The other looks for principles of aging, for a central theme or cause.

This distinction may have been anticipated by the Belgian mathematician Quetelet, considered by some to be the first gerontologist. Quetelet, one of the earliest statisticians, helped discover the concept of the normal distribution. The *normal distribution* curve indicates there is an average or central tendency around which are distributed higher and lower measurements. Quetelet applied this notion to various traits such as hand strength and weight, records of birth and death rates, and the relationship between age and productivity (Birren and Clayton 1975).

Sir Francis Galton, an English statistician responsible for developing the index of correlation, was influenced by Quetelet's work. Galton's fundamental contribution to the study of aging is the data gathered by his Anthropometric Laboratory at the International Health Exhibition in London in 1884 (Freeman 1965). Over nine thousand males and females ranging in age from five to eighty were measured on seventeen different characteristics, including hearing, vision, and reaction time. Galton used these data to show how human characteristics change with age. This was the first large survey related to aging, and the data were still being analyzed in the 1920s.

The Twentieth Century

In the early part of the twentieth century interest in aging involved including old age in a developmental psychology framework (Birren and Clayton 1975). G. Stanley Hall, president of Clark University and founder of the psychology department of Johns Hopkins University, had specialized in childhood and adolescence, but concern with his own retirement led him to write *Senescence, the Last Half of Life,* published in 1922. Although he may have been tempted to characterize the second half of life as a regression occurring along the same lines as development, Hall struck a new note:

As a psychologist I am convinced that the psychic states of old people have great significance. Senescence, like adolescence, has its own feeling, thought, and will, as well as its own psychology, and their regimen is important, as well as that of the body. Individual differences here are probably greater than in youth. (Hall 1922:100)

Hall used questionnaire data to investigate the relationship between religious belief and fear of death. The conventional wisdom at the time was that, with age, fear of death increased and people became more religious in an attempt to reconcile themselves to an uncertain future. Hall argued that religious fervor did not increase with age, nor were old people more fearful of death than were the young. In fact, he said, fear of death seems to be a young person's concern (Freeman 1965).

During the early part of the twentieth century biologists such as Child, Metchnikoff, Minot, Pearl, and Weismann were writing prolifically on aging. An internist at Johns Hopkins University, William Osler, while considering the high frequency of cases of arteriosclerosis among the elderly, discovered that the aging was closely related to the state of the blood vessels, and he saw the impact hardening of the arteries had on brain functioning. Clearly, the locus of aging study was shifting to the United States during this period, although important research was being carried out by Pavlov in Russia and Tachibana in Japan.

A new attitude toward old age had emerged by the 1930s, one that has had enormous impact on the growth of gerontology as a scientific discipline. Stimulated by the changing demographics of modern societies, an increased life expectancy, and an aging population, and perhaps by an economic depression, people began to see old age as a social problem (Maddox and Wiley 1976). Recognizing the prevalence of incapacity, isolation, and poverty among aged citizens, Western society's concern turned toward social action on behalf of the aged (Burgess 1960). Interestingly, this concern as well as the accompanying perceived need for collective social action was reflected not only in legislation (such as the passage of the Social Security Act in 1935) in the United States but also in a new institutional approach to aging as a social scientific problem.

In the late 1930s and early 1940s conferences on aging were sponsored by professional and governmental organizations such as the American Orthopsychiatric Association and the National Institutes of Health. Private foundations, including the Josiah Macy Foundation, also provided assistance in conducting conferences on aging. Many issues raised at these early conferences anticipated some of the current concerns in gerontology: mental health and aging, aging and intellectual functioning, and aging and worker productivity. One of the earliest reports on the implications of the changing demographic structure of society in the United States was initiated by the Social Science Research Council (Pollak 1948).

The Second World War interrupted the continuing development of gerontology. But when the war ended in 1945, gerontologists resumed activity and founded the Gerontological Society. The Society publishes two influential journals in the field of aging: *The Journal of Gerontology* and *The Gerontologist*. Other professional associations soon appeared. The American Psychological Association established a division on maturity and old age in 1946; The American Geriatric Society was founded in 1950. The American Society on Aging, organized initially as the Western Gerontological Society, was founded in 1954.

In 1946 a gerontological unit of the National Institutes of Health was started and resulted in the creation of the National Institute of Aging in 1974. Robert Butler, a psychiatrist and gerontologist, became its first director. The International Association of Gerontology was organized in 1948 and had its first meeting in Liege, Belgium. Today, many other professional societies, including the American Sociological Association and the American Public Health Association, maintain sections for those members with a specific interest in aging.

By the 1950s the volume of gerontological literature had increased dramatically, and it continues to increase unabated. The major journals of gerontology were started between 1946 and the early 1970s. In addition to those mentioned above these include *Geriatrics* (1946), *Gerontologia* (1956), *Experimental Gerontology* (1966), *Journal of Geriatric Psychiatry* (1967), *Aging and Human Development* (1971). An attempt to create a definitive bibliography of biomedical and social science research in aging for the years 1954 to 1974 yielded 50,000 titles (Woodruff and Birren 1975). Many gerontologists express both joy and dismay at this explosive increase in gerontological research. The joy comes with being able to participate in an exciting and growing scientific enterprise; the dismay comes with trying to keep pace with the growth of gerontological knowledge.

Several attempts have been made to synthesize this growing body of literature. Landmarks in this regard are Birren's *Handbook of Aging and the Individual: Psychological and Biological Aspects* (1959), Tibbitts's *Handbook of Social Gerontology: Societal Aspects of Aging* (1960), and Burgess's *Aging in Western Societies* (1960). This effort was later matched in three volumes edited by Matilda W. Riley and her colleagues and supported by the Russell Sage Foundation: *Aging and Society: An Inventory of Research Findings* (Riley and Foner 1968), *Aging and the Professions* (Riley, Riley, and Johnson 1969), and *A Sociology of Age Stratification* (Riley, Johnson, and Foner 1972). More recent reviews of the field are provided in the second editions of the Handbook of Aging Series: *The Biology of Aging* (Finch and Scneider 1985), *The Psychology of Aging* (Birren and Schaie 1985), and *Aging and the Social Sciences* (Binstock and Shanas 1985).

Almost every discipline involved in gerontology has had its pioneer through this modern period, and clearly all cannot be listed here. E. V. Cowdry, whom some consider to be the father of modern gerontology, led the way with his seminal volume, *Problems of Aging*, published in 1939. Early on he recognized the interdisciplinary nature of gerontology, synthesized a variety of materials in his field, and contributed significantly to the establishment of the International Association of Gerontology (Oscar Kaplan, in Schwartz and Peterson 1979). Social psychologist Bernice Neugarten began teaching the psychology of aging at the University of Chicago in the early 1930s. She and her students have contributed immeasurably to the development of gerontology as well as to the broader study of human development. Other outstanding work was produced in psychology by Birren and Schaie, in sociology by Shanas and Rosow, in anthropology by Simmons and Clark, in economics by Kreps, and in history (more recently) by Fischer and Achenbaum. These people and others not named here have also contributed to the development of strong university centers at Chicago, Duke, Brandeis, Southern California, and elsewhere.

The study of aging continues to grow, in part fueled by funding from federal government sources. The National Institutes of Health, including the National Institute of Mental Health and the newer National Institute on Aging, and the Administration on Aging, through state and area offices on aging, provide the primary funding for interdisciplinary research and training in gerontology. Other governmental agencies (the Department of Labor, for example) as well as private organizations such as the American Association of Retired Persons also fund research and training programs related to aging.

If one were to write a more detailed history of the last thirty years in gerontology, an important point to develop would be the extent to which it has been institutionalized on the U.S. academic scene. Courses on aging are taught on almost every college and university campus; students major in gerontology, and professors identify themselves as gerontologists. The Association for Gerontology in Higher Education (AGHE) was established in 1974 for the purpose of advancing gerontology as a field of study within institutions of higher learning. The 1985 AGHE Directory lists 205 formal gerontology programs at member colleges and universities. A formal gerontology program is defined as one offering a degree, certificate, concentration, specialization, emphasis, or minor in gerontology, or is identified as a research or clinical training center in gerontology, geriatrics, or both.

Still, there remains much debate over whether or not gerontology ought to be recognized as a discipline in its own right, as are psychology, physics, and philosophy. Some argue that gerontologists have not really succeeded in creating a body of theory all their own, that gerontology is just a consumer of theories from other sciences, and that gerontologists should be satisfied with the field functioning as an applied social science. One contributing factor in this argument involves the dissension over what constitutes the common core of knowledge in gerontology. A joint committee of the Association for Gerontology in Higher Education (AGHE) and the Gerontological Society has addressed this issue. And, according to the committee, insufficient consensus exists about the common core of knowledge in gerontology. Defining consensus as 90 percent agreement, this committee found that gerontological educators and practitioners agreed on only three topics—the psychology of aging, health and aging, and the biology of aging—for inclusion in an essential content of gerontology (Jacobson 1980). Other topics that came close included demography of aging, sensory change, the sociology of aging, and the environment and aging.

The future of gerontology continues to depend on the willingness of traditional academic departments (for example, psychology, sociology, biology, and so on) to cooperate in the gerontological enterprise. If academic competition becomes the order of the day, the field will surely suffer. If these traditional disciplines make a commitment to interdisciplinary activity, the field will surely flourish. Some of us are optimistic, for we understand that no discipline by itself is capable of providing adequate education in gerontology.

METHODOLOGICAL ISSUES IN AGING RESEARCH

Earlier we defined *gerontology* as the systematic study of the aging process. In addition, gerontology was described as an interdisciplinary study with *major* elements drawn from the physical and social sciences. In this regard, active researchers in gerontology have relied and continue to rely on scientific methods of investigation. Actually, as Popenoe (1983) points out, scientists can take three paths in the pursuit of knowledge. One path, involving reasoning from what is already known in order to discover the unknown, is referred to as the use of *deductive logic.* A second path, which involves what may be described as the direct perception of truth without the encumbrances of reasoning or logic, can be referred to as *intuition.* Gerontologists do not reject deductive logic and intuition as paths to knowledge, but they do rely more heavily on a third path—the empirical method. The *empirical method* involves the use of human senses—sight and hearing, for example—to "observe" the world (Popenoe 1983). This method is public; the observations of one researcher can be checked for accuracy by others using the same process. Gerontological "truths" cannot be accepted solely on the basis of logic or intuition. They must be subjected to empirical investigation.

Most students reading this text have limited experience with empirical research (and, likely, even less experience with such research carried out by gerontologists). Moreover, much of this experience comes from reading research reports required for fulfilling course assignments. Typically, what the student sees is a finished product, which includes a statement of the problem to be investigated, some theoretical justification, discussion of the research methods employed, presentation of the data, and discussion of the findings. Rarely does the student get a chance to observe firsthand the problems involved in carrying out the research process. These include how the project may have changed in the course of the research process and the judgments that the researcher was forced to make as difficulties were encountered (Williamson, Karp, and Dalphin 1977).

The research problems gerontologists encounter are much like those encountered by scientists working in a wide array of scientific disciplines. Common concerns include the appropriateness of research technique and design, the validity and reliability of measurement devices, problems of sampling, data analysis, and so on. The following brief description of the most frequently used methods in gerontological research provides examples from the social sciences (with particular emphasis on sociology and psychology) to show how research is currently carried out in the field of aging.

Field Research

Field research is generally observation-centered. It is most useful in the study of relatively small groups of individuals or well-defined social settings and may allow the researcher to establish and maintain close, firsthand contact with subjects and their actions (Williamson, Karp, and Dalphin 1977). Zelditch (1962) distinguishes among three types of strategies for field research: (1) participant observation, (2) informant interviewing, and (3) enumeration and samples.

Participant observation includes observing and participating in events, interviewing other participants during the events, and maintaining stable relationships in the group. *Informant interviewing* involves interviewing an informant about others in the group and about events that have happened in the past. *Enumerations and samples* include small surveys and structured observations that require a low level of participation in group events.

Field work requires what Smith (1975) describes as "distinctive methodological attitudes." In general, this means that the researcher must be comfortable with the lack of standardization and the unstructured nature of the field research process. Field research must be quite flexible and adaptable to changing environmental conditions as well as to emerging theoretical concerns. In this regard, field methods are much more conducive to description than inferential analysis and more conducive to hypothesis generation than hypothesis testing (Smith 1975).

A significant problem the field researcher faces has to do with the possible influence or affect the research itself may have on the field setting. For example, as Smith (1975) indicates, the more the researcher finds it necessary to participate in the field setting, the more the research role will depend on the ability to establish successful trust relationships with individuals in the field setting. The fact of establishing informant contacts with some subjects and not others may affect the relationships among these subjects. Also, such relationships with informants may bias data collection towards one point of view and away from others.

A number of gerontological researchers have employed field research methods, principally participant observation, with considerable success in the study of retirement communities (Keith 1977, 1982; Jacobs 1974; Hochschild 1973; Johnson 1971), nursing homes (Gubrium 1975), and single-room occupancy (SRO) hotels (Stephens 1976). Keith (1977, 1982) and her husband took an apartment at Les Floralies, a high-rise retirement residence with a planned capacity of 150, which was built by the French national retirement fund for construction workers and is located in a suburb outside of Paris. Residents included those who had worked in the construction trades and their spouses. The average age of residents was seventy-five, almost two-thirds were female, and 90 percent received some form of government assistance to meet the costs of living in the residence. Keith (1977, 1982) immersed herself in the activities of the retirement community:

> In the first few weeks, I participated in every possible aspect of community life, as I tried to outline a map of social relations. Access to organized activities was easy: committee meetings once a week, a weekly sewing and knitting group, daily work with volunteer residents in the kitchen, the laundry or the research office, and the afternoon *belote* game. These activities, as well as the meals at different tables, led to invitations to aperitif or coffee in people's apartments. Neighbors invited us too, and the head of the Communist faction became my knitting teacher, which required frequent visits. (Reproduced by permission from Jennie Keith: *Old people, new lives*, pp. 29–30. Chicago: University of Chicago Press. Copyright 1977, 1982 by The University of Chicago. All rights reserved.)

Les Floralies is not just an apartment house for elderly retirees. Rather, Keith informs us that it is inhabited by people who are engaged together in the process of creating community. This work identifies a number of factors that contribute to the creation of community among these people. First, residents share many characteristics in common in addition to age. These include occupation, educational level, income, ethnicity, and social class. Second, these old people believed that their alternatives were few. Thus, they made considerable financial and emotional investment in the move. Being "here for the rest of our lives" was certainly an important source of identification with the community. Third, they entered this setting in small enough numbers to get to know each other personally; the physical arrangements, in particular those in the dining room, helped promote a greater sense of participation in the residence:

> The small round tables undoubtedly make possible very different social consequences for eating together than the long, institutional tables I have seen in some residences. The table group of four offers a possibility for immediate, primary ties which consistently appear in studies of human groups as essential for linking the individual to a larger community. (Reproduced by permission from Jennie Keith: *Old people, new lives*. Chicago: University of Chicago Press. Copyright 1977, 1982 by The University of Chicago. All rights reserved.)

Keith believes that these factors allowed residents to turn to each other for the fulfillment of their social needs. They supported each other in illness and emergency, just as they laughed and danced together at parties. Further, they were able to evaluate each other in terms of the life they shared in the residence, rather than according to the status system of the outside world. In this regard, they identified themselves as members of a community of age-mates sharing refuge from an outside world fraught with physical, financial, social, and psychological dangers for them.

Although Keith's insightful work involves the study of only one specific retirement community—a fact that makes generalization to other communities problematic—it can be added to a body of field research on retirement communities (for example, Hochschild 1973; Jacobs 1974; Johnson 1971) that suggests that the factors important for community formation among old people in the suburbs of Paris may be the same for communities of old people in the United States.

Use of Existing Records

Examination of existing records of individual behavior or social conditions can serve as a useful method of research for the gerontologist. Such records include personal written accounts, such as diaries or letters; public documents, such as birth, death, marriage, and probate records; and print media, film records, and sound recordings. Another kind of existing record that can be useful to a researcher is the statistical compilation (Palmer 1978). Although the best and most widely used statistical compilations are the official publications of the U.S. Bureau of the Census, other organizations provide additional sources of statistical information. In recent years there has been considerable growth in the number of machine-readable data files available for statistical analysis. Archival organizations have become important in making these data files available to researchers. The two largest machine-readable data archives in the United States serving the general social science community are the Inter-University Consortium for Political and Social Research (ICPSR) at the University of Michigan and the Roper Center (Sinott et al. 1983). Many universities and research institutes serve their social science researchers by providing facilities to order data from these two repositories. Such data can be used for secondary analysis. *Secondary analysis* describes a reanalysis of data produced by someone else and often for other purposes. One problem with secondary analysis is that the current researcher is at the mercy of the original researcher in terms of what questions were asked to collect the data. Nevertheless, secondary analysis can be quite fruitful and, given the prohibitive costs of doing research, is likely to become even more popular in the future.

Researchers who use existing records not provided in some statistical format are likely to engage in some kind of *content analysis*. Here the researcher establishes a number of categories, each of which refers to some repeated or patterned occurrence in the content of the record. Tabulations made of the frequency of each element or combination of elements may constitute the basic data in the research (Palmer 1978). It is important in content analysis that the

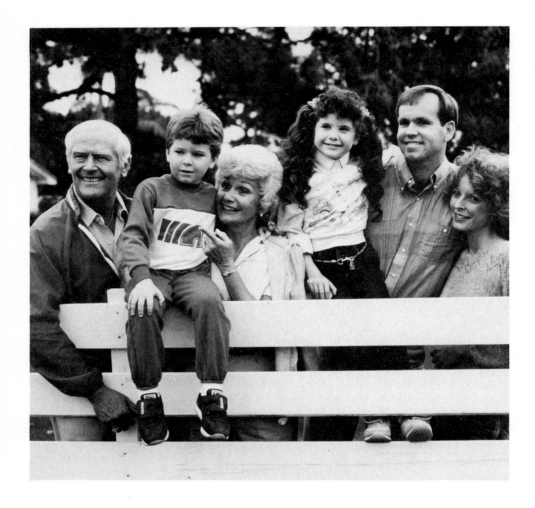

categories used are precisely defined and well tailored to the research problem at hand.

Engler-Bowles and Kart (1983) content analyzed sixty wills sampled from Wood County, Ohio, probate records filed between 1820 and 1967. They were interested in the extent to which inheritance practices reflected changes in the family relationships of older people in a largely rural area of northwest Ohio during this time period. Testamentary documents commend themselves for such use because of their public and permanent accessibility as well as the demands for legal accuracy (Bryant and Snizek 1975). In addition, the will represents a most candid and forthright form of communication. Nevertheless, testamentary records do have some limitations. Systematic bias may be introduced as a result of the number of people who die intestate (without a will).

Also, the wills themselves often do not contain relevant demographic, social, and economic information that is important for addressing certain research questions.

In order to categorize the way elderly testators disposed of their estates, Engler-Bowles and Kart used a typology of inheritance patterns adapted from Rosenfeld (1979) to identify the presence or absence of family obligation. This typology was used to measure the relative degree of that obligation as indicated by the following three categories of inheritance patterns: familistic inheritance, articulated inheritance, and disinheritance.

Familistic inheritance represents the strongest degree of obligation by the testator to family ties. Wills in this category generally distribute the estate among family members only. *Articulated inheritance* is the dual recognition of kin and nonkin, with priority placed on nonkin heirs in testamentary disposition. *Disinheritance* is the total exclusion of family members from testamentary disposition and, therefore, the apparent absence of family obligation as perceived by the testator.

The familistic inheritance pattern dominated the time period explored by Engler-Bowles and Kart. Articulated wills appeared rarely; several wills seemed equally divided between familistic and articulated bequests; and no examples of total family disinheritance were evident in this population of wills. Across this lengthy time span married testators emphasized their conjugal relations, showing the strong emphasis placed on the nuclear family throughout the period. In the early part of this time period direct bequests to children were usually unequal, sometimes reflecting differences in sex and individual circumstances such as advancements made to certain children. Starting in the latter part of the nineteenth century, sons and daughters were equally likely to receive testamentary bequest.

Misconceptions about the family lives of elderly Americans past and present abound. Stereotypical images of alienated families and the isolated aged are popular topics for research and mass media reports. The study by Engler-Bowles and Kart presents a different picture. Their analysis suggests that elderly Wood County, Ohio, testators were active participants in family life and maintained strong ties to their children from the early nineteenth century until the middle of the twentieth century. Still, additional historical research is necessary to determine whether the results of this study are idiosyncratic to a small sample of will writers in rural, northwest Ohio.

Survey Research

Survey research differs from other methods of data collection in two important ways. First, the focus is generally on a representative sample of a relatively large population. Second, data are collected from respondents directly, often at their homes, through the use of interviews or questionnaires or both. The major elements that in combination make up the survey research process include sampling procedures, questionnaire or interview schedule construction and testing, interviews carried out by trained interviewers, and data preparation and analysis (Palmer 1978).

Studies that employ a survey research approach may follow a cross-sectional or a longitudinal design. A *cross-sectional* study is carried out at one point in time and examines the relationships among a set of variables as they occur at that time. A *longitudinal* study involves repeated contacts with the same respondents over a period of time and is particularly attentive to changes that occur with time. This type of research design is frequently referred to as a panel study.

There are important differences between questionnaires and interviews as data collecting tools in survey research. Questionnaires, delivered to respondents at work or school or mailed to them at home, are filled out by the respondents themselves. This permits access to many people who are spread over a large geographical area while saving time and money. Disadvantages include the need for a literate population and the low response rate that can be expected (30 percent is not uncommon). Also, questionnaires must be relatively brief, as respondents may lose interest quickly. Thus, questionnaires often cannot provide an in-depth probing of respondents' attitudes.

Interviews can be carried out either face to face or over the telephone. The latter are less expensive, because interviewer travel time is virtually eliminated. A serious obstacle to the personal interview is the initial resistance to being interviewed. Nevertheless, as Blalock and Blalock (1982) point out, refusals to be interviewed once a contact has been made are relatively rare, and most respondents are cooperative, seem to enjoy the experience, and appear to take it seriously.

The National Council on the Aging, Inc., commissioned the polling firm of Louis Harris and Associates, Inc., to carry out an in-depth survey of public attitudes in the United States toward the elderly. The survey, conducted in the summer of 1974, also documented older citizens' views and expectations of themselves and their personal experiences of old age. Trained interviewers completed over 4,200 in-person household interviews for the study. The sample included a representative cross-section of the U.S. public eighteen years of age and over, selected by random sampling techniques. Additional representative samples of the public sixty-five years of age and over as well as those fifty-five to sixty-four were drawn to allow detailed analysis of these groups. Finally, the sample design included an additional cross-section of blacks aged sixty-five years and over to ensure a detailed look at their conditions and attitudes. All subgroups were weighted back to their true proportions in the U.S. population for the purpose of analysis.

The findings reported in the original study report were organized into eight sections and are too numerous to list here. Sections include "public expectations of most people over sixty-five," the "social and economic contribution of people sixty-five and over," "the media and the image of people over sixty-five," and "the politics of old age." One conclusion of the report is that, although serious problems of inadequate income, fear of crime, poor health, loneliness, lack of medical care, and transportation do indeed exist for certain minorities of older people, they are not as pervasive as the public thinks. More importantly, having a problem should not be confused with *being* one. The report goes on:

> Such generalizations about the elderly as an economically and socially deprived group can do the old a disservice, for they confront older people with a society who sees them merely as a problem and not as part of the solution to any of society's problems. Such problems as the public perceive among the elderly can only generate a sense of guilt and pity among the young, and not a sense of appreciation for the talents and energies that older people can still contribute to society. As a result, older people are not likely to find themselves the recipients of opportunities to pitch in and help solve the problems that affect our society as a whole. As a group for whom there is little social and economic demand, the older population also may lose self-esteem with deleterious effects. (p. 38)

Laboratory Experimentation

Laboratory experimentation, used primarily by psychologists, involves the systematic observation of phenomenon under controlled conditions. In the simplest experiment there is a single independent variable (*I*) and a single dependent variable (*D*), and the research hypothesis is that *I* leads to *D*. As Abrahamson (1983) suggests, the effect of the independent variable upon the dependent variable need not be viewed as causal, although it ordinarily is in experiments. The primary objective of the experimental procedure is to eliminate the possibility that any variable other than the independent variable will affect the dependent variable.

The operationalization of the independent variable acts to define experimental and control groups in the simple laboratory experiment. These groups comprise subjects who are alike in every way except that those in the experimental group are exposed to *I*, whereas those in the control group are not. Assuming initial equality, any observed differences between the two groups on the dependent variable can be attributed to the influence of the experimentally introduced independent variable (Palmer 1978). Numerous variations on this uncomplicated model have been developed and are represented in the gerontological literature. An example follows.

Elderly adults often complain about memory problems, in particular the forgetting of names. Yesavage and his colleagues (1983) devised an experiment to determine the effectiveness of different techniques in helping older people improve their learning of face-name associations. Elderly participants in a retirement fund, invited to join a brief course on memory improvement, were divided into three groups. Initially, members of all groups were taught to remember names by (1) identifying a prominent feature of a person's face (for example, a large mouth); (2) transforming the person's surname into a concrete word (for example, the name "Whalen" becomes "a whale"); and (3) associating the concrete word with the prominent facial feature.

The control group received no further instruction in the encoding of names and faces. A second group received treatment identical to the control group; in addition, however, participants were taught to form a *visual image* incorporating both the prominent facial feature of the person and a concrete transformation of the name. It was emphasized that the images be seen interacting physically (for example, a whale in a person's mouth). This second group will be referred to as the *image group.* Group 3 was treated identically to the image group except that participants were further told to make a *judgment* about the pleasantness or unpleasantness of the visual image association (this group will be referred to as the *image + judgment group).*

Testing materials including faces taken from a high school yearbook. Male and female faces were represented equally, as was the distribution of prominent facial features in each test set. Common surnames were chosen and randomly assigned to the faces. Immediate tests of name recall were given after groups received their instruction and again after a forty-eight–hour delay.

Those in the image + judgment group outperformed all others, whereas those in the image group performed better than control group participants only in immediate recall. The researchers suggest that having the participants make affective judgments increases the image association and enhances both immediate and delayed recall. Still, laboratory experiments are not aimed at replicating the real world. Further research, both inside and outside the laboratory, will be required to determine the effectiveness of such techniques in cognitive training programs for elderly adults.

The Age/Period/Cohort Problem

One methodological issue in particular, referred to as the *age/period/cohort problem* (APC), has preoccupied gerontological researchers for over a decade (Maddox 1979). Interest in this problem first developed among psychologists attempting to understand what happens to intellectual functioning in old age (for example, Schaie 1976) and among political scientists interested in voting behavior across the life cycle (for example, Hudson and Binstock 1976). Both groups of researchers came to realize the importance of conceptually distinguishing among maturational factors (age), biographical factors (cohort), and environmental factors (period of measurement). This realization is now fundamental to all research on matters of the life course.

Age. It is commonly assumed that people change in certain ways as they age. Yet age change may refer to three different aspects of aging: biological aging (sometimes referred to as maturation), psychological aging (including developmental processes related to intellectual functioning and coping), and sociological aging (connoting role changes and social adjustment). It is often difficult to make clear distinctions among these three aspects of aging, especially when one takes the approach (as this book does) that biological and psychological aging can be shaped by social experience. And, as the effects of social experience on individuals are specified with increasing precision, chronological age may come to have less utility as a variable in research.

Period. The period of historical time through which a person lives influences the way that person ages. In addition, two people who experience the same historical point in time at different times in their life cycles may be influenced differently. For example, people who experienced the depression as teenagers may have been affected differently from those who were already middle-aged during that period. Glen Elder, Jr. (1974, 1975), studied the impact of the depression on different individuals and noted that their conditions of life during this period varied greatly according to their age, sex, race, and residence. He found that not everyone suffered economic deprivation. Working-class and self-employed persons as well as "foreigners" were among those most affected by the Great Depression; their deprivation during this period seems to have made a lasting impression on them. As Elder (1974) points out, adults who remember what it was like to have very little in the 1930s appear to be more appreciative of their life situations during the more affluent, secure years of the 1940s and 1950s.

A problem for gerontological researchers is that the notion of *period* usually refers to some environmental context. Most Americans think of the whole society as the environmental context for the depression, but Elder informs us that this was not the case. The depression did not occur everywhere in the United States and did not have the same impact in all those places where it did occur. Maddox (1979) believes that researchers must reach a point where they can specify and then measure relevant environments. This is no simple task because environments may range from large-scale sociocultural contexts (for example, "society") to smaller scale environments such as communities, neighborhoods, and families.

Cohort. The term *cohort* is used to describe a group of persons born at approximately the same time. The value in the concept lies in the ability to define it broadly (for example, persons born within a five- or ten-year period) and use it to describe summarily the size and characteristics of a segment of the population. Unfortunately, the term is often used to describe a broad segment of the life course such as adolescence or old age. This can be misleading. Such life course segments include many cohorts. We all may recognize the differences between twenty-year-old and forty-year-old persons, but we often overlook the same twenty-year difference between those who are fifty-five and those who are seventy-five. Neugarten (1974) makes the distinction between the "young-old" (fifty-five to seventy-four years of age) and the "old-old" (seventy-five years of age and older). The young-old are healthier, wealthier, and more educated than the old-old, and their family and career experiences and ex-pectations are quite different. Clearly, gerontologists must become sensitive to the fact that people with different biographical characteristics all undergo the aging process.

Even Neugarten's dichotomizing of the elderly population is insufficient. There are no theoretical or empirical grounds for treating those fifty-five to fifty-nine years of age and those seventy to seventy-four years as if they were interchangeable. In the final analysis, sensitivity to cohort differences acts to reduce the utility of conceptualizing persons sixty-five years of age and over as *the* elderly (Maddox and Campbell 1985).

As Maddox and Campbell (1985) point out, although conventional defi-nitions of age, period, or cohort effect can be found in diverse sources, the actual practical distinctions among these effects can tend to blur. They offer as example the introduction of vitamin D into milk supplies. This innovation was made instantaneously; thus it can be thought of as a period effect that cuts across all age groups. Yet, certain cohorts of newborns received the benefits of vitamin D supplements in their milk almost immediately from birth, whereas preceding cohorts received the benefits no earlier than the date of introduction. The period effect had potentially different consequences for different cohorts. Some received the vitamin supplements through all of their childhood years; others received the supplements for a smaller proportion of those years. Is this nutritional innovation a period or cohort effect or both?

Concern with age, period, and cohort analyses in gerontology reflects a need to understand the relationship between environmental alternatives and constraints (broadly construed) and individual biological aging. The data sets necessary to address the age/period/cohort problem are beginning to emerge. They include measures at the individual and societal levels across time and nations. It is not clear, though, that the pace of conceptual and theoretical debate in gerontology has kept up with methodological and statistical advances in identifying APC effects (Maddox and Campbell 1985).

SUMMARY

There are several reasons for studying aging, not the least of which is the intrinsic fascination of the field. Students of aging date back several thousand years. Perhaps the most prominent past concern was the quest to prolong life. This is reflected in the antediluvian, hyperborean, and fountain themes, all represented in contemporary times.

The scientific study of the aging process is a recent phenomenon, which arose out of a need to make clear distinctions between myth and history, magic and science. The first full, explicit theory of the causation of aging is found in Greco-Roman medicine and the Hippocratic theory. The Greek influence persisted, and a radical break with earlier modes of thought did not occur until the scientific method was born during the sixteenth and seventeenth centuries.

By the nineteenth century, capacity for scientific research increased; by the latter part of the century a fledgling science of old age could be envisioned. During the early part of the twentieth century the locus of aging study shifted toward the United States. By the 1930s a new attitude toward old age emerged—a perception of old age as a social problem. Recognition of the prevalence of incapacity, isolation, and poverty among elderly people had enormous impact on the growth of gerontology as both a scientific and applied discipline.

In the 1970s gerontology was institutionalized on the U.S. academic scene. There is still much debate over whether or not gerontology can be recognized as a discipline in its own right. Some argue that gerontologists have not created a body of theory of their own and should be satisfied to see gerontology function as an applied social science. Nevertheless, gerontologists today show a strong research orientation and employ a variety of research procedures in their efforts, including field research, use of existing records, survey research, and laboratory experimentation. Gerontologists are also concerned with a number of special methodological issues in aging research—in particular, the age/period/cohort problem—as well as the common concerns shared by scientists in a wide array of scientific disciplines.

STUDY QUESTIONS

1. Describe the antediluvian, hyperborean, and fountain themes of aging. How are these themes reflected in modern society?

2. What are the three main tasks confronting the student of aging?

3. The Hippocratic theory of innate heat was the first explicit theory of aging in the Western world. Describe this theory, explaining why it is considered a breakthrough in the study of aging.

4. Changing attitudes in the 1930s resulted in a major growth of the field of gerontology. Old age was increasingly recognized as a social problem. Can you discuss some social and demographic factors influencing this change in attitude?

5. Discuss the application of field research in the study of gerontology, distinguishing among (1) participant observation, (2) informant interviewing, and (3) enumeration and samples.

6. Explain how survey research differs from other methods of data collection. What are the major elements of the survey research process?

7. Distinguish between cross-sectional and longitudinal research designs.

8. Why is it important to distinguish age, period, and cohort effects in gerontological research?

BIBLIOGRAPHY

Abrahamson, M. 1983. *Social research methods.* Englewood Cliffs, N.J.: Prentice-Hall.

Achenbaum, W.A. 1978. *Old age in the new land.* Baltimore, Md.: Johns Hopkins University Press.

Binstock, R., and Shanas, E. 1985. *Aging and the social sciences* (2nd ed.). New York: Van Nostrand Reinhold Co.

Birren, J. 1959. *Handbook of aging and the individual: Psychological and biological aspects.* Chicago: University of Chicago Press.

———. 1961. A brief history of the psychology of aging. *Gerontologist* 1:69–77.

Birren, J., and Clayton, V. 1975. History of gerontology. In D. Woodruff and J. Birren (eds.), *Aging: Scientific perspectives and social issues.* New York: D. Van Nostrand Co.

Birren, J., and Schaie, W. 1985. *The psychology of aging* (2nd ed.). New York: Van Nostrand Reinhold Co.

Blalock, A.B., and Blacock, H.M., Jr. 1982. *Introduction to social research* (2nd ed.). Englewood Cliffs, N.J.: Prentice-Hall.

Blythe, R. 1979. *The view in winter: Reflections on old age.* New York: Harcourt Brace Jovanovich, Inc.

Bromley, D.B. 1974. *The psychology of human aging* (2nd ed.). Middlesex, England: Penguin Books.

Bryant C., and Snizek, W. 1975. The last will and testament: A neglected document in sociological research. *Sociology and Social Research* 59:219–230.

Burgess, E. 1960. *Aging in Western societies.* Chicago: University of Chicago Press.

Elder, G., Jr. 1974. *Children of the Great Depression.* Chicago: University of Chicago Press.

———. 1975. Age differentiation and the life course. *American Sociological Review* 1:165–190.

Engler-Bowles, C.A., and Kart, C.S. 1983. Intergenerational relations and testamentary patterns: An exploration. *Gerontologist* 23(2):167–173.

Finch, C., and Hayflick, L. 1977. *The biology of aging.* New York: Van Nostrand Reinhold Co.

Freeman, J. 1965. Medical perspectives in aging (12-19th century). *Gerontologist* 5:1–24.

Grant, R.L. 1963. Concepts of aging: An historical review. *Perspectives in Biology and Medicine* 6:443–478.

Gruman, G. 1966. *A history of ideas about the prolongation of life.* Philadelphia, Pa.: American Philosophical Society.

Gubrium, J.F. 1975. *Living and dying at Murray Manor.* New York: St. Martin's Press.

Hall, G.S. 1922. *Senescence, the last half of life.* New York: Appleton and Co.

Hendricks, J., and Hendricks, C.D. 1977. *Aging in mass society: Myths and realities.* Cambridge, Mass.: Winthrop Publishers, Inc.

Henratta, J., and Campbell, R. 1976. Status attainment and status maintenance: A study of satisfaction in old age. *American Sociological Review* 41:981–992.

Hochschild, A.R. 1973. *The unexpected community.* Englewood Cliffs, N.J.: Prentice-Hall.

Hudson, R., and Binstock, R. 1976. Political systems and aging. In R. Binstock and E. Shanas (eds.), *Aging and the social sciences.* New York: Van Nostrand Reinhold Co.

Jacobs, J. 1974. *Fun City: An ethnographic study of a retirement community.* New York: Holt, Rinehart and Winston.

Jacobson, R.L. 1980. Gerontology said to lack identity as an academic discipline. *The Chronicle of Higher Education* March 17:4.

Johnson, S.K. 1971. *Idle Haven: Community building among the working class retired.* Berkeley: University of California Press.

Keith, J. 1977, 1982. *Old people, new lives.* Chicago: University of Chicago Press.

Krause, D. 1987. Careers in gerontology: Occupational fact or academic fancy? *Gerontologist* 27(1):30–33.

Lowenthal, M. 1977. Toward a sociological theory of change in adulthood and old age. In J. Birren and W. Schaie (eds.), *The psychology of aging.* New York: Van Nostrand Reinhold Co.

Maddox, G. 1979. Sociology of later life. *Annual Review of Sociology* 5:113–135.

Maddox, G., and Campbell, R.T. 1985. Scope, concepts and methods in the study of aging. In R. Binstock and E. Shanas (eds.), *Aging and the social sciencies* (2nd ed.). New York: Van Nostrand Reinhold Co.

Maddox, G., and Wiley, J. 1976. Scope, concepts and methods in the study of aging. In R. Binstock and E. Shanas (eds.), *Aging and the social sciences.* New York: Van Nostrand Reinhold Co.

National Council on the Aging. 1976. *The myth and reality of aging in America.* Washington, D.C.: NCOA.

Neugarten, B. 1974. Age groups in American society and the rise of the young-old. *Annals of the American Academy* (September): 187–198.

Palmer, N. 1978. Measurement procedures. In C. Kart (ed.), *Exploring social problems.* Sherman Oaks, Calif.: Alfred Publishing.

Pollak, O. 1948. *Social adjustment in old age: A research planning report.* New York: Social Science Research Council.

Popenoe, D. 1983. *Sociology* (5th ed.). Englewood Cliffs, N.J.: Prentice-Hall.

Riley, M.W., and Foner, A. 1968. *Aging and society: An inventory of research findings.* New York: Russell Sage Foundation.

Riley, M.W., Johnson, M., and Foner, A. 1972. *A sociology of age stratification.* New York: Russell Sage Foundation.

Riley, M.W., Riley, J., and Johnson, M. 1969. *Aging and the professions.* New York: Russell Sage Foundation.

Rosow, I. 1976. Status and role change through the life span. In R. Binstock and E. Shanas (eds.), *Aging and the social sciences.* New York: Van Nostrand Reinhold Company.

Schaie, W. 1976. Quasi-experimental research design in the psychology of aging. In J. Birren and W. Schaie (eds.), *The psychology of aging.* New York: Van Nostrand Reinhold Co.

Schwartz, A., and Peterson, J. 1979. *Introduction to gerontology.* New York: Holt, Rinehart and Winston, Inc.

Sinnott, J.D., Harris, C.S., Block, M.R., Collesano, S., and Jacobson, S.G. 1983. *Applied research in aging: A guide to methods and resources.* Boston: Little, Brown and Co.

Smith, H.W. 1975. *Strategies of social research: The methodological imagination.* Englewood Cliffs, N.J.: Prentice-Hall.

Stephens, J. 1976. *Loners, losers, and lovers: Elderly tenants in a slum hotel.* Seattle: University of Washington Press.

Sussman, M. 1976. The family life of old people. In R. Binstock and E. Shanas (eds.), *Aging and the social sciences.* New York: Van Nostrand Reinhold Co.

Tibbitts, C. 1960. *Handbook of social gerontology: Societal aspects of aging.* Chicago: University of Chicago Press.

Williamson, J.B., Karp, D.A., and Dalphin, J.R. 1977. *The research craft: An introduction to social science methods.* Boston: Little, Brown and Co.

Woodruff, D., and Birren, J. 1975. *Aging: Scientific perspectives and social issues.* New York: D. Van Nostrand Co.

Yesavage, J.A., Rose, T.L., and Bower, G.H. 1983. Interactive imagery and affective judgments improve face-name learning in the elderly. *Journal of Gerontology* 38(2):197–203.

Zelditch, M., Jr. 1962. Some methodological problems of field studies. *American Journal of Sociology* 67:566–576.

CHAPTER 3

THE DEMOGRAPHY OF AGING

There are now more than 27 million people aged sixty-five years and older in the United States. This group represents the fastest growing age group in the U.S. population: if those aged sixty-five years and over were all grouped together, they would make up the most populous state in the nation, exceeding the population of California. Actually, there are more people aged sixty-five and older in the United States than the combined total resident populations of New England (Maine, New Hampshire, Vermont, Massachusetts, Rhode Island, and Connecticut) and the Mountain States (Montana, Idaho, Wyoming, Colorado, New Mexico, Arizona, Utah, and Nevada).

Assessing the circumstances of old people in the United States requires an understanding of how this group is currently composed, how the elderly population has changed from the past, and how it may change in the future. Population attributes—*fertility, mortality, and migration*—influence and are influenced by social and economic conditions. High birth rates in the first decades of the twentieth century have yielded large numbers of elderly sixty-five to seventy-five years later. Progress in public health and medicine has reduced the rates of illness and mortality, especially among infants and the young, allowing more of the population to live to be old. Immigration to the United States has also had an impact on the growth of the elderly population in recent years. Migrants who were young adults at the time of their immigration before World War I increased the numbers of persons in their respective age groups, leading to large numbers of older people decades later.

This chapter presents a systematic study of aged population trends and phenomena in relation to their social setting. Much of the available data in the United States define the elderly as those sixty-five years of age and older. Although 65+ is an imprecise identifier of the older population, it is a useful designation for gerontologists, and we follow it in this chapter. This definition is not universal, however. We all may recognize the differences between twenty-year-old and forty-year-old persons, but we often overlook the same twenty-year difference between those who are fifty-five and those who are seventy-five. Neugarten (1974) makes the distinction between the *young-old* (fifty-five to seventy-four years of age) and the *old-old* (seventy-five years of age and older). Recently, the National Institute on Aging has sought research proposals to study those individuals eighty-five years of age and older. This activity suggests the usefulness of further subdividing the old-old into those seventy-five to eighty-four years (*the elderly*) and those eighty-five years and over (*the very-old*). The young-old are healthier, wealthier, and better educated than the old-old, and their family and career experiences and expectations are quite different.

NUMBER AND PROPORTION
OF THE ELDERLY

The elderly population of the United States has grown consistently since the turn of the century, when about 3.1 million men and women were aged sixty-five and over. By 1990 this population is expected to increase to almost 31.8 million (see Table 3-1), a more than tenfold increase. This is much greater than the rate of increase for the total U.S. population, which is expected to increase little more than three times from 76 to 250 million in the same period.

As Table 3-1 shows, the absolute and proportional increases in the aged population are expected to continue into the twenty-first century, though at a slowed pace until the 2010–2020 decade. Between 1990 and 2000 the projected increase in the aged population is about 3.2 million, or a 10.2 percent decennial

TABLE 3-1   Total Aged Population and Percentage of Total Population That Is Aged, 1950–2020

	1950	1960	1970	1980	Projections			
					1990	2000	2010	2020
65 years and older (thousands)	12,397	16,675	20,087	25,708	31,799	35,036	39,269	51,386
Percent of total population (%)	8.1	9.3	9.9	11.3	12.7	13.1	13.9	17.3
Increase in preceding decade (%)	—	34.5	20.5	28.0	23.7	10.2	12.1	30.9

Note: Based on Middle Series Census Bureau Projections. These projections are based on the following assumptions: (1) an average of 1.9 lifetime births per woman; (2) life expectancy in 2050 of 79.6; and (3) net immigration of 450,000.

Source: Siegel and Davidson (1984, Tables 2.1 and 2.5).

increase. This compares with the 6.1 million or 23.7 percent decennial increase projected between 1980 and 1990. This slowed growth rate in the elderly population is a reflection of the small cohorts caused by the low birth rate during the Great Depression and up to World War II. (All persons born during the

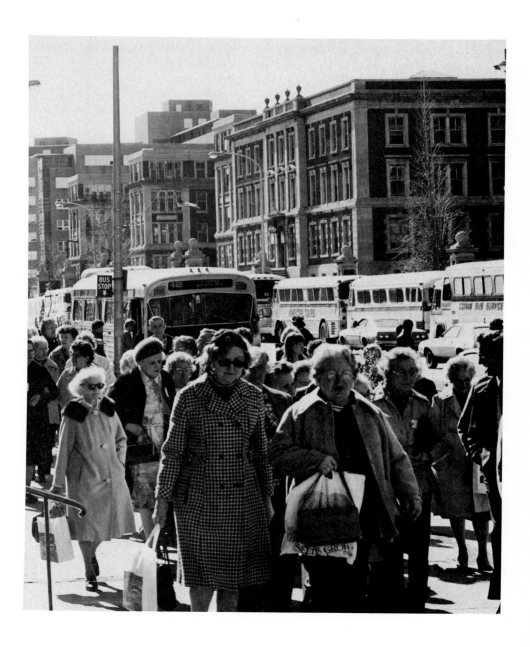

same year who are analyzed as a unit throughout their lifetimes constitute a *cohort* [Petersen 1975].) The earliest of these small cohorts reach age sixty-five during the last decade of this century. When the postwar babies reach age sixty-five shortly after the year 2010, the growth rate in the elderly population will again increase. Table 3-1 shows this; the projected increase in the elderly population between 2010 and 2020 is 30.9 percent. Later, this growth rate will most likely fall, reflecting a decline in birth rates that began in the 1960s.

Demographers have considerable confidence in these projections, because all those who will be elderly by the year 2050 have already been born. The accuracy of these projections will be determined ultimately by how accurately demographers predict mortality among these maturing individuals. This is not an easy task. For a time, demographers employed a single assumption of regular small declines in mortality rates among older adults. Census Bureau demographer Jacob S. Siegel (1979) indicates that this is no longer a safe course to follow. Death rates may decline at different rates in successive periods or may even rise occasionally as they have in the last several decades. Crimmins (1980) suggests that we have entered a new era of mortality decline primarily caused by reduced death rates from cardiovascular diseases and reduced death rates generally at older ages. If this is so, there would be a substantial increase in the number of people over sixty-five in the population.

How accurate have past projections of the older population been? U.S. Census Bureau projections of the population sixty-five years of age and over for 1975 were published at various dates from August 1953 to December 1972 and varied from 20.7 million to 22.2 million. The current figure used is 22.4 million, 7.9 percent above the low estimate and 1.1 percent above the high estimate. As Siegel (1979) points out, the percentage deviation from the current figure declined as the publication date approached 1975. This is what might have been expected. After all, the first projections were made about a future that was twenty-two years away; but in December 1972 this future was only three years ahead.

This phenomenon has already appeared in projections for the year 2000. Until 1975 estimates for the older population of 2000 ranged from 28 million to 29 million range. In 1975 the Census Bureau increased the estimate to about 30.5 million. The latest projection is 15 percent greater, or almost 35.1 million people aged sixty-five and over in the year 2000. According to Siegel, these newly revised estimates reflect lower than anticipated mortality in the 1972–76 period and the use of more favorable mortality rates in making future estimates.

Death rates are expected to continue to decline, though at a less rapid rate than in the past two decades (Siegel and Davidson 1984). Still, there is the possibility of marked future reductions in death rates at the older ages. Such changes in the trends could bring a somewhat larger elderly population and greater increases than are shown by the Census Bureau's middle series of population projections used in this text. As Table 3-1 indicates, the middle series of population projections used by the Census Bureau assumes mortality rates consistent with achieving an *average life expectancy at birth* of 79.6 years in the year 2050. Using the "highest" series of population projections, including the assumption that life expectancy in 2050 will be 83.3 years, the Census Bureau projects 36.6 million elderly in the year 2000 and 57 million by the year 2020. The "highest" series projects an aged population that is 1.6 million or 4.5 percent larger than that projected by the "middle" series for the year 2000 and 5.7 million or 11 percent larger for the year 2020.

What proportion of the total population older people will make up in the future will be determined in great part by fertility (birth rate) levels. The "middle" series of population projections used by the Census Bureau include an assumption of 1.9 lifetime births per woman. As Table 3-1 indicates, under this assumption, the elderly are expected to constitute about 17.3 percent of the total U.S. population by the year 2020. Using a "lowest" series projection, which assumes a fertility rate of 1.6, the Census Bureau estimates the elderly constituting 17.8 percent of the total U.S. population in 2020; with the "highest" series projection, which assumes a rate of 2.3 lifetime births per woman, the elderly would constitute 16.7 percent of the total population in the U.S. in 2020.

AGING OF THE OLDER POPULATION

Not only has the older population of the United States grown in absolute size and proportion of the total population during this century, but it has also aged. Table 3-2 shows that the proportion of the aged who are sixty-five to seventy-four years of age has been getting smaller and will continue to do so until

TABLE 3-2   Percent Distribution of the Population 65 Years and over, by Age, 1950–2020

	1950	1960	1970	1980	1990	2000	2010	2020
65 years and over	100.0	100.0	100.0	100.0	100.0	100.0	100.0	100.0
65 to 69	40.7	37.7	35.0	34.2	31.5	26.0	29.8	32.3
70 to 74	27.8	28.6	27.2	26.6	25.3	24.5	21.9	25.6
75 to 79	17.4	18.5	19.2	18.7	19.6	20.7	17.1	17.0
80 to 84	9.3	9.6	11.5	11.6	12.8	14.2	13.9	10.8
85 and over	4.8	5.6	7.1	8.8	10.9	14.7	17.4	14.3

Note: Based on Middle Series Census Bureau Projections. See Table 3-1 for explanation of assumptions.
Source: Siegel and Davidson (1984, Table 2.6).

2010; the proportion of the elderly aged seventy-five or over has been getting larger, and this trend is also expected to continue. In 1900 the proportion of those aged sixty-five and over who were seventy-five or over was 29 percent. By the year 2000 this figure will be about 50 percent. After the year 2010, the aging trend of the population sixty-five years and over should reverse itself as larger cohorts born in the post–World War II period enter the younger segment (sixty-five to seventy-four years) of the elderly population. The median age of the population is expected to rise to about thirty-eight years by 2030.

The aging of the older population expected to occur over the next two decades or so has important policy implications for local, state, and federal agencies. One example involves the likelihood of an increased need for extended care among the growing number of very old (Siegel and Davidson 1984).

THE DEMOGRAPHIC TRANSITION

The pattern of an increasing number and proportion of elderly persons in the U.S. population is no real surprise to students of demography. In fact, it is predictable from a theory of population change used by many demographers to explain the growth in a society's population. This theory is concerned with the relationship between birth rates and death rates (as well as migration rates) and the resulting effects on the age composition of populations. It allows us to understand and predict changes in the age composition of a society. The theory, which describes a three-stage process whereby a population moves from high fertility and high mortality to low fertility and low mortality, is often called the *demographic transition.*

The first stage of the demographic transition, characterized by high birth rates and high death rates, has been called the *high growth potential* stage because a decline in mortality, in the absence of other changes, implies very high rates of population growth (Matras 1973, 25). Preindustrial societies are examples of populations in the first stage, with their high death rates. They were extremely vulnerable to crop failure and famine, possessed limited environmental health controls, and had no health technologies for caring for the sick and disabled. Individuals in such societies usually had a life expectancy of no more than thirty-five or forty years, on the average. Fertility was also necessarily high as mortality took such a substantial toll. The continued existence of the society required these high birth rates.

The second stage, sometimes called the stage of *transitional growth,* is characterized by continued high birth rates but a declining mortality. In this second stage of demographic transition, the population grows rapidly and also undergoes changes in age composition. Typically, the declining death rates are due to technological changes: increased food production, distribution, and availability; and reduced vulnerability to crop failures and famine. The age composition changes accompanying the technological changes usually involve a slightly increased proportion of the elderly (increased longevity being the likely cause) and a marked increase in the proportion of the population that is young (resulting from a significant decline in infant and child mortality).

The third stage, characterized by low mortality and low or controlled fertility, is most often descriptive of modern Western societies. Populations experiencing this stage are capable of controlling birth rates so that low or no population growth may eventually occur. No population has as yet shown the long-term low fertility rates expected in the third stage. As the demographer Matras (1973) points out, during World War II, France and Belgium had depressed fertility and an excess of deaths over births and thus experienced a decline in population size. Still, several nations are approaching what some consider the completion of the third stage. Donald Bogue has developed an index to measure the extent to which a nation has completed the demographic transition. Applying his index to 1960 data, Bogue (1969) found that the European nations were the furthest along with a median percent of demographic transition completed of 91.4. The USSR was next, with a percentage between 80.0 and 90.0, whereas the nations of North America had a median percent of 79.0. In contrast, the African nations had a median percentage of demographic transition completed of 19.9. Many nations, including the United States, have made substantial moves toward completing the transition since 1960.

Some demographers believe that demographic transition theory is a useful tool only for analyzing population change in the West. William Petersen (1975), for example, argues that today's so-called underdeveloped nations and totalitarian societies exhibit patterns of fertility, mortality, and migration that make them difficult to analyze in terms of a three-stage transition process. Typically, underdeveloped countries interested in rapid development have imported Western health programs and medical technology on a wholesale basis. This has resulted in significant declines in the death rates. Unfortunately, efforts to cut fertility have been less successful, with enormous population growth as a result. In this context, totalitarian societies are peculiar only to the extent to which the state can (and does) intervene while trying to achieve demographic goals. Thus, such policies as family subsidies, state-controlled abortion centers, forced migration, and immigration or emigration restrictions may significantly affect population dynamics.

The Population Pyramid

One graphic technique often employed to depict the demographic transition process is the population pyramid. The population pyramid is a special type of bar graph with the various bars representing successive age categories, from the lowest at the bottom to the highest at the top. The population represented in this graphic device is usually broken down into five- or ten-year intervals, with each bar divided between males at the left and females at the right. The length of the bars represents the population either in absolute figures or as a percentage.

Figure 3-1 shows population pyramids for the United States in 1960 and 1985, and projected to 2010 and 2030. The reason for the basic shape of the pyramid is that among those born in a given year—1920 for example—some have died in each year since then, thus reducing the length of the bars rep-

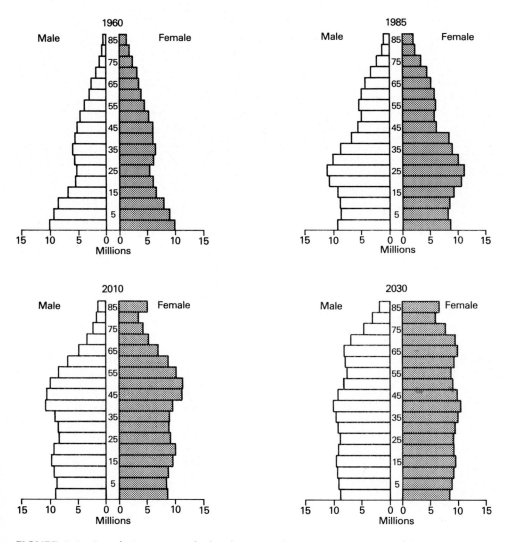

FIGURE 3-1 Population pyramids for the United States, 1960, 1985, 2010, and 2030. *Source: U.S. Bureau of the Census.*

resenting successively higher ages. The shape is not ordinarily pyramidal because birth rates, death rates, and rates of migration all vary from year to year. The base of the 1960 pyramid has been broadened by the baby boomers of the 1950s. The pinched-in waist of the 1960 form reflects the lower birth rates during the Great Depression and through World War II. The 1985 pyramid has a narrower base resulting from lower birth rates beginning again in the 1960s and shows a broader top indicating an increasing proportion of the population that is old.

If we are able consistently to maintain birth and death rates at the low levels required in stage three of the demographic transition, the pyramid would come to look like a rectangle turned on its end, with relatively no population growth over the long term. The relative number of older people is expected to continue to increase over time. Assuming only modest change, the greatest increase will occur between 2010 and 2020 when the projected proportion of elderly increases to about 17 percent as the members of the baby boom turn 65. The pyramid projected for the year 2030 approximates the form of the rectangle turned on its end.

THE DEPENDENCY RATIO

The growth of the elderly population has led gerontologists to look to the demographic relationship between it and the rest of the population. To the degree that the old are to be supported by the society to which they have contributed, this relationship may suggest the extent of social, economic, and political effort a society may be asked to make in support of its elderly.

One measure used to crudely summarize this relationship is known as the *dependency ratio*. Arithmetically, the ratio represents the number or proportion of individuals in the dependent segment of the population divided by the number or proportion of individuals in the supportive or working population. Although the dependent population has two components, the young and the old, students of gerontology have especially concerned themselves with the old-age dependency ratio. Definitions of *old* and *working* are "sixty-five and over" and "eighteen to sixty-four" years of age, respectively. Thus, the old-age dependency ratio is, in simple demographic terms, $65+/18$–64. This does not mean that every person aged sixty-five and over is dependent or that every person in the eighteen to sixty-four range is working. Nevertheless, we use these basic census categories to depict the relationship between these two segments of the society's population.

Table 3-3 shows old-age dependency ratios for the United States from 1930 to 2020. The ratio has increased in this century and is expected to continue to do so until the year 2020, when it is expected to increase dramatically. During the decade between 2010 and 2020, the baby-boom children of the late 1940s

TABLE 3-3   Societal Old-Age Dependency Ratios: 1930–2020

Year	$\text{Ratio} = \dfrac{\text{Population 65 years and over}}{\text{Population 18 to 64 years}} \times 100$
1930	9.1
1940	10.9
1950	13.4
1960	16.8
1970	17.6
1980	18.6
Projections	
1990	20.7
2000	21.2
2010	21.9
2020	28.7

Note: Based on Middle Series Census Bureau Projections. See Table 3-1 for an explanation of assumptions.

Source: Siegel and Davidson (1984, Table 8.14).

and 1950s will begin reaching retirement age, thus increasing the numerator; and a lowered birth rate, such as now exists, means a relatively smaller work force population (eighteen to sixty-four), thereby reducing the denominator (Cutler and Harootyan 1975). The projected old-age dependency ratio of 28.7 in 2020 indicates that every twenty-nine individuals aged sixty-five years or more will hypothetically be supported by one hundred working persons between the ages of eighteen and sixty-four. This constitutes a ratio of between one to three and one to four. In 1930, this ratio was about one to eleven.

Some demographers have begun to distinguish between a *societal* old-age dependency ratio (discussed above) and a *familial* old-age dependency ratio. The familial old-age dependency ratio can be used to illustrate the shifts in the ratio of elderly parents to children who would support them. This ratio is also defined in simple demographic terms: population aged 65–79/population aged 45–49. This does not mean that all persons aged sixty-five to seventy-nine need support or even have children, or that every person in the forty-five to forty-nine age range is willing or able to provide. Yet we use these age categories to depict the ratio of the number of elderly persons to the number of younger persons of the next generation.

Table 3-4 shows familial old-age dependency ratios for the United States from 1930 to 2020. The ratios increased from 1930 to 1980, and then are projected to decline, until the year 2020 when a dramatic increase is expected. In 1930, for every one hundred persons aged forty-five to forty-nine, there were eighty-two persons aged sixty-five to seventy-nine. This figure reached 185 in 1980 and is projected to increase to 220 in the year 2020. Changes in the familial

TABLE 3-4 Familial Old-Age Dependency Ratios: 1930–2020

Year	Ratio $= \dfrac{\text{Population 65 to 79 years}}{\text{Population 45 to 49 years}} \times 100$
1930	82
1940	95
1950	166
1960	129
1970	135
1980	185
Projections	
1990	174
2000	126
2010	126
2020	220

Note: Based on Middle Series Census Bureau Projections. See Table 3-1 for an explanation of assumptions.

Source: Siegel and Davidson (1984, Table 7.9).

old-age dependency ratio result mainly from past trends in fertility. For example, the high ratio in 1980 reflects the combination of high fertility (and in-migration) in the early part of this century (population aged sixty-five to seventy-nine) and reduced birth rates during the 1930s (those aged forty-five to forty-nine). The high ratio expected in the year 2020 results from high fertility during the post–World War II baby-boom years and the lower birth rates of the early 1970s.

Shifts in the societal and familial old-age dependency ratios suggest that support of the aged will become increasingly problematic through the remainder of this century and especially serious after 2010. It would seem that unless future aged are better able to support themselves than are current cohorts of elderly, an increasing burden will fall on the working population, requiring government to play a larger part in providing health and other services to the aged.

Some disagree, though. It may be argued that measuring the dependency burden of the elderly should not occur in a vacuum. And, that the level of the child- or "young-age" dependency ratio should be taken into account, since the share of society's support available for the elderly is affected by the level of young-age dependency (Siegel and Davidson 1984). Table 3-5 presents the old- and young-age dependency ratios for the United States for 1970 and 1980 and projected through the year 2020. The child- or young-age dependency ratio—the number of children under age eighteen per one hundred persons aged eighteen to sixty-four years—is expected to decline from sixty-one in 1970 to thirty-seven in 2020. This results from a continued expectation of reduced

TABLE 3-5   Old- and Young-Age Dependency Ratios, 1970–2020

Year	Ratio = $\dfrac{\text{Population 65 and over}}{\text{Population 18 to 64}} \times 100$	Ratio = $\dfrac{\text{Population under 18}}{\text{Population 18 to 64}} \times 100$	Total Dependency Burden
1970	18	61	78
1980	19	46	65
Projections			
1990	21	42	63
2000	21	41	62
2010	22	36	58
2020	29	37	66

Note: Based on Middle Series Census Bureau Projections. See Table 3-1 for an explanation of assumptions.

Source: Siegel and Davidson (1984, 113).

fertility and implies a generally decreasing burden on the working population. The combination of old- and young-age dependency ratios, representing an overall dependency burden on the working-age population, declined sharply between 1970 and 1980 and is expected to be relatively stable through the year 2020. The total dependency burden in 2020, projected to be sixty-six, is almost precisely the figure (sixty-five) used to describe the total burden in 1980. Between 1980 and 2020, the projected share of the total dependency burden accounted for by those under 18 years of age declines from 71 percent to 56 percent. Presumably, this decline would permit the conversion of some funds and other support resources from use by children to use by the elderly. Support costs for the elderly are generally thought to be greater than for the young and historically more likely to become a public responsibility; in the United States, support for children tends to be a private family responsibility (Clark and Spengler 1978). As a result, despite the expected shift in dependency burden between 1980 and 2020 from the young to the old, government may be expected to play a larger part in providing health and other support services to the aged.

SEX, RACE, AND ETHNIC COMPOSITION

Elderly women outnumber elderly men in virtually all settings within which aging takes place (Cowgill 1972). This occurs despite the fact that the number of male births in a population always exceeds the number of female births (Matras 1973, 145–146). Typically, after the earliest ages, the male excess is reduced by higher male mortality; at the most advanced ages the number of females exceeds the number of males.

In the United States, the number of males for every one hundred females—the *sex ratio*—in the over–sixty-five population has been declining throughout this century. In 1900 the sex ratio was 102; by 1930 it had declined to 100.4. The sex ratio in these years, however, was still heavily influenced by the predominantly male immigration prior to the First World War. As Table 3-6 shows, the 1980 sex ratio in the older population was 67.5 (it was 94.8 for the total population) and is projected to decline further until about 2010. Principally, we continue to explain the sex ratio of the aged population in terms of the higher mortality of males, particularly at the ages below sixty-five. This higher mortality among males reduces the relative number of survivors at the older ages.

The female population aged sixty-five and over has been growing much more rapidly than the male population in this age stratum (Siegel 1975, 34). Siegel notes that between 1960 and 1970 the female population aged sixty-five and over increased 28 percent, whereas the comparable male population increased by about 12 percent; between 1970 and 1980 the projected increase in the aged female population is about 25 percent, while for the aged male population, it is about 18 percent. This differential in growth rates added to the continued excess of males among the newborns yields a proportion of those sixty-five and over among females that is considerably above that for males. For 1980 aged females constitute about 13.0 percent of the total female pop-

TABLE 3-6   Males per 100 Females by Age and Race, 1950–2020

Age and Race	1950	1960	1970	1980	Projections			
					1990	2000	2010	2020
All Races								
All ages	99.3	97.0	94.8	94.8	94.7	94.7	94.8	94.6
65 years and over	89.5	82.6	72.0	67.5	66.1	64.5	65.2	69.1
75 years and over	82.6	75.0	63.3	55.2	53.5	52.5	51.2	53.3
White								
All ages	99.6	98.1	96.3	95.2	95.4	95.5	95.5	95.4
65 years and over	89.1	82.0	71.3	67.2	66.4	65.3	66.4	70.7
75 years and over	81.9	74.2	62.6	54.5	53.3	52.8	52.0	54.4
Black								
All ages	96.5	93.8	91.8	89.6	90.7	91.2	91.7	92.1
65 years and over	95.8	86.5	76.3	68.0	61.7	56.1	54.5	58.2
75 years and over	93.2	82.6	70.5	60.0	53.0	47.9	43.7	43.7

Note: Based on Middle Series Census Bureau Projections. See Table 3-1 for an explanation of assumptions.
Source: Siegel and Davidson (1984, Table 3.1).

ulation, and aged males constitute about 9.3 percent of the total male population. The sex ratio of the elderly population in 1980 corresponds to an excess
of 5 million women, or about 19 percent of the total aged population. Twenty
years earlier, in 1960, the excess was less than 1 million women (accounting
for about 5 percent of the aged population). The latest Census Bureau estimates
for the year 2000 project an excess of 7.6 million women, or about 20 percent
of the total population aged sixty-five years and over (Siegel and Davidson
1984).

Because of enumeration problems, statistics on *minority elderly* should be
viewed with some caution. Black elderly make up about 8.2 percent of the total
elderly population, whereas 11.8 percent of the total U.S. population is black.
In general, the U.S. black population is younger than the population of whites.
The proportion of the black population that is sixty-five years of age and over
is considerably smaller than that of the white population, for both males and
females. Smaller proportions of blacks than whites survive to old age, though
survival rates within old age are quite similar across the races. Siegel and
Davidson (1984) point out that according to *life tables* for 1978, 77 percent of
whites survive from birth to age sixty-five as compared with 65 percent for
blacks; for survival from age sixty-five to eighty-five, the percentages converge
to 34 and 31, respectively.

The key factor in the relative youthfulness of the black population is the
higher fertility among blacks. On average, black women have 3.1 children,
compared with the 2.2 recorded for white women. Whereas approximately 39
percent of all blacks are under age twenty-two, only about 30 percent of all
whites are in this age grouping. The median age of blacks is roughly six years
less than that of whites. In 1981, for example, black women had a median age
of 26.5 years; the comparable figure for white women is 32.5 years.

Next to blacks, *Spanish Americans* make up the largest minority in the United
States. And, this population is quickly growing. In 1980 Spanish Americans
constituted 6.4 percent of the U.S. population or over 14 million people. Officially, this population increased by 50 percent between 1970 and 1980. The
actual rate of growth has probably been higher as a result of illegal immigration.
Some experts forecast that before the year 2000 Spanish Americans will become
the nation's largest minority group (Farley 1982).

The Spanish-American population is a heterogeneous group. About 60
percent are of Mexican origin. One in seven Spanish Americans is of Puerto
Rican background (14 percent), whereas 6 percent are Cuban and 21 percent are of other Spanish heritage. About one-half of the Spanish-American
elderly are foreign-born. Cubans and Puerto Ricans are more recent immigrants
than are Mexican Americans, many of whom are descendants of original settlers
of territories annexed by the United States in the Mexican-American War. The
Spanish-American population is an even younger population than blacks (43
percent under twenty years of age versus 39 percent for blacks). High fertility

and large family size, in addition to immigration of the young and repatriation of the middle-aged, contribute to the youthfulness of this group.

Many *ancestry groups* are represented within the United States population. Table 3-7 presents some data on single-ancestry groups collected through the Ancestry and Language Survey conducted by the Census Bureau in late 1979. Though relatively small in numbers, those who identified themselves as singly of Russian ancestry had the largest proportion of elderly (27.4 percent), followed by the Polish (19.2 percent), English (17.9 percent), and Irish and Italian (16.3). The relative "agedness" of those of Russian and Polish ancestry results from the considerable migration to the United States that occurred early in this century, mostly before 1924. This explanation may similarly work for the Italians. English and Irish migration largely took place in the nineteenth century. Thus, the high proportion of elderly in these groups is likely a result of declining fertility during the twentieth century.

Migration has had great impact on the age distribution of the foreign-born population in the United States. Before World War I, immigration was relatively unrestricted. After the war, changes in policy brought a sharp curtailment to immigration. In 1970, a relatively high proportion of the elderly were themselves foreign-born; among those sixty-five years of age and older, 15.3 percent were born outside the United States. By 1979 this figure had dropped to 11.4 percent. And we can expect the proportion of the elderly population that is foreign-born to continue to decline. In 1979, only 7.7 percent of those aged fifty-five to sixty-four years and 5.1 percent of those aged forty-five to fifty-four years were themselves foreign-born.

TABLE 3-7   Percent of the Population 65 Years and over, for Specified Ancestry Groups, 1979 (single ancestry only)

Ancestry	Number, All Ages (in thousands)	Percent 65 Years and over
German	17,160	14.8
English	11,501	17.9
Irish	9,760	16.3
Afro-American, African	15,057	7.3
Italian	6,110	16.3
Polish	3,498	19.2
Spanish (including Latin America)	9,762	4.6
Russian	1,496	27.4
French	3,047	13.1
All others	19,105	15.6
Total	96,496	13.6

Source: U.S. Bureau of the Census, *Current Population Reports,* Series P-23, No. 116, March 1982.

GEOGRAPHIC DISTRIBUTION

The elderly population, like the total population, is not distributed equally across the United States. Generally, the elderly are most numerous in the states with the largest populations. New York, California, and Florida have the largest elderly populations, with more than 2 million each in 1986. Pennsylvania, Illinois, Ohio, Michigan, and Texas each have over a million aged residents. Together, these eight states account for 48.9 percent of the entire 1986 United States aged population. Table 3-8 presents a listing of the states by percentage of population aged sixty-five and over for 1986.

In all states the aged population increased between 1970 and 1980, and again from 1980 to 1986, though at widely differing rates. Whereas in the District of Columbia the number of persons aged sixty-five and over grew slowly (under 5.0 percent), in Nevada the number of persons sixty-five and over grew by 112.3 percent between 1970 and 1980, and an additional 51.3 percent by 1986. Florida showed the greatest absolute growth between 1970 and 1986—from 985,000 to almost 2.1 million. A cursory review of the states listed in Table 3-8 highlights the relatively higher proportion of aged in states in northeastern, mideastern, and midwestern regions of the United States and the relative scarcity of the aged in the western region.

Residential Mobility. Some of the growth in state elderly populations is due to natural increase, but some is the result of interstate migration. Compared with younger persons, the elderly are much less likely to be residentially mobile.

TABLE 3-8   States by Percentage of Population Aged 65 and over, 1986

17.7	1	Florida
14.5–14.6	4	Pennsylvania, Rhode Island, Iowa, Arkansas
13.0–13.9	11	South Dakota, Missouri, West Virginia, Nebraska, Massachusetts, Oregon, Kansas, Maine, Connecticut, Wisconsin, North Dakota
12.2–12.9	9	District of Columbia, Alabama, Tennessee, Ohio, Arizona, Oklahoma, Minnesota, New York, New Jersey
12.1	1	Montana
11.4–12.0	10	Michigan, Delaware, North Carolina, New Hampshire, Washington, Vermont, Indiana, Mississippi, Illinois, Kentucky
10.0–11.2	8	Georgia, Louisiana, Nevada, Virginia, South Carolina, California, Maryland, Idaho
9.0–9.8	4	Colorado, Texas, Hawaii, New Mexico
8.0–8.4	2	Utah, Wyoming
3.4	1	Alaska
Total	51	

Source: *Aging America, Trends and Projections, 1987–88 Edition* prepared by the U.S. Senate Special Committee on Aging in conjunction with the American Association of Retired People, the Federal Council on the Aging, and the U.S. Administration on Aging. Table 1-7, pp. 31–32.

Whereas 40 percent of those aged four and over lived in a different household in 1979 from that in 1975, only 17.7 percent of those sixty-five to seventy-four years of age exhibited this residential mobility. Only 15.6 percent of those aged seventy-five and over lived in a different household in 1979 from that in 1975. In general, this pattern reflects movement to a different household in the same county. Less than 5 percent of the U.S. elderly population made an interstate move between 1975 and 1980, compared with 10 percent of the total U.S. population (Biggar 1984).

Biggar (1984) points out that twelve states drew more than one-half of the nation's elderly migrants. Five Sun Belt states ranked among the top ten most popular destinations, and Florida, California, Arizona, and Texas were ranked first through fourth, respectively. Florida alone attracted more than one-fourth of the entire nation's elderly migrants (Biggar 1984). Elderly Sun Belt migrants seem to be younger, better educated, more financially secure, and more likely to be married than are migrants to other states. This seems especially the case for Arizona and Florida. California appears to receive the greatest number of poorer migrants. According to Biggar (1984), in states such as Arizona and Florida, the "graying of the Sun Belt" brings increased demands for consumer goods as well as housing, recreational, health, and protective services. For California, the elderly migration increases the demands placed on state and local social and welfare service agencies for the aged.

Where do migrants to the Sun Belt come from? Several major "streams" from noncontiguous states provide a source of migrants to the Sun Belt. Between 1975 and 1980, major streams into Florida came from Connecticut, Indiana, Massachusetts, Michigan, New Jersey, New York, Ohio, and Pennsylvania. From this list, only Michigan also provided a major stream of migrants to Arizona, which also drew from Illinois, Iowa, Minnesota, Washington, and Wisconsin. Migrants to California were drawn from Illinois and Washington. In the central Sun Belt, Texas has become a destination for streams of elderly migrants from Kansas and Missouri. Another newly emerging Sun Belt destination is North Carolina, drawing migrants from Maryland and New Jersey (Biggar 1984).

Often, states with high in-migration rates also have high out-migration rates. This seems especially the case for California and Florida. Between 1975 and 1980, major streams of elderly migrants left Florida for Michigan, New York, Ohio, and Pennsylvania. Longino (1979) has reported that one-third of the national interstate migrating older population residing outside their state of birth in 1965 returned by 1970. Given that the states identified above all provide major streams of elderly migrants to Florida, Biggar (1984) hypothesizes that much of this outmigration involves "returning home" to be near family after a spouse dies or with the onset of problems with health or finances or possibly both.

California may represent a different case of "returning home." States receiving streams of outmigrants from California include Arkansas, Colorado,

Idaho, Missouri, Oklahoma, Utah, and Washington. Only Washington provided a sizable stream into California. Others on this list may represent states
of birth for individuals who migrated to California in early adulthood. Remember, during the first half of the twentieth century California was an important destination for migrants of all ages seeking a "land of opportunity."

Residential Concentration. Increasingly, the elderly have become an urbanized
population, locating in central cities or in places that structurally and functionally are parts of larger metropolitan areas (Golant 1975). In 1980 only one
in four elderly whites and one in five elderly nonwhites were located in rural
areas. According to Golant (1972), the growth in the urban elderly population
is largely the result of younger cohorts aging "in place" and of residential
relocations made earlier in the life span, rather than of relocation made after
retirement. Still, we should remember that twenty-one states have at least 40
percent of their older population in rural areas; and in nine states (Alaska,
Arkansas, Mississippi, North Carolina, North Dakota, South Carolina, South
Dakota, Vermont, and West Virginia), more than half of the older population
is rural. Thirteen states have more than 10 percent of their older populations
living on farms (here, for the moment, we define the elderly as those sixty
years of age and over). This has important policy implications, since so many
government programs are designed to serve an urban population.

In 1980, 31 percent of all elderly in the United States were concentrated in
central cities. Yet during the last decades suburbanization has proceeded rapidly, so that by 1980 the fastest growing site for the elderly population was
the suburbs. In 1960 only about 17 percent of all elderly citizens were living
in the urban fringe around central city areas; by 1980 this proportion exceeded
28 percent. This pattern reflects less the migration of those sixty-five and over
than the aging of suburban populations.

SUMMARY

The elderly population of the United States has been increasing since 1900. Changes
in fertility, mortality, and migration have all contributed to this growth. The absolute
number of the elderly and the proportion of the population they constitute are expected
to increase further in this century, though at a slowed pace. In addition, the aged
population is itself aging. By the year 2000, approximately 50 percent of the aged will
be seventy-five years of age or over.

The old-age dependency ratio is a measure often used to summarize the demographic relationship between the elderly and the rest of the population. It is expected
to increase in the coming years. Continued expectations for reduced fertility during this
same period should allow for a projected decline in the young-age dependency ratio.
Thus, the total dependency burden over the next thirty to forty years should be relatively
stable.

Elderly women outnumber elderly men, a difference that has been increasing for
the past several decades. Because of enumeration problems, data on minority elderly

must be evaluated cautiously. Blacks constitute the largest group of nonwhite elderly, although they represent a smaller proportion of the total elderly population than of the total general population. Some experts forecast that before the year 2000 Spanish Americans will become the nation's largest minority group. This population, though, is even more youthful than the black population.

In general, the elderly population is concentrated in the largest states. Some growth in state populations of elderly is due to interstate migration. Sun Belt states rank among the most popular destinations for elderly migrants. Streams of elderly migrants seem to come to the Sun Belt principally from the Northeast and Midwest. Recently, gerontologists have identified streams of outmigrants returning home from the Sun Belt states. For individual elderly, this may be a consequence of widowhood or the onset of problems with health, or finance, or both.

Like the rest of the U.S. population, the elderly have become increasingly urbanized. Still, in nine states more than one-half of the older population is rural. These patterns reflect the aging in place of populations that may have relocated earlier in life more than they do migration of those over sixty years of age.

STUDY QUESTIONS

1. Discuss the roles fertility, mortality, and migration have played in the growth of the aged population in the United States during the twentieth century.

2. Should we have confidence in Census Bureau projections of the growth in numbers and proportion of the elderly population in the United States in the future? Why?

3. What is a dependency ratio? Distinguish between the *societal* old-age dependency ratio and the *familial* old-age dependency ratio. How is the "mix" of old-age and young-age dependency ratios expected to change in the future and what is the significance of this change?

4. Define *sex ratio*. Applying the concept to the elderly population, how has the sex ratio changed since the beginning of the twentieth century? Why has it changed?

5. Why is recognition of minority elderly issues likely to increase in the future? Why may the importance of ancestry groups diminish among the elderly in this same future?

6. Describe the residential mobility patterns of the elderly in the contemporary United States. What role do the Sun Belt states play in elderly migration? In this context, what do we mean by "returning home?"

7. How has the residential concentration of the elderly population changed in recent decades? Why?

BIBLIOGRAPHY

Biggar, J.C. 1984. *The graying of the Sun Belt*. Washington, D.C.: Population Reference Bureau, Inc.

Bogue, D.J. 1969. *Principles of demography*. New York: Wiley.

Clark, R.L., and Spengler, J.J. 1978. Changing dependency and dependency costs: The implications of future dependency ratios and their composition. In B. Herzog (ed.), *Aging and income: Programs and prospects for the elderly.* New York: Human Sciences Press.

Cowgill, D. 1972. A theory of aging in cross-cultural perspective. In D. Cowgill and L. Holmes (eds.), *Aging and modernization.* New York: Appleton-Century-Crofts.

Crimmins, E.M. 1980. Implications of recent mortality trends for the size and composition of the population over 65. Paper presented at the Annual Meeting of the Gerontological Society of America, November.

Cutler, N., and Harootyan, R. 1975. Demography of the aged. In D. Woodruff and J. Birren (eds.), *Aging: Scientific perspectives and social issues.* New York: Van Nostrand Reinhold Co.

Farley, J.E. 1982. *Majority-minority relations.* Englewood Cliffs, N.J.: Prentice-Hall.

Golant, S.M. 1972. The residential location and spatial behavior of the elderly. Research Paper 143, University of Chicago, Department of Geography.

———. 1975. Residential concentrations of the future elderly. *Gerontologist* 15:16–23.

Longino, C.F. 1979. Going home: Aged return migration in the United States 1965–70. *Journal of Gerontology* 34(5):736–745.

Matras, J. 1973. *Populations and societies.* Englewood Cliffs, N.J.: Prentice-Hall.

Neugarten, B. 1974. Age groups in American society and the rise of the young-old. *Annals of the American Academy* (September):187–198.

Petersen, W. 1975. *Population* (3d ed.). New York: Macmillan.

Siegel, J.S. 1975. Some demographic aspects of aging in the United States. In A. Ostfeld and D. Gibson (eds.), *Epidemiology of aging.* Bethesda, Md.: National Institutes of Health.

———. 1979. *Perspective trends in the size and structure of the elderly population, impact of mortality trends and some implications.* Current Population Reports, Special Studies Series P-23, No. 78. Washington, D.C.: U.S. Department of Commerce, Bureau of the Census.

Siegel, J.S., and Davidson, M. 1984. *Demographic and socioeconomic aspects of aging in the United States.* Current Population Reports, Special Studies Series P-23, No. 138. Washington, D.C.: U.S. Department of Commerce, Bureau of the Census.

PART II

BIOMEDICAL ASPECTS OF AGING

CHAPTER 4

WHAT ARE THE RESULTS OF AGING?

CHAPTER 5

WHY DO WE BECOME OLD?

CHAPTER 6

HEALTH STATUS OF THE ELDERLY

CHAPTER 4

WHAT ARE THE RESULTS OF AGING?

Cary S. Kart, Eileen S. Metress, and Seamus P. Metress

The physician Alexander Leaf (1973) quotes Frederic Verzar, the Swiss gerontologist, as saying: "Old age is not an illness. It is a continuation of life with decreasing capacities for adaptation." Some students of aging disagree. It has been a popular view that, if old age is not an illness in and of itself, there is at least a strong relationship between biological aging and pathology. This view posits that biological deterioration creates a state of susceptibility to disease and susceptibility to particular diseases leads to death.

One way out of this disagreement may be to distinguish between biological and pathological aging (Blumenthal 1968). It may be difficult to say at what point in life a person is old, but it is clear that everyone becomes so. Everyone ages. Genetic and other prenatal influences set the stage for the aging sequence, and factors in the postnatal environment (demographic, economic, psychological, and social) act to modify this sequence (Sobel 1966; Wilson 1974). The changes that accompany aging occur in different people at different chronological ages and progress at different rates. Changes in physical appearance are the most easily recognized; it is also well known that some physical capabilities diminish. These changes may be placed in the category of biological aging.

Disease is another matter. As individuals grow older, they are more likely to become afflicted with certain diseases, many of which prove fatal. Changes that occur as a result of disease processes may be categorized as pathological aging.

We begin this chapter by discussing recent progress in mortality and life expectancy among the elderly. This is followed by description of the results of biological aging—those important bodily changes that occur as age increases. Current theories or explanations of biological aging are evaluated in Chapter 5.

Disease processes related to pathological aging are reserved for discussion in Chapter 6.

For those who wonder why a social gerontologist needs to know so much about biology, the gerontologist Robert Atchley has an answer. As he so aptly points out, understanding the physiological changes that accompany aging is important for the social gerontologist "because they represent the concrete physiological limits around which social arrangements are built" (Atchley 1972, 47). Broadly interpreted, Atchley's statement means that changes fundamental to aging do not occur in isolation. Psychological and social changes both affect and are affected by the physiological changes taking place. The social gerontologist who is ignorant about the biological aspects of aging cannot hope to comprehend the important relationships among the physical, psychological, and social changes that accompany aging.

MORTALITY

Gerontologists use the term *senescence* to describe all postmaturational changes and the increasing vulnerability individuals face as a result of these changes. Senescence describes the group of effects that leads to a decreasing expectation of life with increasing age (Comfort 1979). Strehler (1962) distinguishes senescence from other biological processes in four ways: (1) its characteristics are universal; (2) the changes that constitute it come from within the individual; (3) the processes associated with senescence occur gradually; and (4) the changes that appear in senescence have a deleterious effect on the individual.

Is senescence a fundamental, inherent biological process? Comfort (1979) is doubtful. He believes that attempts to identify a single underlying property that explains all instances of senescent change are misplaced. Yet, there does appear to be some pattern to our increased vulnerability through the life course. Roughly speaking, it appears that the probability of dying doubles every eight years.

This phenomenon has been recognized since 1825 when Benjamin Gompertz observed that an exponential increase in death rate occurred between the ages of ten and sixty. After plotting age-specific death rates on a logarithmic scale and finding an increase that was nearly linear, Gompertz suggested that human mortality was governed by an equation with two terms. The first accounted for chance deaths that occur at any age; the second, characteristic of the species, represented the exponential increase with time. These observations, sometimes referred to as Gompertz's law, seem reasonably to described human mortality in many human societies (Fries and Crapo 1981). Nevertheless, although we can accept the principle that the probability of our dying increases with age, it is important to emphasize that the probabilities themselves differ for males and females by race and change through time.

During 1985 an estimated 2.1 million deaths occurred in the United States. The preliminary death rate for that year was 8.7 deaths per 1,000 population; the 1982 rate of 8.5 deaths per 1,000 population was the lowest annual rate ever recorded in this country. The majority of these deaths involved elderly people. Over 1.2 million (or about 60 percent) of the deaths occurred among individuals who had passed their sixty-fifty birthday.

The leading cause of death among the elderly is heart disease, which accounts for about 44 percent of all deaths in old age. Malignant neoplasms (cancer) account for another 18 percent of the deaths (19 percent for men, 16 percent for women); cerebrovascular diseases account for 13 percent of deaths among the elderly. Together, these three account for 75 percent of all deaths of elderly people and over 50 percent of the deaths of those under sixty-five in the United States. Obviously, the high proportion of the deaths of elderly people resulting from these three causes is an expression of vulnerability to these afflictions, which begins earlier in the life cycle.

Figure 4-1 shows the pattern of death rates for five leading causes of death among the elderly between 1950 and 1979. Death rates for the elderly have declined overall since 1950, although most of the decline has been since about 1968. The age-adjusted death rate for the population sixty-five years of age and over fell by 27 percent since 1950, and the decline for females was twice as great as that for males. The death rate for elderly men was considerably higher than that of elderly women (almost 70 percent in 1975), though this continues a long-term trend. The sex differential in death rates was 34 percent higher for elderly men in 1950.

As Figure 4-1 indicates, the death rates for two of the three leading causes of death, heart disease and stroke (cerebrovascular disease), have declined significantly between 1950 and 1979. The death rate for cancer, the second leading cause of death in 1979, has increased slowly over the years (13 percent in the 1950–1979 period). Sex differences are quite pronounced for cancer, especially lung cancer, for which male mortality is about four times greater than female mortality. Since 1960, however, there have been large annual increases in lung cancer mortality for older women, associated with cigarette smoking. The percent change from 1960 to 1982 in mortality rates from lung cancer among women aged sixty-five to seventy-four is 390.2. This compares with a 15.3 percent increase in mortality rates from breast cancer for comparably aged women over the same time period. In 1982, for women aged sixty-five to seventy-four, the death rate from lung cancer was higher than that from breast cancer (Metropolitan Life Insurance Company 1985).

Most elderly people die as a result of some long-standing chronic condition which is sometimes related to personal habits (for example, smoking, drinking, poor eating habits) or environmental conditions (for example, harsh work environments, air pollution) that go back many years. Preventing illness and death from these conditions must begin before old age. Some deaths, such as those from accidents, have declined significantly. The death rate from accidents

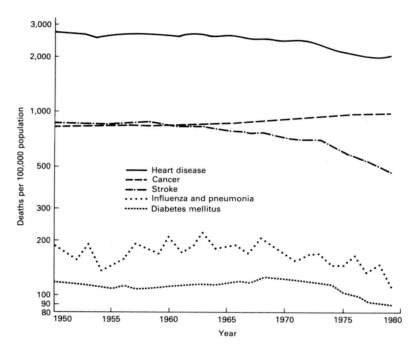

FIGURE 4-1   Age-adjusted death rates for persons 65 years of age and over, according to leading causes of death, United States, 1950–1979. *Source: National Center for Health Statistics; computed by the Division of Analysis from data compiled by the Division of Vital Statistics.* (Note: Causes of death are assigned according to the International List of Causes of Death. Because of the decennial revisions and changes in rules for cause-of-death selection, there may be some lack of comparability from one revision to the next. The beginning dates of the revisions are 1949, 1958, 1968 and 1979.)

(and violence) for white males aged sixty-five years and over in 1982 was 32 percent lower than that in 1960; the comparable decline for aged white females during this period was 47 percent.

Sex Differences in Mortality

As can be seen from Table 4-1, comparisons by race show that men have higher death rates than do women in every age category. Some of this difference is almost certainly attributable to biological factors. For example, the larger proportion of males who die in infancy is apparently not explainable by any systematic variation in physical or social environmental factors. For most adults, however, it may be difficult to distinguish between biological and environmental contributors to death. Male–female differences in mortality may be due, in part, to sex differences in the use of physician services. Typically, women

TABLE 4-1   Age-Specific Death Rates, by Race and Sex, 1980

| | Deaths per 1,000 | | | |
| | White | | Black | |
Age	Male	Female	Male	Female
All ages	9.8	8.1	10.3	7.3
Age-adjusted	7.5	4.1	11.1	6.3
Under 1	12.3	9.6	25.9	21.2
1–4	0.7	0.5	1.1	0.8
5–9	0.3	0.2	0.5	0.3
10–14	0.4	0.2	0.5	0.3
15–19	1.4	0.5	1.4	0.5
20–24	1.9	0.6	2.9	0.9
25–29	1.7	0.6	3.7	1.3
30–34	1.7	0.7	4.6	1.7
35–39	2.1	1.1	5.9	2.5
40–44	3.2	1.7	8.1	4.1
45–49	5.2	2.8	12.0	6.3
50–54	8.7	4.5	17.6	9.1
55–59	13.8	7.0	24.6	13.1
60–64	21.4	10.8	33.8	18.6
65–69	33.1	16.4	44.8	25.4
70–74	50.2	25.9	60.5	37.6
75–79	74.7	41.9	80.9	52.4
80–84	112.7	72.4	115.5	80.3
85 +	191.0	149.8	161.0	123.7

Source: National Center for Health Statistics, Advance Report of Final Mortality Statistics, 1980, *Monthly Vital Statistics Report,* vol. 32, no. 4 (1983), Tables 1 and 9.

report using health services more frequently than men do. This may result in earlier and more effective treatment of their illnesses and may contribute to lower death rates relative to men (Marcus and Siegel 1982). The childbearing experience of females and the overrepresentation of males in dangerous occupations are two additional factors that make it difficult to determine the relative effect on mortality of biological and environmental or sociocultural factors.

Francis Madigan (1957) attempted to differentiate between biological and environmental factors in mortality. His classic study compared the mortality experience of Catholic brothers and nuns who were members of teaching communities. Madigan argued that the life patterns of these two groups are quite similar, and that, over time, brothers and nuns are subjected to the same sociocultural stresses. Of particular importance here is the absence of gender-linked activities that are relevant to mortality—namely, childbearing for females and participation in dangerous occupations for males. Madigan found that the difference in death rates between brothers and nuns was greater than between males and females in the population as a whole and that this difference had been increasing during the decades under study. From this he argued that biological factors are more important than sociocultural ones. Further, he hypothesized that the death rate advantage enjoyed by women was bound up in their greater constitutional resistance to the degenerative diseases (Madigan 1957).

Such a hypothesis is difficult to test empirically. Table 4-2 presents ratios of male-to-female death rates for the population sixty-five years of age and over, by age and race, from 1940 to 1980. In general, the table shows increasing male–female mortality differences throughout this period, though there are still important differences in these ratios by age. Whereas among people aged sixty-five to sixty-nine the male death rate is about twice that of females, the death rate of men in the group aged eighty-five years and older is only 27 percent higher than that of women.

TABLE 4-2   Male-to-Female Death Rate Ratios Among the Elderly, by Age and Race, 1940–80

Race and Year	Death Rate Ratio, by Age				
	65–69	**70–74**	**75–79**	**80–84**	**85 +**
All Races					
1940	1.34	1.25	1.20	1.15	1.08
1950	1.58	1.40	1.29	1.21	1.13
1960	1.83	1.62	1.42	1.26	1.11
1970	2.02	1.82	1.61	1.41	1.15
1980	1.98	1.90	1.76	1.55	1.27
White					
1940	1.36	1.26	1.19	1.14	1.07
1950	1.62	1.42	1.29	1.20	1.12
1960	1.88	1.65	1.43	1.27	1.12
1970	2.10	1.86	1.62	1.42	1.16
1980	2.02	1.94	1.78	1.56	1.27
Other Races					
1940	1.20	1.20	1.28	1.33	1.25
1950	1.28	1.23	1.28	1.30	1.20
1960	1.47	1.37	1.30	1.30	1.18
1970	1.52	1.46	1.47	1.33	1.12
1980	1.74	1.58	1.53	1.45	1.32

Sources: Robert D. Grove and Alice M. Hetzel, *Vital Statistics Rates in the United States, 1940–1960* (Washington, D.C.: National Center for Health Statistics, 1968), Table 55; National Center for Health Statistics, *Vital Statistics of the United States, 1970*, vol. 2, *Mortality*, Part A (1974), Table 1-8; Advance Report of Final Mortality Statistics, 1980, *Monthly Vital Statistics Report*, vol. 32, no. 4 (1983), Table 1.

The general increase in mortality differences between the sexes very likely reflects a major shift in the cause pattern of mortality. During the twentieth century, the contribution of infectious and parasitic diseases and maternal mortality to overall mortality rates has diminished relative to that of the chronic degenerative diseases such as diseases of the heart, malignant neoplasms, and cerebrovascular diseases (Siegel 1979). Nevertheless, changes in recent decades in the male–female mortality ratio appear to be more associated with social and environmental factors than with biological ones. For example, according to Petersen (1975), the age-adjusted death rate from cancers was 65 percent higher for females than males in 1900, about equal between the sexes in 1947, and 20 percent higher for males by 1963. This changing pattern would seem to have more to do with technological advancements than with innate biological factors. The diagnosis and cure of cancers most frequent among females, breast and uterine, have improved at a more rapid rate than those for cancers most frequent among males, those of the lung and digestive system.

Can the pattern of increasing male-to-female death rate ratios among the elderly continue? Among those of all races and whites aged sixty-five to sixty-nine, ratios have actually fallen between 1970 and 1980. According to Zopf (1986), this deceleration suggests that the death rate differential between older men and women will not increase in the future as it has in the past. This is especially the case for the young-old, though increases in the mortality differential by sex are likely to continue for the old-old and for blacks.

Race Differentials in Mortality

The large racial differential in mortality rates does not often receive the attention it deserves because it is a hidden factor. If we return to Table 4-1 and look across the first row ("All ages") we observe that the death rate of black males is slightly higher than that of white males (10.3 versus 9.8), whereas the death rate for black females is slightly lower than that for white females (7.3 versus 8.1). Nevertheless, because of higher birthrates, blacks have a younger age structure, and this factor tends to mask true mortality. If we examine mortality across the second row ("Age-adjusted") and in individual age groups, the full impact of race emerges. For example, infant mortality in the United States in 1980 was 121 percent higher among black than white females (21.2 versus 9.6) and 111 percent higher among black than white males (25.9 versus 12.3). Death rates among young adults twenty-five to twenty-nine years of age are 118 percent greater for black males and 117 percent greater for black females. It is only at age eighty-five that the racial differential in death rates tends to disappear. According to the demographer Donald Bogue (1969, 595–596), "[T]hroughout almost all of the ages when great progress in death control has been accomplished, death rates for blacks are about double those of whites."

Although there has been some long-term progress in reducing the racial differential in mortality, this has slowed to a standstill recently. In 1960, the age-adjusted death rate for blacks was 32 percent higher than the comparable figure for whites. For 1970 this differential was 35 percent, and by 1980 it was 33 percent.

The race differential in mortality is greater for females than for males. As Table 4-1 shows, in 1980 black males had an age-adjusted death rate that was 48 percent higher than the rate for white males in 1980 (11.1 versus 7.5); this differential for females was 54 percent (6.3 versus 4.1). Also, the sex differential in mortality is smaller for blacks on a proportional basis than for the white population. Among whites, males have an age-adjusted death rate that is 83 percent higher than that among females; among blacks this difference is 76 percent. It appears that black women have not been able to achieve as large a share of the available advancements to prevent death as have black men (Bogue 1969, 596–597).

Two additional points need be stressed when dealing with racial differentials in mortality. First, there is no reason to believe that blacks in particular or nonwhites in general are biologically less fit than whites in their capacity to survive. What this point emphasizes is that racial differentials in mortality reflect unnecessarily high mortality among nonwhites. Second, other factors, not the least of which is socioeconomic status, confound mortality data. Kitagawa and Hauser (1973) have shown the age-adjusted mortality rates for Japanese Americans to be about one-third the corresponding rates for whites and one-half as large as the rate for blacks. Their analysis of median family income among these groups suggests that socioeconomic status may account for a considerable proportion of the race differentials in mortality.

How does low socioeconomic status contribute to the higher mortality rates prevalent among blacks? Their lack of access to high quality medical care is one reason. According to the U.S. Office of Health Resources (1979), black people receive considerably fewer preventive health services, on the average, than do white people. Also, medical treatment of blacks is often delayed until the onset of later stages of disease (Gonnella, Louis, and McCord 1976).

Although we are unable to say precisely whether biological or social factors are more important contributors to mortality differentials among different population groups in our society, we recognize that aging, even biological aging, does not occur in a social vacuum. Age-adjusted death rates in our total population are, for example, only about one-third what they were at the beginning of this century. Additionally, even when considering those who as a group are already chronologically old, there has been a significant decline in death rates since 1960; for males aged sixty-five to seventy-four years, for example, the reduction from 1960 to 1983 is 20 percent; for comparably aged females, the reduction is 27 percent. These reductions in the death rates of our population reflect at least four factors, all of which involve attempts begun in the nineteenth century to increase control over the environment (Dorn 1959): (1) increased food supply; (2) development of commerce and transportation; (3) changes in technology and industry; and (4) increased control over infectious disease.

LIFE EXPECTANCY

Progress in the reduction of mortality is also reflected in figures for average life expectancy at birth. Average life expectancy at birth, defined as the average number of years a person born today can expect to live under current mortality conditions, has shown great improvement since 1900. It rose from 49.2 years in 1900–02 to 73.9 years in 1980–81 (Table 4-3). This change constitutes a 50 percent increase in life expectancy at birth, or an average annual gain of more than 0.3 years in this period. Still, just as there are significant sex and racial differentials in mortality, there are similar differentials in life expectancy. As Table 4-3 shows us, the population group with the highest life expectancy at birth in 1980–81 is the white female (78.4 years); nonwhite males have the lowest life expectancy (65.7 years). All groups have substantially increased life expectancies since 1900. Better sanitary conditions, the development of effective public health programs, and rises in the standard of living are three additional factors often cited with those listed above to explain increased life expectancy in this century.

Life expectancy at birth is a function of death rates at all ages. Thus, the statistic does not tell us at what specific ages improvement has occurred. We are particularly interested in judging progress in "survivorship" for those aged sixty-five and over. One technique for judging such progress is to look at actual survivorship rates. For example, in 1900–02, 40.9 percent of newborn babies could be expected to reach age sixty-five; in 1983 the figure has almost doubled to 78.4 percent. The proportion of persons surviving from age sixty-five to age eighty-five has more than doubled between 1900 and 1984. In 1900–02, 14.8 percent of those aged sixty-five could expect to survive to age eighty-five; in

TABLE 4-3   Years of Life Expectancy at Birth, by Race and Sex, 1900–02 to 1980–81

Years	All Groups	White		Other Races	
		Male	Female	Male	Female
1900–02*	49.2	48.2	51.1	32.5	35.0
1909–11*	51.6	50.3	53.7	34.2	37.7
1919–21*	56.5	56.6	58.6	47.2	47.0
1929–31	59.3	59.2	62.8	47.5	49.5
1939–41	63.8	63.3	67.2	52.4	55.4
1949–51	68.2	66.4	72.2	59.1	63.0
1959–61	68.9	67.6	74.2	61.5	66.5
1969–71	70.7	67.9	75.5	61.0	69.1
1980–81	73.9	70.8	78.4	65.7	74.8

Sources: National Center for Health Statistics, *Vital Statistics of the United States, 1978,* vol. 2, sec. 5, *Life Tables* (1980), Tables 5-A and 5-5; Annual Summary of Births, Deaths, Marriages, and Divorces: United States, 1981, *Monthly Vital Statistics Report,* vol. 30, no. 13 (1982), pp. 3–4 and 15.
* Death-registration states only.

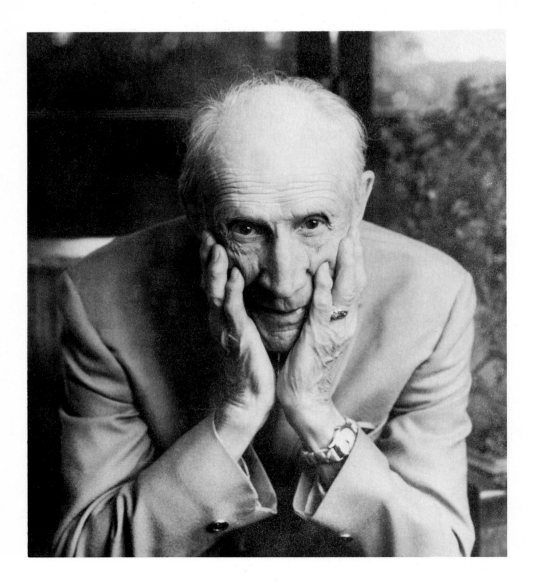

1984 this figure was 37.4 percent, though 46.1 percent of women aged sixty-five could expect to survive to age eighty-five (Metropolitan Life Insurance Company 1985, 1987).

   A second technique for measuring changes in survivorship involves looking at changes in age-specific life expectancy. Table 4-4 presents life expectancies at various elderly ages by sex and race in the United States for 1900–02 and 1980. Life expectancy at age sixty-five has moved ahead more slowly than has

TABLE 4-4   Years of Life Expectancy at Various Elderly Ages, 1900–02 and 1980

Year and Age	White		Black	
	Male	Female	Male	Female
1900–02*				
65	11.5	12.2	10.4	11.4
70	9.0	9.6	8.3	9.6
75	6.8	7.3	6.6	7.9
80	5.1	5.5	5.1	6.5
85	3.8	4.1	4.0	5.1
1980				
65	14.2	18.5	13.5	17.3
70	11.3	14.8	11.1	14.2
75	8.8	11.5	8.9	11.4
80	6.7	8.6	6.9	9.0
85	5.0	6.3	5.3	7.0

Sources: National Center for Health Statistics, *Vital Statistics of the United States, 1978,* vol. 2, sec. 5, *Life Tables* (1980), Table 5-4; Advance Report of Final Mortality Statistics, 1980, *Monthly Vital Statistics Report,* vol. 32, no. 4 (1983), Table 2.

* Death-registration states only.

life expectancy at birth since 1900 (4.8 versus 24.7 years). The small increase of "expectation" values for those sixty-five and over between 1900–02 and 1980 is in part a function of the relative lack of success the health sciences have had in reducing adult deaths caused by heart disease, cancer, and cerebrovascular diseases. These have been the leading causes of death among persons sixty-five years and over since 1950. Although some modest progress in reducing death rates caused by heart disease and cerebrovascular diseases has been made in the last quarter of a century, the death rate from malignant neoplasms (cancer) has increased by about 13 percent since 1950.

AGE-RELATED
PHYSIOLOGICAL CHANGES[1]

It is important to recall that, although all people age, not everyone does so at the same rate. Some individuals show symptoms of aging before they are chronologically old. Others, who are chronologically old, do not yet show all of the results of senescence. According to Alexander Leaf (1973, 52), the average

---

[1] Materials presented in this section are adapted from Kart, Metress, and Metress (1988).

individual of seventy-five, compared with the same person at age thirty, will have 92 percent of his or her former brain weight, 84 percent basal metabolism, 70 percent kidney filtration rate, and 43 percent maximum breathing capacity. Still, the loss of function reflected in these figures does not occur at the same rate in every individual. More important, these changes do not in and of themselves bring dysfunction. Yet, these figures do provide empirical support for something many of us (even those under seventy-five) have long suspected: We are not the people we once were.

What happens to us physiologically as we age? What are the specific results of senescence?

The Skin

To most people the condition of the skin, hair, and connective tissue collectively represents the ultimate indicator of age. People are often judged to be of a certain age on the basis of visible wrinkles or the degree of graying of the hair. Many older people (as well as younger people) invest in so-called miracle creams and hair dyes in an attempt to disguise these signs of age. Although perceptions of age, like those of beauty, are in the eyes of the beholder, our outward appearance does change as we age. These alterations in appearance are due, for the most part, to subcutaneous fat loss, loss of functioning cells that contribute to pigmentation, atrophy of sweat and oil-secreting glands, and a decrease in the number of blood vessels that supply the skin.

The speed and degree of some of the age-associated skin changes are related to a number of factors such as heredity, hormone balances, nutrition, and exposure to sun, wind, or chemicals. In fact, long-term exposure to sunlight accelerates time's metamorphosis of the skin and is a major factor contributing to diseases of the aging skin. Thus, one's occupation may play an important role in age-associated skin changes. People who spend a considerable amount of time in the sun, such as fishermen, farmers, construction workers, and even dedicated sunbathers, generally show a hastening of age-associated skin changes.

Most of these skin changes are not life threatening. For the most part they are cosmetic and benign in nature. For some, however, even these changes will be disconcerting. These are the changes that many in this highly youth-oriented society characteristically equate with dreaded old age. In this regard, such changes, cosmetic and benign (as they are described here), may affect an individual's self-concept. Older people have pride in their appearance, and such concerns should not be dismissed because of their age.

The skin is a marvelous organ that generally serves its owner well throughout life, including old age. Its elasticity, suppleness, and musculature allow us freedom of movement and expression. It also serves to protect us against various physical and chemical injuries while serving as an important heat regulator and sensory device. As a protective sheath it limits water loss and prohibits the entrance of countless numbers of disease-causing microorganisms. These various functions of the human skin are aided by the presence of subcutaneous fat tissue, sweat- and oil-secreting glands, pigment cells, and blood vessels. Changes in these structures lead to various age-associated changes in the form and function of the skin.

Certainly wrinkling is the most obvious age-associated skin change. Wrinkling, which begins during one's twenties and continues throughout life, is influenced by several factors. The human face, because of its musculature, is capable of tremendous movement and expression of emotions. Indeed, facial expressions represent an extremely important component of human communication. Smiles, laughter, frowns, disappointment, anger, rage, and surprise are all recorded. The hand of time captures our expressions and outlines them on our faces. The lines that begin to form in areas of greatest movement proliferate and become deeper as the years pass. By the age of forty, most of us bear the typical lines of our expressions.

Much of the wrinkling is caused by a loss of subcutaneous fat tissue as well as by a loss of skin elasticity. The loss of fat tissue is generalized but is usually most obvious in the face and the upper and lower extremities. The entire body becomes wrinkled and thus changed in appearance. Diminished subcutaneous fat tissue is also largely responsible for the characteristic emaciated look of old age. A once filled-out form gives way to a frame that seems to exhibit many of the constituents of which it is made. The hands prominently display the bones, tendons, and blood vessels that constitute their being. Likewise, bony prominences and vessels of the face, trunk, and extremities become more apparent.

A loss of padding, which is normally provided by subcutaneous fat tissue, also serves to predispose many older persons to the development of pressure sores. These sores develop in areas between bony prominences and overlying skin areas when pressure is unrelieved. These serious lesions represent an important problem in the health care of older persons.

The loss of subcutaneous fat tissue alters certain normal functions of the skin. Subcutaneous fat serves as an important insulator of the body; as it is lost, greater amounts of body heat escape, often leaving an individual feeling chilly. Older persons often complain of being cold when others around them are comfortable. An older person may tend to turn up the heat so much as to make a room too warm for younger individuals. Complaints of being cold are caused largely by a loss of body insulation and partially by a diminished blood flow to skin and extremities.

Older persons are also more likely to suffer from heat exhaustion because of changes in their capacity to perspire as a result of atrophy of the sweat glands. Thus, elderly individuals should avoid being in hot, stuffy rooms, spending too much time in the sun on a warm day, and overexerting themselves. Furthermore, atrophic changes in the sweat glands make the use of deodorants and antiperspirants unnecessary for many older people.

As has already been noted, aging is accompanied by a reduction of blood flow to the skin. The diminished blood supply contributes to the coolness of the surface of the aged skin as well as to thickened fingernails and toenails and a generalized loss of body hair, including a reduction of head hair.

The hair also grays with age—one of the most noted age-associated physical changes. Loss of hair color as well as loss of one's previously characteristic skin color occurs as a result of a decrease in the number of functioning pigment-producing cells. As if to compensate for their loss, some pigment cells of the skin enlarge. These enlarged areas are responsible for many of the pigmented blotches seen on aged skin.

Various factors contribute to increased skin infections in the elderly. They are blood vessel changes, an altered immune response, and atrophy of the sebaceous or oil-secreting glands. Blood vessels supply our bodies with the nutrients and chemicals that help to repair tissue and combat foreign invaders such as infectious microorganisms. If blood flow is decreased, so is the important supply of these substances. Furthermore, skin may dry and crack because of the atrophy of the oil-secreting glands. Cracks and breaks in the skin not only lead to discomfort but can serve as portals of entry for bacteria, viruses, and fungi.

The elderly are susceptible to the same skin disorders as are persons in younger age groups. Still, there are certain skin disorders that are more common among older persons, such as senile pruritus (itching), keratosis (a localized thickening of the skin), skin cancer, and pressure sores.

The Skeletomuscular System

Together our bones and muscles provide us with support, protect vital organs, give stability to the body and preserve its shape, and allow us freedom of movement and locomotion. These provisions of the skeletomuscular system are ones that we take very much for granted. As we age, however, we find that many of these functions become limited and, on occasion, denied. Joint changes, along with diminished bone and muscle mass, can give way to increased fractures and falls, stooped posture and shortened stature, loss of muscle power, misshapen joints, pain, stiffness, and limited mobility. Arthritis and allied bone and muscular conditions are among the most common of all disorders affecting people sixty-five years of age and over. In fact, joint and muscular aches and pains and stiffness are often expected in old age. Frequently, all such symptoms are lumped together as discomforts of arthritis or rheumatism. Such a practice can be dangerous. The stiff limbs of Parkinson's disease and the bone pain of osteomalacia may be dismissed and needed medical attention delayed. Chronic, recurrent muscular and joint pain is *not* natural; in response to such symptoms, people of all ages should seek prompt medical attention.

Bone and muscle changes are significant in that they can greatly alter an individual's lifestyle by making certain tasks of daily living much more difficult.

It should be emphasized that even though certain degenerative changes occur, they need not necessarily be disabling if proper diagnosis, treatment, and maintenance are given. Changes or disease states of the skeletomuscular system rarely serve directly to shorten the lifespan. Nevertheless, if a person is bed-ridden and immobilized as result of pain and stiffness or falls or fractures, complications can result that lead to death.

Arthritis is a generic term that refers to an inflammation or a degenerative change of a joint. It has occurred all over the world and throughout time, being one of the oldest known diseases. Indeed, the cartoon image of Neanderthal man as a stooped brute with a bent-knee gait represents a caricature of an arthritic relative who lived over 40,000 years ago. This condition is still very much with us today; it represents the number one crippler of all age groups in the United States.

Osteoarthritis, the most common joint disease, is a degenerative joint change that takes place with aging. Its cause is not definitely known. It is also known as "wear and tear arthritis" and "degenerative joint disease." With this con-dition there is a gradual wearing away of joint cartilage. The resultant exposure of rough underlying bone ends can cause pain and stiffness. Bony outgrowths known as osteophytes may appear at the margin of the affected bone. Long-standing osteoarthritis can also do damage to the internal ligaments, resulting in abnormal movements of the bones and joint instability or disorganization. The joints reflecting such involvement are most generally those associated with weight bearing.

Although osteoarthritis affects more people (perhaps as many as 40 million in the United States), *rheumatoid arthritis* is the more serious and carries the greatest potential for pain, disfigurement, and crippling. It may commence at any age, but persons most commonly develop initial symptoms somewhere between the ages of twenty and fifty years. The disease is not typically a condition of old age per se; most people carry it into old age.

Rheumatoid arthritis is a chronic, systemic, inflammatory disease of con-nective tissue that is two to three times more common among women than men. This condition is most-commonly characterized by persistent and pro-gressive joint involvement leading to disorganized joints and great pain and discomfort. Symptoms include malaise, fatigue, weight loss, fever, joint pain, redness, swelling, stiffness, and deformity. Many joints are affected. Extra-articulated tissue—especially that of the heart, lungs, eyes, and blood vessels—is also involved. The disease is characterized by acute episodes or flares and remissions or periods of relative inactivity. Within ten to fifteen years, most rheumatoid arthritis victims will develop moderate to marked decline in func-tional capacity.

The cause of rheumatoid arthritis is not fully understood. It is now viewed as an autoimmune disease, that is, one that results from the production of antibodies that work against the body's own tissues. The autoantibody known as rheumatoid factor (RF) is apparently present in 85 percent of rheumatoid arthritis patients. Multiple factors that probably lead to the development of this condition include possible previous exposure to an infectious agent and genetic factors that program a given immune response.

Associated with the aging process is a gradual loss of bone that reduces skeletal mass without disrupting the proportions of minerals and organic materials. This general loss of bone, known as *osteoporosis*, has been recognized for many years since it was first described by German anatomists. The quantitative decrease in bone mass can result in diminished height, slumped posture, backache, and a reduction in the structural strength of bones, making them more susceptible to fracture. For many persons, however, bone loss is asymptomatic.

Osteoporosis can involve most bones of the body; those most critically involved, however, include the vertebrae, wrist, and hip. Some diminution in the density of the vertebral column eventually occurs in most individuals beyond a certain age, resulting in vertebral compression and an age-associated shortening of the trunk and loss of stature. Osteoporosis of the spine is a common cause of backache in the elderly, with symptoms of vertebral involvement ranging from minor to acute back pain. A more severe consequence of osteoporosis is a femoral neck fracture. The neck of the femur is forced to bear much weight, and osteoporosis can so diminish its mechanical integrity that a fracture results. It is now believed that many of the falls and associated hip fractures of old age actually represent an osteoporotic femoral neck that broke under its weight-bearing task. In fact, radiographic evidence indicates that approximately three out of four of those elderly individuals who suffer from a broken hip express evidence of osteoporotic involvement of the femoral neck. So significant is the mortality associated with a hip fracture among the elderly that osteoporosis is listed as the twelfth leading cause of death in the United States.

The Neurosensory System

The nervous system is important in controlling the functioning of the body— including activities such as smooth and skeletal muscle contractions—and in receiving, processing, and storing information. The special senses of vision, hearing, taste, smell, and touch provide an individual with a link to the outside world. Neurosensory changes that can influence an individual's functioning, activities, response to stimuli, and perception of the world do occur with age. It is also true that the world's perception of an individual may be unduly influenced by neurosensory changes that he or she has undergone. For example, the older person with impaired hearing or vision may be labeled as stubborn, eccentric, or even senile.

Nerve cells, or neurons, are lost during the process of aging. The number of the basic functioning units begins to decline around the age of twenty-five. Associated with this decline is a decreased capacity for sending nerve impulses to and from the brain. Conduction velocity decreases, voluntary motor movements slow down, and the reflex time for skeletal muscles is increased. Degenerative changes and disease states involving the sense organs can alter vision, hearing, taste, smell, and touch.

The Gastrointestinal System

The gastrointestinal tract is the product of millions of years of biocultural evolution. Our species evolved from primate ancestors who were primarily vegetarian but were capable of omnivorous alimentation. The omnivorous nature of the species helped it expand and evolve to fit a wide variety of ecological conditions. Judging from the development of a great variety of cultural traditions with dissimilar eating customs, it seems that the gastrointestinal system has served the species well.

The gastrointestinal system, like other body systems, is subject to the aging process. Age-associated changes include atrophy of the secretion mechanisms, decreasing motility of the gut, loss of strength and tone of the muscular tissue and its supporting structures, changes in neurosensory feedback on such things as enzyme and hormone release, innervation of the tract, and the diminished response to pain and internal sensations. Although the indisputable evidence for the relationship between these changes and aging is still not overwhelming, there is certainly enough circumstantial evidence to warrant a consideration of the possibilities.

Gastrointestinal symptoms such as indigestion, heartburn, and epigastric discomfort increase with age, although identifying and evaluating these symptoms are difficult. Many symptoms are caused by normal functional changes in the tract. With increasing age, however, they often are associated with serious pathologic conditions such as cancer. The threat or fear of cancer can exert a great deal of psychological pressure on individuals. Stress of this type not only affects mental health but can also affect other body systems to cause or exacerbate problems such as hypertension and chronic respiratory disease.

The signs and symptoms often associated with one part of the gastrointestinal tract may actually be associated with another part of the tract. This is caused by the phenomenon of referral, as well as by the fact that the organs are part of an integrated system and thus are interrelated. The tract includes the mouth, esophagus, stomach, small intestine, gall bladder, liver, pancreas, and large intestine. Discomfort perceived as originating in the stomach may actually be coming from the lower gastrointestinal tract. An organ-based survey of the gastrointestinal system and its age-related problems is beyond the scope of this chapter. Still, several caveats are in order. Health professionals who deal with gastrointestinal disorders of the aged must be flexible in their approach. Disorders should be carefully evaluated before being dismissed as functional manifestations. If evaluation indicates a functional disorder, an effort should be made to explain the problem to the patient in clear, jargon-free terms. A sympathetic attitude and a face-to-face discussion of the situation can sometimes do more for people than medical intervention.

The Cardiopulmonary System

Generally, the anatomical and physiological changes that take place in the aging heart still allow it to function adequately if the coronary artery system is not greatly damaged by disease. Because coronary artery disease is such a prevalent condition among older Americans, however, it is difficult to determine the extent to which the heart ages independently of the disease. In the absence of disease the heart tends to maintain its size and in some individuals may become smaller with age. In particular, the left ventricular cavity, the chamber of the heart that sends oxygenated blood to the body, may decrease in size because of a reduction in activity and physical demands in old age. In addition, older people who are malnourished, confined to bed, or experiencing extended illness may show additional atrophy of the heart. Accompanying this reduction in heart size is a reduction in heart muscle strength and cardiac output. Still, without disease or additional alteration in heart function, cardiac output should be quite adequate as the body's requirements are reduced because of the atrophy of other body tissues and a decreased basal metabolism rate.

The heart valves tend to increase in thickness with age, and certain valves may be the sites of calcium salt deposits. These changes are not clinically significant unless there is a modification in the normal closing of a heart valve, which may stimulate more serious heart disease. Blood pressure also tends to increase with age. Systolic pressure—associated with that phase of the cardiac cycle when the heart contracts, expelling blood—tends to stabilize at approximately seventy-five years of age. Diastolic pressure, involving that phase of the cardiac cycle during which the heart relaxes and its chamber fills with blood—tends to stabilize at age sixty-five and then may gradually decline.

Coronary artery disease increases in incidence with age and represents the major cause of heart disease and death in older Americans. The disease represents a condition in which there is a deficiency of blood to the heart tissue because of the narrowing or constricting of the cardiac vessels that supply it. Tissue denied an adequate blood supply is called *ischemic;* hence, coronary artery disease is also known as *ischemic heart disease.*

The factors responsible for the narrowed and constricted arteries are not definitely known. What is known is that an overwhelming number of persons living in industrialized nations develop a condition known as *atherosclerosis.* In atherosclerosis the large arteries in particular undergo a narrowing of their passageways as a result of the development of plaques on their interior walls. These plaques, which contain an accumulation of smooth muscle cells and fat and cholesterol crystals in combination with calcium salts, connective tissue, and scar tissue, serve to reduce the size of the passageway in such a manner that the vessel may eventually become totally closed off. The closing of an artery can cause ischemic heart tissue.

Arteriosclerosis is a generic term referring to the loss of elasticity of the arterial walls; it is sometimes popularly called "hardening of the arteries." This condition, which occurs in all populations, is progressive and age related.

Ultimately, this age-associated loss of elasticity of arteries can contribute to reduced blood flow to an area. Unfortunately, this term is often confused or used interchangeably with atherosclerosis. Whereas arteriosclerosis is a general aging phenomenon, atherosclerosis is variable in individuals and populations.

A number of aging changes collectively exert an effect on the respiratory system. These changes, which serve to reduce maximum breathing capacity, are significant in that they cause an elderly person to become fatigued more easily than would a younger person. Nevertheless, these changes are not sufficient to cause apparent symptoms at a resting state. In the absence of disease they do not significantly affect the lifestyle of an older individual. Changes do occur, but they are not necessarily incapacitating.

The airways and tissues of the respiratory tract, including the air sacs, become less elastic and more rigid with age. Osteoporosis may alter the size of the chest cavity as a result of the downward and forward movement of the ribs. Also, the power of the respiratory muscles becomes reduced along with that of the abdominal muscles, which can hinder the movement of the diaphragm.

Respiratory diseases are more prevalent in older individuals than in the general population. The threat of serious respiratory infection increases with age, as does the threat of the obstructive conditions of chronic bronchitis, emphysema, and lung cancer. Some researchers believe the threat of respiratory infection is related to age-associated reductions in resistance to infectious microorganisms. Nevertheless, obstructive pulmonary conditions and lung cancer are not solely the results of inherent age factors. Environmental conditions such as exposure to cigarette smoke and polluted air play an important role in their development. Recently data from the Department of Health and Human Services show that death rates from lung cancer increase fourfold throughout the adult life of a nonsmoker. Nevertheless, the risk of developing lung cancer in an elderly moderate smoker (one-half to a full pack of cigarettes a day) is ten times as great. With additional increase in the degree of exposure to tobacco, the risk increases still further.

The Urinary System

The bladder of an elderly person has a capacity of less than half (250 milliliters) that of a young adult (600 ml) and often contains as much as 100 ml of residual urine. Moreover, the onset of the desire to urinate, often referred to as the *micturition reflex,* is delayed in older persons. Normally this reflex is activated when the bladder is half full, but in the elderly it often does not occur until the bladder is near capacity. The origin of this alteration of the micturition reflex is unclear, but it may be related to age changes in the frontal area of the cerebral cortex or to damage associated with a cerebral infarction or tumor. Reduced bladder capacity coupled with a delayed micturition reflex can lead to problems of frequent urination and extreme urgency of urination. These conditions, even if they do not render an individual incontinent, are an annoyance to an older person.

There appears to be a decrease in average renal function with age. This may result from a loss of nephrons, the basic cell unit in the kidneys. With increasing age the kidneys themselves are found to be smaller, and the nephrons are smaller in size and fewer in number. Despite these apparently dramatic changes, loss of renal tissue is probably secondary in importance to the structural vascular changes that occur in the kidney with age. In general, the arterial tree atrophies, and blood flow to the kidneys is reduced, decreasing the functional efficiency of the system. These vascular changes likely contribute to the loss of nephrons, and this is especially significant when the kidney is seriously malfunctioning or when severe atherosclerosis is superimposed on the aging process.

SEXUALITY AND AGING
Late-Life Sexuality: Myths and Reality

The reputedly "long-lived" Abkhasians attribute their longevity to their practices in sex, work, and diet (Benet 1971). They normally do not begin regular sexual relations before the age of thirty, the traditional age of marriage. They believe such self-discipline is necessary to conserve energy, including sexual energy, in order to enjoy prolonged life. The anthropologist Sula Benet (1971) reports that one medical team investigating the sex life of the Abkhasians concluded that many men retain their sexual potency long after the age of seventy, and almost 14 percent of the women continue to menstruate after the age of fifty-five.

Although there is no "hard evidence" to link Abkhasian sexual practices with longevity, it is fair to say that the relationship between sexuality and age expressed in Abkhasian society is quite different from the norm in our own. In our society, sex and aging are often linked to negative humor that is filled with disdain and often contains an apprehensiveness about growing older. Popular themes for such humor often include the impotence of older men and the unquestioned unattractiveness of older women. Examples abound:

> An eighty-five-year-old man was complaining to his friend, "My stenographer is suing me for breach of promise." His friend answered, "At eighty-five, what could you promise her?" (Adams 1968).

> It may be that life begins at forty but everything else starts to wear out, fall out, or spread out. (*Reader's Digest* 1972)

To the extent that such jokes may reflect basic attitudes, thoughts, and feelings that are not commonly stated, we must ask, "Why are attitudes generally so negative about sex in later life?" Certainly some of this reflects negative feelings about old people and aging in general, what we have referred to in this book as *ageism*. Ageism includes among its stereotypes the myth of de-sexualization: If you are old (or getting old), you are alleged to be finished with sex. This myth is part of what Butler and Lewis (1976) refer to as the "aesthetic narrowness" about sex that prevails in our society. Stated simply, there is a widespread assumption in the United States (and in most of the western world) that sex is only for the young and beautiful. Unfortunately, it is not just the young who believe this but many older people as well.

Misinformation surrounds the issue of late-life sexuality. For example, there is a common presumption that sexual desire diminishes with age, but this is not necessarily the case. Verwoerdt and his colleagues at Duke University (Verwoerdt et al. 1969a, 1969b) found the following:

1. The incidence of sexual interest does not show an age-related decline—interest may persist into the eighties.

2. The incidence of sexual activity declines from a level of more than 50 percent in the early sixties to a level between 10 percent and 20 percent for people in their eighties.

3. The sexual behavior patterns of the later years correlate with those of the younger years—if there were interest and satisfying activity in the early years, there are likely to be interest and satisfying activity in the later years as well.

Sexual interest, capacities, and functions change with age. For the most part, like many biological and psychological functions discussed in this book, these dimensions of sexuality decline with increasing age. This decline can be seen as part of the normal aging process, but it does *not* mean that older men and women in reasonably good health should not be able to have an active and satisfying sex life.

Age-Related Changes in the Genital System[2]

The genital system is characterized by a number of age-related changes in physiology and anatomy. On the whole, few age-specific disorders are associated with this body system. Most of the problems of sexuality and aging are sociogenic or psychogenic.

The Male Genital System. The male reproductive system continues to produce germ cells (*sperm*) and sex hormones (*testosterone*) well into old age. Production of both declines with advancing age, although testosterone production is main-

---

[2] This part relies heavily on Katchadourian (1972) and Fulton (1988).

tained at a higher level longer than is estrogen production in women. The decrease of testosterone has definite effects on older men, including a possible waning of sexual desire, though other physiological changes such as decreased sensitivity of the penis may be even more responsible for the decline.

A number of major physical changes occur in the genital system. The size and the firmness of the testes decrease. Sperm production takes place within the testes in seminiferous or sperm-bearing tubules, which thicken and decrease in diameter with age. This reduces sperm production, although abundant spermatozoa are found even in old age. The production of sex hormones also takes place in the testes but is independent of the sperm-producing structures. The cells responsible for hormone production, located between the seminiferous tubules in proximity to blood vessels, are called *interstitial cells*. Age-related fibrosis, involving an increase in the amount of fibrous connective tissue in the testes, constricts the blood supply and reduces production capacities of the sperm and hormone-producing structures.

Fibrosis may also affect the penis, the male organ for sexual intercourse and for the delivery of semen for reproductive purposes. The penis has no bone and no intrinsic muscles; its components are sheathed in fibrous coats and enclosed within a loose skin. Erection is a purely vascular phenomenon, and age-related increase in fibrous tissue can affect blood supply.

Secretions of the prostate gland account for much of the volume of semen as well as its characteristic odor. The prostate gland often enlarges in older men. The ejaculatory duct, which empties into the urethra (the tube that leads out of the bladder), and the urethra itself traverse the prostate gland. Thus, prostatic enlargement often has the dual effect of making ejaculatory contractions less forceful and urination more difficult. Cancer of the prostate is a frequent neoplasm among older men. All older men should have regular physical examinations to monitor the condition of the prostate.

Masters and Johnson (1970) have translated these physical changes into their impact on the sexual functioning of the older male. Summarized, these effects include the following:

1. It takes an older man longer to achieve a full erection, which may not be as full or as firm as for a younger man.

2. It usually takes an older man longer to achieve orgasm. The force and amount of the ejaculation are reduced, and fewer genital spasms are experienced.

3. In an older man, erection subsides more rapidly after ejaculation.

4. It takes an older man longer than a younger man to have a second erection and orgasm.

The Female Genital System. The female reproductive system becomes less efficient with age, with a reduction in secretion of sex hormones (estrogen and progesterone), less ovulation, and a declining ability of the uterine tube (where fertilization occurs) and uterus (womb) to support a young embryo.

Many physical changes occur in the female genital tract. The external genitalia of the female, known as the *vulva,* include the major and minor lips, the clitoris, and the vaginal orifice. With age, the fold of the major and minor lips become less pronounced and the skin becomes thinner. Vascularity and elasticity decrease, and the area becomes more susceptible to tissue trauma and the development of pruritus (itching). Glands decrease in number, as does the level of secretion, leading to shrinking and drying of the area.

Among internal female reproductive organs, the uterus decreases in size, becomes more fibrous, and has fewer endometrial glands. The cervix or lower portion of the uterus is reduced in size, and the cervical canal (which is surrounded by the upper end of the vagina) decreases in diameter. The uterine tubes (where ova pass and are fertilized) become thinner, and the ovary takes on an irregular shape. Ovulation becomes irregular and finally stops, and there is a drastic reduction in the production of female hormones.

The latter changes, along with irregular or absent menstruation, often characterize *menopause,* a term used to describe the conclusion of a twenty- to thirty-year period of change in the female genital system that progresses differently in each individual. Approximately 50 percent of all women go through menopause between the ages of forty-five and fifty years, about 25 percent before age forty-five, and about 25 percent after age fifty (Hafez 1976). The age of onset can be accelerated by debilitating disease, endocrine disorder, or both.

A number of symptoms are associated with menopause, although they appear to be less common than is popularly thought. These include irritability, anxiety, depression, loss of appetite, insomnia, and headache. Some of these symptoms have more of a psychological than a physiological base. It has been observed that these symptoms are found more often in women with a history of psychotic behavior. Hot flashes, patchy redness on the face and chest, and sweating are associated with vasomotor instability, which causes irregularity in blood vessel diameter and thus irregularity of blood flow to the surface. There is a tendency to deposit fat in the abdominal and pelvic areas. Pubic hair becomes abundant, and breasts may atrophy. The nipples become smaller and less erectile. Still, postmenopausal women can continue to be interested and active sexually.

How do these changes affect female functioning in sexual relations? According to Masters and Johnson (1970):

1. Older women take a longer time to respond to sexual stimuli.
2. Lubrication takes longer and is generally less effective than in younger women.
3. The vagina has reduced elasticity and expansive qualities. The tissues lining the vagina are more easily irritated.
4. In the older women, the clitoris is reduced in size, though still responsive to stimulation.
5. Orgasms are generally less intense and of shorter duration.

The changes described above are a normal part of aging, but individual variations should be recognized. Individuals should understand these age-related changes and not be alarmed when they occur. With proper education, the aging individual may be assured that competent sexual function and fulfillment can continue into the later years.

Sexual dysfunction is certainly not an inevitable result of the aging process. The same factors that lead to sexual problems in the younger years are also important in the elderly, especially when superimposed on the changing genital system. These factors include drug abuse, fatigue, emotional problems, disease, urogenital surgery, alcoholism, overeating, and sociocultural pressures. In the elderly these factors are compounded by fear of failure and society's expectations concerning sexual behavior and the older adult.

A special note is in order about disorders of the female genital system. The uterus and breast are frequent sites of cancer. Breast cancer is the leading cause of death among women between the ages of forty and sixty. Cervical cancer peaks during these same ages, whereas uterine cancer does so at about sixty-five years of age. Cancer of the vulva is more a disease of older women; over 50 percent of the cases occur in those over sixty. These are all good reasons that sex organs should not be cloaked in myth and mystery. All these disorders give early warnings, which should be taken seriously. Not every swelling of the breast indicates breast cancer, and not every vaginal discharge is evidence of carcinoma. These are some of the early signs of cancer, however, and are *not* normal age-related changes. Women can be alert to them without becoming preoccupied. Often, the difference between alertness and ignorance may be one of life and death.

SUMMARY

Senescence describes the effects that lead to the increasing vulnerability individuals face with increasing age. Is senescence an inherent biological process? That may be difficult to say, yet as long ago as 1825 Gompertz identified a pattern to our increased vulnerability through the life course.

A variety of factors influence when we become old and, in particular, the time when we show the kind of vulnerability to aging processes that results in mortality. These include not only differences in biological potential, but also social and environment factors that may limit the expression of biological potential. The leading cause of death among the elderly is heart disease, followed by cancer and stroke. Death rates differ significantly by sex and race. Average life expectancy at birth has increased about 50 percent since the turn of the century. And, survivorship rates to old age have improved even more dramatically. In 1983, the proportion of newborn babies expected to reach age sixty-five was 78.4 percent, almost twice the figure in 1900–02. Age-specific life expectancy at sixty-five years has moved ahead more slowly than has life expectancy at birth during the twentieth century.

What are the specific results of senescence? Age-related physiological changes affect the skin and the skeletomuscular, neurosensory, gastrointestinal, cardiopulmonary, and urinary systems.

Misinformation surrounds the issue of sexuality and aging. Some people may experience declines in sexual desire and activity with advancing age. Such a decline can be seen as part of the normal aging process. Nevertheless, older people in reasonably good health should be able to have an active and satisfying sex life.

STUDY QUESTIONS

1. Distinguish between *biological aging* and *pathological aging*. Define senescence. How can it be distinguished from other biological processes?

2. Taking biological and socioenvironmental factors into consideration, explain the impact of sex on mortality rates. What role do socioeconomic factors play in the racial differences in mortality rates observed in the United States today?

3. Explain the following: (a) increased life expectancy at birth in this century; (b) the small increase in life expectancy from age sixty-five in this century.

4. Discuss those changes in the form and function of the skin that are associated with the aging process.

5. Define and distinguish osteoarthritis, rheumatoid arthritis, and osteoporosis. Describe the resulting complications for those afflicted with these conditions.

6. How is the neurosensory system subject to aging? The gastrointestinal system?

7. Discuss coronary heart disease, making the distinction between *atherosclerosis* and *arteriosclerosis*.

8. Why are attitudes generally so negative about sex in later life? Discuss the impact of physical changes associated with the aging process on the sexual functioning of the older male. Do the same for the older female.

BIBLIOGRAPHY

Adams, J. 1968. *Joey Adams' encyclopedia of humor.* New York: Bonanza Books.

Atchley, R. 1972. *Social forces in later life.* Belmont, Calif.: Wadsworth Publishing Co., Inc.

Benet, S. 1971. Why they live to be 100, or even older in Abkhasia. *New York Times Magazine* (December 26).

Blumenthal, H.T. 1968. Some biomedical aspects of aging. *Gerontologist,* 8:3–5.

Bogue, D.J. 1969. *Principles of demography.* New York: John Wiley and Sons, Inc.

Butler, R., and Lewis, M. 1976. *Love and sex after sixty.* New York: Harper and Row.

Comfort, A. 1979. *The biology of senescence* (3d ed.). New York: The New American Library Inc.

Dorn, H. 1959. Mortality. In P. Hauser and O. Duncan (eds.), *The study of population.* Chicago: University of Chicago Press.

Fries, J.F., and Crapo, L.M. 1981. *Vitality and aging.* San Francisco: W.H. Freeman and Company.

Fulton, G.B. 1988. Sexuality in later life. In C. Kart, E. Metress, and S. Metress (eds.), *Aging, Health and Society.* Menlo Park, Calif.: Jones and Bartlett Publishers, Inc.

Gonnella, J.S., Louis, D.Z., and McCord, J.J. 1976. The staging concept: An approach to the assessment of outcome of ambulatory care. *Medical Care* 14:13–21.

Hafez, E. 1976. Aging and reproductive physiology. Ann Arbor, Mich.: Ann Arbor Science Publishers.

Kart, C., Metress, E., and Metress, J. 1978. *Aging and health: Biologic and social perspectives.* Menlo Park, Calif.: Addison-Wesley Publishing Co., Inc.

Kart, C., Metress, E., and Metress, S. 1988. *Aging, health and society.* Menlo Park, Calif.: Jones and Bartlett Publishers, Inc.

Katchadourian, H. 1972. *Human sexuality: Sense and nonsense.* New York: W.W. Norton and Company, Inc.

Kitagawa, E.M., and Hauser, P.M. 1973. *Differential mortality in the United States: A study in socioeconomic epidemiology.* Cambridge, Mass.: Harvard University Press.

Leaf, A. 1973. Getting old. *Scientific American* 299(3):44–52.

Madigan, F.C. 1957. Are sex mortality differentials biologically caused? *Milbank Memorial Fund Quarterly* 35(2):202–223.

Marcus, A.C., and Siegel, J.M. 1982. Sex differences in the use of physician services: A preliminary test of the fixed role hypothesis. *Journal of Health and Social Behavior* 23:186–196.

Masters, W., and Johnson, V. 1970. *Human sexual response.* Boston: Little, Brown and Company.

Metropolitan Life Insurance Company. 1985. Slight gains in U.S. longevity. *Statistical Bulletin* 66(3):20–23.

———. 1987. Trends in longevity after age 65. *Statistical Bulletin* 68(1):10–17.

Petersen, W. 1975. *Population* (3d ed.). New York: Macmillan.

Reader's Digest. 1972. *Treasury of American humor.* New York: American Heritage Publishing Co., Inc.

Shock, N. 1961. Physiological aspects of aging in man. *Annual Review of Physiology* 23:97–122.

———. 1962. The physiology of aging. *Scientific American* 206(1):100–111.

Siegel, J.S. 1979. *Prospective trends in the size and structure of the elderly population, impact of mortality trends, and some implications.* Current Population Reports, Special Studies Series P-23, No. 78. Washington, D.C., U.S. Department of Commerce, Bureau of the Census.

Sobel, H. 1966. When does human aging start? *Gerontologist* 6:17–22.

Strehler, B. 1962. *Time, cells and aging.* New York: Academic Press, Inc.

U.S. Office of Health Resources Opportunity. 1979. *Health status of minorities and low-income groups.* DHEW Pub. No. (HRA) 79-627. Health Resources Administration, Washington, D.C., U.S. Government Printing Office.

Verwoerdt, A., Pfeiffer, E., and Wang, H.S. 1969a. Sexual behavior in senescence. I. Changes in sexual activity and interest of aging men and women. *Journal of Geriatric Psychiatry* 2:163–180.

———. 1969b. Sexual behavior in senescence. II. Patterns of change in sexual activity and interest. *Geriatrics* 24:137–154.

Wilson, D.L. 1974. The programmed theory of aging. In M. Rockstein (ed.), *Theoretical aspects of aging.* New York: Academic Press, Inc.

Zopf, P.E., Jr. 1986. *America's older population.* Houston, TX: Cap and Gown Press, Inc.

CHAPTER 5

WHY DO WE BECOME OLD?

Cary S. Kart and Eileen S. Metress

Why do we become old? Potential answers to this question are being researched at both the cellular and physiological levels. According to Comfort (1979), there are four classical hypotheses that attempt to explain the mechanism of aging. These include the beliefs that vigor declines as a result of the following: (1) changes in the properties of multiplying cells; (2) loss of, or injury to, non-multiplying cells (for example, neurons); and (3) primary changes in the non-cellular materials of the body (for example, collagen). A fourth hypothesis locates the mechanism of aging in the "software" of the body—"in the overall program of regulation by which other aspects of the life cycle are governed" (Comfort 1979, 17). These hypotheses are not mutually exclusive. After all, aging is a complex phenomenon. Different explanations may be required for different aspects of the aging process; diverse phenomena may act together to account for biological aging. As Comfort has pointed out, though some of these hypotheses have been around for 200 years, none has yet been eliminated by convincing experimental data. The alert reader may recognize these classic hypotheses in the brief summaries of research in biological aging that appear below.

Differentiating between normal aging and superimposed disease is vital to understanding why we become old. The ultimate cause of the majority of deaths in older adults is physiological decline that increases the risk of disease. Mortality results when the ability to withstand the challenge of disease is overwhelmed. For instance, the increased risk of death from pneumonia among older persons is associated with age-related declines in the body's immune defense and reduced pulmonary reserve and function (Rothschild 1984).

Unlocking the mystery of aging and extending the human life span has been the dream of many. As noted in Chapter 2, efforts at prolonging life have been in the written and oral records of societies dating back many thousands of years. Research efforts in biogerontology continue. There are no magic potions to "cure" aging, despite the fact that books on longevity and its promotion have appeared on best-seller lists in recent years.

What follows is an overview of some of the important research in the biology of aging. We distinguish cellular theories of aging from physiological theories of aging. The goal of this research, regardless of whether it is aimed at understanding aging from the cellular or organismic level, is not to grant immortality but to understand the aging process and improve the quality of life for the growing numbers of us who are being added to the ranks of the aged.

CELLULAR THEORIES OF AGING

In the early part of this century it was widely believed that, if some cells were not immortal, at the very least they could grow and multiply for an extended time. Child (1915) "showed" that senescence in planarians (small flatworms that move by means of cilia) is reversible, and Carrel (1912) "demonstrated" that tissue cells taken from adult animals could be propagated indefinitely *in vitro* (in a test tube or other artificial environment). In the same vein, Bidder (1925, 1932) "identified" a number of instances in fish where the life span was not believed to be fixed—that is, general vigor appeared to persist indefinitely.

Recent experiments, particularly those observing cell growth and development in tissue culture, suggest that this earlier research was inaccurate. Still, this work had a significant impact on the field of gerontology. During most of the first half of the twentieth century aging was not considered a characteristic of cells (Cristofalo 1985).

Since the late 1950s, Leonard Hayflick has shown that fibroblast cells (that give rise to connective tissue) from human fetal tissues cultured *in vitro* undergo a finite number of divisions and then die. Across several experiments, Hayflick and Moorhead (1961) observed that such cells undergo an average of fifty divisions *in vitro*, with a range from about forty to about sixty, before losing the ability to replicate themselves. In 1965 Hayflick reported that fibroblasts isolated from human adult tissue undergo only about twenty divisions *in vitro*. On the basis of these and other studies, he argued that (1) the limited replicative capacity of cultured normal human cells is an expression of programmed genetic events and that (2) the limit on normal cell division *in vitro* is a function of the age of the donor. It is now generally believed that there is an inverse relationship between the age of a human donor and the *in vitro* cell division capacity of fibroblasts derived from the skin, lung, and liver (Hayflick 1977).

Although it appears that normal cells have a finite lifetime, this is not the case for "abnormal cells." Such cells, which are distinguishable from normal cells in structure, by genetic makeup, or by both factors, are capable of unlimited division. Cancer cells, for example, are able to divide indefinitely in tissue culture. A famous line of human cancer cells named HeLa (after Henrietta Lacks, the woman from whom they were taken after her death in 1951) is still being cultured for use in standardized cancer cell studies (Gold 1981). Whatever causes noncancerous cells to gradually lose the ability to divide appears to be lacking in cancer cells. The study of cancer may yet reveal what limits the ability of normal cells to divide indefinitely.

Tissue culture studies have limitations and, almost certainly, these experiments do not literally replicate the aging process. Yet, the experiments have been analyzed by many investigators. All confirm the findings. Fries and Crapo (1981) report that in 1962 Hayflick froze many vials of embryo cells that had completed several divisions. Each year since that time, some vials have been thawed and cultured; they always go on to complete their natural growth to the same roughly fifty divisions (Fries and Crapo 1981).

Do humans age solely because their cells have an intrinsically limited capacity to reproduce? This seems unlikely. Nerve and muscle cells do not divide at all in adult life, though they do show deterioration with age.

Researchers continue to suggest that aging may be genetically programmed into cells. Bernard Strehler has hypothesized that programmed loss of genetic material might cause aging. As Strehler (1973) points out, most cells contain hundreds of repetitions of the same DNA (the molecule of heredity in nearly all organisms) for the known genes they contain. This simply means that the cell does not have to rely upon a single copy of its genetic blueprint for any one trait. In experiments done on beagles, Strehler found that, as cells age, a considerable number of these repetitions are lost (Johnson, Crisp, and Strehler 1972). This is especially true for brain, heart, and skeletal muscle cells. How the loss occurs is not specifically known, although there is some speculation that it results from age-related changes in cell metabolism. Strehler suspects that cells may be programmed, at a fixed point in life, to start manufacturing a substance that inhibits protein synthesis.

Another school of thought claims that senescence is largely a result of the accumulation of accidental changes that occur to cells over a period of time. Sinex (1977) thinks that random mutations may produce aging by causing damage to DNA molecules. Although the cell has DNA repair mechanisms, it is likely either that some mutational changes are too subtle for the repair process to detect or that mutations occur too rapidly for them all to be repaired. It is theorized that as mutations accumulate in the body's cells, these cells begin to lose their ability to function, including even a loss of the ability to divide.

Orgel (1963, 1973) has also hypothesized that random errors or mutations might show up in the transcriptions of DNA into RNA (ribonucleic acid, which carries instructions from the DNA) or through errors in the translation of RNA into proteins. He suggests that random errors in the synthesizing of information-carrying proteins might lead to a cascade of other errors. This "error cascade" (sometimes referred to as an "error catastrophe") results in cell deterioration. This hypothesis has not been confirmed experimentally. No one has yet been able to detect errors at the protein level, though efforts continue to be made (Fries and Crapo 1981). This error or mutation theory may not be incompatible with the genetic programmed theory. It is certainly possible that a shutoff of cellular repair mechanisms is a programmed genetic event.

Another explanation of aging involves the belief that *free radicals,* highly unstable molecules containing an unpaired electron (Sanadi 1977), reduce cellular efficiency and cause an accumulation of cellular waste. Free radicals may be produced by radiation, extreme heat, or oxidation reactions. They may also be created in small quantities as part of normal cell metabolism. According to Sanadi (1977), the hypothesis that excessive numbers of free radicals, regardless of source, may damage cellular membranes and other cellular components merits further consideration. Such damage could accelerate aging and bring about the premature death of an organism. Some believe that the fatty "age pigment" lipofuscin, which accumulates to an appreciable extent in neurons and cardiac and skeletal muscle cells, may be an end product of cellular membrane damage caused by free radicals. It should be emphasized, however, that current thinking holds that lipofuscin is an indicator rather than a cause of aging.

Harman (1961, 1968), among others, has done work attempting to reduce the source of free radicals. Certain chemicals, called *antioxidants* (a common one is BHT, the food preservative), have been used to combine with and "disarm" free radicals. Harman reported that the inclusion of antioxidants in the diet increased the average life span of experimental animals by 15 to 30 percent. The animals receiving the antioxidants showed lower weight, suggesting the possibility that dietary restriction itself may prolong average life span. Another effect of adding antioxidants to the diet of experimental animals was the reduction in tumor production (Harman 1968).

A well-known antioxidant is vitamin E. Although there is some evidence that vitamin E deficiency reduces the life expectancy of experimental animals, no experimental evidence is available to show that supplementing the diet with vitamin E extends average life expectancy (Tapple 1968). In addition, there is no current evidence to support the idea that dietary supplementation of other vitamins (A and C) and minerals (silenium, for example) with antioxidant properties can prevent cancer or extend human life (Ames 1983; Schneider and Reed 1985; Willet and MacMahon 1984).

Higher organisms do possess sophisticated biochemical systems for scavenging free radicals. The enzyme *superoxide dismutase* is a part of such a system. A relationship has been noted between superoxide dismutase activity and life span in varying species and species strains (Bartosz, Leyko, and Fried 1979; Kellogg and Fridovich 1976; Munkres, Rana, and Goldstein 1984; Tolmasoff, Ono, and Cutler 1980). It is possible that the regulation of superoxide dismutase is under the control of the same genes that dictate the life span of a particular species (Schneider and Reed 1985). Superoxide dismutase tablets have been touted for their "anti-aging effect." Nevertheless, there is no evidence that oral administration of the enzyme prolongs life. In fact, one report demonstrates that blood and tissue levels of this enzyme are not affected by its ingestion (Zidenburg-Cherr et al., 1983).

The above mentioned theories are concerned with aging at the cellular (and molecular) level; nevertheless, it is a long leap from cell biology to studying aging in the total organism. Several physiological theories attempt to relate aging to the performance of the total organism, and these deserve our attention.

PHYSIOLOGICAL THEORIES OF AGING

One physiological theory of aging involves the autoimmune mechanism. This theory postulates that many age-related changes can be accounted for by changes in the immune response. Normally, the immune system, through the action of special immune cells and the production of antibodies, serves to protect us from material that the body reads as foreign, including cancer cells. With age, immune cell function declines, and increased levels of autoantibodies are found in the blood (Goidl, Thorbecke, and Weksler 1980; Walford, 1982; Weksler 1982). Autoantibodies are substances produced against host tissues. In usual circumstances the body's immune system is able to distinguish between host body cells and foreign substances subject to attack.

The significance of age-associated increases in autoantibodies is not well understood, but they are believed to contribute to inefficiencies in physiological functioning. Why these antibodies are produced against one's own tissues is not known. Perhaps, once-normal body cells begin to look different as a result of accumulated changes resulting from mutation or free-radical damage. If immune cells undergo similar changes, this might cause production of aberrant antibodies. Also, body constituents may break down from disease or other damage and appear as "new" substances that the body's defense mechanism will not tolerate. Potentially, all these factors may interact to produce autoimmunity.

Diminished immunocompetence has been established as an age-related change. Schneider and Reed (1985) suggest that the decline in immune function may have evolved as a protective mechanism against the ravages of autoimmunity. Presumably, a vigorous immune reaction might allow for an even greater production of autoantibodies.

The immune system is not organ-specific. It is in constant contact with all body cells, tissues, and organs. Any alteration in the immune system may be expected to exert an effect on all body systems (Kay and Baker 1979; Kay and Makinodan 1982). Thus, as immune competence decreases, the incidence of autoimmunity, infection, and cancer can be expected to increase (Good and Yunis 1974; MacKay, Whittington, and Mathews 1977).

In humans, the immune system begins to decline shortly after puberty. This decline includes beginning atrophy of the thymus, the gland thought by many to be the structure central to the aging of the immune system. Thymic hormone influences immune functioning. Its progressive age-related loss is associated with declines in the reactivity of certain immune cells. The percentage of immature immune cells increases in association with the lack of thymic hormone. Other substances, termed lymphokines, are also important in activating and maintaining the immune response. One lymphokine, interleukin-2 (IL-2), undergoes limited production with age (Thoman 1985).

Thompson and his associates (1984) recently reported on the immune status of a group of healthy centenarians. This study population had withstood the risk of cancer and an assortment of other diseases for at least one hundred years. Their immune systems appeared to function in a fashion similar to the immune systems of much younger individuals. These researchers were left asking (1) when changes in the immune cells of these centenarians began; (2) whether these changes represent irreversible programmed aging that simply began later in this group; and, (3) whether other "outside" factors are responsible for immune decline.

Another theory with a long history is the "wear and tear" theory of aging. In effect, this theory posits an inverse relationship between "rate of living" and length of life—that is, those who live too hard and fast cannot expect to live very long. In the early part of this century, Rubner (described in Comfort 1979) carried out calorimetric experiments to determine the energy requirements necessary for the maintenance of body metabolism. He suggested that senescence might reflect the expenditure of fixed amounts of energy used to complete particular chemical reactions. An important question then arises: Can an individual live a life that causes a speedup or slowdown in the expenditure of such energy?

Many theorists using this model employ machine analogies to exemplify the theory's underlying assumption that an organism wears out with use. Nevertheless, these analogies often fail to take into account two important characteristics of living organisms: (1) living organisms have mechanisms for self-repair not available to machines; and (2) functions in a living organism may actually become more efficient with use.

Hans Selye's work on stress has been used by some to support the wear and tear theory. Selye (1966) has identified three stages of responses to continued stress, based on his experiments with animals. Each stage of response parallels a phase of aging. Stage one is characterized by an alarm reaction in which the body's adaptive forces are being activated but are not yet fully operational. This stage is reminiscent of childhood in which adaptability to stress is growing but in which adaptability is still limited. Stage two is the stage of resistance—mobilization of the defensive reactions to stress is completed. This phase parallels adulthood, during which the body has acquired resistance to most stress agents likely to affect it. Stage three, the stage of exhaustion, eventually results in a breakdown of resistance and eventual death. This last stage parallels the process of senescence in human beings.

Though it makes intuitive sense that an old animal is less able to withstand the same stress that can be tolerated by a young animal, there is little empirical evidence that accumulated stress is the cause of aging. Selye's work has been and continues to be important in showing the relationship between stress and disease. Nevertheless, it has not yet been helpful in attempts to specify the mechanisms of aging.

Collagen, an extracellular component of connective tissue, has also been implicated in age-related changes in physiological functions. Collagen, widely scattered throughout the body, is included in the skin, blood vessels, bone, cartilage, tendons, and other body organs. With age, collagen shows a reduction in its elastic properties as well as an increase in cross-linkages. Cross-linkage is a process whereby proteins in the body bind to each other.

According to the cross-linkage theory of aging, alteration in collagen plays an important role in impairing functional capacities. For example, the reduced efficiency of cardiac muscle may be the result of increasing stiffness. Connective tissue changes in small blood vessels may lead to the development of hypertension. Less elastic vessels may likewise have altered permeability, thereby affecting nutrient transport and waste removal. Such changes can have far-reaching effects on all body organs.

Diabetics may be susceptible to excessive cross-linking. They undergo many complications that are similar to age-related changes, such as cataract formation and atherosclerosis. Diabetes is often referred to as a model for studying the aging process. Elevated blood sugar levels promote cross-linkage formation (Cerami 1985). It is presently believed that many of the long-term complications of diabetes are related to glucose-induced cross-linking, especially the cross-linking of collagen. Future work will likely provide greater insight into the possible role of glucose as a mediator of aging. Researchers at Rockefeller University are presently studying a drug that prevents blood sugar from promoting protein cross-linking. It is hoped that the drug can be used in the future treatment of diabetic complications. Perhaps its most provocative use in the distant future might be the treatment of "aging" disorders in the nondiabetic (Wechsler 1986).

Nathan Shock, a noted gerontologist, has recently suggested that there is sufficient evidence for us to entertain the possibility that aging results from some breakdown or impairment in the performance of endocrine and neural control mechanisms (Shock 1961, 1962, 1974). Studies carried out by the National Institutes of Health's Gerontology Research Center show that age-related declines in humans are greater for functions that are complex and require the coordinated activity of whole organ systems. Measurements of functions related to a single physiological system, like nerve conduction velocity, show considerably less age decrement than do functions such as maximum breathing capacity, which involve coordination between systems (in this case between the nervous and muscular systems).

The relationship between age and task performance also shows greater age-related decline that is most likely associated with task complexity. For example, simple motor performance, as demonstrated by the time it takes an individual to push a button in response to a signal of light, increases only modestly across the human life span. Complex motor performance, on the other hand, does show significant decrement with age. Complex motor performance can involve having an individual select one of several possible responses after the presentation of a complex stimulus. Although simple motor performance involves the transmission of nerve impulses over short distances and through relatively few synapses, complex motor performance requires transmission through many synapses and is influenced by other factors in the central nervous system. Interestingly, though, the aged often show significantly improved motor performance with practice (Botwinick 1973).

PROLONGEVITY

Some information presented in this and previous chapters may lead readers to believe that length of life has been increased and will continue to increase almost automatically as a by-product of technological and social changes. Whether or not this is really so is unclear and illustrates the necessity of distinguishing between the concepts "life expectancy" and "life span." Whereas life expectancy refers to the average length of life of persons, life span refers to the longevity of long-lived persons. Life span is the extreme limit of human longevity, the age beyond which no one can expect to live (Gruman 1977, 7). Gerontologists estimate the life span at about 110 years; some have argued that it has not increased notably in the course of history.

Is the human life span an absolute standard? Or can (should) we expect a significant extension of the length of life? Some have always shared the view that human life should be lengthened indefinitely. These are proponents of *prolongevity*, defined as the significant extension of the length of life by human action (Gruman 1977, 6). Others believe that new treatments and technology as well as improved health habits may continue to increase life expectancy but that human life span is unlikely to increase.

Prolongevitists often point to the "long-lived" peoples in mountain regions of Ecuador (the Andean village of Vilacabamba), Pakistan (the Hunza people of Kashmir), and the Soviet Union (the Abkhasians in the Russian Caucasus) as examples of populations that have already extended the human life span (Leaf 1973). Each of these groups purportedly shows a statistically higher proportion of centenarians in the population, with many individuals reaching 120,

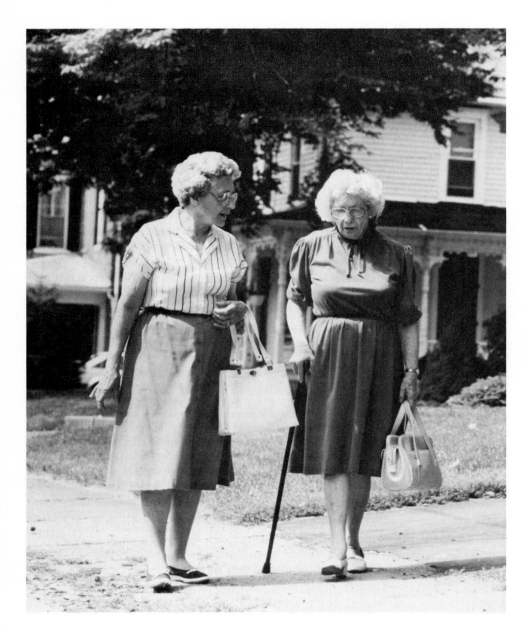

130, or even 150 and 160 years. Unfortunately, there are many reasons for doubting the validity of these claims (Kyncharyants 1974; Mazess and Forman 1979; Medvedev 1974, 1975). The Russian gerontologist Medvedev says that none of these cases of superlongevity is scientifically valid. He offers the following case as explanation of why many in the Caucasus claim superlongevity:

> The famous man from Yakutia, who was found during the 1959 census to be
> 130 years old, received especially great publicity because he lived in the place
> with the most terrible climate. . . . When . . . a picture of this outstanding man
> was published in the central government newspaper, Isvestia, the puzzle was
> quickly solved. A letter was received from a group of Ukrainian villagers who
> recognized this centenarian as a fellow villager who deserted from the army
> during the First World War and forged documents or used his father's. . . . It
> was found that this man was really only seventy-eight years old (Medvedev
> 1974, 387).

There continues to be interest—even mass interest—in increasing human
longevity. A good part of this interest originates in the antediluvian theme
found in tradition and folklore that people lived much longer in the distant
past. Noah, after all, supposedly lived to be 950 years old.

What are the prospects for continued reduction in death rates and life
extension? As we have already shown, death rates have declined and are likely
to continue to do so. Nevertheless, some research suggests there is little room
for improvement, unless some significant breakthrough eliminates cardiovascular diseases. In any case, small improvements seem to be attainable. According to Siegel (1975), if the lowest death rates for females in the countries
of Europe are combined into a single table, the values for life expectancy at
birth and at age sixty-five exceed those same values for the United States by
4.3 and 1.4 years respectively. Table 5-1 shows average life expectancy at birth,
according to sex, for selected countries in the years 1979 to 1982. Whereas the
United States has experienced gains in life expectancy during the twentieth
century, it is clear that Canada, France, Netherlands, Sweden, Switzerland,
Australia, and Japan have life expectancies at birth for both males and females
that exceed those of the United States.

Most elderly people die as a result of some long-standing chronic condition,
which is sometimes related to personal habits (for example, smoking, drinking
alcohol, poor eating habits) or environmental conditions (for example, harsh
work environments, air pollution) that go back many years. Attempts to prevent
illness and death from these conditions must begin before old age. But, what
if we could prevent death from these conditions? Table 5-2 gives a partial answer
to this question, using life table data for 1969 to 1971. The elimination of all
deaths in the United States caused by accidents, influenza and pneumonia,
infective and parasitic diseases, diabetes mellitus, and tuberculosis would increase life expectancy at birth by 1.6 years and at age sixty-five by 0.6 years.
Even the elimination of cancer as a cause of death would result in only a 2.5-
year gain in life expectancy at birth and little more than half that (1.4 years)
at age sixty-five. This is because cancer affects individuals in all age groups.
If the major cardiovascular-renal diseases were eliminated, there would be an
11.8-year gain in life expectancy at birth, and even an 11.4-year gain in life

TABLE 5-1 Life Expectancy at Birth by Sex, for Selected Countries

Country and Year	Male	Female
North America		
Canada (1980–82)	71.9	78.9
United States (1979–81)	70.1	77.6
Europe		
Denmark (1980–81)	71.1	77.2
Finland (1981)	69.5	77.8
France (1981)	70.4	78.5
Netherlands (1981)	72.7	79.3
Sweden (1981)	73.1	79.1
Switzerland (1981–82)	72.7	79.6
United Kingdom: England and Wales (1980–82)	71.1	77.1
Other Areas		
Australia (1981)	71.4	78.4
Israel (1981)	72.7	75.9
Japan (1981)	73.8	79.1

Source: Metropolitan Life (1986).

expectancy at age sixty-five. These diseases are not likely to be eliminated in the near future, although death rates as a result of them may be reduced.

There is substantial room for improvement in death rates and life expectancies in the United States among men and nonwhites. As has already been pointed out in Chapter 4, the death rate for aged men is considerably higher than those rates for aged women and, controlling for sex, the death rates for elderly blacks are higher than those for their white counterparts.

TABLE 5-2 Gain in Life Expectancy if Various Causes of Death Were Eliminated

Various Causes of Death	Gain in Years	
	At Birth	At Age 65
1. Major cardiovascular-renal diseases	11.8	11.4
2. Malignant neoplasms	2.5	1.4
3. Motor vehicle accidents	0.7	0.1
4. Influenza and pneumonia	0.5	0.2
5. Diabetes mellitus	0.2	0.2
6. Infective and parasitic diseases	0.2	0.1

Source: U.S. Public Health Service data of life tables by cause of death for 1969–71, U.S. Bureau of the Census, *Current Population Reports*, Series P-23, No. 59, January 1978 (revised).

Much more discussion of biogerontological research on prolongevity is needed. Improving death rates and life expectancies in the United States along the lines suggested above would still not achieve an extension of the life span. Should people live to be 120 or 130 years of age? When thinking about your answer, assume first that this would involve more than a simple increase in time at the end of life. Imagine that researchers could alter the rate of aging in such a way as to give extra years to all the healthy and productive stages of life. Under these conditions, extra years might be difficult to turn down. But, what if a longer life meant a longer "old age"? Many of you, while thinking of answers to the question of whether we should extend the human life span, will think about pollution, overpopulation, dwindling energy resources, retirement policies, social security benefits, and the like. The list of negative implications is a long one and may simply reflect your negative characterization of old age. If you think of old age in terms of the continuation of productive possibilities, then you may very well accept these extra years, however and whenever they come.

SUMMARY

Answers abound to the question, "Why do we become old?" They reflect the commitment of biogerontologists to aging research at both the cellular and organismic levels. Clearly, more research is needed to understand biological aging and improve the quality of life for increasing numbers of the aged. Attempts should be made to test the relative merits of genetic programmed theory and mutation theory, autoimmune theory, cross-linkage theory, and stress theory, among others. Also, perhaps we should discard the expectation that there is one overall theory of biological aging. After all, aging is a complex phenomenon, and it may well be that different explanations are required for different aspects of the aging process.

Finally, what will be the effect of a solution to the riddle of biological aging? Should we welcome prolongevity? And, have we thought sufficiently about its potential impact on individuals as well as on society as a whole?

STUDY QUESTIONS

1. List the four classical hypotheses, identified by Comfort, that attempt to explain the mechanisms of aging. Can you link any of the theories of biological aging discussed in this chapter with these classical hypotheses?

2. Which cellular theories suggest that aging may be genetically programmed into cells? Which cellular theories of aging appear to implicate diet or nutrition in the aging process?

3. Identify the following physiological theories of aging: (a) autoimmune theory; (b)

wear and tear theory; (c) collagen theory. How may a breakdown in endocrine or neural mechanisms influence the aging process?

4. Define prolongevity. Distinguish between life expectancy and life span. Can we be sure that the Abkhasians of the Russian Caucasus really live as long as they claim?

5. Compare the life expectancy at birth of people in the United States with citizens of other industrialized nations. Which groups in the United States seem to show the greatest potential for improvement in the values of life expectancy and death rates?

6. How much gain in life expectancy in the United States can be realized through the elimination of certain diseases? Where would the greatest gain come from?

7. Eliminating certain diseases and, thus, extending life expectancy would seem to be an inherently positive thing. Is the idea of extending the human life span equally as positive? Explain your answer.

BIBLIOGRAPHY

Ames, B. 1983. Dietary carcinogens and anticarcinogens: Oxygen radicals and degenerative disease. *Science* 221:1256–1264.

Bartosz, G., Leyko, W., and Fried, R. 1979. Superoxide dismutase and life span of Drosophila melanogaster. *Experientia* 35:1193.

Bidder, G.P. 1925. The mortality of Plaice. *Nature* 115:495.

———. 1932. Senescence. *British Medical Journal* 115:5831.

Botwinick, J. 1973. *Aging and behavior*. New York: Springer.

Carrel, A. 1912. On the permanent life of tissues. *Journal of Experimental Medicine* 15:516.

Cerami, A. 1985. Hypothesis: Glucose as a mediator of aging. *Journal of American Geriatrics Society* 33:626–634.

Child, C.M. 1915. *Senescence and rejuvenescence*. Chicago: University of Chicago Press.

Comfort, A. 1979. *The biology of senescence* (3d ed.). New York: The New American Library Inc.

Cristofalo, V. 1985. The destiny of cells: Mechanisms and implications of senescence. *Gerontologist* 25:577–583.

Fries, J.F., and Crapo, L.M. 1981. *Vitality and aging*. San Francisco: W.H. Freeman and Co.

Goidl, E., Thorbecke, G., and Weksler, M. 1980. Production of auto-anti-idiotypic antibody during the normal immune response. *Proceedings of National Academy of Science* 77:6788.

Gold, M. 1981. The cells that would not die. *Science 81* 2(3):28–35.

Good, R., and Yunis, E. 1974. Association of autoimmunity, immunodeficiency and aging in man, rabbits and mice. *Federation Proceedings* 33:2040–2050.

Gruman, G. 1977. *A history of ideas about the prolongation of life*. New York: Arno Press, Inc.

Harman, D. 1961. Prolongation of the normal lifespan and inhibition of spontaneous cancer by antioxidants. *Journal of Gerontology* 16:247–254.

———. 1968. Free radical theory of aging. *Journal of Gerontology* 23:476–482.

Hayflick, L. 1977. The cellular basis for biological aging. In C. Finch and L. Hayflick (eds.), *Handbook of the biology of aging*. New York: Van Nostrand Reinhold Co.

Hayflick, L., and Moorhead, P.S. 1961. The serial cultivation of human diploid cell strains. *Experimental Cell Research* 25:585–621.

Johnson, R., Crisp, C., and Strehler, B. 1972. Selective loss of ribosomal RNA genes during the aging of postmitotic tissues. *Mechanisms of Aging and Development* 1.

Kay, M., and Baker, L. 1979. Cell changes associated with declining immune function: Physiology and cell biology of aging. In A. Cherkin, C. Finch, N. Kharasch, T. McKinodan, F. Scott, and B. Strehler (eds.), *Aging*, Vol. 8. New York: Raven Press.

Kay, M., and Makinodan, T. 1982. The aging immune system. In A. Viidik (ed.), *Lectures on gerontology, Vol. 1: On biology of aging, part A.* London: Academic Press.

Kellogg, E., and Fridovich, I. 1976. Superoxide dismutase in the rat and mouse as a function of age and longevity. *Journal of Gerontology* 31:405–408.

Kyncharyants, V. 1974. Will the human life-span reach one hundred? *Gerontologist* 14:377–380.

Leaf, A. 1973. Getting old. *Scientific American* 299(3):44–52.

MacKay, I., Whittington, S., and Mathews, J. 1977. The immunoepidemiology of aging. In T. Makinodan and E. Yunis (eds.), *Immunity and Aging*. New York: Plenum Press.

Mazess, R., and Forman, S. 1979. Longevity and age exaggeration in Vilacabamba, Ecuador. *Journal of Gerontology* 34:94–98.

Medvedev, Z.A. 1974. Caucasus and Altay longevity: A biological or social problem? *Gerontologist* 14:381–387.

———. 1975. Aging and longevity: New approaches and new perspectives. *Gerontologist* 15:196–210.

Metropolitan Life Insurance Company. 1986. Recent international changes in longevity. *Statistical Bulletin* 67(1):16–21.

Munkres, K., Rana, R., and Goldstein, E. 1984. Genetically determined conidial longevity is positively correlated with superoxide dismutase, catalase, glutathione peroxidase, cytochrome peroxidase and ascorbate free radical reductase activities in Neurospora crass. *Mechanisms of Aging and Development* 24:83–100.

Orgel, L.E. 1963. The maintenance of the accuracy of protein synthesis and its relevance to aging. *Proceedings of the National Academy of Sciences* 49:517.

———. 1973. The maintenance of the accuracy of protein synthesis and its relevance to aging. *Proceedings of the National Academy of Sciences* 67:1496.

Rothschild, H. 1984. The biology of aging. In H. Rothschild (ed.), *Risk factors for senility*. New York: Oxford University Press.

Sanadi, D.R. 1977. Metabolic changes and their significance in aging. In C. Finch and L. Hayflick (eds.), *Handbook of the biology of aging*. New York: Van Nostrand Reinhold Co.

Schneider, E., and Reed, J. 1985. Life extension. *New England Journal of Medicine* 312:1159–1168.

Selye, H. 1966. *The stress of life* (2nd ed.). New York: McGraw-Hill, Inc.

Shock, N. 1961. Physiological aspects of aging in man. *Annual Review of Physiology* 23:97–122.

———. 1962. The physiology of aging. *Scientific American* 206(1):100–111.

———. 1974. Physiological theories of aging. In M. Rockstein (ed.), *Theoretical aspects of aging*. New York: Academic Press, Inc.

Siegel, J.S. 1975. Some demographic aspects of aging in the United States. In A. Ostfeld and D. Gibson (eds.), *Epidemiology of aging*. Bethesda, Md.: National Institutes of Health.

Sinex, F.M. 1977. The molecular genetics of aging. In C. Finch and L. Hayflick (eds.), *Handbook of the biology of aging*. New York: Van Nostrand Reinhold Co.

Strehler, B. 1973. A new age for aging. *Natural History*, February.

Tapple, A.L. 1968. Will antioxidant nutrients slow aging processes? *Geriatrics* 23:97.

Thoman, M. 1985. Role of interleukin-2 in the age-related impairment of immune function. *Journal of American Geriatrics Society* 33:781–787.

Thompson, J., Wekstein, D., Rhoades, J., Kirkpatrick, C., Brown, S., Rozman, T., Straus, R., and Tietz, N. 1984. The immune status of healthy centenarians. *Journal of American Geriatrics Society* 32:274–281.

Tolmasoff, J., Ono, T., and Cutler, R. 1980. Superoxide dismutase: Correlation with life span and specific metabolic rate in primate species. *Proceedings of the National Academy of Sciences* 77:2777–2781.

Walford, R. 1982. Studies in immunogerontology. *Journal of American Geriatrics Society* 30:617.

Wechsler, R. 1986. Unshackled from diabetes. *Discover* 7:77–85.

Weksler, M. 1982. Age-associated changes in the immune response. *Journal of American Geriatrics Society* 30:718.

Willet, W., and MacMahon, B. 1984. Diet and cancer—an overview. *New England Journal of Medicine* 310:633–638, 697–703.

Zidenberg-Cherr, S., Keen, C., Lonnerdal, B., and Hurley, L. 1983. Dietary superoxide dismutase does not affect tissue levels. *American Journal of Clinical Nutrition* 37:5–7.

CHAPTER 6

HEALTH STATUS OF THE ELDERLY

Human organs gradually diminish in function over time, although not at the same rate in every individual. By itself, this gradual diminution of function is not a real threat to the health of most older people; diseases are another matter. Diseases represent the chief barriers to extended health and longevity. And, when they accompany normal changes associated with biological aging, maintaining health and securing appropriate health care becomes especially problematic for older people.

Two additional factors contribute to the difficulty older persons face in maintaining their health status. One has to do with the basic orientation of modern medicine, the other with the attitudes and expectations that older people themselves, family and friends, and health-care providers have about what aging means.

THE MEDICAL MODEL

According to the logic of both contemporary medical diagnosis and the disease model, attention is aimed at obtaining a diagnosis of a condition and developing a treatment regimen for its cure. Efforts are almost always geared at identifying just one condition or dysfunction. Among the elderly in ill health, however, a single condition is unusual. More often, elderly patients have multiple conditions, including degenerative changes associated with biological aging and diseases associated with pathological aging. These multiple changes may lead to confusion in trying to diagnose accurately and to difficulty in generating an appropriate treatment plan. Chest pain may be a signal for any number of serious conditions, including heart disease (or an impending heart attack), gastrointestinal disorders, and esophageal problems. If the symptoms are less specific, certain disease states may be overlooked. Pathy (1967) has reported that 13 percent of elderly patients suffering acute myocardial infarction (heart attack) present mental confusion as the major symptom. Yet mental confusion is a major symptom in the elderly under conditions of metabolic imbalance, depression, malnutrition, the presence of a tumor, cirrhosis, diminished cardiac output, vascular syndromes, fever, and chronic lung disease (Libow 1973).

The World Health Organization defines *health* as "a state of complete physical, mental, and social well-being," not merely the absence of disease. This definition extends beyond biological considerations. To the extent that modern medicine has been concerned with "what went wrong" biologically, it has sacrificed recognition of the broader social and emotional elements that contribute to health.

> Seventy-year-old Mr. Hernandez went directly from the hospital to his city-project apartment—where he lived alone—after cataract surgery. When the public health nurse arrived a week later, she found him weak from hunger. The refrigerator was empty, and there were but a few cans of food in the cupboards. In addition, the apartment was dirty and cluttered with garbage and soiled clothes. The patient's limited eyesight and recent hospitalization had left him disoriented and unsure of himself in his own home. He was afraid to brave the stairs or elevator leading from his apartment to pick up his Social Security check in the mailbox, let alone to go shopping, do his laundry, or throw out the garbage. He could neither cook nor tend to his personal hygiene. And he had no friends or family near (Luke 1976, p. 26).

Although no one would challenge Mr. Hernandez's need for cataract surgery, many would debate whether he was "healthier" before or after medical intervention. Health care extends beyond the doors of the health-care institution. Understanding the factors that contribute or detract from health may be less dramatic than developing "miracle cures," but no less important. Until organized medicine shifts its focus and identifies those conditions that enable people to thrive rather than merely survive, older people like Mr. Hernandez will continue to be "doing better and feeling worse" (Daedulus 1977).

ATTRIBUTION OF ILLNESS

Health is as much a subjective as an objective phenomenon. Individuals assess their health on the basis of various factors, including their own expectations about how people like themselves should feel. People experiencing changes in usual body functioning try to make sense of their experiences, often by hypothesizing about the possible causes of symptoms. A central issue in most perceptions of causality is whether to attribute a given experience to internal or external states (Freedman, Sears, and Carlsmith 1978). *External* attribution ascribes causality to anything external to the individual, such as the general environment, role constraints or role losses, stressful tasks being worked on, and so on. *Internal* causes include such factors as disease states, biological aging, personality, and mood and motivation (Freedman, Sears, and Carlsmith 1978).

Potentially, the development of illness attribution and misattribution can be affected by many factors internal and external to the individual. These include the perceived seriousness of symptoms, the extent of disruption of normal activities involved, the frequency and persistence of the symptoms, the amount of pain and discomfort to which a person is accustomed, the medical knowledge of the person, the need to deny the illness, the nature of competing needs, the availability of alternative explanations, and the accessibility of treatment (Mechanic 1978). Sex (Nathanson 1975), social class (Koos 1954; Andersen, Anderson, and Smedby 1968; Osborn 1973), and the presence of a community referral system (Freidson 1960, 1961) also affect how symptoms are evaluated and defined.

According to Jones and Nisbett (1971), actors and observers tend to make different causal attributions. Actors usually see their behavior as a response to an external situation in which they find themselves; typically, observers attribute the same response to factors internal to the actor. This difference between an actor's and an observer's attributions can lead to misunderstanding and, perhaps, especially so in a health-care context. Patients and their physicians may see the same event from different perspectives. The patient attributes his response to environmental factors (for example, stress at home) that are out of the purview of the physician, but the physician attributes the patient's response to internal physical processes—disease states or biological aging. These internal processes are, for the most part, the only causal explanations available to the physician, who may be handicapped by a lack of information about those factors to which the patient is responding in the environment.

This is the basis for problems in the doctor–patient relationship. The noncompliant patient may be deemed uncooperative or recalcitrant by the physician—"the patient has a personality problem"—whereas the patient may attribute noncompliance to situational factors—"the medication made me sick" (Janis and Rodin 1979).

The elderly themselves seem overly ready to make attributions to internal physical processes rather than to the environment (Janis and Rodin 1979). Their perceptions often include grossly exaggerated notions of what happens during normal aging. Too many associate pain and discomfort, debilitation, or decline in intellectual function with aging in itself. These are not normal accompaniments of aging. Unfortunately, such associations are supported by significant others ("What do you expect at your age?") as well as by physicians. In fact, the relationship between an aged patient and the doctor may be a *special case* of actor–observer interaction, when both agree that events are attributable to internal physical processes (for example, biological aging). This consensus may reinforce a set of consequences that are essentially negative. First, elderly individuals may assume that aging has had a greater impact on them than it really has. For example, Kahn and his associates (1975) found that only a small amount of memory loss was evident in an elderly sample; yet patients perceived a high degree of loss. These perceptions were highly correlated with depression. Second, they attribute all negative changes in health and mood to aging per se. Chest pain as a warning signal of heart disease may be considered another attack of heartburn; bone pain, which may herald a fracture or bone cancer, may be ascribed to age-related rheumatism. A change in bowel habits is a well-known danger signal of cancer. Such an alteration may easily be ignored by an older person who seems to be plagued by bowel problems. Even rectal bleeding may be attributed to hemorrhoids.

Attributing illness or biological changes to "normal aging" may incorrectly focus an elderly person (and his physician) away from situational and social factors that are stress-inducing and affect health. Much gerontological literature is concerned with the impact on health status of retirement, widowhood, and changing living environments, among other factors.

In general, no social science support has been found for the notion that retirement is detrimental to health. Yet, as Butler and Lewis (1982) point out, reconciling social science and clinical data may be difficult because individuals get lost in the mass of data. Butler (1975) has used the term "retirement syndrome" to describe the fact that retirement may be pathogenic to some individuals. Ellison (1968) suggests that some retirees become "ill" because they define illness as a more legitimate role than being retired. Simon and Cahan (1963) reported that patients with reversible (acute) brain syndromes were likely to have fewer family ties, and their retirement tended to occur before age sixty-five.

It is well established that the mortality rate for many causes of death is much higher among widows and widowers than among married persons of the same age (Parkes 1964). Kraus and Lilienfeld (1959) showed that the effects of widowhood (grief and accompanying environmental changes) are the most likely causes of this increased mortality. Informative studies having to do with widowhood and morbidity are scarce. One noteworthy report published forty years ago indicated that the physical reactions to grief experienced by older people included stomach distress, shortness of breath, lack of strength, and "subjective distress" (Lindemann 1944). Several more recent studies also show increases in physician visits during the first year of bereavement, especially for psychological symptoms (Clayton 1973).

The relationship of environmental change to mortality and morbidity has been investigated in mental hospitals, nursing homes, and homes for the aged. Moving the older person from a familiar setting into an institution, or even into surroundings similar to his or her own home, has been reported to cause psychological disorganization. Verwoerdt (1976) offers the case of the 74-year-old recluse who lived in an old shack in filth and constant danger of being burned. After great effort, the old man was persuaded to move to a more modern facility. Shortly after the move, the social worker was called to the facility. She found him in a disoriented state with evidence of incontinence all about. These had not been problems prior to the move. Although some researchers might emphasize the stress of relocation involved in the above anecdote, others might focus on environmental discontinuity or the degree of change between a new and old environment. Lawton (1974) believes the newly institutionalized elderly are in double jeopardy in this regard. He argues that individuals with health-related incapacities are less capable than the healthy to adapt to new environmental situations.

Clearly, when individuals exaggerate the effects of normal aging and attribute all negative changes to inevitable aging processes, actions that might be beneficial are not undertaken. This is the case whether the misattribution ignores real disease processes or environmental factors. Sometimes misattribution can have tragic consequences. Unfortunately, reeducating aged individuals about the effects of normal aging may not be effective in correcting incorrect attributions. Data from studies by Ross, Lepper, and Hubbard (1975) show that incorrect attributions tend to persevere. Although this research was not carried out in a health context, it suggests the importance of early education about the effects of normal aging. This may be the only effective device for reducing illness misattribution to aging among the elderly.

TRENDS IN HEALTH
Morbidity and Disability

Generally, there has been a reduction in the incidence of infectious diseases in the United States and an increase in the importance of chronic conditions. Today, chronic conditions represent the key health problems affecting middle-aged and older adults. In fact, when compared with younger age groups, middle-aged and older adults show lower rates of acute conditions, including infective and parasitic conditions, respiratory conditions, conditions of the digestive system, and injuries (U.S. Bureau of the Census, 1985, Table 186).

Chronic conditions are long lasting, and their progress generally causes irreversible pathology. Data recently made available by the National Center for Health Statistics show that almost 26 percent (25.9 percent) of all office visits to physicians made by aged individuals were related to conditions of the circulatory system, including heart conditions. Another 9.4 percent of the office visits made by those sixty-five years and over involved a diagnosis of disease of the nervous system or sense organs, including hearing and vision impairments; 9.3 percent of office visits involved diseases of musculoskeletal systems and connective systems, a category that includes arthritis and rheumatism. Thus, three disease categories dominated by chronic conditions accounted for 44.6 percent of all physician office visits of older people in 1975.

Table 6-1 presents data on chronic conditions among four age groups of people, according to type of condition and sex. The age groups include individuals under eighteen, eighteen to forty-four, forty-five to sixty-four, and sixty-five years and over. Generally, the prevalence of chronic conditions among the elderly is higher than among younger persons. The reported prevalence rates among the elderly for heart conditions, hypertension, varicose veins, arthritis, diabetes, diseases of the urinary system, visual and hearing impairments, and deformities or orthopedic impairments show the most substantial differences when compared with the prevalence rates of chronic conditions among those in the younger age groups. For hemorrhoids, respiratory conditions (bronchitis, asthma, sinusitis, and hay fever), skin conditions (dermatitis and diseases of the sebaceous glands), and migraines, the elderly show comparable or even lower prevalence rates than is the case for those in younger age groups.

Women appear to be more likely to be troubled by hypertension, varicose veins, hemorrhoids, chronic sinusitis, dermatitis, arthritis, diabetes, migraines, and diseases of the urinary system. Men are more troubled by visual and hearing impairments. Heart conditions show almost no sex differentiation in prevalence rates. This is the case as well for respiratory conditions (excluding chronic sinusitis) and deformities or orthopedic impairments. The sex-differentiated patterns of prevalence of chronic conditions described above generally hold among the elderly. Women live longer than men, on the average, so they are more likely to suffer from a variety of chronic (and disabling) diseases. It should also be pointed out, though, that sex-role typing may make older women more ready to report chronic illness during the household interviews used to collect data reported in Table 6-1.

The relationship between family income and the prevalence of chronic conditions is worthy of some discussion. For some specific conditions, arthritis, for example, there does appear to be a linear relationship between income and prevalence; the higher the family income, the lower the prevalence rate of arthritis (Kart 1985). For other conditions, the pattern is not so clear-cut. Still, for most chronic conditions, those elderly with low family income (less than $5,000) show a prevalence rate that is higher than that for the total sixty-five years and over population, whereas those elderly with higher family income ($15,000 or more) show a prevalence rate below that for the total elderly population (Kart 1985). Most older people with low incomes had lower incomes before old age. Thus, their access to medical care and their capacity to generate a favorable living environment have likely been reduced for a long period of time. This may result in higher rates of disease, as well as in earlier death. Also, some people suffer reduced incomes because of illness and disability.

The actual presence of a chronic condition is often not as important to people as the impact the condition has on their ability to carry out usual

TABLE 6-1   Persons With Selected Chronic Conditions, by Sex and Age: 1982

Chronic Condition	Persons with Condition (1,000)	Rate per 1,000 Persons						
		Total	Male	Female	Under 18 Years	18–44 Years	45–64 Years	65 Years and over
Heart conditions	16,926	74.5	73.6	75.4	17.2	34.7	136.8	256.8
High blood pressure (hypertension)	26,542	116.9	101.3	131.4	2.9*	58.9	245.7	390.4
Varicose veins of lower extremities	6,880	30.3	11.5	47.8	—*†	21.9	64.1	77.7
Hemorrhoids	10,449	46.0	40.0	51.6	.8*	54.0	75.5	76.5
Chronic bronchitis	7,709	33.9	31.4	36.3	33.7	24.5	44.2	52.0
Asthma	7,899	34.8	36.5	33.2	40.1	29.0	36.3	40.8
Chronic sinusitis	27,644	121.7	104.3	138.0	43.0	138.9	179.1	151.7
Hay fever, allergic rhinitis without asthma	19,323	85.1	83.8	86.2	55.1	109.3	87.5	64.6
Dermatitis, including eczema	8,652	38.1	30.5	45.2	40.0	40.3	38.2	24.9
Diseases of sebaceous glands‡	6,079	26.8	26.6	27.0	26.5	38.4	13.5	7.2
Arthritis	30,207	133.0	96.8	166.7	2.7*	55.3	276.2	495.8
Diabetes	5,767	25.4	22.0	28.6	1.4*	9.2	57.6	88.9
Migraine	7,640	33.6	18.0	48.2	7.8	47.0	49.9	19.2
Diseases of urinary system	5,917	26.1	11.4	39.7	6.6	24.3	40.0	56.6
Visual impairments	8,699	38.3	48.2	29.1	13.1	31.2	53.4	101.1
Hearing impairments	19,776	87.1	103.7	71.5	19.7	48.8	142.7	299.7
Deformities or orthopedic impairments	22,522	99.2	98.9	99.5	31.8	106.5	139.0	168.5

Source: U.S. Bureau of the Census (1985, Table 187).

* Figure does not meet standards of reliability or precision.

† —represents zero.

‡ Acne and sebaceous skin cyst.

activities. Chronic illness can be burdensome, as Figure 6-1 shows in terms of bed days, hospital days, and doctor visits for selected conditions. Arthritis and rheumatism are particularly interesting examples. Though accounting for relatively few hospital days, these conditions are responsible for 16 percent of days spent in bed by older people, nearly as much as for heart disease, and 6 percent of doctor visits, more than for cancer. Just as the prevalence rates for chronic conditions increase with age, so does limitation of activity. Figure 6-2 presents data on the extent and seriousness of limited activity caused by chronic conditions among those twenty-five years and older in the United States for 1981.

Twenty-four percent of those aged forty-five to sixty-four and 47 percent of those aged sixty-five years and over had some limitation of activity. Almost one in five (18 percent) elderly reported being unable to carry on a major activity such as working or keeping house: 7 percent of those aged forty-five to sixty-four reported similarly. Although females show higher prevalence rates for many chronic conditions, they report lower rates of activity limitation than

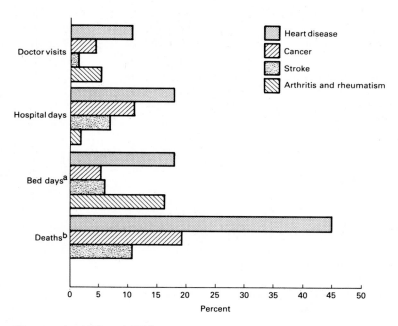

ᵃAverage for 1979 and 1980.
ᵇProvisional data.

FIGURE 6-1   Burden of illness for persons 65 years of age and over, according to selected conditions, United States, 1980. *Source: National Center for Health Statistics: Division of Health Care Statistics, Division of Health Interview Statistics, and Division of Vital Statistics.*

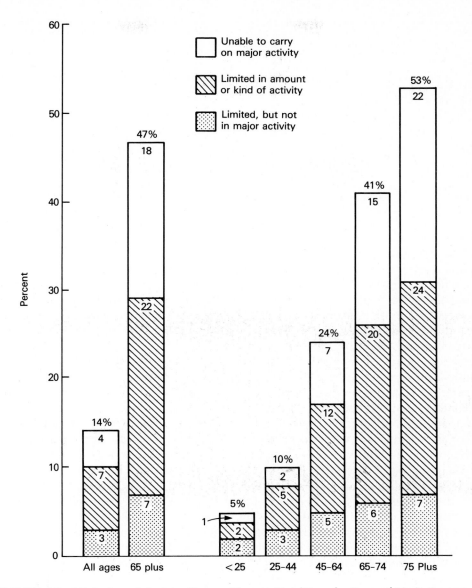

FIGURE 6-2   Limitation of Activity Due to Chronic Conditions by Type of Limitations and Age, 1981. *Source: National Center for Health Statistics, 1981 Health Interview Survey, unpublished.*

TABLE 6-2   Proportion of Population Aged 65 and Over, Bedfast, Housebound, and Ambulatory with Difficulty, in Seven Countries

Country	Percentage Bedfast	Percentage Housebound	Percentage Ambulatory with Difficulty
Denmark	2	8	14
Britain	3	11	8
United States	2	6	6
Israel	2	13	n.a.
Poland	4	6	16
Yugoslavia	3	4	20
Japan	4	16	n.a.

Source: Palmore (1975); Shanas, Townsend, Wedderburn, Friis, Milhøj, and Stehouver (1968).

males do (Kart 1985: Table 8-1). This may be because traditionally women have played social roles that are less physically demanding, so that chronic conditions did not prevent them from meeting obligations. Another explanation may be that the roles played by women (wife, mother, grandmother, socioemotional leader of the family) are so important they *must* be carried out. Under such conditions, women (even older women) can ill afford to be reporting limitations in activity, even in the presence of chronic illness.

Some data are available for making cross-national comparisons on activity limitations among the aged of comparably developed countries. Table 6-2 presents data on the proportion of aged who are bedfast, homebound, and ambulatory with difficulty in Denmark, Britain, Israel, Poland, Yugoslavia, Japan, and the United States. Combining the bedfast and household categories, only Yugoslavia has a lower proportion of its aged citizens so limited in activity than does the United States. Two important factors must be considered when observing these data. First, cultural considerations may be at play in the reporting of these data. Shanas et al. (1968), for example, suggest that "old people in the United States, more than old people in Europe, seem to feel that to admit incapacity is somehow psychologically wrong." Palmore (1975) points out that the high proportion of Japanese aged who are homebound (16 percent) may simply reflect their greater willingness to report being housebound. Finally, these data compare *only* the most disabled portion of the aged population of the selected countries, not the health of the great majority of aged persons in these seven lands.

Chronic Illness

A *chronic illness* is an illness or disease of a long-lasting nature. Three chronic illnesses that cause a great deal of morbidity, activity limitation, and mortality among the elderly (and other age groups as well) are heart disease, cancer,

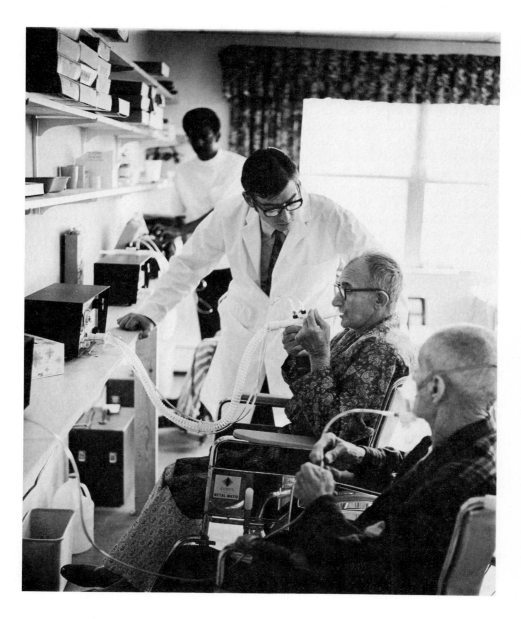

and cerebrovascular disease. These conditions are briefly discussed in this section.

Heart Disease. Heart disease has already been identified as the principal cause of death among the elderly. In addition, heart disease accounts for a great deal of morbidity, disablement, and inactivity in older people. The dominant cause or form of heart disease is ischemia, closely followed by hypertension; in third place are mixed cases where both these diseases are present (Brocklehurst and Hanley 1981). Ischemic heart disease is a category that represents conditions in which there is a deficiency of blood to the heart because of the narrowing or constricting of the cardiac vessels that supply it.

A common form of ischemic heart disease is myocardial infarction, or heart attack. In time, if a deficient blood supply to the heart persists, heart tissue will die. The dead area is known as an infarct. The extent of heart tissue involved determines the severity of the episode. Most often, only a small portion of heart muscle is affected, and cardiac reserves allow the work of the heart to be continued. In some older persons there may not be sufficient heart reserve to withstand the attack.

Brocklehurst and Hanley (1981) point out that in virtually all aspects heart disease is no different in old age than it is in youth. The symptoms and presentation of myocardial infarction may be an exception. They indicate, for example, that although complete absence of chest pain is very rare in acute myocardial infarction up to middle age, it is a "mundane occurrence" in old people. In fact, only about one-third of elderly patients present with a classical prolonged episode of chest pain. Other atypical presentations (representing about another one-third of the cases) include (1) development of acute brain failure; (2) severe breathing difficulty; (3) severe fall in blood pressure; (4) formation of an arterial embolism or clot in the area of the infarction; and (5) vomiting and weakness.

Some myocardial infarcts in the aged are completely "silent" and may be discovered only with an electrocardiograph (Brocklehurst and Hanley 1981). This may be more likely to occur in the very old, who show a greater prevalence of chronic brain disorder.

Exton-Smith and Overstall (1979) believe that the elderly patient with an infarct "probably does as well at home as in (the) hospital." This, no doubt, presumes the availability of home services and community support. They point out that an optimistic attitude and early mobilization are important in maintaining the patient's morale. And, in most cases, regaining independence is a reasonable goal.

A significant number of elderly individuals have hypertension, or high blood pressure. Defined as diastolic pressure greater than 100 mm Hg, as many as one in four older people have high blood pressure (Steinberg 1976). Studies of large groups of individuals show that both systolic and diastolic blood pressure continue to rise throughout adult life to old age. Brocklehurst and Hanley (1981) argue that a systolic pressure exceeding 200 mm Hg and a diastolic of 110 mm Hg or more may be compatible with normal health.

Still, each patient warrants individual consideration. Kotchen and Ernst (1976) offer the clinician's perspective in defining hypertension as "that level of arterial pressure at which therapeutic intervention has an impact on cardio-vascular morbidity and mortality.''

The most important causes of hypertension in older persons are arterio-sclerotic and atherosclerotic changes. Such changes decrease the diameter, dis-tensibility, and capacity of the arteries. Hence, the heart has to work that much harder to maintain blood flow through these vessels to supply the body with nourishment. In general, what can result is reduced blood flow to vital organs, with impaired circulation to the brain, heart, and kidneys being especially important. Death can result as a consequence of hypertension and the heart failure, stroke, and kidney failure it can cause.

Kidney damage may be either a consequence of or a cause of high blood pressure. It is more often the case, though, that the kidney is a victim of high blood pressure. Inelastic and occluded renal arteries lead to ischemic renal tissue. When there is inadequate blood flow to the kidneys, they can no longer remove sufficient fluid from the blood for urine output. Hence, the volume of fluid in the blood further increases the work load of the heart and increases blood pressure. Vascular changes and hypertension can significantly reduce kidney function and can lead to kidney failure. Injury to the brain may be manifested in dull headaches, impaired memory, and disoriented and confused behavior. In serious cases, cerebrovascular accident or stroke can result.

Blood pressure can be controlled with the use of drug therapy, though Brocklehurst and Hanley (1981) indicate that current medical opinion is gen-erally antagonistic to antihypertensive therapy in the old. This is largely because of the possible side effects of the treatment, not the least of these being cerebral thrombosis and heart failure. Much evidence shows how treatment of hyper-tension reduces morbidity and mortality from myocardial infarction and stroke among middle-aged individuals. These authors simply suggest that it is not safe to extrapolate such findings to the aged, in particular those aged seventy-five years and older.

Elderly patients require a cautious approach when treatment of hyperten-sion is initiated. Exton-Smith and Overstall (1979) recommend aiming for a gentle reduction in blood pressure over several weeks. They indicate a lack of firm rules and suggest physicians be guided by the individual response to treatment.

Cancer. Cancer is the second leading cause of death in the United States. Over 440,000 Americans died of cancer in 1983. The incidence of cancer increases with age such that the death rate in 1983 among those aged seventy-five to eighty-four years of age is almost one hundred times that among those aged twenty-five to thirty-four and about seven times that among those aged forty-five to fifty-four years of age. In part, these facts reflect two important un-derstandings that have been developed about the etiology of cancer (Wright et al. 1976): (1) Most forms of cancer have a long latent period, and initiating

factors start during youth; and (2) increasing age and the accompanying physiological changes make the patient more susceptible to the actions of
carcinogens.

The death rate from cancer for older women is about 56 percent that for
aged men in 1983. Table 6-3 shows the differences in death rates from cancer
for persons sixty-five years and older by sex and the site of cancer in this year.
Primary sites of cancer for men involve the lungs (respiratory), digestive organs,
and genital and urinary organs; primary sites among women include the digestive and respiratory systems, breast, and genital (cervical) area.

The onset and management of many cancers do not vary greatly in the
old and young (Brocklehurst and Hanley 1981). Prevention is still the order of
the day regarding cancer. Where possible, known causes of cancer should be
avoided and removed from the environment. As Wright and her colleagues
(1976) point out, this includes (1) avoiding unnecessary exposure to ionizing
and ultraviolet radiation, (2) implementing hygienic measures in occupations
involving exposure to cancer-producing chemicals and dusts, and (3) avoiding
exposure to tobacco and cigarette smoke.

Older people should be encouraged to have periodic preventive medical
examinations. Physicians should take corrective and preventive measures with
regard to any predisposing factors or premalignant conditions. Older persons
and health-care personnel must not misattribute such factors or conditions to
old age. Even in the oldest patients, cancer can be cured if it is detected early
and diagnosed at a localized stage.

Stroke. Just as heart tissue can be denied adequate blood supply, changes in
blood vessels that serve brain tissue, cerebral infarction, or cerebral hemorrhage
can reduce nourishment carried to the brain and result in a malfunction or

**TABLE 6-3 Death Rates From Cancer, by Sex and Selected
Type, for Persons 65 Years and over: 1983**

	Males	Females
Total U.S. rate	209.6	170.1
Total 65+	1383.6	791.0
Respiratory, intrathoracic	459.2	122.9
Digestive organs, peritoneum	360.0	249.8
Breast	1.6	121.0
Genital organs	202.1	83.6
Lymphatic and hematopoietic tissues		
(excl. leukemia)	64.4	47.6
Urinary organs	77.5	30.1
Lip, oral cavity, pharynx	26.7	9.7
Leukemia	50.0	29.3

Source: U.S. Bureau of the Census (1986, Table 118).

death of brain cells. Such impaired brain tissue circulation is referred to as *cerebrovascular disease.*

When a portion of the brain is completely denied blood, a cerebrovascular accident (CVA), or stroke, results. The severity of the accident is determined by the particular area affected as well as by the total amount of brain tissue involved. A stroke may affect such a small area of the brain that it goes unnoticed or such a large area that it causes death. Cerebrovascular disease is the third leading cause of death in the United States today.

Cerebral thrombosis is a main cause of stroke in the elderly and occurs when a formed clot becomes lodged in an already narrowed artery. There may be no transient symptoms before the stroke occurs, or there may be what Brocklehurst and Hanley (1981) describe as a *stroke-in-evolution.* In the latter case, the stroke may develop over hours or even days. Symptoms may appear within minutes or hours after the onset of a stroke. A cerebral embolism may also be responsible for a CVA. In this instance, the thrombus does not form locally but is derived from elsewhere in the body and travels to obstruct a vessel supplying the brain. In such cases, the stroke and its damage appear almost instantly.

When a stroke does occur, varying degrees of damage may result. Exton-Smith and Overstall (1979) list disorders of motor function, disturbances of sensation, visual disturbances, aphasia (speech disorders), apraxia, and mental symptoms, among others, as possible clinical features of a CVA. Rehabilitation efforts should begin immediately, and family members and health workers must be sensitive to the needs of the stroke patient; they should try to put themselves in the patient's position. Sometimes this is difficult. Rehabilitation of the stroke patient is a neglected area in most medical schools, and all too often the patient may be regarded as an embarrassment for whom the doctor can do nothing (Exton-Smith and Overstall 1979). Still, the effort must be made.

Sometimes a CVA may occur while a person is sleeping. Imagine how traumatic it would be to awaken and find yourself unable to move a part of your body and possibly unable to speak or to understand what is said to you. *Aphasia* is a term used to denote impaired ability to comprehend or express verbal language and is a clinical feature of stroke in many elderly victims. The condition is emotionally disturbing to the victim, especially to those persons who were very verbal before a stroke, as well as to family members and friends. In *receptive aphasia* a person has difficulty processing external stimuli. Because of damage within the speech center of the brain, the individual may not understand others' speech or what is read; also, familiar objects may become unrecognizable. When a person understands what is said but cannot form the words or gestures to respond to stimuli, *expressive aphasia* has resulted. Frequently, an aphasiac suffers from a mixed condition.

Tragically, aphasia may be incorrectly associated with mental deterioration. In such cases, people may assume that comprehension is impaired when it is not, and the patient may be infantilized—treated as a child—while being fully aware of the situation. Patients should be encouraged to speak, and those around them should listen patiently. They should not be rushed or cut off in the middle of their attempts. Such behavior on the part of a listener can cause the patient to feel awkward and self-conscious. And, it may foster depression and withdrawal.

The extent of the damage and the degree of deficit that has taken place determine to what extent functional language skills can be regained. Unless the aphasia lasts but a few days, it may be difficult for geriatric patients to ever regain their former level of articulation. This is not to say that they cannot reestablish functional language patterns but that they and their families should not set goals too high. Every attempt should be made at language rehabilitation, and every gain should be recognized. The success of small forward steps should not be discounted because of failure to meet great expectations. A paternalistic or overly helpful attitude toward the stroke victim, although well intended, may slow recovery and make the patient feel helpless or even useless. Any gain in independent living can only enhance a person's sense of self-worth and dignity.

MENTAL HEALTH

Estimates vary as to the proportion of the elderly population with mental health problems. According to Pfeiffer (1977), approximately 15 percent of the elderly population in the United States suffer from significant, substantial, or moderate psychopathological conditions. Gurland and Toner (1982) argue that 15 percent may represent only that proportion of the elderly with clinically significant depression. Roybal (1984) states that as many as 25 percent of the elderly have significant mental health problems. Presumably this percentage includes both long-term care facility and community residents.

Blazer (1980) reports that the rate of severe impairment of subjects in various studies ranges from 4 to 18 percent of community-dwelling elders and 32 to 47 percent of those elderly persons residing in long-term care institutions. Among the specified diagnoses, organic brain syndromes, depressive disorders, schizophrenia, and alcohol disorders account for high rates of patient care episodes in outpatient psychiatric services for old people in the United States. The same list applies to inpatient facilities. Over 600,000 nursing home residents in the United States in 1973 to 1974 were diagnosed as senile. More recently, 15 to 70 percent of those found in various sorts of long-term care institutions showed symptoms of dementia (Blazer 1980).

Figures on the mental health status of the elderly must be viewed with some caution. The epidemiology of psychopathological conditions is beset by conceptual and methodological difficulties. Even under careful conditions of assessment, diagnosing schizophrenia or depression is often difficult. Different doctors, using different definitions and criteria and varying widely in their competence as well as in their understanding of aging processes, should make us suspicious of the adequacy of their diagnoses. For example, there has been a tendency to overestimate the incidence of dementia among the old, while underestimating that of depression. The symptoms of these disorders are similar, and correct diagnosis can also be confounded by attitudes toward the elderly (Butler and Lewis 1982; Eisdorfer and Cohen 1982). In addition, as Libow (1973) reminds us, much of the early mental change shown by elderly persons can be explained by changes in the environment. A National Institute of Mental Health study of healthy male volunteers, whose average age was seventy at the start of the study and who were followed for eleven years, found a strong relationship between survival and the organization of a subject's daily behavior (Bartko and Patterson 1971). The greater the complexity and variability of a day's behavior, the greater the likelihood of survival.

Sampling error also contributes to the generation of inaccurate estimates of the incidence of mental health problems among the aged. If samples are drawn from lists of present users of mental health services, then older people will be underrepresented. According to Kermis (1986), the belief is that, since older people do not use mental health services, it must be because they do not need them. If samples are drawn from a community at large, older people with mental health problems are also underrepresented because many of them reside in group or institutional settings (Kermis 1986).

Despite the conceptual and methodological difficulties involved in determining the degree and extent to which psychopathological conditions are distributed among the elderly, it is quite clear that some older people do have mental health problems. And, these problems are often categorized according to the degree of actual impairment in brain functioning.

Depression appears to be the most common of the functional psychiatric disorders in the later years, yet it is not often recognized in older people (Kermis 1986). Depression can vary in duration and degree; it may be triggered by loss of a loved one or by the onset of a physical disease. A depressed individual may show any combination of psychological and physiological manifestations. Core symptoms include abject and painful sadness, generalized withdrawal of interest and inhibition of activity, pervasive pessimism, decreased self-esteem, and poor self-prognosis (American Psychological Association 1980). Kermis (1986) lists some atypical clinical features that further confuse diagnosis including pseudodementia (apathy and slowness of cognition resembling dementia) and somatic complaints without obvious mood changes.

Depression in older persons is a treatable syndrome. If untreated it may become chronic and lead to social dysfunction, drug use, and physical morbidity (Gurland and Toner 1982). Drug therapies are popular. Other treatment modalities are available, although as Butler and Lewis (1982) indicate, many professionals view the elderly as "poor candidates" for the psychotherapies.

Suicidal thoughts often accompany depression. Gardner, Bahn, and Mack (1964) found in their research that the majority of older persons who committed suicide had been depressed. According to the U.S. Center for Health Statistics, the suicide rate among the elderly in 1983 was 58 percent higher than that among the total population. This statistic may present a conservative picture. Many doctors do not report suicides because they think it stigmatizes the surviving family members; family members themselves often hide or destroy suicide notes—usually unnecessarily—to try to ensure payments by life insurance companies.

Table 6-4 presents suicide rates by sex, race, and age group for 1983. Aged white males show the highest suicide rate of any group. Their rate is almost three times that of aged black males, more than five times that of aged white females, and about twenty-nine times that of aged black females. Aged females in the United States have among the lowest suicide rates in the world. Aged American males fall in the middle of the range represented by selected countries. Male elderly have higher suicide rates in Austria, Denmark, France, West Germany, and Japan; countries in which the elderly have lower suicide rates than is the case in the United States include England and Wales, Australia, Canada, Italy, and Poland, among others (U.S. Bureau of the Census 1986, Table 1443).

Two additional common functional psychiatric disorders in the later years are paranoia and hypochondriasis. *Paranoia* is a delusional state that is usually persecutory in nature. It often involves attributing motivations to other people that they simply do not have. Paranoia is more common in individuals suffering from sensory deficits such as hearing loss (Post 1980). Some paranoia may be "caused" by changes in life situation, such as relocation or other stresses. Kermis (1986) describes a seventy-two-year-old woman hospitalized while recovering from major heart surgery. She had a persistent delusion that CIA agents were spying on her. She recorded these occurrences and reported them to the staff, who discovered that her CIA visits corresponded to security guards' checks of the floor.

TABLE 6-4   Suicide Rates, by Sex, Race, and Age Group: 1983

	Male		Female	
	White	**Black**	**White**	**Black**
All ages (years)	20.6	9.9	5.9	2.0
5–14	.9	.5	.3	.6
15–24	20.6	11.5	4.6	2.7
25–34	26.2	19.1	7.2	2.9
35–44	23.2	14.0	8.2	3.5
45–54	25.5	12.1	9.9	3.0
55–64	27.4	11.6	9.1	1.7
65 and over	40.2	14.2	7.2	1.4

Source: U.S. Bureau of the Census (1986, Table 121).

Characteristically, the initial premise of the paranoid is irrational, although the rest of the delusional system often follows logically. Kermis (1986) notes, if the paranoid's basic premise is accepted, the rest of the delusion often makes sense. Most paranoids have a fairly focused problem and are not impaired in their daily functioning. If the disorder remains chronic, however, social and psychological function may be negatively affected (American Psychiatric Association 1980).

Hypochondriasis is an overconcern for one's health, usually accompanied by delusions about physical dysfunction, disease, or both. The conventional wisdom is that hypochondriacs displace their psychological distress onto the body. A number of observers have emphasized the utility of the condition—after all, it is far more acceptable in this society to be physically ill than it is to be emotionally or mentally disabled (Pfeiffer and Busse 1973). Hypochondriacs will diligently seek medical help, yet treatment of the disorder is difficult because they are not predisposed to psychological explanations of their condition.

The 1980 edition of the American Psychiatric Association's *Diagnostic and Statistical Manual of Mental Disorders* (DSM III) makes the distinction between *organic brain syndromes* (OBS) and *organic mental disorders* (OMD). "Organic brain syndrome" is used to refer to a group of psychological or behavioral signs and symptoms without reference to etiology; "organic mental disorder" designates a particular OBS in which the etiology is known or presumed (APA 1980). OBS can be grouped into six categories, the most common of which are delirium, dementia, and intoxication and withdrawal. Perhaps as many as one-half of the aged population with mental disorders have OBS (Kramer, Taube, and Redick 1973; Redick, Kramer, and Taube 1973); the prevalence rate of OBS appears to increase with age (Kramer, Taube, and Redick 1973), although onset usually occurs in the seventh to ninth decades and is more common in women than in men (Fann, Wheless, and Richman 1976).

Primary degenerative dementia of the Alzheimer type may be the single most common OBS. According to the DSM III, between 2 and 4 percent of the entire population over the age of sixty-five may have this dementia. Alzheimer's disease has an "insidious onset and gradually progressive course" (American Psychiatric Association 1980). It brings a multifaceted loss of intellectual abilities, including memory, judgment, and abstract thought, as well as changes in personality and behavior. The clinical picture may also be clouded by the presence of depression, delusions, or, more rarely, delirium.

Initially, the Alzheimer's victim experiences minor symptoms that may be attributed to stress or physical illness. With time, however, the person becomes more forgetful. Things get misplaced, routine chores take longer, and already answered questions are repeated. As the disease progresses, memory loss as well as confusion, irritability, restlessness, and agitation are likely to appear. Judgment, concentration, orientation, writing, reading, speech, motor behavior, and naming of objects may also be affected. Even when a loving and supportive family is available, the Alzheimer's victim may ultimately require institutional care (U.S. Department of Health and Human Services 1984).

At the present time, there is no cure for Alzheimer's disease. What are the possible causes of this debilitating disease? Since the 1970s, research scientists have been studying the evidence of a significant and progressive decrease in the activity of the enzyme choline acetyltransferase (ChAT) in the brain tissue of Alzheimer's patients. ChAT is an important ingredient in neurotransmissions involved with learning and memory. There appears to be a link between changes in this neurochemical activity and changes in cognition and the physical appearance of the brains of Alzheimer's patients (U.S. Department of Health and Human Services 1984). Additional research is needed to determine whether accumulations of trace metals in the brain (such as aluminum) are a primary cause of Alzheimer's disease or if other factors like slow-acting transmissible viruses might combine with environmental factors to trigger the onset of the disease (U.S. Department of Health and Human Services 1984).

Some scientists see an inherited predisposition or genetic marker to Alzheimer's disease. Zubenko and his colleagues at the University of Pittsburgh have discovered an abnormality in the blood that may predict the later onset of Alzheimer's. This abnormality was found in blood platelets, particles vital to the process of blood clotting. The blood platelets of Alzheimer's patients show less rigidity in their structural membranes, though this abnormality does not impair blood platelet functioning. Such an alternation would not likely have any direct causal effect bearing on Alzheimer's, but scientists speculate that the gene that does cause this change may have different, as yet unidentified, effects on brain cells (Schmeck 1987). The platelet abnormality was not found in people with depression or mania, conditions sometimes confused with Alzheimer's disease. Interestingly, when the platelet was found in an Alzheimer's patient, it was 3.5 to 11 times more likely to appear in close relatives of the patient than in the general population at large. Family studies have already found that first-degree relatives of Alzheimer's patients are at a significantly higher lifetime risk of developing dementia, especially if the affected family member is a parent and the age of onset occurs before age seventy (Schmeck 1987).

Do social or psychological experiences contribute to the cause or development of Alzheimer's disease? Too little research has been aimed at this question. For the most part, social and behavioral scientists have focused on the development of diagnostic tests, the changes in language use that results from brain dysfunction, and the need for special support for the families of disease victims (U.S. Department of Health and Human Services 1984).

The descriptions of the organic brain syndromes presented in DSM III are clear and straightforward and give the impression that their recognition and diagnosis are equally so. The core manifestations of the disorders are described above. Although these symptoms may indeed be classic for advancing OBS, not every patient with this set of symptoms has OBS (Wells 1978).

There is some reliable evidence to demonstrate that OBS is overdiagnosed

(Clark 1980; Fox, Topel, and Huckman, 1975; Glassman 1980; Kaercher 1980; Marsden and Harrison 1972; Seltzer and Sherwin 1978; Wells 1978). For example, Duckworth and Ross (1975) compared psychiatric diagnoses given to patients over the age of sixty-five in Toronto, New York, and London. They found that organic brain disorders were diagnosed with more than 50 percent greater frequency in New York than in either Toronto or London. Though variation in patient populations may account for some of this difference, Wells (1978) suggests that in Toronto and London a greater emphasis is placed on recognizing functional disorders in the aged and, thus, elderly patients are more likely to be labeled correctly.

Libow (1973) has used the term "pseudosenility" to refer to conditions that may manifest themselves as senility and thus cause misdiagnosis or mislabeling of OBS. Causes of pseudosenility include drug interactions, malnutrition, and fever. When these conditions are treated, the senility often goes away. While admittedly there are no definitive studies identifying the frequency of pseudosenility, a task force sponsored by the National Institute on Aging suggests that 10 to 20 percent of all older people diagnosed with mental impairments have these reversible conditions (National Institute on Aging 1980).

The importance of organic brain syndromes, in both numerical and personal terms, is being recognized increasingly. This recognition is reflected in gerontological and popular literature that points out that many curable physical and psychological disorders in the elderly produce intellectual impairments that may be difficult to distinguish from OBS. More importantly, this growing body of literature states clearly, if not emphatically, that normal aging does not include the symptoms of OBS; these are diseases, not the inevitable accompaniments of aging.

SELF-ASSESSMENT OF HEALTH

The high prevalence of chronic conditions including psychopathological conditions and the relatively high levels of limitation of activity may give the impression that elderly people view themselves as being in poor health and unable to function. This is not the case. According to the National Health Interview Survey, Supplement on Aging, carried out in 1984, the majority (67.5 percent) of people sixty-five years of age and older assess themselves as being in excellent, very good, or good health when compared with other people their own age. Self-assessment does not differ substantively between older men and women. Older whites offer more positive assessments of their health than do older blacks; almost 69 percent of older whites assess their health as excellent, very good, or good while about 50 percent of older blacks do similarly. Table 6.5 presents data on the self-assessment of health by the elderly according to family income range for 1984. The proportion of the elderly with self-reported fair or poor health diminishes as family income increases. Only about 22 percent

TABLE 6-5   Self-Assessment of Health by Family Income Range, Persons 65 Years and Older, 1984

Health Status	Family Income			
	Less Than $10,000	$10–14,999	$15–24,999	$25,000+
Excellent or very good	29.9%	33.7%	39.1%	48.4%
Good	28.4	35.9	33.7	30.0
Fair	25.6	20.8	19.7	14.5
Poor	16.1	9.6	7.5	7.1
Total	3755	1923	2199	1691
	(100.0%)	(100.0%)	(100.0%)	(100.0%)

Source: National Center for Health Statistics. 1984 National Health Interview Survey, Supplement on Aging, unpublished data.

of aged individuals with incomes of $25,000 or more assessed their health as fair or poor; 42 percent was the comparable figure among those with incomes of less than $10,000.

Self-assessment of health may be as important as actual medical status in predicting general emotional state and behavior (Maddox and Douglas 1973). As well, self-assessed health status correlates with other measures of health status and health behavior (Ferraro 1980). For example, data from the 1984 National Health Interview Survey, Supplement on Aging, show that among the aged the more positive the self-report of health status, the greater the perceived control over health, and the more positive is a person's assessment of the job he or she is doing in taking care of his or her own health.

SUMMARY

Disease is the chief barrier to extended health and longevity in older people. Yet the orientation of modern medicine and the attitudes and expectations of many old people contribute to the difficulty of maintaining health in later life. The elderly along with health-care professionals may be too ready to attribute illness or biological changes to "normal aging."

Today chronic illnesses, including heart disease, cancer, and stroke, represent the key health problems affecting middle-aged and older adults. The prevalence of chronic conditions varies by age, sex, race, and income. Chronic illness can be burdensome in terms of days spent in bed, hospital stays, and doctor visits. Although about 47 percent of all aged persons report some limitation in activity resulting from a chronic illness, only about one in five indicate being unable to work or keep house.

Estimates vary as to the proportion of the elderly population with mental health problems. Perhaps as many as 25 percent of the elderly have some mental health problems. Depression, paranoia, and hypochondriasis are common functional psychiatric disorders in the later years. Suicidal thoughts often accompany depression. In 1983 the suicide rate among the elderly was 58 percent higher than that among the total population, though much of this difference is attributable to the very high suicide rate among aged white males.

Alzheimer's disease is the most common organic brain syndrome. At the present time there is no cure for Alzheimer's disease; little is known about the extent to which social and psychological experiences may contribute to the onset of the disease.

The majority of older people assess themselves as being in excellent or good health compared with other people their own age.

STUDY QUESTIONS

1. Explain the medical model as it is applied to the elderly. What are its primary limitations?

2. How does the attribution (or misattribution) of illness to the normal aging process pose serious health and social problems for older individuals?

3. How does the prevalence of chronic conditions among the elderly vary by sex and income? To what extent do chronic conditions interfere with the activity levels of aging men and women?

4. Discuss the dominant causes or forms of heart disease and their impacts on the elderly.

5. What understandings have developed about the etiology of cancer? Describe the death rate differences from cancer between older men and women. Which are primary sites of cancer for men? For women?

6. What social and psychological problems does aphasia create for the stroke victim?

7. Identify and describe the common functional psychiatric disorders in the later years. How do suicide rates vary by sex and race among the elderly?

8. Distinguish between *organic brain syndrome* and *organic mental disorder*. What are the diagnostic problems in determining the prevalence rate of these and other mental disorders afflicting the elderly?

9. What is Alzheimer's disease? Describe its symptoms. What do we know about the causes and cures for this disease?

10. What is the relationship between the high prevalence of chronic conditions among the elderly and the way this population assesses its health? How does self-assessment of health by the elderly vary by sex, race, and income?

BIBLIOGRAPHY

American Psychiatric Association. 1980. *Diagnostic and statistical manual of disorders* (3d ed.). Washington, D.C.: American Psychiatric Association.

Andersen, R., Anderson, O., and Smedby, B. 1968. Perceptions of and response to symptoms of illness in Sweden and the U.S. *Medical Care* 6:18–30.

Bartko, J., and Patterson, R. 1971. Survival among healthy old men: A multivariate analysis. In S. Granick and R. Patterson (eds.), *Human aging II. An 11-year follow-up.* Washington, D.C.: U.S. Government Printing Office.

Blazer, D. 1980. The epidemiology of mental illness in late life. In E. Busse and D. Blazer (eds.), *Handbook of geriatric psychiatry.* New York: Van Nostrand Reinhold Co.

Brocklehurst, J.C., and Hanley, T. 1981. *Geriatric medicine for students.* Edinburgh: Churchill Livingstone.

Butler, R. 1975. *Why survive? Being old in America.* New York: Harper and Row.

Butler, R., and Lewis, M. 1982. *Aging and mental health* (2d ed.). St. Louis: The C.V. Mosby Co.

Clark, M. 1980. The scourge of senility. *Newsweek* September 15:85–86.

Clayton, P. 1973. The clinical morbidity of the first year of bereavement: A review. *Comprehensive Psychiatry* 14:151–157.

Daedulus. 1977. *Doing better and feeling worse: Health in the U.S.*, Vol. 106.

Duckworth, G.S., and Ross, H. 1975. Diagnostic differences in psychogeriatric patients in Toronto, New York and London, England. *Canadian Medical Association Journal* 112:847–851.

Eisdorfer, C., and Cohen, D. 1982. *Mental health care of the aging: A multidisciplinary curriculum for professional training.* New York: Springer.

Ellison, D. 1968. Work, retirement and the sick role. *Gerontologist* 8:189–192.

Exton-Smith, A.N., and Overstall, P.W. 1979. *Geriatrics.* Baltimore: University Park Press.

Fann, W., Wheless, J.C., and Richman, B.W. 1976. Treating the aged with psychotropic drugs. *Gerontologist* 16:322–328.

Ferraro, K.F. 1980. Self-ratings of health among the old and old-old. *Journal of Health and Social Behavior* 21:377–383.

Fox, J.H., Topel, J.L., and Huckman, M.S. 1975. Dementia in the elderly–A search for treatable illnesses. *Journal of Gerontology* 10:557–574.

Freedman, J., Sears, D., and Carlsmith, J. 1978. *Social psychology* (3d ed.). Englewood Cliffs, N.J.: Prentice-Hall.

Freidson, E. 1960. Client control and medical practice. *American Journal of Sociology* 65:374–382.

———. 1961. *Patients' view of medical practice.* New York: Russell Sage Foundation.

Gardner, E., Bahn, A., and Mack, M. 1964. Suicide and psychiatric care in the aging. *Archives of General Psychiatry* 10:547–553.

Glassman, M. 1980. Misdiagnosis of senile dementia: Denial of care to the elderly. *Social Work* 25:288–292.

Gurland, B.J., and Toner, J.A. 1982. Depression in the elderly: A review of recently published studies. In C. Eisdorfer (ed.), *Annual review of geriatrics and gerontology.* New York: Springer.

Janis, I., and Rodin, J. 1979. Attribution, control and decision making: Social psychology and health care. In C.G. Stone, F. Cohen, and N.E. Adler (eds.), *Health psychology— A handbook.* San Francisco: Jossey-Bass.

Jones, E., and Nisbett, R. 1971. *The actor and the observer: Divergent perceptions of the causes of behavior.* Morristown, N.J.: General Learning Press.

Kaercher, D. 1980. Senility: A misdiagnosis. *Better Homes and Gardens* November:27–32, 34–37.

Kahn, R., Zarit, S., Hilbert, N., and Niederehe, G. 1975. Memory complaint and impairment in the aged. *Archives of General Psychiatry* 32:1569–1573.

Kart, C.S. 1985. *The realities of aging* (2nd ed.). Boston: Allyn and Bacon.

Kermis, M.D. 1986. *Mental health in late life: The adaptive process.* Boston: Jones and Bartlett.

Koos, E. 1954. *The health of Regionville.* New York: Columbia University Press.

Kotchen, T., and Ernst, C. 1976. Detecting and treating arteriosclerotic renovascular hypertension. *Geriatrics* 31:83–89.

Kramer, M., Taube, C.A., and Redick, R.W. 1973. Patterns of use of psychiatric facilities by the aged: Past, present and future. In C. Eisdorfer and M. Lawton (eds.), *The psychology of adult development and aging.* Washington, D.C.: American Psychological Association.

Kraus, A., and Lilienfeld, A. 1959. Some epidemiologic aspects of the high mortality rate in the young widowed group. *Journal of Chronic Diseases* 10:207–217.

Lawton, M.P. 1974. Social ecology and the health of older people. *American Journal of Sociology* 64:257–260.

Libow, L. 1973. Pseudo-senility: Acute and reversible organic brain syndrome. *Journal of the American Geriatrics Society* 21:112–120.

Lindemann, E. 1944. Symptomatology and management of acute grief. *American Journal of Psychiatry* 101:141–148.

Luke, B. 1976. Good geriatric nutrition is a lifelong nursing matter. *RN* (July):24–26.

Maddox, G., and Douglas, E. 1973. Self-assessment of health, a longitudinal study of elderly subjects. *Journal of Health and Social Behavior* 14:87–92.

Marsden, C.D., and Harrison, M.J.G. 1972. Outcome of investigation of patients with presenile dementia. *British Medical Journal* 2:249–252.

Mechanic, D. 1978. *Medical sociology* (2nd ed.). New York: The Free Press.

Nathanson, C. 1975. Illness and the feminine role: A theoretical review. *Social Science and Medicine* 9:57–62.

National Institute on Aging. 1980. Treatment possibilities for mental impairment in the elderly. *Journal of the American Medical Association* 244:259–263.

Osborn, R. 1973. Social rank and self-health evaluation of older urban males. *Social Science and Medicine* 7:209–218.

Palmore, E. 1975. *The honorable elders.* Durham, N.C.: Duke University Press.

Parkes, C. 1964. Effects of bereavement on physical and mental health—A study of the medical records of widows. *British Medical Journal* 2:274–279.

Pathy, M. 1967. Clinical presentation of myocardial infarction in the elderly. *British Heart Journal* 29:190.

Pfeiffer, E. 1977. Psychopathy and social pathology. In J. Birren and K. Schaie (eds.), *Handbook of the psychology of aging.* New York: Van Nostrand Reinhold Co.

Pfeiffer, E., and Busse, E. 1973. Mental disorders in later life: Affective disorder, paranoid, neurotic and situational reactions. In E. Busse and E. Pfeiffer (eds.), *Mental illness in later life*. Washington, D.C.: American Psychiatric Association.

Post, F. 1980. Paranoid, schizophrenia-like and schizophrenia states in the aged. In J.E. Birren and R.B. Sloane (eds.), *Handbook of mental health and aging*. Englewood Cliffs, N.J.: Prentice-Hall.

Redick, R., Kramer, M., and Taube, C. 1973. Epidemiology of mental illness and utilization of psychiatric facilities among older persons. In E. Busse and E. Pfeiffer (eds.), *Mental illness in later life*. Washington, D.C.: American Psychiatric Association.

Ross, L., Lepper, M., and Hubbard, M. 1975. Perseverance in self-perception and social perception: Biased attributional processes in the debriefing paradigm. *Journal of Personality and Social Psychology* 32:880–892.

Roybal, E.R. 1984. Federal involvement in mental health care for the aged. *American Psychologist* 39:163–166.

Schmeck, H.M. 1987. Blood abnormality may predict the onset of Alzheimer's disease. *New York Times* October 29:12.

Seltzer, B., and Sherwin, I. 1978. Organic brain syndromes: An empirical study and critical review. *The American Journal of Psychiatry* 135:13–21.

Shanas, E., Townsend, P., Wedderburn, D., Friis, H., Milhoj, P., and Stehouver, J. 1968. *Old people in three industrial societies*. New York: Atherton Press.

Simon, A., and Cahan, R. 1963. The acute brain syndrome in geriatric patients. In W. Mendel and L. Epstein (eds.), *Acute psychotic reaction*. Washington, D.C.: Psychiatric Research Reports.

Steinberg, F.U. (eds.). 1976. *Cowdry's the care of the geriatric patient*. St. Louis: C.V. Mosby.

U.S. Bureau of the Census. 1985. *Statistical abstract of the United States, 1986*. Washington, D.C.: U.S. Government Printing Office.

U.S. Bureau of the Census. 1986. *Statistical abstract of the United States, 1987*. Washington, D.C.: U.S. Government Printing Office.

U.S. Department of Health and Human Services. 1984. *Progress report on Alzheimer's disease, Vol. 2*, National Institutes of Health Publication No. 84-2500. Washington, D.C.: U.S. Government Printing Office.

Verwoerdt, A. 1976. *Clinical geropsychiatry*. Baltimore: The Williams and Wilkins Co.

Wells, C.E. 1978. Chronic brain disease: An overview. *The American Journal of Psychiatry* 135:1–12.

Wright, J.C., Mersheimer, W., Miller, D., and Rotman, D. 1976. Cancer. In F.U. Steinberg (ed.), *Cowdry's the care of the geriatric patient*. St. Louis: The C.V. Mosby Co.

PART III

AGING IN PSYCHOLOGICAL AND SOCIAL PERSPECTIVE

CHAPTER 7

**PSYCHOLOGICAL ASPECTS
OF AGING**

CHAPTER 8

SOCIAL ASPECTS OF AGING

CHAPTER 9

**SOCIOLOGICAL THEORIES
OF AGING**

CHAPTER 7

PSYCHOLOGICAL ASPECTS OF AGING

In perhaps the first book on aging written by a psychologist, G. Stanley Hall (1922) divided life into five stages: (1) childhood; (2) adolescence; (3) middle life—or "the prime," ranging from age twenty-five to age forty or forty-five and comprising the "best" years; (4) senescence—beginning in the early forties "or before in woman"; and (5) senectitude, constituted by "old age proper." Hall was seventy-eight years old when the book was published and, according to his biographer (Ross 1972), resented every moment that moved him further from youth. We might have guessed as much; after all, Hall placed the onset of senescence at age forty-five. Apparently, the noted psychologist associated growing older with declining physical and mental vitality. His concern for the latter, however, was clearly related more to others than to himself.

The physical changes that accompany aging have already been discussed in some detail. This chapter deals with the study of aging with respect to mental vitality—the psychology of aging. The psychology of aging is a broad field, including, among other substantive areas, personality development, intelligence functioning, and sensory and motor processes.

In some contexts it is difficult to distinguish between biological and psychological aspects of aging. Biological changes do affect an individual's psychological state of being, and psychological and psychosocial changes may affect biological functioning. Almost fifty years ago the philosopher–educator John Dewey (1939) addressed the problems of aging and made this very point:

> Biological processes are at the root of the problem and of the methods of solving them, but the biological processes take place in economic, political, and cultural contexts. They are inextricably interwoven with these contexts so that one reacts upon the other in all sorts of intricate ways. We need to know the ways in

which social contexts react back into biological processes as well as to know the ways in which the biological processes condition social life.

Not long ago a former president of the American Psychological Association suggested that since Dewey wrote these words, "[W]e have made little progress in coming to know the ways in which psychosocial and biological processes interact in the production of age-correlated changes" (Jarvik 1975). Some disagree. This chapter provides a perspective on some psychological aspects of aging that lends support to the view that the psychology of aging has matured markedly in recent years.

HUMAN DEVELOPMENT ACROSS THE LIFE SPAN

Social scientists have accumulated enormous amounts of data on specific features of adult life. This book is filled with statistics on health, illness, life expectancy, death rates, income, and occupation. Curiously, however, the extensive information we have on adult life has provided relatively little toward identifying some basic developmental principles of adulthood. In fact, only recently have mature adulthood and old age been placed within a developmental framework, unlike childhood and adolescence, for which the developmental perspective has helped identify principles that affect us all as we pass through these life-periods.

The different rates of development of child psychology and the psychology of adulthood are a function of several factors. First, there are enormous conceptual and methodological difficulties involved in studying whole lives, not the least of which involves the fact that concepts and measures used by a researcher in a longitudinal study may be relevant at one age ("young adulthood") but not at a later age ("old age").[1] This has resulted, until quite recently, in a scarcity of empirical research on the psychology of middle and later adulthood. Second, the work of Sigmund Freud has influenced and continues to influence the development of a psychology of adulthood.

Freud had a theory of the origins of personality that emphasized how development in the early years significantly influenced one's later life (Lidz 1976). For Freud, personality problems of the adult years could be understood largely in terms of what had happened in infancy and early childhood. Infants and children could be expected to pass through a series of stages of psychosexual development—oral, anal, and genital—each involving the experience of

---

[1] Methodology itself becomes an issue in understanding the relationship between intelligence and aging. This is discussed later in this chapter and, at that time, the longitudinal study is further defined.

bodily pleasure through these "erogenous" zones of the body, assuming all went well. If things did not go well, if parents were overly anxious, or if there was a failure to achieve gratification through other channels, the child could become "fixated" on securing pleasure through oral or anal modes. Such fixations could activate personality attributes. Thus, some persons become "oral types," overeating and otherwise gaining satisfaction through the mouth. Others become "anal types," hoarding and behaving in a constricted, constipated way (Clausen 1986).

Freud was perhaps the first theorist to recognize important processes of early emotional development. Yet he regarded adulthood as a theater in which the dramas of unconscious childhood conflicts are acted out and reenacted. Adulthood, then, is not for further development! As a result, several prominent theories of life cycle development have used Freud's psychosexual stages as a point of departure. A number of these theories include a personality dimension. It may be useful to consider these theories briefly in order to see how they conceptualize the relationships among life-cycle development, personality, and aging.

Conceptions of the Life Cycle

An early pioneer of developmental psychology was Charlotte Buhler. As head of the Vienna Research Center in Child Psychology, she was interested mainly in the psychology of childhood and adolescence. In the early 1930s she began to extend this work to include the rest of the life span. Buhler's (1933) early work is as interesting for its methodology as it is for its conceptualization of the course of the life span. Her book, *Der Menschliche Lebenslauf als psychologisches Problem,* is based on analyses of 250 individual lifespans; 50 of these case histories were gathered retrospectively from aged people, and the rest were taken from biographies and autobiographies.

Buhler did not confine herself to the analysis of diverse life histories; she tried to detect similarities and regularities in the structure of behavior and thought across the diverse life histories of different individuals (Filipp and Olbrich 1986). She suggests that five major phases or periods in the life course can be identified, and that the psychological curve of life parallels the biological curve of ascent and decline, although these curves do not necessarily proceed synchronously. The phases are as follows (Frenkel-Brunswick 1963):

1. In the first phase the child lives at home and his or her life centers around family and school.

2. The second phase begins at about age fifteen and is characterized by entrance into independent activity. This period lasts until the latter half of the third decade. Often, the turning point for this phase can be placed at

the time the young person leaves the home of his or her family. Preparation for career and the acquisition of personal relations also mark this phase.

3. The third phase begins between the twenty-sixth and the thirtieth years of life. It is representative of the most fruitful and creative aspects of life. Definitive career choices are made; marriage and the establishment of home and family are other likely accomplishments.

4. A decrease in the amount of one's activities as well as "negative dimensions" characterize the fourth and fifth phases, which begin at about age fifty. Illness, loss of associates, death of relatives and friends, and reduction in social activities are more noteworthy in the fourth phase. Psychological crises, discontent, and unrest are often evident in this phase.

5. The fifth period is often introduced by complete retirement from work (at about age sixty-five). There is an obvious further decrease in social activities; retrospection and life review are characteristic of this period. Sickness and death are preeminent in these years.

Although Buhler has attempted to identify and determine the regularity with which the various phases of life succeed one another, not all the experiences mentioned here are expected to be present in every individual. For example, some people may not experience as negative the reduction in physical and social activities that accompanies movement from the third to the fourth phase. They may not seek their measure in "physical efficiency" but, rather in a continued mental vitality that brings new interests and attitudes.

The psychoanalytic theorists have dealt most explicitly with the personality dimension as it relates to age. Yet, as has been indicated, much of this work involves developmental theories of childhood and adolescence. Stated tersely, the psychoanalytic theories regard adult personality as stable (Neugarten 1977). Jung (1933) is an exception. He begins his discussion of the stages of life with youth—a period extending from after puberty to about age thirty-five. In general, this period involves giving up childhood and widening the scope of one's life. The next stage begins at about age thirty-five and continues to old age. He characterizes this stage as follows:

> At first it is not a conscious and striking change; it is rather a matter of indirect signs of a change which seems to take its rise in the unconscious. Often it is something like a slow change in a person's character; in another case certain traits may come to light which had disappeared since childhood; or again, one's previous inclinations and interests begin to weaken and others take their place. Conversely—and this happens very frequently—one's cherished convictions and principles, especially the moral ones, begin to harden and to grow increasingly rigid until, somewhere around the age of fifty, a period of intolerance and fanaticism is reached. It is as if the existence of these principles were endangered and it were therefore necessary to emphasize them all the more. (Jung 1971)

Jung sees significant personality changes in old age. The individual's attention may turn inward in an attempt to find meaning in life. Often, he says, individuals will change into their opposites. He argues: "[W]e cannot live the afternoon of life according to the programme of life's morning; for what was great in the morning will be little at evening and what in the morning was true will at evening have become a lie" (Jung 1971).

The most important exception to the general thrust of psychoanalytic theory has been the theories of Erik Erikson (1950, 1963, 1968). Erikson outlines eight ages of humanity stretching from birth to death, each representing a choice or a crisis. Intrinsically social or *psychosocial*, these crises occur within the context of relationships with other people. If decisions are made well during one age, then successful adaptation can be made in the subsequent age. Whereas Freud believed a person became fixated at a particular stage, Erikson sees each stage as reworking elements of the prior stage. Thus people could act as their own therapists and rework difficult areas of their personalities (Kermis 1986). Each age leads to further differentiation of the personality, and each new accomplishment is integrated into experiences and may be drawn upon in later years (Clausen 1986).

Erikson's first five ages rely heavily on the work of Freud and deal largely with childhood development. The last three ages focus on adult development. The eight ages are as follows:

1. In early infancy, the development of a sense of basic *trust* versus a sense of mistrust

2. In later infancy, when some anal muscular maturation has occurred, a growing sense of *autonomy* versus a sense of shame and doubt

3. In early childhood, a developing sense of *initiative* versus a sense of guilt

4. In the middle years of childhood, a sense of *industry* versus a sense of inferiority

5. In adolescence, a sense of *ego identity* (involving certainty about self, career, sex role, and values) versus role confusion

6. In early adulthood, the development of *intimacy* (including more than simply sexual intimacy) versus a sense of ego isolation

7. In middle adulthood, the development of *generativity* (achieving a sense of productivity and creativity) versus ego stagnation

8. In late adulthood, a sense of *ego integrity* (including a basic acceptance of one's life as having been appropriate and meaningful) versus a sense of despair

The sense of ego integration generated in late adulthood is very much a function of what has taken place in the previous ages. Erikson contends that good adjustment in this age comes only when important matters have been placed in proper perspective and when the successes and failures of life have been seen as inevitable. According to Erikson (1963):

> Only in him who in some way has taken care of things and people and has adapted himself to the triumphs and disappointments adherent to being, the originator of others or the generator of products and ideas—only in him may gradually ripen the fruit of these seven stages.

A lack in this accumulated ego integration is often characterized by a failure to accept one's life and ultimately by fear of death.

Not all agree with Erikson. Butler (1975), for one, finds the idea that we are in old age a function of what we were before to be potentially regressive. He argues that, although it is important to recognize the basic foundation of one's identity, it is equally important to recognize the existence of continuing possibilities. Butler quotes the art historian Bernard Berenson, who at age eighty-three stated: "I for one have never touched bottom in self, nor even struck against the surface, the outlines, the boundaries of this self. On the contrary, I feel the self as an energy which expands and contracts" (Berenson in Butler 1975, 401).

Still, Butler (1963) has provided us with a concept, *life review,* which seems integral to carrying out the tasks of Erikson's eighth age. All people reminisce. Yet, according to Butler, this is not an idle process. Rather, life review occurs naturally so that unresolved conflicts may be given attention and resolved. Old age and, perhaps, impending death highlight this process. If conflicts are not resolved, there may be a failure in adjustment, resulting in what Erikson describes as "despair."

Peck (1968) has attempted to refine Erikson's theory, paying special attention to the crucial issues of middle and old age. He describes four developmental tasks of middle age:

1. Valuing wisdom over physical powers
2. Socializing versus sexualizing in human relations
3. Becoming emotionally flexible versus emotionally impoverished
4. Developing mental flexibility in place of mental rigidity

Peck sees three issues as central to old age. First, the individual must establish a wide range of activities so that adjustment to the loss of accustomed roles such as those of worker or parent is minimized (ego differentiation versus work-role preoccupation). Second, because nearly all elderly individuals suffer physical decline or illness, activities in the later years should allow them to transcend their physical limitations (body transcendence versus body preoccupation). Finally, although death is inevitable, individuals may in various ways make contributions that extend beyond their own lifetimes; this may provide meaning for life and overcome despair that one's life was meaningless or should have been other than it was (ego transcendence versus ego preoccupation).

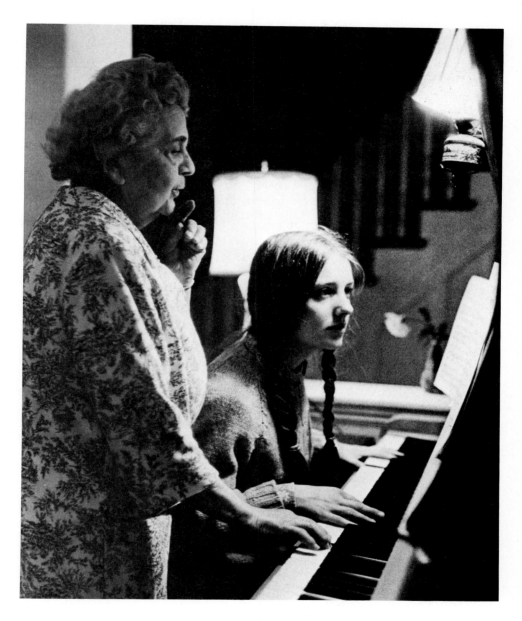

More recently, Levinson and his colleagues (1978), based on their research on men aged thirty-five to forty-five years, have come to view the life cycle as evolving through a sequence of *eras*, each lasting approximately twenty to twenty-five years. In the broadest sense, each era is a "time of life" with its own distinctive qualities. As in Erikson's psychosocial theory, personal crises and developmental tasks characterize each era. In contrast to Erikson, however, Levinson believes that relationships and personal commitments through which tasks of one period are accomplished may *not* serve the needs of the individual beyond that period. Figure 7-1 shows Levinson's developmental periods in early and middle adulthood. A primary developmental task of late adulthood (which begins at about age sixty) is to find a new balance between involvement with society and with the self. It is during this era (according to Levinson) that Erikson's final age (ego integrity versus despair) occurs.

Employing the same extensive biographical interviewing used to study men, Levinson has recently turned his attention to women aged thirty-five to forty-five (Brown 1987). Studying homemakers, businesswomen, and women from academia, Levinson found that women go through the same sequence of periods at the same ages as men. One substantial difference between men and

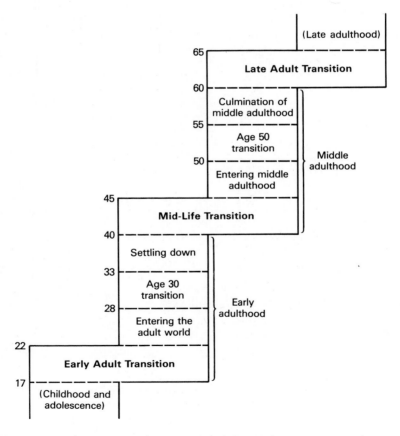

FIGURE 7-1   *From The Seasons of a Man's Life by Daniel J. Levinson et al. Copyright © 1978 by Daniel J. Levinson. Reprinted by permission of Alfred A. Knopf, Inc.*

women, and between groups of women, concerns the life plans envisioned between the ages of twenty-two and twenty-eight. Typically, young men organize a "tentative life structure" around occupation. Young women have more difficulty forming their plans for the life course. According to Levinson, "everything in society supports men having an occupational dream, but for a woman, there is still a quality of going into forbidden territory" (Brown 1987, 23). For many women, the themes of career and family are viewed as two mutually exclusive choices. As Levinson points out, there is no preponderance of cultural wisdom to aid women with these choices. In many respects, they are pioneers.

It is difficult to move away from a discussion of life cycle development without making some mention of Gail Sheehy's (1976) best-selling book of the 1970s, *Passages: Predictable Crises of Adult Life*. In answer to the question, "Is there life after youth?" Sheehy outlines a set of developmental stages, beginning with late adolescence, which she believes most if not all individuals must pass through. The precise age at which each passage is encountered is less important than the sequence of the stages. Catchy phrases are employed as brief descriptions of each stage: "pulling up roots," "the trying twenties," "catch-30," "rooting and extending," "the deadline decade," and "renewal or resignation." The central theme of adult development appears to be one of abandonment; each of us and those around us are forever "growing up and going away." Interestingly, the last stage, including the "after-fifty" years, is presented in the most positive of terms. Somehow, only in late middle-life are we able to build an "authentic life structure," to become warm and mellow. Sheehy suggests that the appropriate motto for this stage of life be "No more bullshit!"

Personality Theory

Although most psychologists of the life cycle have dealt more or less implicitly with the relationship between personality and aging, there is no theory useful to gerontologists that explicitly conceptualizes this relationship. Scientific methods for studying personality have not been very successful and are still in somewhat of an elementary state (Neugarten 1977). Havighurst (1968) suggests that what we need is a theory of the relationship between personality and successful aging.

Thomae (1980) raises several methodological issues important to the study of personality and aging, not the least of which has to do with the selectivity of study samples. For example, studies of elite population groups such as centenarians or the survivors in longitudinal studies are much more likely to show homogeneity of personality characteristics than are samples from normal aging or even institutionalized aging population groups. Thomae suggests that the particular personality pattern an individual shows may depend on a complex interaction of ten factors influential for longevity and survivorship. These factors are as follows:

1. The person at the beginning of the process

2. Recent changes in the individual's biological systems
3. Recent changes in the social system in which the person lives
4. The individual's socioeconomic status and ecologic situation
5. Consistency or change in the individual's cognitive functioning
6. Consistency or change in the individual's personality (including measurable change in activity, interest, mood, creativity, adjustment, or ego-control)
7. The individual life-space of the person
8. The individual's life satisfaction.
9. The person's capacity for restoring balance to his or her life by coping actively
10. The person's social competence

Unfortunately, most researchers have not taken these factors into account in their research designs. In reading below, it may be useful to remember the complexity of factors that may influence personality patterns across the life course.

Reichard, Livson, and Peterson (1962) studied eighty-seven elderly working men in the San Francisco area, forty-two retired and forty-five not retired. They rated these respondents on 115 personality variables and, after a "cluster analysis," identified five types of "agers." Three of these types were judged on the basis of additional analysis to be well adjusted to the aging process; two types were rated as low on adjustment-to-aging measures. Those elderly men judged as successful in aging were labeled the "mature," "rocking-chair," and "armored," respectively; those judged unsuccessful were the "angry" and the "self-haters." The mature group took a constructive view of life, whereas the rocking chair group was more dependent. The armored men did not accept dependency; many of them protected themselves from it by avoiding retirement. The angry men directed hostility at the world, which they blamed for all that was wrong in their lives. Finally, the self-haters blamed themselves for their difficulties.

These men were making quite different behavioral adjustments to aging. As Reichard and her colleagues point out, however, these personality patterns did not likely emerge for the first time in old age. For most men, they were carryovers of adjustment and coping styles from the younger years. Some achieved successful aging through activity; others achieved it through disengagement. In general, those whose personal adjustment was high were effective in overcoming frustrations; they were able to resolve conflicts and remain socially active and accepted. The poorly adjusted, however, were unhappy, fearful of contact with others, withdrawn, and incompetent.

Havighurst (1968) and his colleagues conducted their search for a personality theory of successful aging by studying women and men. The Kansas City Study of Adult Life rated 159 healthy middle- and working-class individuals on forty-five personality dimensions. The researchers used a factor analysis to extract eight personality types, as follows:

1. Reorganized
2. Focused
3. Successfully disengaged
4. Holding-on
5. Constricted
6. Succorance-seeking
7. Apathetic
8. Disorganized

Group 1 reorganize their lives by substituting new activities for lost ones, whereas Group 2, the focused, are more selective about their activities. They focus time and energy on gaining satisfaction from one or two roles. Group 3 have low levels of activity yet are highly satisfied. They have accepted withdrawal from social interaction and are content. Group 4 shows a holding-on pattern. As long as they are able to continue the activities of middle age, they are satisfied with life. Group 5, in contrast, reduce their activity levels as do the focused, but they differ from the focused in being much more defensive about their aging. Group 6, the succorance-seeking, are dependent on others for support. To the extent that they are successful in obtaining this support, they are satisfied with the level of activity they are able to maintain. Group 7 are apathetic and have a low level of participation in activities; life satisfaction for this group is not high. Group 8, the disorganized, have difficulty in maintaining themselves in the community. Intellectual functioning has declined; generally speaking, group members show reduced control over their lives.

According to Havighurst (1968), these eight personality types are probably established by middle age. That is, patterns of adjustment and overall personality in later adulthood probably reflect the individual's adjustment and personality in youth. It should be remembered, though, that the individual's personality often develops along the lines of the demand for adaptation he or she receives from the social environment. Changes in the social environment may require changes in personality. In this regard, personality should not be seen as a fixed system that is completed in early childhood. Personality and personality changes in adults should be considered in terms of long-range developmental changes in, among other things, motivations, intellectual functioning, and the social environment.

One personality study, carried out by Douglas and Arenberg (1978), attempted to measure such changes with longitudinal and cross-sectional research designs. Over 300 males (N = 336) from the highly select group of participants in the Baltimore Longitudinal Study (Stone and Norris 1966), ranging in age from twenty to eighty-one, were tested with the Guilford-Zimmerman Temperament Survey (GZTS), and then were retested an average of seven years later. The GZTS provides an assessment of ten personality traits. Five of the scales showed significant change between the first and second testing, but only two scales were interpreted as showing age effects: (1) Beginning at age fifty, preference for rapidly paced activity declined; and (2) at all ages, men declined in masculine interests. The three other scales showing declines attributed to sociocultural changes include friendliness, thoughtfulness, and personal relations.

Schaie and Parham (1976) also carried out a test–retest study of nineteen personality traits over a seven-year period. They concluded that "stability of personality traits is the rule rather than the exception." Still, they point out that such stability cannot be equated with lack of change after adolescence, as many personality theorists believe. Rather, it is likely that much change does in fact take place. The direction it takes may be a function of early socialization experiences, cohort differences, and social change (Schaie and Parham 1976).

Life-Span Developmental Psychology

The last ten years or so have seen dramatic growth in developmental psychology. In particular, after an extended gestation period, there has been increasing recognition of the value of a life-span developmental perspective (Baltes 1983). Life-span developmental psychology claims the entire life course as its unit of analysis (Fillip and Olbrich 1986). From this perspective, emphasis on a particular age group or life phase, such as old age, is misplaced. Changes experienced by individuals during adulthood may not show the same characteristics as changes experienced during childhood.

Interestingly, the life-span developmental perspective has emphasized the importance of biological, social, and psychological factors contributing to development and has diminished the importance of chronological age itself as an explanatory variable. The life-span perspective places explicit emphasis on the temporal interrelatedness of earlier and later components of the human life course. Thus, at any point in time, an individual's behavior is conceptualized not only as the result of interactions between present biological, social, and psychological factors, but also as a result of their interactions with earlier (and, perhaps, later) experiences and processes (Fillip and Olbrich 1986).

Because the entire life span is the unit of analysis for this perspective, developmental psychology has had to be open to the contributions of other disciplines and scientific approaches, including biology and sociology, among others. Developmental psychology has had impact on these other disciplines as well. As developmental psychology becomes "truly" developmental, we can expect the life-span perspective to gain in scientific status and make a greater contribution to our understanding of the varieties of human development.

AGE-RELATED PSYCHOLOGICAL CHANGES

This section deals with age-related changes in sensory processes and psychomotor response, the relationships between age and intelligence, and memory and learning. The more common forms of intrapersonal and interpersonal psychopathology observed in later life were discussed in Chapter 6.

In more primitive societies, old people have often been found to be held in high esteem. In many cases, however, this lasted only as long as they were able to retain their faculties and a semblance of their previous strength. Old people who lost their sight or hearing, their speed of hand or foot—who became less able to pull their own weight and contribute to the group—were more likely to be neglected, abandoned, or even killed outright. Barash (1983) points out that although such treatment seems harsh, even vicious, to us, it reflects the hard realities of primitive life, not the hardness of the hearts of primitive people.

The anthropologist John Moffat once found an old Hottentot woman left by herself in the South African desert. She spoke as follows:

> Yes, my children, three sons and two daughters, are gone to yonder blue mountain and have left me to die. I am very old you see, and am not able to serve them. When they kill game, I am too feeble to help in carrying home the flesh. I am not able to gather wood and make a fire and I cannot carry their children on my back as I used to. (Barash 1983, 178)

Why was this old woman abandoned by her children? It was, as Barash indicates, for the same reason a resident of this country might discard any possession that was worn out and no longer worked. Many of us recognize this attitude in ourselves when it comes to old things. But what about our attitude toward old people who do not work quite as well as they once did?

Sensory Processes[2]

The nervous system is important in controlling body functioning—especially in controlling smooth and skeletal muscle contractions—and in receiving, processing, and storing information. The senses of vision, hearing, taste, smell, and touch provide links with the outside world. Neurosensory changes that influence an individual's functioning, activities, response to stimuli, and perception of the world do occur with age. Similarly, the world's perception of an individual may be influenced by age-related neurosensory changes that he or she has undergone. Witness, for example, the older person with impaired hearing or vision who may be labeled as stubborn, eccentric, or senile.

---

[2] Materials on sensory processes were adapted from Chapter 8 in Kart, Metress, and Metress (1988).

Nerve cells, or neurons, are lost during the process of aging. The number of the basic functioning units begins to decline around the age of twenty-five. This decline brings a decreased capacity for sending nerve impulses to and from the brain, a decrease in conduction velocity, a slowing down of voluntary motor movements, and an increase in reflex time for skeletal muscles. In addition, degenerative changes and disease states (for the most part involving the sense organs) may alter the sensory processes.

Vision. Many persons maintain near-normal sight well into old age. Still, surveys of the incidence of blindness and problems of visual acuity in different age groups show that these problems of vision are associated with older age. The incidence of visual impairment increases more than threefold per 1,000 persons when comparing those aged eighteen to forty-four years and those aged sixty-five years and over (U.S. Bureau of the Census, 1986, Table 166). The incidence of poorer visual acuity as defined by conventional clinical standards also increases with age (Anderson and Palmore 1974). According to a recent National Health Survey report, whereas about 40 percent of those aged sixty years who were surveyed had visual acuity of 20/20 or better, this declined to about 25 percent at seventy years of age and 10 percent of those eighty years of age. Degenerative changes and eye disorders, which become more frequent with age, contribute to the poorer visual acuity incurred by older people.

Presbyopia is not a disease but a degenerative change that occurs in the aging eye. With this condition the lens loses its ability to focus upon near objects. Visual accommodation or focusing is normally permitted by the ability of the lens to change shape or to accommodate for distant and near vision. This ability is at a maximum around the age of ten years and is almost nonexistent in most persons by the age of fifty-five years. Because of presbyopia, the majority of individuals need reading glasses or bifocals by the time they are in their forties or fifties. The glasses mechanically compensate for the loss of accommodation and allow the individual to focus on objects both near and far.

Changes in the lens lead to farsightedness. Thus, there is a marked tendency for older persons to hold things at a distance in order to see them. The playbill or recipe card may be held at arm's length because the print cannot be discriminated at closer range. Reading glasses allow the individual to discern objects that are in the field of near vision.

With presbyopia, there is a tendency for the lens of the eye to undergo a yellowing effect. This change is significant in that it becomes more difficult for the person to discern certain color intensities, especially the cool colors (blue, green, and violet), which are filtered out. Warm colors (yellow, red, and orange) are generally seen more easily, thus it is advisable to mark objects such as steps and handrails with these colors.

Cataracts are the most common disability of the aged eye. It has been said that all of us would develop them, even if only to a mild degree, if we lived long enough. They represent an opacity and frequently a yellowing of the normally transparent lens of the eye. The opaqueness of the lens interferes with the passage of light to the retina. Depending upon the degree of cataract development, an individual will suffer blurred and dimmed vision. A person may need brighter light to read and may need to hold objects extremely close in order to be able to see them. As the cataract advances, useful sight is lost. Surgical removal of the opaque lens provides safe and effective treatment for cataracts. Eyeglasses, contact lenses, or intraocular lens implants are used to compensate for the loss of the lens.

Glaucoma is the second leading cause of blindness in adults in the United States and the first cause among blacks (Leske 1983). The disease generally develops somewhere between the ages of forty and sixty-five years in response to increased pressure within the eyeball. The increase in pressure is caused by a buildup of aqueous humor, a nutrient fluid that circulates in the anterior chamber of the eye. If this fluid is formed faster than it can be eliminated, an increase in eye pressure results. This pressure can lead to irreparable damage to the optic nerve and to total blindness.

A gradual loss of peripheral vision is one of the earliest indications of glaucoma. This loss of side vision may cause its victim to bump into things or not see passing cars in the next highway lane. In time so much of the normal range of vision becomes eliminated that the victim is said to suffer from "tunnel vision." Left untreated, this limited field of sight will also disappear, leaving the person totally blind.

Before chronic glaucoma develops to such an extent, an individual will express other warning signs. Included in the symptoms of glaucoma are severe headache, nausea, blurred vision, dull eye pain, tearing of the eyes, and the appearance of halos around objects of light. Thus, street lights, house lights, and stars may appear to be surrounded by rings of light.

Senile macular degeneration (SMD) is the leading cause of registered blindness among adults in the United States. As the name implies, the condition involves damage to the macular area of the retina, which ordinarily permits an individual to discriminate fine detail. The majority of those legally blind as a result of SMD have a neovascular or exudative form of the disease. In the latter condition, abnormal blood vessels form within the retina, with resultant hemorrhaging and distortion of vision (Ferris, Fine, and Hyman 1984). Of all the risk factors, increasing age is most strongly associated with SMD. Research also suggests that familial and genetic factors are important.

Age-related visual impairment may produce alterations in behavior as well as in feelings of self-esteem. The visually impaired older person may suffer from serious communication problems. Vision represents one of our most important links with the outside world. During a lifetime an individual becomes dependent upon vision for receiving and processing information about the world and for functioning in his or her surroundings. Information about the local and world scenes comes to us through newspapers, magazines, books, and television. Carrying out activities of daily living involves the ability to master various chores that characteristically depend on visual acuity: sewing on a button, turning on the stove, stirring the sauce until it appears thick and bubbly, getting dressed in the morning, matching the same color socks. A person may be hesitant to perform tasks, especially new ones, because of self-consciousness about the situation.

Special efforts can and should be carried out to help make independent living possible among visually impaired older adults. Coding schemes can be employed in the home setting to help make independent living possible. Fluorescent tape around electric outlets, light switches, door handles, and keyholes can make things much easier for someone who suffers some visual impairment.

An older person who is sent home from a hospital or a neighborhood pharmacy with a vial of medicine may not be able to read the dosage instructions printed on it. All too often such a situation and its possible consequences are not comprehended. Large-print instructions can sometimes help to solve the problem. Many older persons take a number of different drugs, and impaired vision may make it difficult to differentiate one bottle of pills from another. Taping different-colored pieces of paper to the various medicine vials might help to alleviate the problem. For persons not able to discriminate the colors, other coding methods can be employed. The medicine with the piece of sandpaper on the cap can be identified as the pain reliever; the one with the felt-cap top might be the antihypertensive medication.

A final point that is useful for family members, friends, and health-care workers to remember is that persons who have been blind since birth have had a lifetime to adjust to living in a world that assumes everyone can see. For those who suffer visual impairments after having depended on their sight for many years, the adjustments may be quite difficult.

Hearing. Although most persons past sixty-five years of age retain hearing sufficient for normal living, the elderly individual is six times more likely to display a significant loss of hearing than is a young or middle-aged adult. Data from the National Center for Health Statistics indicate that the ratio of hearing impairments for persons eighteen to forty-four years of age is 49.8 per 1,000 persons; this ratio increases to 314.8 per 1,000 for persons sixty-five years and over (U.S. Bureau of the Census 1986, Table 166).

Presbycusis is the most common cause of sensorineural hearing deficit in older adults (Olsen 1984). It is estimated that approximately 13 percent or more of those aged sixty-five years and older would show advanced signs of presbycusis, if tested (Corso 1987). At first, the loss of the ability to perceive higher frequencies does not involve normal speech patterns; but as the condition progresses, conversation does become affected. Because consonant sounds are typically those in the higher frequencies and vowel sounds are those in the lower frequencies, speech discrimination becomes poor. Speech can be heard, but words cannot be detected.

Presbycusis is most frequently the result of changes in important structures of the inner ear. In the inner ear, sound vibrations are transformed into nerve impulses by the cochlea. This complicated spiral cavity houses the organ of Corti, which possesses delicate hair cells. Hair cell stimulation produces nerve impulses that are carried by the auditory or eighth cranial nerve. The auditory nerve transmits the sensations to the brain, where they are then perceived as sound. Aging itself, combined with exposure to loud noise, certain drugs, and disease, can rob the cochlea of functioning hair cells. It is believed that the loss of these hair cells in the organ of Corti is the most common cause of presbycusis. Presbycusis can be ameliorated by the use of a hearing aid, but it must be emphasized that hearing aids do not represent a perfect substitute for normal hearing. They cannot restore the full frequency range of more severe losses.

Hearing loss can also result from interrupted conduction. The middle ear contains a series of delicate bones: the malleus or hammer, the incus or anvil, and the stapes or stirrup. It is the function of these bones to receive vibrations that have entered the external ear through the external auditory meatus or ear canal. The eardrum, which essentially demarcates the outer ear from the middle ear, receives vibrations and moves them along the chain of bones in the middle ear. Vibrations move from the middle ear to the oval window in the delicate membrane separating the middle from the inner ear. Wax can build up in the ear and interfere with proper conduction and contribute to impaired hearing. Fortunately, this common cause of conductive impairment in the older adult is reversible. The ears of the elderly individual should be checked for the collection of wax. Irrigation of the ear canal can remove collected wax and contribute to a restoration of hearing in many persons. Otosclerosis or a hardening of the stapes can also result in conductive hearing loss, a condition that can often be corrected by surgery.

Factors that can lead to hearing loss of a perceptive or conductive nature include genetic conditions, exposure to environmental noise, the use of certain drugs, and chronic ear infections. In industrialized societies we have almost come to take for granted an age-associated loss of hearing as well as the differential sex manifestation of hearing loss. Men in the United States have suffered from a loss of hearing with age to a greater degree than have women. Workplace noise has likely contributed to this pattern. Perhaps, as noise exposure becomes more uniform, we will see less gender-based difference in hearing decline.

Use of hearing aids can compensate for some of these changes in hearing. This is especially the case if the aids are balanced to correct for each ear (Welford 1980). According to Welford (1980), if they are not balanced, or if only one aid is used, differences of phase and intensity, which enable the location of sounds to be identified, will be lost. If the ability to locate sound is lost, then wanted and unwanted sounds may combine together in confused noise. This is what the hearing aid wearer is describing by the complaint that "all it does is bring in noise."

Taste, Smell, and Touch. Loss of taste is a common complaint among the elderly. Some researchers have suggested that people have fewer taste buds with aging (Arey, Tremaine, and Monzingo 1936). There are small but clearly measurable increases in both detection thresholds (concentration at which subjects can first detect a difference between a stimulus and water) and recognition thresholds (concentration at which subjects can first recognize a quality such as sweet). Still, conclusions about the relationship between taste sensitivity and age must be viewed cautiously. Methodological problems abound. Not all experiments verify the relationship, and intervening factors such as disease, medications, and smoking habits need to be evaluated for their impact on taste sensitivity (Engen 1977).

There is a general decline in olfactory functioning with age (Schiffman 1987). Diminished smell perception among the elderly can result from a variety of anatomic and physiological losses that are a consequence of normal aging (Schiffman, Orlandi, and Erickson 1979). Medical conditions, pharmacological agents, and smoking habits may also play a role in diminished smell perception among the elderly (Schiffman 1983).

Loss of touch sensitivity has been reported to occur in a small proportion of the aged population. Birren (1964), in reviewing this scarce literature, concluded that "touch sensitivity remains unchanged from early adulthood through about age fifty to fifty-five, with a rise in threshold thereafter." In an often cited study, Thompson, Axelrod, and Cohen (1965) had young adult (eighteen to thirty-four years) and older adult (sixty to seventy-seven years) subjects touch a variety of objects without looking at them. The task was to identify the objects with those represented on a visual display. The older adults did less well than the younger group did, although the researchers attributed this as much to decline in visual acuity as to a decline in touch sensitivity.

There is some clinical evidence that old people do not feel pain as intensely as do younger people. Yet, subjective sensory complaints are very common in old age (Botwinick 1973). Part of the inconsistency in the literature lies in the fact that a subject's response to noxious stimuli has cognitive and motivational components as well as a sensory component (Melzack 1973). Thus, as Gelfand (1964) points out, the way a subject views an experimental situation, the experimenter, and even the instructions given may affect the outcome of laboratory experiments on pain threshold and pain tolerance.

Psychomotor Responses

Psychomotor response is more complex than simple sensation and perception. If the concept of psychomotor response could be diagrammatically presented, it would show the organism taking in sensory input (or information), giving meaning to this new information through perceptual and integrative processes, determining whether or not this new information calls for any action, sending instructions to the appropriate activity center (a muscle, for example), and activating the appropriate response. Psychomotor performance may be limited by a weakness at any point in this chain of events. It may be limited by changes in the sensory threshold, in the processes dealing with perception, in the translation from perception to action, in the strength of the sensory signal, and in muscular output.

Psychomotor performance changes as an individual ages. Evidence of the slowing of behavioral responses with age has been accumulating for decades (Birren, Woods, and Williams 1980). This relationship is complicated by a number of factors. The nature of the stimulus and the complexity of the response appear to affect reaction time. When tasks are simple and little decision making is required, the increase in reaction time observed in the elderly is slight. When choice is required, the task becomes more complex, and reaction time slows. The particular motor skills involved and the familiarity of the task also make assessments of the relationship between reaction time and age difficult. Botwinick (1973) points out that practice at a task and exercise may reduce the effects of a slowing in reaction time. It should be remembered also that psychosocial variables such as motivation will affect reaction time.

Older people show slower speed of movement than do the young. Precision of response also declines with age. Some research suggests that older individuals are willing to sacrifice speed for accuracy (Botwinick 1967; Welford 1959). This seems to indicate that, without the pressures of time, older people are as capable of performance as their younger counterparts.

Age decrements in performance seem to relate to cerebral cortex functioning rather than to any loss of ability to move. Circulatory deterioration, reduced cerebral metabolism, and suppressed brain rhythms tend to produce slower reaction times (Hendricks and Hendricks 1977). Botwinick and Storandt (1974) point out that cardiovascular problems may also serve to depress reaction time in a way that cannot be overcome by exercise.

The impact of an age-related decline in psychomotor performance on social functioning should be obvious. In general, such decline—especially in combination with sensory and perceptual decline—reduces the aged individual's ability to exert control over his or her environment. Tasks that were formerly nonproblematic such as driving a car or using a sewing machine may become hazardous with advancing age. Some work activities may also suffer, mainly in jobs relying on exceptionally speedy reactions or responses to incoming information. Activities directly related to health maintenance and care may also become more difficult to carry out. Also, as Atchley (1977, 49) indicates, the nature of the decline in psychomotor performance is such that it is difficult to offset mechanically in the way glasses or hearing aids can be used to offset declines in sensory processes.

Intellectual Functioning

The conventional view is that aging brings with it a decline in intelligence, but most researchers today agree that there are a great many problems associated with this assumption. Botwinick (1977) identifies five areas of concern that must be dealt with in evaluating the conventional view that age brings intellectual decline: (1) what age period are we looking at; (2) what tests do we use; (3) how do we define intelligence; (4) what sampling techniques are employed; and (5) what are the problems associated with specific research methods?

Intelligence can only be surmised from performance scores; therefore, problems of measurement and testing affect outcomes. The most popular tool used to study age-related changes in intelligence has been the Wechsler Adult Intelligence Scale (WAIS). Results of studies with the WAIS often describe a "classic aging pattern" that shows a plateau reached in the twenties, maintenance of performance on verbal subtests, such as vocabulary and comprehension, until the sixties, but early adult decline on performance tests such as block design and object assembly (Botwinick 1977).

Critics of the WAIS argue that the test measures mental skills and abilities that are currently being emphasized by the educational system. This makes it a more appropriate tool for determining the intelligence of younger people (Atchley 1977; Hendricks and Hendricks 1977). These critics and others argue that testing procedures that reflect the intellectual functioning required in everyday life should be used to test the relationship between age and intelligence; after all, intelligence is only one of the important ingredients necessary in carrying out successful behavior. This has been done to a limited extent. Demming and Pressey (1957) measured intellectual functioning in three task-related ways. They asked if respondents could (1) use the telephone directory, (2) understand some common legal terms, and (3) secure social services that might be required. Middle-aged and older adults scored higher as a group on these performance measures than younger respondents did. Fisher (1973) suggests that the concepts of social competence and effectiveness should be used in place of intellectual functioning when evaluating the aged.

Baltes and Labouvie (1973) argue that intelligence is not a single factor but consists of many abilities. In an extensive literature review, they report on many studies that conceptualize intelligence as a complex of mental abilities. The relationship between age and intelligence presented in these studies varies depending on which mental abilities are stressed.

Research design appears to strongly influence the results of studies of age and intelligence. By and large, cross-sectional studies show early intelligence decrements, whereas longitudinal studies show stability of intelligence into late adulthood. Cross-sectional research is conducted at one point in time; the effect of age is determined by comparing people of different ages at the time the research is carried out. Longitudinal research involves observing the same people over an extended period of time. Because cross-sectional studies sample respondents from different age cohorts or generations and longitudinal studies sample respondents from a single cohort or generation, comparable outcomes should not be expected. Generations differ as to their genetic potential and historical experiences (Baltes and Labouvie 1973). Many people who are old today did not have the advantage of long years of formal education. This may be especially the case for women. This intellectual underdevelopment is sometimes confused with a lack of intelligence. Schaie (1965) and Baltes (1968) propose the use of both cross-sectional and longitudinal studies to attempt to disentangle these genetic and experiential components.

Another factor that must be considered in the relationship between age and intelligence is health status. Birren (1968) argues that the average person growing older in our society need not expect to show a typical deterioration of mental functioning in the later years. Rather, "limitation of mental functioning occurs precipitously in individuals over the age of sixty-five or seventy and is closely related to health status." Particularly problematic are vascular diseases, which affect the cerebral cortex and probably influence the brain's capacity to store information. Related to this are the results of several studies that show a relationship between intelligence decline and survival among elderly subjects. Five years after an initial survey of elderly subjects in good health, Birren (1968) compared survivors and nonsurvivors with respect to their WAIS scores. It was primarily the verbal skills tests that distinguished them; nonsurvivors had significantly lower verbal scores at the time of initial survey. Eleven years after the initial survey, Granick (1971) reported both low verbal *and* low performance scores to be associated with early death.

Health practitioners and others should be aware that intelligence differences among individuals are great enough so that use of conventional ideas in this area is problematic. Although aging influences intellectual functioning to some extent, careful observation and evaluation of each elderly person is in order before conclusions can be drawn. An individual should not be underestimated in these matters simply because he or she is old. Intellectual decline before the late fifties is probably pathological rather than normal. From the early sixties on there is decline in some but not all abilities, for some but not all individuals. Data from the Seattle Longitudinal Study (Schaie 1983, 1984) shows that, over a seven-year period, about 67 percent of the "young-old" and 50 percent of the "old-old" were able to maintain their functional level of intelligence.

As we point out again in later chapters on old age institutions and alternatives to institutionalization, the impact of the environment (psychosocial and physical) in which the elderly person resides also deserves careful evaluation. The possibility that environmental considerations are constraining intellectual functioning in some of the aged should not be ignored. Finally, the pace of sociocultural change has been rapid. As a result, many older people (including the "young-old") suffer from what can only be described as "obsolescence" effects and compare poorly with younger peers, even though they may function as well as they ever have (Schaie 1980).

Memory and Learning

Memory and learning are functions of the central nervous system. In general, age-related changes in learning ability appear to be small, even after the keenness of the senses has begun to decline. Impairment in learning is often due to an associated condition—some prior incapacity or a debilitating change in the individual. Arteriosclerosis and senile brain changes in old age have been linked to the dulling of memory and learning disability. In the presence of dulled memory or impaired learning, it should not be assumed that some typical process of normal aging is at work.

There appears to be a greater loss with age in recent memory than in old memory. Also, as age increases, the retention of things heard becomes increasingly superior to the retention of things seen (Atchley 1977). Some suggest that new learning interferes with recall of old material, but there seems to be little support for either this proposition or the proposition that old memory interferes with new learning.

Does learning ability decline with advancing age? The research literature indicates two tendencies: As a group, older adults tend to be slower at learning new material than they were when younger and in comparison with younger cohorts, but some of their decline is explainable by learning-related and individual difference-related variables other than chronological age (Poon 1987).

Attitudes toward learning may change with age as well. The older individual may be less ready to learn than he or she was as a youth. Aged individuals may be more likely to attempt to solve problems on the basis of what they already know, rather than learn new solutions (Poon 1985).

SUMMARY

Psychological aspects of aging are tied up with biological and social processes—and these are often difficult to tease out.

Social scientists have collected a great deal of data on adult life. Little of it has been useful for developing a psychology of the life cycle. A number of different conceptions of life cycle development have been put forth in the last fifty years or so—including those of Buhler, Jung, Erikson, and Levinson and his colleagues. More research is needed, and methodological difficulties involved in studying adult development must be overcome. Personality theory remains an underdeveloped area for psychologists of aging. Yet much research suggests that styles of coping and adjustment carry over from the younger to the later adult years.

Age-related sensory changes in individuals affect the quality and quantity of their interaction with the world at large. Degenerative changes and eye disorders that increase with age are contributing factors in the poorer visual acuity experienced by many older people. Cataracts, glaucoma, and senile macular degeneration are the most common eye disorders among the elderly. Impaired hearing is also associated with aging. There is a small diminishment of the perception of taste and smell among the elderly that is a consequence of normal aging. Loss of touch sensitivity has been reported to occur in some elderly individuals.

Psychomotor response changes as an individual ages. Speed and precision of response decline with age, although some of this decrement may be disease- and not age-related.

The relationship between intelligence and aging is a complex one, although a "classic aging pattern" appears to exist. Verbal skills hold up better than performance scores across the life cycle. Health status is an important intervening variable. Still, whether health status affects intelligence functioning or whether intellectual decline is a precursor of ill health or even mortality is subject to debate.

Learning capacity per se appears to be relatively unaffected by age. Attitude toward learning may change more significantly with age. This is the case as well with old memory; recent memory shows greater loss with age.

STUDY QUESTIONS

1. Explain why the development of a psychology of adulthood has been slowed. How is Freud's theory of the origins of personality implicated?

2. Describe Erikson's conception of the life cycle. List the eight ages. In attempting to refine Erikson's theory, Peck pointed out three issues as central to old age. Briefly describe each issue.

3. How have methodological issues contributed to the way the relationship between personality and aging has been conceptualized to date? List the ten factors identified by Thomae as influential for longevity and survivorship.

4. List and explain each of the five types of "agers" identified by Reichard and her associates in their study of working men in San Francisco.

5. Discuss the sensory deprivations that occur with the aging process. What are the social–psychological implications for elderly individuals experiencing visual and hearing impairments?

6. Identify the "classic aging pattern" that emerges from tests of the relationship between intelligence and aging. Discuss the weaknesses and strengths of intelligence testing with the elderly. What factors should be considered when administering and evaluating intelligence tests to this age group?

7. To what extent does the aging process influence memory? Learning?

BIBLIOGRAPHY

Anderson, B., and Palmore, E. 1974. Longitudinal evaluation of ocular function. In E. Palmore (ed.), *Normal aging*. Durham, N.C.: Duke University Press.

Arey, L., Tremaine, M.J., and Monzingo, F.L. 1936. The numerical and topographical relations of taste buds to human circumvillate papillae throughout the life span. *Anatomical Record* 64(1):9–25.

Atchley, R. 1977. *Social forces in later life* (2nd ed.). Belmont, Calif.: Wadsworth Publishing Co. Inc.

Baltes, P.B. 1983. Life-span developmental psychology: Observations on history and theory revisited. In R.M. Lerner (ed.), *Developmental psychology: Historical and philosophical perspectives*. Hillsdale, N.J.: Lawrence Erlbaum Associates.

———. 1968. Longitudinal and cross-sectional sequences in the study of age and generation effects. *Human Development* 11:145–171.

Baltes, P.B., and Labouvie, G. 1973. Adult development of intellectual performance: Description, explanation and modification. In C. Eisdorfer and M.P. Lawton (eds.), *The psychology of adult development and aging.* Washington, D.C.: American Psychological Association.

Barash, D. 1983. *Aging: An exploration.* Seattle, Wash.: University of Washington Press.

Birren, J. 1964. *The psychology of aging.* Englewood Cliffs, N.J.: Prentice-Hall.

———. 1968. Psychological aspects of aging: Intellectual functioning. *Gerontologist* 8(1, Part II):16–19.

Birren, J., Woods, A., and Williams, M.V. 1980. Behavioral slowing with age. In L.W. Poon (ed.), *Aging in the 1980s.* Washington, D.C.: American Psychological Association.

Botwinick, J. 1967. *Cognitive processes in maturity and old age.* New York: Springer Publishing Co., Inc.

———. 1973. *Aging and behavior.* New York: Springer Publishing Co., Inc.

———. 1977. Intellectual abilities. In J. Birren and K. Schaie (eds.), *Handbook of the psychology of aging.* New York: Van Nostrand Reinhold Co.

Botwinick, J., and Storandt, M. 1974. Cardiovascular status, depressive effect and other factors in reaction time. *Journal of Gerontology* 29(5):543–548.

Brown, P.L. 1987. Studying seasons of a woman's life. *New York Times* September 14: 23.

Buhler, C. 1933. *Der menschliche Lebenslauf als psychologisches Problem.* Leipzig: Hirzel.

Butler, R. 1963. The life review: An interpretation of reminiscence in the aged. *Psychiatry* 26:65–76.

———. 1975. *Why survive? Being old in America.* New York: Harper and Row.

Clausen, J. 1986. *The life course: A sociological perspective.* Englewood Cliffs, N.J.: Prentice-Hall.

Corso, J.F. 1987. Hearing. In G.L. Maddox (ed.), *The encyclopedia of aging.* New York: Springer.

Demming, J., and Pressey, S. 1957. Tests 'indigenous' to the adult and older years. *Journal of Counseling Psychology* 2:144–148.

Dewey, J. 1939. Introduction. In E.V. Cowdry (ed.), *Problems of aging.* Baltimore, Md.: The Williams and Wilkins Co.

Douglas, K., and Arenberg, D. 1978. Age changes, cohort differences, and cultural change on the Guilford-Zimmerman Temperament Survey. *Journal of Gerontology* 33(5):737–747.

Engen, T. 1977. Taste and smell. In J. Birren and K. Schaie (eds.), *Handbook of the psychology of aging.* New York: Van Nostrand Reinhold Co.

Erikson, E. 1950. *Childhood and society.* New York: W.W. Norton and Co.

———. 1963. *Childhood and society* (2nd ed.). New York: W.W. Norton and Co.

———. 1968. *Identity: Youth and crisis.* New York: W.W. Norton and Co.

Ferris, F., Fine, S., and Hyman, L. 1984. Age-related macular degeneration and blindness due to neovascular maculopathy. *Archives of Ophthalmology* 102:1640–1642.

Fillip, S., and Olbrich, E. 1986. Human development across the life-span: Overview and highlights of the psychological perspective. In A. Sorensen, F.E. Weinert, and L.R. Sherrod (eds.), *Human development and the life course: Multidisciplinary perspectives.* Hillsdale, N.J.: Lawrence Erlbaum Associates, Publishers.

Fisher, J. 1973. Competence, effectiveness, intellectual functioning and aging. *Gerontologist* 13:62–68.

Frenkel-Brunswick, E. 1963. Adjustments and reorientation in the course of the life-span. In R. Kuhler and G. Thompson (eds.), *Psychological studies of human development* (rev. ed.). New York: Appleton-Century-Crofts.

Gelfand, S. 1964. The relationship of experimental pain tolerance to pain threshold. *Canadian Journal of Psychology* 18:36–42.

Granick, S. 1971. Psychological test functioning. In S. Granick and R. Patterson (eds.), *Human aging II: An eleven-year follow-up biomedical and behavioral study.* Washington, D.C.: U.S. Government Printing Office.

Hall, G.S. 1922. *Senescence, the last half of life.* New York: Appleton-Century-Crofts.

Havighurst, R. 1968. Personality and patterns of aging. *Gerontologist* 8:20–23.

Hendricks, J., and Hendricks, C. 1977. *Aging in a mass society.* Cambridge, Mass.: Winthrop Publishers, Inc.

Jarvik, L.F. 1975. Thoughts on the psychobiology of aging. *American Psychologist* (May):576–583.

Jung, C. 1933. *Modern man in search of a soul.* New York: Harcourt, Brace and World.

———. 1971. The stages of life. In J. Campbell (ed.), *The portable Jung.* New York: The Viking Press, Inc.

Kart, C., Metress, E., and Metress, J. 1988. *Aging, health and society.* Boston: Jones and Bartlett.

Kart, C., Metress, E., and Metress, J. 1978. *Aging and health.* Menlo Park, Calif.: Addison-Wesley Publishing Co., Inc.

Kermis, M.D. 1986. *Mental health in late life: The adaptive process.* Boston: Jones and Bartlett.

Leske, M.C. 1983. The epidemiology of open-angle glaucoma: A review. *American Journal of Epidemiology* 118:166–191.

Levinson, D.J., Darrow, C.N., Klein, E.B., Levinson, M.H., and Mckee, B. 1978. *The seasons of a man's choice.* New York: Alfred A. Knopf, Inc.

Lidz, T. 1976. *The person: His or her development throughout the life cycle* (2nd ed.). New York: Basic Books.

Melzack, R. 1973. *The puzzle of pain.* New York: Basic Books.

Neugarten, B. 1977. Personality and aging. In J. Birren and K. Schaie (eds.), *Handbook of the psychology of aging.* New York: Van Nostrand Reinhold Co.

Olsen, W. 1984. When hearing wanes, is amplification the answer? *Postgraduate Medicine* 76:189–198.

Peck, R. 1968. Psychological developments in the second half of life. In B. Neugarten (ed.), *Middle age and aging: A reader in social psychology.* Chicago: The University of Chicago Press.

Poon, L.W. 1987. Learning. In G.L. Maddox (ed.), *The encyclopedia of aging*. New York: Springer.

———. 1985. Differences in human memory with aging: Nature, causes and clinical implications. In J. Birren and K. Schaie (eds.), *Handbook of the psychology of aging* (2nd ed.). New York: Van Nostrand Reinhold Co.

Reichard, S., Livson, F., and Peterson, P.G. 1962. *Aging and personality*. New York: John Wiley and Sons, Inc.

Ross, D. 1972. *G. Stanley Hall: The psychologist as prophet?* Chicago: University of Chicago Press.

Schaie, K.W. 1984. Midlife influences upon intellectual functioning in old age. *International Journal of Behavioral Development* 7:463–478.

———. 1983. *Longitudinal studies of adult psychological development*. New York: Guilford Press.

———. 1980. Intelligence and problem solving. In J.E. Birren and R.B. Sloane (eds.), *Handbook of mental health and aging*. Englewood Cliffs, N.J.: Prentice-Hall.

———. 1965. A general model for the study of developmental problems. *Psychological Bulletin* 64:92–107.

Schaie, K.W., and Parham, I.A. 1976. Stability of adult personality traits: Fact or fable? *Journal of Personality and Social Psychology* 34(1):146–158.

Schiffman, S.S. 1987. Smell. In G.L. Maddox (ed.), *The encyclopedia of aging*. New York: Springer.

———. 1983. Taste and smell in disease. *New England Journal of Medicine* 308:1275–1279, 1337–1343.

———. 1979. Changes in taste and smell with age: Psychological aspects. In J.M. Ordy and K. Brizzee (eds.), *Sensory systems and communication in the elderly: Vol. 10, Aging*. New York: Raven Press.

Schiffman, S.S., Orlandi, M., and Erickson, R.P. 1979. Changes in taste and smell with age: Biological aspects. In J.M. Ordy and K. Brizzee (eds.), *Sensory systems and communication in the elderly: Vol. 10, Aging*. New York: Raven Press.

Sheehy, Gail. 1976. *Passages: Predictable crises of adult life*. New York: E.P. Dutton & Co., Inc.

Stone, J.L., and Norris, A.H. 1966. Activities and attitudes of participants in the Baltimore Longitudinal Study. *Journal of Gerontology* 21:575–580.

Thomae, H. 1980. Personality and adjustment to aging. In J.E. Birren and R.B. Sloane (eds.), *Handbook of mental health and aging*. Englewood Cliffs, N.J.: Prentice-Hall.

Thompson, L.W., Axelrod, S., and Cohen, L.D. 1965. Senescence and visual identification of tactual-kinesthetic forms. *Journal of Gerontology* 20(2):244–249.

U.S. Bureau of the Census. 1986. *Statistical abstract of the United States, 1987*. Washington, D.C.: U.S. Government Printing Office.

Welford, A. 1959. Psychomotor performance. In J. Birren (ed.), *Handbook of aging and the individual*. Chicago: University of Chicago Press.

———. 1980. Sensory, perceptual, and motor processes in older adults. In J.E. Birren and R.B. Sloane (eds.), *Handbook of mental health and aging*. Englewood Cliffs, N.J.: Prentice-Hall.

CHAPTER 8

SOCIAL ASPECTS OF AGING

This chapter introduces the concept of the *life course* and contrasts it with life-stage and life-span developmental approaches identified in the previous chapter. The life course, a schedule or sequence of roles and group memberships that individuals are expected to follow as they move through life, is socially prescribed. Thus, basic anthropological and sociological concepts are useful for describing and understanding its structure. In a second section, we use such concepts as *social role* and *role transition* to help explain the sequencing of the life course. Finally, although the life course may have predictable, socially recognized transitions to it, most of us experience events and circumstances over which we have little or no control. Coping with change or stress and developing successful strategies for adaptation are important elements in the life course. We conclude with a review of some work on life stress and adaptation. Chapter 9 deals in specific terms with sociological theories of aging.

THE LIFE COURSE PERSPECTIVE

In Chapter 7 you were introduced to life-stage and life-span developmental approaches to understanding the changes people experience as they age. The work of Erikson and Levinson represent examples of the *life-stage* approach. And, as we observed, these frameworks appear to contend that development proceeds through a set pattern of sequential stages that most individuals experience. As Levinson and his colleagues (1974) summarize this approach:

> We are interested in generating . . . hypotheses concerning *relatively universal,*

genotypic, age-linked, adult developmental periods within which variations occur.
. . . (p. 244; italics in original)

A second perspective is found in the growing body of work on *life-span* developmental psychology. This approach was originally developed as a counterpoint to life-stage or life-cycle theories that posited irreversible, unidirectional, age-determined change through the lifetime (Bush and Simmons 1981). Life-span developmental psychology is devoted to "the description and explication of ontogenetic (age-related) behavioral changes from birth to death" (Baltes and Goulet 1970, 12). Although proponents of the life-span approach can be accused of focusing a good deal of attention on intrapsychic phenomena, it is fair to say that in recent years researchers have shifted some focus to environmental determinants of behavior. Thus, as Bush and Simmons (1981) point out, many life-span researchers now emphasize the interaction of individual and social characteristics in explanations of behavioral change.

The life course perspective "concentrates on age-related transitions that are *socially created*, *socially recognized*, and *shared*" (Hagestad and Neugarten 1985, 35; italics in original). Life course researchers focus on the ways in which social norms and definitions influence the pattern or sequence of role changes and role transitions in the life course. Generally speaking, intraindividual or biological phenomena are excluded from analysis. This is especially the case after the individual reaches adulthood or biological maturation. Table 8-1 compares the life-stage, life-span, and life course perspectives.

All societies divide the lifetime into recognized seasons of life—what Zerubavel (1981) describes as a *sociotemporal order*—that regulate the structure and dynamics of social life. Passing from one "season" to another often marks multiple changes in social identity. The way lifetime is divided or segmented differs in different cultures. Typically, periods of life are identified and defined; age criteria are used to channel people into positions and roles. Rights, responsibilities, privileges, and obligations are assigned based on these culturally specific definitions (Hagestad and Neugarten 1985). The St. Lawrence Island Eskimos exemplify a culturally defined life course typology. Among these people, age is used simply to separate boys from men, and girls from women; as men and women mature, they "continue doing what (they have) always done as long as possible," then finally enter old age (Hughes 1961).

Linton (1942) suggested that the minimal number of age groupings in a society must be four—infancy, childhood, adulthood, and old age. Jennie Keith (1982) reports studying sixty traditional societies and finding a range of two to eight categories or age-grades used to "slice" up the life course. Cowgill (1986) identifies at least ten age grades in contemporary America: infancy, preschool age, kindergarten age, elementary school age, intermediate school age, high school age, young adult, middle aged, young old, and old old.

Early in the seventeenth century, Shakespeare's character Jaques in *As You*

TABLE 8-1   Conceptualizations of Change and Individual Development through the Lifetime According to Life-Stage, Life-Span and Life-Course Perspectives

Change Issues	Amount of Change Possible	Abruptness of Change	Direction of Change	Universality of Change	Origin of Change
Perspectives:					
Life Stage	Change between stages; little change within	Abrupt between stages	Unidirectional	Universal	Largely internal
Life-Span	Change throughout life but amount varies depending upon individual characteristics, life experiences, history	Varies	Reversible	Relative	Internal and external, emphasis on latter
Life Course	Change throughout life but amount varies depending upon individual experiences, age norms, cohort effects, and history	Varies	Reversible	Relative	Internal and external, much emphasis on latter

Source: Bush and Simmons (1985, p. 153).
From *Social psychology: sociological perspectives*, edited by Morris Rosenberg and Ralph H. Turner. Copyright © 1981 by the American Sociological Association. Reprinted by permission of Basic Books, Inc., Publishers.

Like It limited life's script to seven acts or ages:

> All the world's a stage,
> And all the men and women merely players.
> They have their exits and their entrances,
> And one man in his time plays many parts,
> His acts being seven ages.
> (act 2, sc. 7, lines 139–143)

The seven acts or ages (applicable to a woman's life script as well) constitute the sequence of roles that make up a life course, each role symbolizing age-appropriate behaviors.

> . . . At first the infant,
> mewling and puking in the nurse's arms.
> Then the whining schoolboy, with his satchel
> And shining morning face, creeping like snail
> Unwillingly to school. And then the lover,
> Sighing like furnace, with a woeful ballad
> Made to the mistress' eyebrow. Then a soldier,
> Full of strange oaths, and bearded like the pard,
> Jealous in honor, sudden and quick in quarrel,
> Seeking the bubble reputation
> Even in the cannon's mouth. And then the justice,
> In fair round belly with good capon lined,
> With eyes severe and beard of formal cut,
> Full of wise saws and modern instances;
> And so he plays his part. The sixth age shifts
> Into the lean and slippered pantaloon,
> With spectacles on nose and pouch on side;
> His youthful hose, well saved, a world too wide
> For his shrunk shank; and his big manly voice,
> Turning again towards childish treble, pipes
> And whistles in his sound. Last scene of all,
> That ends this strange eventful history,
> Is second childishness and mere oblivion,
> sans teeth, sans eyes, sans taste, sans everything.
> (act 2, sc. 7, lines 143–166).

For Shakespeare, life begins with a helpless dependency and ends absent the sensory capabilities that make it worth living. The course between these end points is described in terms of social roles. But understanding how the "mewling, puking infant" becomes the lover, the soldier, the justice, and finally enters "second childishness" and "mere oblivion" requires some familiarity with the process of socialization.

SOCIALIZATION AND SOCIAL ROLES

The human animal is distinguished by its capacity to learn, and this capacity underlies the efforts in human society to develop and institutionalize modes of instruction to better prepare individuals to function as members of society. Stated more succinctly, human behavior is primarily learned. The learning process is called *socialization* and involves the transmission, by language and gesture, of the culture into which we are born. As Clausen (1987, 17) reminds us, socialization is a lifelong process, "the process of transmitting the skills and knowledge needed to perform roles that one will (or may) occupy as one moves along the life course."

Much socialization effort is directed toward the developing child. The function of early socialization is to present a single world of meaning as the only possible way to organize perceptions (Berger and Luckman 1966). But socialization goes on long after physical maturity has been achieved. Early socialization is insufficient to prepare a person for the many different roles of adulthood in a modern industrial society. When focused on the adult life course, socialization stresses the importance of the demands that institutions and other members of the society make on the individual (Brim 1968). These demands shape attitudes, interests, and opinions. They require *desocialization* (learning to give up a role) and *resocialization* (learning new ways to deal with the old role partners). Such changes carry with them the potential for major reorganization of the self (Hess, Markson, and Stein 1988).

The concept of *social role* describes the expectations we have for individuals who occupy a given social position or status. Each distinctive social status has a set of role, or behavioral, expectations attached to it. It is the concept of social role that leads us to expect that college students submit their assignments on time, that accountants are familiar with current tax law, and that police officers are responsive to citizens in distress. It is also the concept that helps us understand how the same individual can juggle the different expectations associated with being a mother, professor, community volunteer, friend, spouse, and theatre patron all in the same day.

Roles are not acted out in a social vacuum. They are usually defined in the context of interacting social roles performed by others. Thus, expectations I fulfill in my role as a professor are often carried out in association with someone else fulfilling the role of student. Only with the cooperation of two individuals fulfilling their roles of daughter and son, respectively, have I been able to carry out the expectations associated with being a father. Many social roles come in pairs or sets, like those described above (for example, professor–student; father–child). Such role pairs or sets are known as *complementary roles*, since they require that the behavior of two or more persons interact in specific ways.

Social roles, including complementary roles, are not defined in specific or uniform terms throughout a society. Some of this lack of uniformity comes from variation in actual performance across individuals. One professor may befriend students and provide advice and counsel on personal matters, whereas another may focus strictly on duties related to the coursework at hand. In one family, the father may play a strong role as decision-maker, whereas in another the mother may take responsibility for most decisions. Generally speaking, to operate effectively, the roles people assume must complement the roles of those with whom they interact most of the time.

Social roles are a significant component of the social structure. They allow us to anticipate the behavior of others and to respond or pattern our own actions accordingly. The individual acquisition of social roles is a key element in the socialization process. Although Freud presumably never used the concept of role, the end-product of psychosexual development appears to be male and female sex roles (Sales 1978).

Piaget's concern with the development of cognitive and interpretive capabilities seems to stem from the presumption that social roles require such capabilities (Bush and Simmons 1981). Piaget (1970; Piaget and Inhelder 1969) posits three broad stages of cognitive development: sensorimotor, concrete operations, and formal operations. Movement through these stages represents, in part, the shift from being self- or ego-centered to being decentered, and from understanding concrete objects or pairs of objects to comprehending complex relationships. As a result, by about age thirteen or fourteen, the adolescent is presumed capable of grasping social and physical changes without ever seeing the relevant material reality. This ability is crucial because, among other things, "it enables the individual to have affective relationships in which she/he not only realizes that others may have different perspectives from her/his own, but she or he is able to coordinate other's perspectives with her or his own as well" (Bush and Simmons 1981, 139).

George Herbert Mead's (1934) theory of the development of the self also highlights the importance of social roles. According to Mead, the self comprises two parts: the "I" and the "me." The "I" is the spontaneous part of self, the active responder; the "me" is the person's conception of self. How does this differentiated self become a whole? Basically, Mead argues that the self evolves as a function of social interaction with others—social interaction in which the individual takes the role of the other and comes to understand how the social roles encountered are related to one another. For Mead, understanding social roles and being able to assume the role of the other is a basic component of socialization.

While social interaction with others represents external stimuli, internal stimuli may also affect how we learn or acquire social roles. According to Brim (1968), the internal demands of self may be as important as the demands of others and society:

> There may be small but incremental shifts from time to time in what an individual asks of himself, and the resultant day-to-day alterations in his behavior,

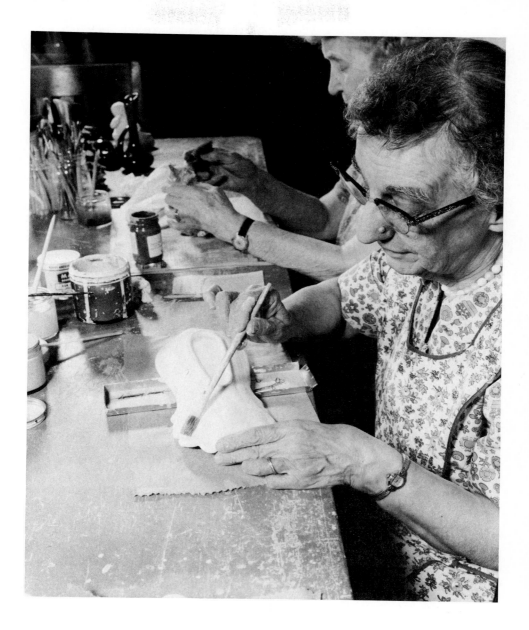

rewarded by himself, lead to a cumulative change which over the years makes him much different from what he was when he was younger . . . until one day he finds himself a person quite different from that of a decade earlier, without knowing how the change occurred. (pp. 191–192)

Old Age and Social Roles

Is old age a social role? Do we have behavioral expectations for those who achieve old age? These are difficult questions to answer. Some have suggested that old age is a formal status or position in our society and that expectations for behavior are attached to that position. Others, arguing that the problems of older people in our society center around the absence of expectations we have for them, have characterized old age as the "roleless role." Clearly, when people become old, when they achieve some chronological or even functional definition of old age, they continue to occupy many of the social roles they occupied during the life course. They continue to be family members, community members and volunteers, and some continue to be employed. Perhaps a more appropriate strategy, then, is to ask, "How does age affect the social roles we occupy?"

As Keith (1982) points out, in many societies, when people can no longer work, they are defined as old; in the United States, the situation is reversed—when people are defined as old, they can no longer work. Thus, in the United States, chronological age is used to mark the border between work and retirement. Age is employed as an eligibility criterion for social roles. At the same time, it makes us ineligible to work but eligible to occupy the status of retiree.

Age also influences our ideas about the appropriateness of certain behaviors. Neugarten (1980), for example, has argued that perceptions in the United States about behaviors appropriate at given ages have relaxed considerably:

> There is no longer a particular year—or even a particular decade—in which one marries or enters the labor market, or goes to school or has children. . . . It no longer surprises us to hear of a 22-year-old mayor or a 29-year-old university president—or a 35-year-old grandmother or a retiree of 50. No one blinks at a 70-year-old college student or at the 55-year-old man who becomes a father for the first time—or who starts a second family. I can remember when the late Justice William Douglas, in old age, married a young wife. The press was shocked and hostile. That hostility would be gone today. People might smirk a little, but the outrage has vanished. (p. 66)

Still, a relaxation of age norms should not be equated with the absence of age norms. As Karp and Yoels (1982) indicate, Americans have fairly rigid ideas concerning who may have intimate sexual relationships with whom. Discrepancies in age between sexual partners is frequently a premise for ridicule. And Justice Douglas notwithstanding, if Grandpa Joe came home one evening and announced his intention to marry a twenty-five-year-old woman he met at the local dance club, he might be facing an institutional commitment hearing by morning!

The age norms that develop in age-homogeneous communities can be quite distinctive. Keith (1977, 1982) lived for one year in Les Floralies, a French retirement residence. An amusing moment came in her fieldwork when she overheard commentary by several French men and women on a patronizing article in the daily newspaper on the benefits of sex for the elderly. This idea was not considered to be revolutionary among the residents of Les Floralies. Not only was sex an acceptable topic for discussion, it was considered an appropriate *activity* for those who wanted it. Further, men and women who shared an apartment, appeared together in public, and were presumed to have a sexual relationship were "married" in the eyes of other residents, even if not in the eyes of French law.

ROLE TRANSITIONS

The Mesakin of the Sudan are obsessed with witchcraft (Nadel 1952). An older man is almost always the alleged witch accused of attempting to harm a younger man. The Mesakin explain this in terms of older men's resentments of the young. One important reason why "old" Mesakin men may be resentful of the young is that they are not chronologically old. In fact, the Mesakin have only three age-grades, and men enter the oldest one in their late twenties. The change in expected behavior when the new grade is entered is quite abrupt. The privileges of youthful vigor—wrestling, spear-fighting, and living in cattle camps—are given up absolutely while the men are physically and chronologically so very young. The abruptness with which men are to make the behavioral changes would seem another reason why there is conflict between Mesakin old and young.

In theory at least, anticipatory socialization can cushion the shock associated with a role or status change such as that just described. *Anticipatory socialization* describes a socialization prior to or preparation for successfully taking on a new role. The concept has been applied to the transition to occupational and professional careers. Medical sociologists, for example, have used the concept to speak to the "training for uncertainty" (Fox 1957) and "loss of idealism" (Becker et al. 1961) experienced by those preparing for entry into the medical profession.

But what good is anticipatory socialization if the behavioral expectations associated with the future role are not visible or clear? Rosow (1974) has argued that many of the problems faced by the old in adjusting to their new roles are caused by the lack of clarity in these roles. Whereas there is much prescribed activity associated with other life transitions, there is little prescribed activity that attends to old age.

Some literature suggests that negative effects of role or status transitions like those experienced by Mesakin men can be offset by rites of passage. *Rites of passage* are rituals that help individuals move from one known social position to another and provide signals to the rest of society that new expectations are appropriate. Ceremonial rituals can be used to mark losses or gains in privilege, responsibility, influence, or power. Typical status passages marked by cere-monial ritual in our own society include that from child to adult (confirmation or bar or bat mitzvah), from high school to college student (graduation), from single to married person (wedding), from worker to retiree (retirement party), and from living person to ancestor (funeral).

Are status changes in our society (like those itemized above) made easier by rites of passage? Foner and Kertzer (1978) offer that most of the evidence for the advantage of such rites of passage comes from studies of non-Western cultures, although some of their own work with African societies shows that the absence of firm rules of transition encourages conflict over the timing of such transitions. Thus, those in powerful positions may attempt to delay cer-emonial rites of passage because they do not want to give up their privileges; those who will gain from the transition make effort to hasten the rites of passage.

Keith (1982, 30) argues that the most distinctive characteristics of rites of passage for old people in the United States is in their absence or incompleteness.

> At most, an older person and the others who have social ties to him or her are offered *exit* signs. The separation phase of a rite of passage may be there in retirement parties or gold watches, but there is no clear pathway back to social reincorporation.

The lack of public ceremonial ritual to mark transitions experienced by the old may be further evidence of their roleless roles. Older people themselves, how-ever, may be creating transition rituals. This is exemplified by the extended retirement trip, which makes it easier to change expectations on return, or the change in residence, which also makes it easier for some to face changed expectations.

The Timing of Role Transitions

In most societies, there appears to be a timetable for the ordering of life events and (almost by definition) role transitions. Describing empirical studies begun by Neugarten and her colleagues in the 1950s, Neugarten and Hagestad (1976) report that interviewees were easily able to respond to questions such as, "What is the best age for a man to marry?" or "What is the best age for a woman to become a grandmother?" There was greatest agreement in response to questions dealing with the timing of major role transitions. For example, most middle-class men and women agreed that the best age for a man to marry was from twenty to twenty-five; most men should be settled in a career by twenty-four to twenty-six; they should hold their top jobs by forty; and, be ready to retire by sixty or sixty-five (Neugarten and Hagestad 1976).

The timing of role transitions is not static. Cohort differences and historical period effects have contributed to changes in the timing of role transitions.

Table 8-2 shows the average age of selected critical life events in the early stages of the family life cycle of ever-married white mothers in five birth cohorts between 1900 and 1949. The mean age at marriage of the 1900 to 1909 cohort is 1.5 years higher than that of the 1940 to 1949 cohort. The average age of a mother at the time of the birth of a first child declined by 2.4 years across these five birth cohorts. These cohorts also completed their childbearing at very different ages. In part, this is explained by differences in the number of children born on average to women in these cohorts. Nevertheless, the fact that these cohorts completed their childbearing in different historical periods cannot be overlooked. Women born between 1940 and 1949 finished childbearing in the 1970s and had, on average, 2.4 children; women born between 1900 and 1909 finished their childbearing in the depression years and averaged 3.0 children.

Schoen and his colleagues (cited in Siegel and Davidson 1984) have developed some measures of important events occurring in later segments of the family life cycle (see Table 8-3). Comparing cohorts born from 1908 to 1912 to those born from 1938 to 1942, they observed a decline in the average duration of a first marriage that is slightly greater for men (28.7 years versus 26.1 years) than for women (29.5 years versus 27.4 years). This decline for men and women is clearly a function of an increase in the proportion of first marriages ending in divorce. Whereas 25 percent of men born between 1908 and 1912 had their first marriage end in divorce, almost 40 percent of those born between 1938 and 1942 had a first marriage end in that fashion.

The mean age at widowhood has increased more dramatically for men (64.5 versus 68.4 years) than for women (64.7 years versus 66.1 years), but the average duration of widowhood has remained about the same (6.6 years for men and 14.3 years for women). It should be remembered that much smaller proportions of husbands outlive their wives than is the case for wives who outlive their husbands. Increases in the mean age at widowhood just described are likely a function of the greater increase in longevity of women over men experienced in the period in question. In addition, to date, the percentage of first marriages

TABLE 8-2   Average Age at Which Selected Critical Life Events Occurred for Ever-Married White Mothers Born between 1900 and 1949

Life Cycle Event	Birth Cohort				
	1940–49	1930–39	1920–29	1910–19	1900–1909
Age at first marriage	20.2	20.6	21.4	22.2	21.7
Age at birth of first child	21.8	22.3	23.6	24.6	24.2
Age at birth of last child	25.4	29.1	31.2	32.5	30.8
Mean number of children	2.4	3.4	3.3	3.0	3.0

Source: Spanier and Glick (1980). Data from June 1975 Marital History Supplement of the Current Population Survey.

TABLE 8-3   Measures of the Marital Life Cycle of Men and Women, for Selected Birth Cohorts: 1908–12 to 1938–42

Item (years)	Males Cohort (year of birth)				Females Cohort (year of birth)			
	1908–12	1918–22	1928–32	1938–42	1908–12	1918–22	1928–32	1938–42
Average age at first marriage	26.2	25.0	23.8	23.3	23.3	22.3	21.1	21.2
Average duration of first marriage	28.7	28.9	28.5	26.1	29.5	29.2	29.7	27.4
Outcome of first marriage (%)								
Divorce	25.1	29.3	33.2	39.4	23.8	27.3	31.5	36.7
Widowhood	22.8	21.1	19.6	17.6	53.0	50.3	48.5	45.1
Death	52.0	49.6	47.3	43.0	23.2	21.2	19.9	18.3
Mean age at								
Widowhood	64.5	66.7	67.8	68.4	64.7	65.6	66.0	66.1
Divorce	40.7	39.7	40.1	38.7	37.4	36.5	37.1	36.5
Mean duration of								
Widowhood	6.6	6.7	6.7	6.6	14.4	14.3	14.4	14.3
Divorce	4.4	4.4	4.5	4.2	8.9	8.7	9.7	9.6

Source: Siegel and Davidson (1984, Table 7-8, p. 97).

ending in widowhood has declined. While 53 percent of women born from 1908 to 1912 had their first marriages end in widowhood, only 45.3 percent of women born from 1938 to 1942 had their marriages end in a similar fashion.

Changes in the timing of role transitions make it more difficult to assess the importance of being "on-time" or "off-time" in taking on new roles or disengaging from old ones. This assessment is further exacerbated by the problem of what Roth (1963) described as "an interacting bundle of career time-tables." This may best be observed in early adulthood where a veritable traffic jam of transitions takes place. Around college campuses in May or June of any year, this compression is highly visible. In a matter of a few short weeks, any number of individuals can be found who are completing an education, marrying, embarking on a career path, settling into a new community, and becoming active in volunteer or civic roles. Presumably such people use the remainder of the life course to rest up from this whirlwind of personal change!

Some authors have suggested that being "off-time" (early or late) in taking on new roles or exiting old ones may create additional stresses. The source of such stresses may be *internal*, emanating from the individual's internalization of age norms, or *external*, from the reactions of peers and or friends (Sales 1978). Blau (1961) found that women who were widowed relatively early and men who retired earlier than their colleagues had greater disruptions in their social relationships than did those women and men for whom the events occurred on time. Unanticipated role displacement also complicates the transition process. Postretirement adjustment is generally more problematic when the withdrawal from work is unexpected (see, for example, Streib and Schneider 1971).

In opposition to the hypothesis that being off-time is stressful, several authors have offered evidence of the benefits of being off-time. Nydegger (1973), for example, has shown that men who were fathers relatively late in life were more effective and more comfortable in the role than those who entered the role early or on-time. One explanation for the greater comfort and effectiveness of these "late" fathers is that the demands of parenthood did not compete with the demands of early career building. Along similar lines, Neugarten and Hagestad (1976) cite interviews carried out by Likert with women returning to school in their middle years. These women saw themselves as having an advantage over younger women because they were "taking one thing at a time" and had fewer role changes to negotiate.

LIFE STRESS AND ADAPTATION

Much of the discussion about the social aspects of aging highlights the stresses associated with role transitions and changing behavioral expectations. The age-linked role transitions that are of particular interest to us here are major life transitions: changes in parent roles as children leave home, grandparenthood, retirement, and widowhood, among others. Coping with the stresses of such transitions and adapting more or less successfully to them is an important element in the life course generally, as well as in achieving successful aging. There are various modes of defending against stressors and various modes of coping. *Coping* describes the behaviors individuals use to prevent, alleviate, or respond to stressful situations (George 1980).

Coping strategies generally take one of two forms: behavioral strategies and cognitive/emotional strategies. Behavioral coping strategies include a wide array of actions that individuals can employ to change or alleviate stress. Personal resources, including finances, health, education, and social supports, provide reserves or aids that individuals may draw upon in a stressful situation. Cognitive/emotional strategies refer to ways in which individuals may employ social psychological mechanisms to deal with stress. Clausen (1986) points out that, although coming to grips with a problem and finding ways of overcoming it tend to have more favorable consequences for the individual, we are beginning to learn that defensive maneuvers such as denial may be quite useful. Thus, he suggests that denial of some deficits brought on by old age may be less problematic for the person than dwelling on those deficits about which nothing can be done.

Pearlin and Schooler (1978) have analyzed the coping strategies individuals employ when they face problems in four areas of life: marriage, parenthood, household economics, and occupational goals and activities. Three broad categories of coping responses were identified: (1) responses that modify situations; (2) responses that are used to reappraise the meaning of problems; and (3) responses that help individuals to manage tension. The researchers found that coping responses employed were often specific to an area of life. Reappraisal was the response of choice in the area of household economics where changes in values or goals were required. In the areas of marriage or parenthood, direct action responses were seen as more valuable and effective.

Are specific coping skills or responses associated with old age? It is generally believed that, throughout adulthood, "individuals develop and refine a repertoire of workable coping strategies that are compatible with their personal dispositions and lifestyles" (George 1980, 34). A number of researchers have put forth specific models of adjustment or adaptation in later life. Several of these are worthy of our attention.

Lieberman and Tobin (Lieberman 1975; Tobin and Lieberman 1976) have examined adaptation to changes in living arrangements among older, impaired people. They suggest that change in residence causes *subjective* stress experienced as a sense of loss and *objective* stress experienced as a disruption of customary behavior patterns. The elements of this conceptual model are depicted in Figure 8-1. The model begins with an assessment of personal resources and current functioning. Three adaptive outcomes are possible: (1) enhanced

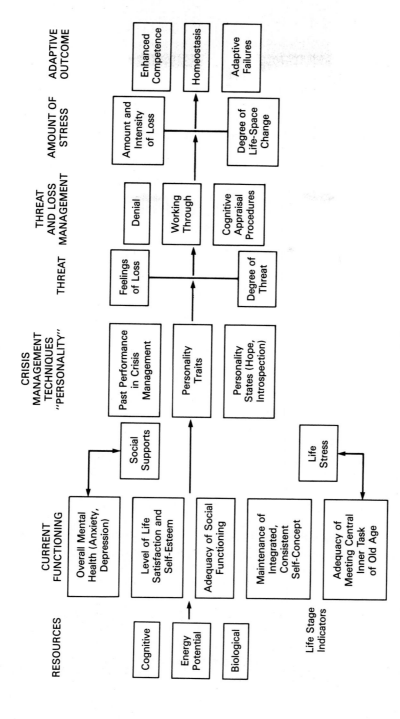

FIGURE 8-1 Lieberman and Tobin's model of adaptation to life crises. *From Adaptive processes in late life, by M. Lieberman. In N. Datan and L. H. Ginsberg (eds.), Life-Span Developmental Psychology: Normative Life Crises. Copyright 1975 by Academic Press, Inc. Reprinted by permission of the publisher.*

competence, in which functioning is improved after a crisis; (2) homeostasis, in which functioning is at the same level before and after a crisis; or (3) adaptive failure, in which functioning is impaired as a result of the crisis. The basic model was applied in four residential relocation studies. Across all the studies, 48 to 56 percent of the subjects experienced adaptive failure. The authors found the degree of environmental change generated by the relocation to be the most important predictor of adaptive outcome: the greater the change, the greater the decline in health or social or psychological functioning among the residents. Perceptions of stress, personal resources, and coping skills seem relatively irrelevant to the adjustment or adaptation process.

Residential relocation is only one event an individual experiences that requires adaptation to change. What if someone experiences other losses or events requiring change in addition to a necessary relocation? According to the *life events model of adaptation* "the normal state of the individual is one of homeostasis and . . . life events that require change are crises to the extent that they require time and energy to return to a steady state of functioning" (Whitbourne 1985, 597). From this perspective, stress is a mediator between an event and adaptation to the event and therefore causes physical and psychological damage in direct proportion to the disruption of an individual's usual life routine. The life events scales have been used to research variation in the impact of events, including having children move out, death of a spouse, and illness, typically experienced by older adults. Age, sex, and socioeconomic status, as well as other personal and social resources, have had a mediating role between such life changes and illness (for example, Pearlin 1980).

The Social Readjustment Rating Scale (SRRS) has become the basic tool to measure stress of life events (Holmes and Rahe 1967). It is a checklist of forty-three events that have been rated with regard to their intensity and the length of time needed to accommodate to them. Scores on the SRRS have generally correlated at a low to moderate level with physical illness and emotional disturbance. Whitbourne (1985) has itemized a series of criticisms of the life events approach, not the least of which has to do with whether life events have differing significance to individuals as they move through the life course.

According to Clausen (1986), the nearest approach to a theoretical statement of the importance of adaptation across the life course is given by Vaillant (1977). Vaillant's essential argument is that "if we are to master conflict gracefully and to harness instinctual striving creatively, our adaptive styles must mature." The devices we employ to protect ourselves as children from painful experiences will not serve us well in adulthood. We must develop mature ways of coping with unacceptable or painful feelings. Thus, each person can be expected to create a unique set of coping strategies to maximize personal happiness and effective functioning. We still know too little about the cumulative effects of stress and the costs and benefits of particular coping strategies employed across the life course.

SUMMARY

The life course perspective is introduced and compared with life-stage and life-span developmental approaches. The life course perspective concentrates on age-related transitions that are socially created, socially recognized, and shared. Life course researchers emphasize the ways in which social norms and definitions influence the sequence of role changes in the life course.

All societies divide the lifetime into different periods of life. Typically, age criteria are used to place people into positions and roles. How many periods or age grades there are in a society may depend on its level of modernization.

Human behavior is primarily learned through a process of socialization. This is a lifelong process that involves transmitting skills and knowledge needed to perform social roles across the life course. The concept of social role describes the expectations we have for individuals who occupy a given social position or status. Is old age a social role in the United States? Some disagreement exists on this point. Age is employed as a criterion for certain social roles, including employment and retirement. Age also influences the ideas we have about the appropriateness of certain behaviors.

In most societies, social role transitions are ordered along a timetable. And the timing of these transitions changes as a function of cohort or historical effects. Role transitions can be stressful, although stresses may be reduced by anticipatory socialization and rites of passage. Keith has argued that the most distinctive characteristics of rites of passage for older people in the United States is in their absence or incompleteness.

Being off-time in taking on new roles or disengaging from old ones may create additional stresses. The source of such stress may be internal or external, personal or social. Several authors have offered evidence of the benefits of being off-time, however.

Coping with transitions and adapting to them are important elements of the life course. There are various modes of defending against stressors and various strategies for coping, although generally these take one of two forms: behavioral or cognitive/emotional. Some coping strategies are problem-specific.

Models of adaptation seem relatively primitive to date. Lieberman and Tobin emphasize the detriment associated with a single significant environmental change. The life events approach emphasizes the aggregate effect of life changes. Vaillant argues for the need for coping strategies to develop or mature as we move through the life course.

STUDY QUESTIONS

1. Distinguish the life course perspective from the life-stage and life-span developmental approaches.

2. Define socialization. Why is early life course socialization insufficient to prepare a person for the role and transitions of adulthood?

3. Freud and Piaget almost certainly did not use the concept of social role. Mead certainly did. Nevertheless, the three major theorists likely would have agreed on the importance of the concept. Why? What is the importance of the concept of social role?

4. Is old age a social role? How does age affect the social roles we occupy?

5. How are status changes in our society made easier by *anticipatory socialization* and *rites of passage*? What does Keith argue is the most distinctive characteristic of rites of passage for old people in the United States? Why?

6. Provide several examples to show that the timing of role transitions is not static in the United States. How do such timing changes make it more difficult to assess the importance of being "on-time" or "off-time" in assuming new roles or exiting old ones?

7. Are specific coping skills associated with old age? What is the importance of environmental change in the Lieberman and Tobin work on adaptation during residential relocation?

8. What is the life events model of adaptation? Do specific life events have the same importance whenever they occur in the life course? What is Vaillant's view of change in adaptive styles through the life course?

BIBLIOGRAPHY

Baltes, P.B., and Goulet, L.R. 1970. Status and issues of a life-span developmental psychology. In L.R. Goulet and P.B. Baltes (eds.), *Life-span developmental psychology.* New York: Academic Press.

Becker, H., Greer, B., Hughes, E.C., and Strauss, A. 1961. *Boys in white: Student culture in medical school.* Chicago: University of Chicago Press.

Berger, J., and Luckman, T. 1966. *The social construction of reality.* Garden City, N.Y.: Doubleday.

Blau, Z. 1961. Structural constraints on friendships in old age. *American Sociological Review* 26:429–439.

Brim, O.G. 1968. Adult socialization. In J.A. Clausen (ed.), *Socialization and society.* Boston: Little, Brown and Co.

Bush, D.M., and Simmons, R.G. 1981. Socialization processes over the life course. In M. Rosenberg and R.H. Turner (eds.), *Social psychology: Sociological perspectives.* New York: Basic Books.

Clausen, J.A. 1986. *The life course: A sociological perspective.* Englewood Cliffs, N.J.: Prentice Hall.

Cowgill, D.O. 1986. *Aging around the world.* Belmont, Calif.: Wadsworth Publishing.

Foner, A., and Kertzer, D. 1978. Transitions over the life course. *American Journal of Sociology* 83:1081–1104.

Fox, R.C. 1957. Training for uncertainty. In R.K. Merton, G. Reader, and P.L. Kendall (eds.), *The student-physician.* Cambridge, Mass.: Harvard University Press.

George, L.K. 1980. *Role transitions in later life.* Monterey, Calif.: Brooks/Cole Publishers.

Hagestad, G.D., and Neugarten, B.L. 1985. Age and the life course. In R.H. Binstock and E. Shanas (eds.), *Handbook of aging and the social science* (2nd ed.). New York: Van Nostrand Reinhold Co.

Hess, B., Markson, E., and Stein, P. 1988. *Sociology* (3d ed.). New York: Macmillan.

Holmes, T.H., and Rahe, R.H. 1967. The Social Readjustment Rating Scale. *Journal of Psychosomatic Research* 11:213–218.

Hughes, C. 1961. The concept and use of time in the middle years: The St. Lawrence Island Eskimo. In R.W. Kleemeier (ed.), *Aging and leisure.* New York: Oxford University Press.

Karp, D.A., and Yoels, W.C. 1982. *Experiencing the life cycle: A social psychology of aging.* Springfield, Ill.: Charles C Thomas.

Keith, J. 1982. *Old people as people: Social and cultural influences on aging and old age.* Boston: Little, Brown and Co.

Keith, J. 1977. *Old people, new lives: Community creation in a retirement residence.* Chicago: University of Chicago Press.

Levinson, D.J., Darro, C.M., Klein, E.B., Levinson, M.H., and McKee, B. 1974. The psychosocial development of men in early adulthood and the mid-life transition. In D.F. Ricks, A. Thomas, and M. Roth (eds.), *Life history research in psychotherapy.* Minneapolis, Minn.: University of Minnesota Press.

Lieberman, M.A. 1975. Adaptive processes in late life. In N. Datan and L.H. Ginsberg (eds.), *Life-span developmental psychology: Normative life crises.* New York: Academic Press.

Linton, R. 1942. Age and sex categories. *American Sociological Review* 7:589–603.

Mead, G.H. 1934. *Mind, self, and society.* Chicago: University of Chicago Press.

Nadel, S.F. 1952. Witchcraft in four African societies. *American Anthropologist* 54:18–29.

Neugarten, B. 1980. Acting one's age: New rules for the old. *Psychology Today* April:66–74, 77–80.

Neugarten, B., and Hagestad, G. 1976. Age and the life course. In R.H. Binstock and E. Shanas (eds.), *Handbook of aging and the social sciences.* New York: Van Nostrand Reinhold Co.

Nydegger, C. 1973. Late and early fathers. Paper presented at the annual meeting of the Gerontological Society, Miami Beach, Florida, October 1973.

Pearlin, L. 1980. Life strains and psychological distress among adults. In N.J. Smelser and E.H. Erikson (eds.), *Themes of work and love in adulthood.* Cambridge, Mass.: Harvard University Press.

Pearlin, L., and Schooler, C. 1978. The structure of coping. *Journal of Health and Social Behavior* 19:2–21.

Piaget, J. 1970. *Structuralism.* New York: Basic Books.

Piaget, J., and Inhelder, B. 1969. *The psychology of the child.* New York: Basic Books.

Rosow, I. 1974. *Socialization to old age.* Berkeley, Calif.: University of California Press.

Roth, J. 1963. *Timetables.* Indianapolis: Robbs-Merrill.

Sales, E. 1978. Women's adult development. In I.H. Frieze, J.E. Parsons, P.B. Johnson, D.N. Ruble, and G.L. Zellman (eds.), *Women and sex-roles: A social psychological perspective.* New York: Norton.

Siegel, J., and Davidson, M. 1984. *Demographic and socioeconomic aspects of aging in the*

United States. Current Population Reports, Special Studies Series P-23, No. 138. Washington, D.C.: U.S. Department of Commerce, Bureau of the Census.

Spanier, G.B., and Glick, P.C. 1980. The life cycles of American families: An expanded analysis. *Journal of Family History* 5(1):98–111.

Streib, G., and Schneider, C.J. 1971. *Retirement in American society: Impact and process*. Ithaca, N.Y.: Cornell University Press.

Tobin, S., and Lieberman, M.A. 1976. *Last home for the aged*. San Francisco, Calif.: Jossey-Bass.

Vaillant, G. 1977. *Adaptation to life*. Boston, Mass.: Little, Brown and Co.

Whitbourne, S.K. 1985. The psychological construction of the life span. In J.E. Birren and K.W. Schaie (eds.), *Handbook of the psychology of aging* (2nd ed.). New York: Van Nostrand Reinhold Co.

Zerubavel, E. 1981. *Hidden rhythms: Schedules and calendars in social life*. Chicago: University of Chicago Press.

CHAPTER 9

SOCIOLOGICAL THEORIES OF AGING

The field of social gerontology has been criticized for its emphasis on the practical issues and problems confronting the elderly. Many scholars believe that this concern, admirable as it may be, has grown at the expense of the development of statements of a theoretical orientation. As a result, these scholar–critics contend, no current comprehensive theoretical framework exists within which to address the question, "What happens to human beings socially as they grow old?"

This is not to say that there have been no attempts to answer this important question. This chapter presents some answers—theoretical statements that we have placed in two broad categories: (1) theories that attempt to conceptualize the adjustment of individuals to their own aging; and (2) theories that deal with the relationship between a society's social system and its older members. Some of these approaches show considerable overlap and often differ only in emphasis.

Readers may have difficulty identifying with the overconcern for theory expressed by gerontologists, perhaps because of a misunderstanding of theory. Most students are accustomed to thinking of theory as boring and not down to earth. Just the opposite is true, however. Theory is the way we accumulate knowledge and make sense of the world. It allows us to see more clearly and logically what we sometimes only vaguely perceive. Strictly speaking, theory differs from vague perception in that it is presented in the form of a generalized statement (or set of systematically organized statements) that can be tested through empirical research.

Theories are created to be rejected. A theory that in principle cannot be rejected is of little use because its acceptance must be on faith. A rejected theory advances the state of the art by reducing the number of possible answers by one. Those theories that survive the rejection process provide, for the present at least, the best answer to a question. In this regard, a theory is never really proven; the next empirical test might always disprove it.

Theorizing in social gerontology has a long way to go. Some of the theories we examine in this chapter are not theories in the strictest sense. Few, for example, are presented in the form of a set of systematically organized statements. Some are more descriptive than explanatory; these might more accurately be referred to as orientations or perspectives rather than theories. None has been sufficiently tested so as to be completely rejected. Each suggests some important factor or set of factors that may be related to aging. In doing so the theories act as continuing guides to further research. The continuation of such research increases the potential for theory building in social gerontology.

AGING AND THE INDIVIDUAL
Role Theory

The earliest attempt in social gerontology to understand the adjustment of the aged individual was placed within a role theory framework (Cottrell 1942). Generally speaking, research done within this framework was concerned with the consequences of role change among older people. The changes individuals undergo in the aging process fall into two categories: the relinquishment of social relationships and roles typical of adulthood; and their replacement by retirement and the acceptance of social relationships typical of the later years, such as dependency on offspring (Cavan et al. 1949).

In an example of empirical research carried out within the role theory framework, Phillips (1957) has shown the relationship between role loss and adjustment to old age. In his study of almost 1,000 individuals aged sixty and over, the retired when compared with the employed, the widowed when compared with the married, and people over seventy when compared with those aged sixty to sixty-nine showed significantly more maladjustment to old age. Maladjustment is measured by self-reports on the amount of time spent daydreaming about the past, thinking about death, and being absent-minded.

Another important variable used by Phillips is labeled "identification as old." This item, a measure of self-image, simply asks, "How do you think of yourself as far as age goes—middle-aged, elderly, old?" Individuals who perceive themselves as elderly or old are significantly more maladjusted than are those who perceive themselves as middle-aged. In addition, age identification appears to reverse the relationship between role loss and maladjustment. Thus, for example, those who are employed but identify themselves as old are more likely to be maladjusted than are those who are retired but identify with middle age. The means by which some elderly individuals, even those who have suffered role loss, identify with middle age are still open to empirical investigation.

Recently, several researchers have looked at the relationship between sex roles and life satisfaction in old age. Sex role differentiation has traditionally been quite strong in U.S. society. Men are expected to be aggressive and independent whereas women are expected to be passive-dependent and nurturant. Sinnott (1977), after reviewing many studies on middle and old age, came to the conclusion that survival and satisfaction in old age often accompany flexibility in sex roles.

Reichard, Livson, and Peterson (1962) studied how eighty-seven men between the ages of fifty-five and eighty-four adjusted to aging. The best adjusted exhibited personalities *not* dominated by male traits. Reichard and her colleagues concluded that growing old may make it possible for a man to integrate formerly unacceptable feminine traits (for example, nurturance or passivity) into his personality. Their research shows that those most able to make the integration are rewarded by a more successful old age. Similarly, Neugarten and her associates (1964) found older men and women who were the most satisfied with life to be those who had best achieved an integration of traits culturally defined as masculine with traits culturally defined as feminine.

While studying the structure of self-concept, Monge (1975) found certain continuities as well as discontinuities across the life cycle. Over 4,000 male and female subjects, aged nine to eighty-nine and recruited from diverse sources, rated the concept "My Characteristic Self" on twenty-one polar adjective pairs (for example, leader–follower or strong–weak). Four factors emerged for all age groups: achievement/leadership; congeniality/sociability; adjustment (the self-perception of health and energy); and, masculinity/femininity. Figure 9-1 shows the mean component scores for these four factors by age group and sex. Monge's results suggest that, as men and women become older, they become more *androgynous*—more alike and, perhaps, more accepting of opposite sex traits in themselves.

For example, as Figure 9-1b depicts, congeniality/sociability is higher at all points in the life-span for women than for men, though both show a decrease at midlife and a subsequent increase in later adulthood. Importantly, men and women are most alike in terms of mean scores on this factor (and all others) in old age. The increase in late adulthood, steeper in men, may reflect the lifting of certain burdens of concern in the area of work responsibilities and may allow more time for social interaction.

Clearly, more research on sex role change across the life course needs to be carried out. In particular, we need to learn more about the blurring of sex roles in old age. Some of the aforementioned research suggests that certain aspects of sex role identification may be less integral to adult personality in later life than may be the case for early adulthood.

Activity Theory

One theory of aging related to role theory has appeared implicitly in much gerontological research. This theory, referred to here as *activity theory* but often called the *implicit theory of aging,* states that there is a positive relationship

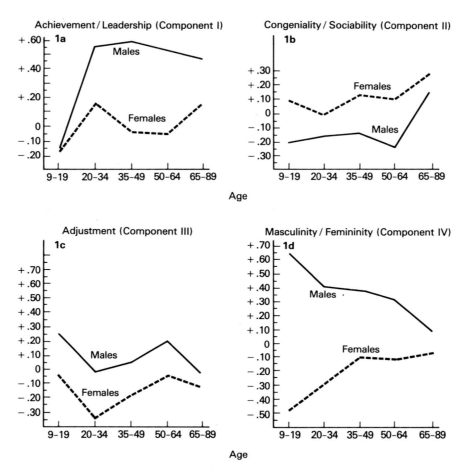

FIGURE 9-1   Factors of self-concept across the adult life span: Mean component scores on four components by age group and sex. *Source: Monge, R.H. 1975. Structure of the self-concept from adolescence through old age. Experimental Aging Research 1(2):281–291.* © *Beech Hill Publishing Company (formerly EAR, Inc.).*

between activity and life satisfaction. This theory holds that, although aging individuals face inevitable changes related to physiology, anatomy, and health status, psychological and social needs remain essentially the same. Those who adopt this view recognize that the social world may withdraw from older people, making it more difficult for them to fulfill these needs. Yet the person who ages optimally is the one who stays active and manages to resist the withdrawal of the social world (Havighurst 1968). According to this theory, the individual who is able to maintain the activities of the middle years for as long as possible will be well adjusted and satisfied with life in the later years.

This person will find an avocation to substitute for work and will replace the old friends and loved ones who have died with new ones.

Lemon, Bengtson, and Peterson (1972) have attempted a formal and explicit test of the activity theory. Using a sample of 411 potential in-movers to a southern California retirement community, and distinguishing among informal activity (with friends, relatives, and neighbors), formal activity (participation in voluntary organizations), and solitary activity (maintenance of household), they found that only social activity with friends was significantly related to life satisfaction. Knapp's (1977) study of fifty-one elderly people residing in the south of England lends support to these findings. Within this sample, there was a strong positive relationship between "the number of hours spent in a typical week with friends and relatives (informal activity)" and life satisfaction. In addition, several measures of formal activity were also found to be strongly related to life satisfaction.

Recently, Longino and Kart (1982) reported on the results of a formal replication of the work on activity theory carried out by Lemon and his team. Using probability samples from three distinct types of retirement communities (N = 1,209), they found support for the positive contribution made by informal activity to the life satisfaction of respondents. Interestingly, they observed formal activity to have a *negative* effect on life satisfaction. Longino and Kart speculated that participation in formal activities may damage self-concept and lower morale through the development of status systems that tend to emerge in formal activity settings. Invidious comparisons that can lead to dissatisfaction are less likely to operate in primary relationships with family and friends than in secondary ones limited to formal organizational settings.

Activity theory is often presented in juxtaposition with the disengagement theory of aging, which will be discussed at some length. Such a presentation leads to comparison of the theories and often causes students to overlook problems that may be internal to the theory. There are several theoretical problems inherent in the activity approach, which deserve some mention here.

First, the activity perspective assumes that individuals have a great deal of control over their social situations. It assumes that people have the capacity to construct—or, more appropriately, reconstruct—their lives by substituting new roles for lost ones. Clearly, this may be the case for the upper-middle class individual whose locus of control has always been internal and whose social and economic resources allow for such reconstruction. But the retired individual who suffers a dramatic decline in income, or the widow who faces an equally dramatic decline in her social relationships, may find it difficult, even with sufficient motivation, to substitute an avocation for work or to replace old friends and loved ones who have died.

Second, the activity perspective emphasizes the stability of psychological and social needs through the adult phases of the life cycle. This makes considerable sense if one thinks about these needs developing in a stable social and physical environment. But what about the person whose environment changes at a particular age, for example, when he or she retires, is deprived of status, or is widowed? Might this individual's social and psychological needs change in the face of the substantial change in environment? Many would answer yes. A no answer smacks of a biological or psychological determinism, which many social scientists (including gerontologists) find unacceptable.

Finally, an important problem in activity theory is the expectation that activities *of any kind* can substitute for lost involvement in areas of life such as work, marriage, and parenting. Weiss (1969), in his study of the Parents Without Partners (PWP) organization, dubbed this the "fund of sociability" hypothesis. According to this idea, people require a certain *quantity* of interaction with others and may achieve this in a variety of ways—through one or two intense relationships or perhaps through a larger number of lesser relationships. Weiss was not able to substantiate this hypothesis. He found that the "sociability" that accrued to a person through participation in the PWP organization did not necessarily compensate for the marital loss. This suggests that substitutability for different losses may be governed by different considerations. Filling a particular role may not do. Fulfillment of those particular needs may be accomplished only through specific role substitution or, perhaps, through the alteration of a person's entire configuration of roles. Whichever is the case, the emphasis here is on the quality rather than the quantity of such interaction.

Disengagement Theory

Disengagement theory, put forth by Cumming and Henry (1961), stands in contrast to the role theory and activity theory approaches. Using data based on 275 respondents ranging in age from fifty to ninety, all of whom resided in Kansas City and were physically and financially self-sufficient, these authors characterized the decreasing social interaction they observed to come with old age as a *mutual withdrawal* between the aging individual and others in the social system to which he or she belongs. Under the terms of the disengagement theory, the aging individual accepts—perhaps even desires—the decreased interaction. In addition, the proponents of this theory argue that gradual disengagement is functional for society, which would otherwise be faced with disruption by the sudden withdrawal of its members. As Cumming (1963) has stated it:

> The disengagement theory postulates that society withdraws from the aging person to the same extent as the person withdraws from society. This is, of course, just another way of saying that the process is normatively governed and in a sense agreed upon by all concerned.

In its original form, the disengagement theory was concerned with the modal case in the United States. Important disengagements included the departure of children from families and retirement for men or widowhood for women. It was not concerned with nonmodal cases—early widowhood or late retirement—nor was it concerned with the special effects of poverty or illness. In 1963, Elaine Cumming, one of the originators of disengagement theory, published a paper in which she discussed the relationship between personality (or what she called "temperament") and disengagement. She wrote that all people have a style of adaptation to the environment, and she went on to identify two different modes of interacting with the environment: the "impinging" mode and the "selecting" mode. The impinger is an activist, willing to try out his or her style of adaptation on others, whereas the selector is more measured in his or her ways. Each may react differently to disengagement. As Cumming (1963) describes it, the impinger's judgment may not be as good as it was, but he is likely to be viewed as an unusual person for his age.

> Ultimately, as he becomes less able to control the situations he provokes, he may suffer anxiety and panic through failure both to arouse and to interpret appropriate reactions. His problem in old age will be to avoid confusion.

The selector can be expected to be more measured in his or her ways. As a youth, this individual may have appeared to others as withdrawn. With age, this style seems more appropriate.

> In old age, because of his reluctance to generate interaction, he may, like a neglected infant, develop a kind of marasmus. His foe will be apathy rather than confusion. (Cumming 1963)

Finally, in summarizing the disengagement theory it is useful to point out that in the initial presentation of the theory Cumming and Henry argued that the process of disengagement was both *inevitable* and *universal*. All social systems, if they were to maintain successful equilibrium, would necessarily disengage from the elderly. Disengagement was seen as a prerequisite to social stability. "When a middle-aged, fully engaged person dies, he leaves many broken ties, and disrupted situations. Disengagement thus frees the old to die without disrupting vital affairs" (Cumming 1963, 384–385).

The disengagement theory has generated much critical discussion. Many have found the theory wanting and indefensible, yet others defend it quite strenuously. Through the 1960s and 1970s, most research efforts were unable to offer empirical support for the theory. Youmans (1967) found that a sample of the rural aged did not in general experience disengagement. Palmore (1968) interviewed 127 individuals who were an average age of seventy-eight. He found little to support the notion that disengagement necessarily increases with age. Other researchers have suggested possible modifications of the disengagement theme. For example, Tallmer and Kutner (1970) found that physical and social stress, rather than aging per se, often produces disengagement. Atchley's (1971) study of emeritus professors showed that individuals could disengage socially without psychological disengagement.

The controversy surrounding disengagement continues. Hochschild (1975) has examined the theory and found three problems that she believes continue to fire the controversy. First, Hochschild argues that the disengagement theory allows no possibility for counterevidence. She points out that in their original work, entitled *Growing Old,* Cumming and Henry offered four types of "back door" explanations to handle cases that did not fit the theory. These types included "unsuccessful" disengagers, those whose disengagement was "off schedule," exceptional individuals who had reengaged, and those who were offered as examples of "variation in the form" of disengagement.

Second, the major variables in the theory —age and disengagement—turn out to be "umbrella" variables which are divisible into numerous other promising variables. Earlier, we made reference to one study that distinguished between social and psychological disengagement. Carp (1969) distinguishes among types of social disengagement, including disengagement from family, friends, social activities, and material possessions. Similarly, in discussing psychological disengagement, one can differentiate among personal adjustment, ego energy, "affect intensity," mastery, and so on. As Hochschild points out, one consequence of this continual fission is that theoretical propositions that once appeared quite simple grow into something much more complex.

Third, the disengagement theory essentially ignores the aging person's own view of aging and disengagement. Behavior that looks like disengagement to the observer may have a completely different meaning for the aging person. Based on his exploratory study of retirement among ninety-nine English couples, Crawford (1971) advances three types of meaning that men attribute to retirement: retiring *back to* something, retiring *from* something, and retiring *for* something. In the first and third types, men view their retirement in terms of continued engagement with new involvements—in the latter case, discarding past obligations to work and building a new social life outside of work; in the former, giving up work and returning to the family. Despite the objective disengagement (retirement), the men attribute different means to the event.

The activity and disengagement perspectives have dominated the theoretical discussion for the last twenty years in social gerontology, but several alternative perspectives have recently been put forth. Three somewhat related theories that deserve mention are the socioenvironmental theory, the exchange theory of aging, and symbolic interactionism. None of the three has as yet received the research attention required for determining its explanatory power.

Socioenvironmental Theory

Socioenvironmental theory directs itself at understanding the effects of the immediate social and physical environment on the activity patterns of aged individuals. The chief proponent of this theory is Jaber Gubrium (1973, 1975). Although other gerontologists have clearly concerned themselves with the environments of old people, Gubrium concerns himself with the meaning old people place on life and with the effect different physical and social contexts may have on that meaning. This approach is based on the understanding that persons respond to the social meaning of events rather than to some "absolute" aspect of these events. Moreover, the responses of persons to the same event might easily be different if the social meaning placed on the event by one varies from the meaning placed on that event by the other.

According to Gubrium (1973), two factors that affect the meaning old people place on events—and, thus, their interaction patterns—are the physical proximity of other persons and the age-homogeneity of an environment. A substantial body of literature supports the importance of these two variables in affecting social interaction among both young and old. For example, Rosow's (1967) seminal work on the aged in Cleveland shows that old people residing in apartment buildings with a high concentration of aged people were more likely to develop friendships with neighbors than was the case for old people residing in buildings with a low concentration of elderly.

A number of studies show the relationship between age-homogeneity and friendship patterns. Bultena and Wood (1969) found that with a population of elderly retired males, friendships occurred primarily among persons of the same age. Messer (1967) found that the elderly, in age-homogeneous public housing projects in Chicago, interacted more frequently than did elderly living in age-heterogeneous settings.

On the basis of the possible contributions of the two variables, physical proximity and age homogeneity, Gubrium (1973) developed a typology of social contexts, each of which, he suggests, has differential impact on social interaction. Figure 9-2 presents this typology.

Socioenvironmental theory posits that Type I social contexts have the highest degree of age-concentration and are thus quite conducive to social inter-

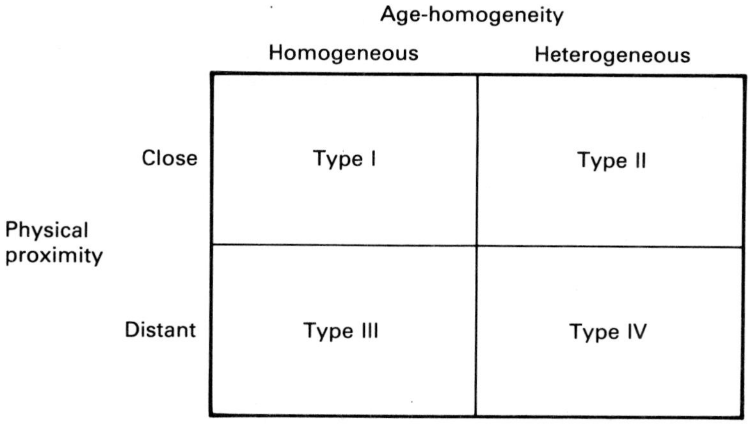

| | Age-homogeneity | |
	Homogeneous	Heterogeneous
Close	Type I	Type II
Distant	Type III	Type IV

(Physical proximity)

FIGURE 9-2   Types of Social Contexts. *Source: Gubrium, J. The Myth of the Golden Years: A Socio-Environmental Theory of Aging, p. 31, 1973. Courtesy of Charles C Thomas, Publisher, Springfield, Illinois.*

action. Residential apartment buildings for the elderly are the Type I variety. Individuals living in such environments hold age-linked behavior expectations for each other. Type IV social contexts are the least age-concentrated and offer reduced opportunity for initiating interaction. These social contexts include age-heterogeneous neighborhoods of single homes. Type II contexts, represented by age-heterogeneous apartment buildings, and Type III contexts, represented by retirement communities commonly found in Florida and California, fall between Types I and IV in terms of their conduciveness to social interaction.

Of utmost importance to the socioenvironmental theory is the recognition that different social contexts generate different sets of activity norms for aged people. To the extent such norms place behavioral demands on individuals, it becomes clear that different social contexts place different demands on the elderly. Gubrium suggests that individuals who have the resources (health, financial solvency, and social support) to meet the demands of the environment will show high morale and self-satisfaction. Incongruence between environmental expectations and activity resources leads to low morale and diminished life satisfaction.

Exchange Theory

An abundance of gerontological literature has consistently shown that older Americans receive regular support from family, friends, and neighbors in carrying out activities of daily living (Shanas 1979; Stoller and Earl 1983; Sussman 1976). This support may be task-oriented and includes help with housework, shopping, transportation, and the like. Support may also take the form of social or emotional assistance provided in times of stress or illness. This literature also reminds us that older people may themselves be support providers, helping family members or neighbors deal with instrumental or emotional problems (Riley and Foner 1968; Sussman 1976).

Informal helping or social support networks, especially those that involve a "reciprocal flow of valued behavior between the participants" (Emerson 1976), may easily be placed within an exchange approach to social interaction. Such an approach views social interaction as governed by rules of fairness or "justice." Gouldner (1960) identified one rule of exchange as the "norm of reciprocity." According to him, this norm establishes a set of reciprocal demands and obligations that lend stability to social systems. One component of the norm of reciprocity is that "people should help those who have helped them" (Gouldner 1960, 171).

Gouldner recognized that the norm of reciprocity requiring an exchange of good for good is not the only rule regulating social interaction. In fact, he proposed what could be described as a norm of beneficence which requires that individuals help others as necessary without thought to what the others have done or can do in return. Gouldner is not alone in recognizing that such nonrational impulses are important components in the broader social intercourse. Almost by definition, there are groups in society who are identified by their incapacity to engage in strict exchange. The mentally handicapped represent one such group. For them, beneficence supersedes reciprocity as the prevailing norm.

Recently, Dowd (1984) has suggested that in our relations with the very old, the requirements of reciprocity may have been superseded by those of beneficence. This shift, he argues, results from a redefinition of age strata that itself has emerged from a need to reallocate scarce policy resources in the society at large. In effect, Dowd believes that the norm of reciprocity will still apply to younger-old people, who receive in social policy terms what is perceived to be something in balance with the value of their current social worth. Policy treatment of the very old, Dowd expects, will be regulated by a principle of beneficence—every person or household will receive as much as is needed, regardless of the value attached to their current social worth.

Homans (1958, 1974) suggests another rule of exchange. He argues that social exchange is governed by a rule of "distributive justice." This rule is defined in terms of the relationship between actors' rewards and costs: the greater the costs, the greater the rewards. Actors are seen as trying to strike a balance, or achieve proportionality, in social exchange. As Homans indicates, "Persons that give much to others try to get much from them, and persons that get much from others are under pressure to give much to them. This process of influence tends to work out at equilibrium to balance in the exchanges." According to Homans, when individuals experience imbalance or distributive injustice, when they give more than they get (or get more than they give), they are offended and experience dissatisfaction.

Dowd (1975, 1978, 1980) has attempted to place aging within an exchange framework. He believes that the problems of the aged in twentieth-century industrial societies are in reality problems of decreasing power. Dowd argues that in social exchanges between the aged and society the aged gradually lose power until all that is left is the capacity to comply. The shift in balance of power between the aged and society reflects the economic and social dependency of the elderly. More than any other event, the phenomenon of retirement seems to exemplify this decline in power. The worker who once exchanged his or her skill for wages must comply with retirement in exchange for pension and health-care benefits.

Recently, Kart and Longino (1987) carried out what they believe to be a definitive test of distributive justice within the context of aged social exchange networks. In 1977, 1,346 persons residing in diverse settings were interviewed in the Social Security Administration's Midwestern Retirement Community Study (Longino 1980). Respondents were asked to list all the persons who were important in their lives, up to as many as fifteen persons. The respondents were then asked what each of these persons did on a more or less regular basis that the respondent really appreciated. Next the relationship was reversed, and the respondents were asked what they themselves did for each person on the list, on an ongoing basis, that was important to the latter.

Students of social support research have suggested that many researchers emphasize the *amount* of support at the expense of the *types* of support being received and given (Thoits 1982). Thus, supportive activities, given and received, were coded into one of three possible categories: emotional, social, and instrumental. In addition, each individual was assigned a score based on responses to thirteen items drawn from the Life Satisfaction Scale B (Neugarten, Havighurst, and Tobin 1961). Finally, each respondent was asked to summarize his or her relationships in terms of how obligated they felt generally toward others.

Initially, Kart and Longino examined the amount of support given and received as they separately predict life satisfaction and feelings of obligation. The amount of support the respondents *received* as well as the support *given*, regardless of type, had little apparent effect upon feelings of obligation to others. Correlations between the support measures and life satisfaction showed a different pattern. Low inverse correlations were present between all types of support given, emotional and social support received, and life satisfaction. Thus, the more support given *or* received, the lower the life satisfaction.

The reciprocal supportive relationship between the respondent and each primary relation was also examined. Within each support type, a ratio of support given to support received was calculated. The retirement community residents, as a whole, had a ratio above 1.0 for each type of support, indicating that they tended to receive more support than they gave. The associations between support ratios and feelings of obligation, however, were weak to nonexistent, nor did the reciprocal imbalance seem to affect the level of life satisfaction.

Kart and Longino conclude that, when actual reciprocal exchange relationships are examined, the exchange paradigm does not operate as straightforwardly between older people and those significant to them as other exchange theorists might have predicted (see Dowd 1978, for example). Only the support *given* by older respondents in their primary relationships seems to be systematically and inversely related to life satisfaction. And, even here, the correlations were quite modest by any standard. One conclusion to draw from these empirical results is quite simply that the exchange theory fails to explain the relationship between support systems and the well-being or life satisfaction of older persons. Of course, leaping to such a conclusion may throw out the baby with the bath water. As Ward (1985) points out, the literature on the contributions of support systems to well-being in later life is equivocal. For example, Conner and his colleagues (1979) found that both the number and frequency of social ties were unrelated to life satisfaction among the elderly. Ward and his associates (1984) reported only a weak relationship between access to instrumental and expressive supports (through involvement with kin, friends, and neighbors) and overall morale.

When attempting to explain the contributions of social support systems to the life satisfaction of older people, the exchange theory makes good sociological as well as intuitive sense. In part, this is because it dovetails nicely with at least two other long-standing sociological traditions that address the relationship between social support and feelings of well-being. Both symbolic interactionism (see below) and Durkheimian anomie theory posit that social interaction with others can provide a basis for psychological good feeling (Thoits 1982). An advantage of formalizing theory is that it facilitates replication and reformulation by other researchers. More seems to be gained at this point by encouraging additional replications and reformulations of exchange theory in a gerontological context than by premature rejection of the theory.

Aging and Symbolic Interactionism

According to Herbert Blumer (1969), the theoretical framework known as *symbolic interactionism* is based on the premise that people behave toward objects (including other people) according to perceptions and meanings developed through social interaction. From this perspective, individuals are seen as conscious actors in the world who adapt to situations and events on the basis of the perceptions and meanings they have constructed for these situations and events. It is important to note that perceptions and meanings are not constructed in a vacuum. Rather, as Blumer (1969) points out, they arise out of social interaction with others:

> Human beings in interacting with one another have to take account of what each is doing or is about to do; they are forced to direct their own conduct or handle their situations in terms of what they take into account. Thus, the activities of others enter as positive factors in the formation of their own conduct; in the face of actions of others one may abandon an intention or purpose, revise it, check or suspend it, intensify it, or replace it. The actions of others enter to set what one plans to do, may oppose or prevent such plans, may require a revision of such plans, and may demand a very different set of such plans. One has to *fit* one's own line of activity in some manner to the actions of others. (p. 8)

The importance of social interaction cannot be exaggerated for the symbolic interactionist. The emphasis in this theoretical perspective is on the human capacity for *socially* constructing reality.

In recent years, symbolic interactionism has been seen as having important implications for the study of aging. At one level, it may provide a basis for understanding how older people perceive and assign meaning to the experience of "old age" in U.S. society (or in any other society, for that matter). Ward (1984), for example, sees the symbolic interactionist perspective as essential to recognizing the importance of change in the social and symbolic worlds of the aging. He argues that role losses, residential mobility, health problems, and other age-related changes pull the elderly from familiar groups and situations. Thus, they may become alienated from past worlds and identities and, at the same time, be granted the potential for new worlds and new identities. This creates the possibility of satisfying personal change and growth, but also may result in stress, marginality, and unhappiness (Ward 1984, 360).

Spence (1986) has explored the implications of the symbolic interactionist perspective for understanding developmental issues of later life. From his view, this perspective is unique because it emphasizes the subjective and focuses on process and change in identity as one develops. Where one is going is secondary to the processes of getting there (Spence 1986). Marshall (1979) has applied the symbolic interactionist perspective to aging through his use of the concept of *status passage*. To speak of aging as a status passage is to suggest the image of an individual negotiating a passage from one age-based status to another (and, perhaps, to others), finally coming to the end of the passage through life, at death.

A status passage may have both an objective as well as a subjective reality. Objectively, any status passage can be defined in terms of a series of dimensions, including the following: physical or social time and space; duration; and the extent to which it is desirable or undesirable, inevitable or optional, voluntary or involuntary. Subjectively, as Marshall indicates, awareness of any of the above properties of the passage may vary. Thus, people may differ in their degree of awareness that they are even undergoing a passage. For the symbolic interactionist, the objective and subjective dimensions of the status passage set the parameters within which the lives of individuals (in this context, aging individuals) will be shaped by themselves. The degree of control over the passage becomes of central importance for aging persons. This is particularly the case for this status passage because, unlike others, it offers no exit from the passage except through death. Other passages in life involve preparation for something to come. Here, however, the passage is all there is. As Marshall (1979) indicates, "No future lies beyond the passage, only the passage and its termination become relevant. . . ."

One theme of this status passage, according to Marshall, is that preparation for death involves the attempt to make sense of death itself as well as to make sense of one's life. This theme appears in psychoanalytic theory and in Butler's concept of *life review* (see Chapter 7). An important difference for symbolic interactionists is their recognition that control over one's own biography involves reconstruction of the past through reminiscence. Marshall (1979) argues this process is most successful when it is conducted socially. Unfortunately, as Marshall sees it, "socializing agents," such as institutional settings (including hospitals, nursing homes, and retirement communities), may severely threaten an aged person's ability to maintain control of the status passage. Too often, status passage control becomes a dilemma for the aging individual who must choose between allowing others to shape their passages, on the one hand, and isolation on the other. This decision is most obvious in cases where others employ criteria for desired behavior that contradict the attempts of the aging person to maintain personal control (Marshall 1979).

Much more empirical research must be done to determine fully the utility of the symbolic interactionist paradigm in social gerontology. Still, we can be optimistic about any framework that suggests that older people retain the human capacity to construct and share meanings and the human tendency to attempt to assert control over their own lives.

AGING AND SOCIETY
The Subculture of the Aging

In an attempt to clarify the nature of relations between older persons and the rest of society, Rose (1965) offered the concept of an *aged subculture*. A subculture may develop when particular members of a society interact with each other significantly more than they do with others in the society. This pattern of interaction may develop when group members have common backgrounds and interests and are excluded from interaction with other population groups in the society. Rose believed that both circumstances exist for the large proportion of older people in U.S. society.

In addition, Rose outlines a variety of demographic, ecological, and social organizational trends that contribute to the development of an aged subculture. These include the growing number and proportion of persons who live beyond the age of sixty-five; the self-segregation of older persons in inner cities and rural areas (caused by migration patterns of the young); the decline in employment of older people; and the development of social services designed to assist older people. Each of these trends either improves the opportunities for older people to identify with each other or separates them from the rest of society.

Rose recognized that not all the distinctive behavior of the elderly can be attributed to the aged subculture. Biological changes, society's expectations for the elderly, and generational differences in socialization all contribute to making the elderly more segregated from other age categories than is true for the rest of society.

What of the content of this aged subculture? According to Rose, the status system among the elderly is only partially a carryover from that of the general society. Wealth carries over from the general culture, as do occupational prestige, achievement, and education, although with some lessening in importance. Physical and mental health and social activity, usually taken as given by younger people, have special value in conferring status among the elderly.

What are the consequences of the development of an aged subculture? Rose discusses two areas: the aging self-conception and aging group consciousness. Rose argues that many Americans suffer a change in self-conception as they

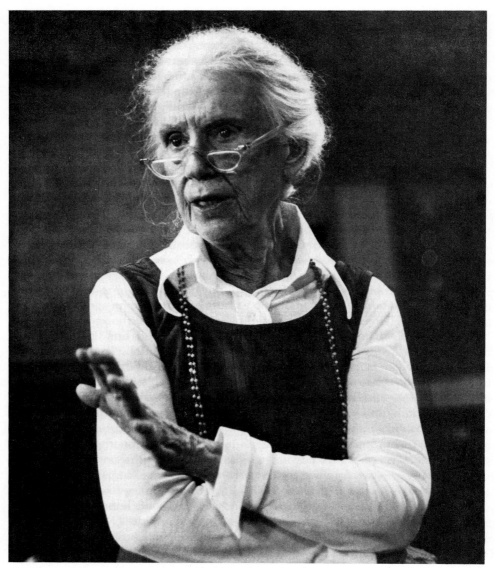

Maggie Kuhn, convenor and founder of the Gray Panthers

grow older, largely as a consequence of the negative evaluation of old age in U.S. culture. Unfortunately, the development of an aged subculture does not necessarily combat this negative evaluation. Rather, it may simply facilitate identification as old. This is a negative consequence of the development of an aged subculture. On the positive side, development of an aged subculture may stimulate a group identification and consciousness, with potential for social action. Rose envisioned older people becoming a voting bloc that exerts political power either within the existing political party structures or on its own.

Despite some debate in the gerontological literature about whether or not the elderly fit a traditional definition of a subculture (Streib 1965), the notion of an aged subculture has served as a useful descriptive guide to the relationship between older persons and the rest of U.S. society. Nevertheless, its predictive power generally has been found wanting (Hendricks and Hendricks 1986). Recently, however, one research team has attempted to test Rose's aged sub-culture hypothesis. Longino, McClelland, and Peterson (1980) compared elderly residents of eight midwestern retirement communities (five age-segregated res-idential settings and three age-concentrated neighborhoods) with a shadow sample of elderly respondents drawn from the Harris general population survey discussed in Chapter 2. The shadow sample involved a random selection of older people in such a way as to replicate or shadow the characteristics of residents of the retirement communities. For example, for every widowed black woman over age seventy-five with an elementary school education and living on less than $2,000 a year in a retirement community, a person with the same profile was placed in the shadow sample. Comparisons were made using mea-sures of social participation, preferences for age-based interaction, general per-ceptions of elders, and self-conception.

The study provided partial support for Rose's subculture of aging theory. On the whole, residents of the retirement communities show a distinctive pattern of responses to the measures of comparison employed. In matters of social participation, differences show up more in quality than quantity. The social life of retirement community residents appears no more strenuous than elsewhere, but residents find this level of activity more satisfying. Problems of being lonely and bored and not feeling needed seem easier to avoid in retire-ment communities than in more age-integrated settings. The self-conceptions of retirement community residents are mixed. Although the residents tend to have significantly greater self-regard than do their shadow samples in judging their own characteristics, they do not surpass shadow sample respondents in judging themselves as useful members of their communities. Community res-idents are also significantly more likely to say that older people get just the right amount of respect, or even too much. In effect, this suggests that retire-ment community residents see themselves in less positive terms than they think the society sees them. Finally, according to the authors of this study, evidence for the development of an aging group political consciousness, at least as Rose envisioned it, was nowhere to be found.

Although Longino, McClelland, and Peterson admit that aging group con-sciousness exists in some local settings among the elderly, they point out that it may not necessarily arise in response to age-segregated residence. Further, they suggest that, as applied to retirement communities, aged subculture theory may need modification to take account of this essentially retreatist phenomenon.

Modernization Theory

In the book *Aging and Modernization,* Cowgill and Holmes (1972) developed a theory of aging in cross-cultural perspective. As the theory emerged, and subsequently in revision (Cowgill 1974), it described the relationship between modernization and the changes in role and status of older people. The theory was originally expressed in twenty-two propositions. Stated tersely, however, it held that with increasing modernization the status of older people declines. This declining status is reflected in reduced leadership roles, power, and influence, as well as increased disengagement of older people from community life.

In the initial presentation of the theory, the definition of modernization was somewhat elusive. Later, Cowgill (1974, 127) put forth an explicit definition of the concept:

> Modernization is the transformation of a total society from a relatively rural way of life based on animate power, limited technology, relatively undifferentiated institutions, parochial and traditional outlook and values, toward a predominantly urban way of life based on inanimate sources of power, highly developed scientific technology, highly differentiated institutions matched by segmented individual roles, and a cosmopolitan outlook which emphasizes efficiency and progress.

In addition, Cowgill argued that no part of the society is left untouched, and that all change, although not uniform, is unidirectional (that is, it always moves from the rural form to the urban form).

Four subsidiary aspects of modernization were identified as salient to the conditions of older people in a society: (1) scientific technology as applied in economic production and distribution; (2) urbanization; (3) literacy and mass education; and (4) health technology. Each of these aspects of modernization helps produce the lower status of older people in society (Cowgill 1974).

Figure 9-3 presents, in schematic form, the modernization theory as revised by Cowgill. Briefly, the causal sequences depicted in the figure can be described as follows:

1. The application of health technology—including public health measures, nutrition, and all aspects of curative and surgical medicine—dramatically affects the age structure of a society so that there is an aging of the population. This comes about through a prolongation of adult life as well as a decline in the birth rate. The theory argues that within the context of an industrialized society with emphasis on youth and new occupations, the extension of adult life leads to an intergenerational competition for jobs. Therefore, older people are forced out of the labor market; they retire. Because they are denied participation in the work ethic, the elderly experience reductions in monetary income, prestige, and honor, and thus decrement in status.

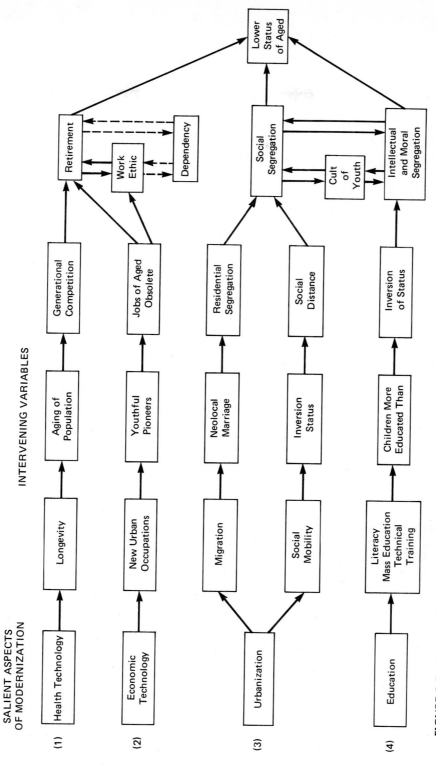

FIGURE 9-3 Aging and modernization. *Source: Cowgill, D. Aging and modernization: A revision of the theory, in Gubrium, J., ed., Late Life: Communities and Environmental Policies, 1974. Courtesy of Charles C Thomas, Publisher, Springfield, Illinois.*

2. The application of economic and industrial technology leads to new occupations located increasingly in an urban setting. Geographically and socially mobile youth migrate to these jobs. Older people are left in positions that are less prestigious and often obsolete. The lack of opportunities for retraining (especially in rural areas) leads to early retirement. This retirement, accompanied by loss of income, may also bring a reversal of traditional family and community roles. Formerly, the young were dependent on the old; now the old suffer dependency.

3. Urbanization, including the separation of work from home and the geographical separation of youthful urban migrants from their parental homes, profoundly changes the nature of intergenerational relations. Residential segregation of the generations changes the bonds of familial association, increases social distance between generations, and, with upward mobility among the young, leads to a reduced status of the aged. This effect is compounded by retirement and dependency.

4. The promotion of literacy and education (almost always targeted at the young in modernization efforts) generates a situation in which children are more literate and have greater skill than their parents do. This imbalance has the effect of inverting roles in the traditional society: The child's generation has higher status than the parents', and children occupy positions in the community formerly held by their parents. The increasing social change brought by that modernization widens the gap between the generations, thus causing an intellectual and moral separation or segregation of the generations. Youth comes to symbolize progress, and the society directs its resources toward the young and away from the old, accentuating the decline in status of the aged.

The Coast Salish Indians of western Washington state and British Columbia represent a challenge to the view that modernization is detrimental to the old (Amoss, 1981). They live on the same wooded coasts and valleys inhabited by their forebears, although their social, economic, and cultural world has changed dramatically. Still, contemporary Coast Salish elders enjoy rank comparable to that of the old people in times before contact with white society. The prestige accorded modern elders, as for their forebears, is based on a recognition of their contribution to the group; the contribution, however, has changed.

In the precontact era, elders were held in high esteem for their special skills in food procurement and processing as well as in canoe building. They made important contributions to group solidarity by maintaining the extended-family household. Modern old people do little of this. The nuclear household is the unit of production and consumption, and the skills of the elderly are of no economic importance. Yet old men and women are held in high standing because of their knowledge of old religious ritual practices and because the people believe that elders control a special spiritual power.

In particular, tribal elders play a central role in aboriginal-style spirit-dancing rituals carried out in winter, when the individual spirit guardians return and inspire tribal members to song and dance. The elders are essential to these ritualistic gatherings in three ways (Amoss 1981). First, because the old-style rituals were not performed for many years, the elders are the only ones who know how things should be done. Second, old people, though generally poor, contribute directly to the ritual occasions by giving goods and money. Third, elders control the initiation process that is the only route to full participation in the winter-dancing ceremonial system. Old people also have status in the group as a function of the monopoly they hold over ritual roles that control the welfare of others. Shamans, who have the power to inflict fatal illness, and mediums, who see ghosts and officiate at funerals, are all old men or women.

The work of Erdman Palmore has generally supported the modernization theory. Palmore and Whittington (1971) found that the status of the aged was lower than that of the younger population on a series of socio-economic measures and had declined significantly from 1940 to 1969. More recently, Palmore and Manton (1974) explored the relationship between modernization and the economic status of the aged in thirty-one countries. Indicators of modernization included the gross national product (GNP) per capita, the percentage of the labor force engaged in agriculture, the change in the proportion of the labor force engaged in agriculture, the percentage of literate adults, the percentage of people aged five to nineteen in schools, and the percentage of the population in higher education. The relative status of the aged was measured by indexes that compared the differences in employment and occupation of the older population (sixty-five and over) with those age twenty-five through sixty-four. In general, correlation between the indicators of modernization and measures of the status of the aged demonstrated the theory. The relative status of older people was lower in the more modernized nations. Interestingly, Palmore and Manton discovered some patterns within their data that imply that the status of the aged decreases in the early stages of modernization (exemplified by nations such as Iran, El Salvador, and the Philippines), but that, after a period of modernization, status may level off and even rise some (exemplified by New Zealand, Canada, and the United States).

Finally, Palmore (1975) has used the case of Japan to show how culture may mitigate the impact of modernization on the status of the aged. According to Palmore, the social and ethnic homogeneity of the Japanese population, the attitude of the Japanese toward time, the tradition of respect for the aged reflected in filial piety, and the prominence of ancestor worship have all helped maintain the relatively high status and integration of older Japanese. Palmore quotes from Japan's 1963 National Law for the Welfare of the Elders, a law comparable in the United States to The Older Americans' Act of 1965: "The elders shall be loved and respected as those who have for many years contributed toward the development of society, and a wholesome and peaceful life shall be guaranteed to them." The Older Americans' Act of 1965 makes no mention of love and respect for the aged, nor does it *guarantee* a wholesome and peaceful life.

The modernization theory has its critics, a number of whom point out how often the term *modernization* is used as synonym for development, change, progress, and westernization—suggesting that the concept is often used because of its vagueness. Two historians, Achenbaum and Stearns (1978), who have written on old age in historical perspective, believe the concept of modernization is worth pursuing in gerontology only with the following stipulations:

1. There should be clear agreement on when the modernization process began. For example, David Hacket Fischer, author of *Growing Old in America*, believes that America's shift from a gerontophilic to a gerontophobic society took place between 1770 and 1820. These dates precede the beginning of the fundamental aspects of modernization Cowgill finds so salient for influencing the status of older people.

2. We should recognize that modernization is not necessarily a linear process. It may proceed in stages, some of which are protracted. Each stage may have a different impact on the status of the elderly.

3. The elderly in preindustrial society demonstrated great diversity of situation. Some owned property and wielded considerable power; others suffered severe degradation. We must recognize that, inevitably, the situation for some improved with modernization, as it deteriorated for others.

4. Finally, we must acknowledge that the process of modernization has affected different age groups in different ways. This is particularly interesting in light of the societal transformations that necessitated the invention of "adolescence" and redefined childhood. Today, we distinguish among young-old and old-old. Each may modernize in a different way, with different degrees of success.

Age Stratification

Age stratification is less a formal theory than a conceptual framework for viewing societal processes and changes that affect aging and the state of being old. Matilda White Riley (1971, 1977; Riley, Johnson, and Foner 1972) and Anne Foner (1975) are the architects of this conceptual framework.

Society is divided into strata not only by social class but by age. Members of the age strata differ in the social roles they are expected to play and in the rights and privileges accorded them by society. This is similarly the case for members of different social classes, who also have different societal expectations for behavior as well as differential access to rewards granted by society. Age stratification and class stratification approaches have much in common. In fact, Riley (1971) argues that two concepts central to class stratification theory, *social class* and *social mobility*, are analogous to two concepts central to age stratification, *age strata* and *aging*. She suggests that sociologists of age stratification use those questions that are important to class stratification theorists to stimulate thinking about age strata and aging. Four sets of these questions are reproduced below.

First, how does an individual's location in the class structure channel his attitudes and the way he behaves? Here there is much evidence that, for example, a person's health, his desire to achieve, his sense of mastery over his own fate, or the way he relates to his family and to his job depend to a considerable extent upon his social class.

Second, how do individuals relate to one another within and between classes? Within class lines, many friendships are formed, marriages often take place, and feelings of solidarity tend to be widespread. Between classes, relationships, even if not solidary, are often symbiotic, as people of unlike status live harmoniously in the same society. However, there seems to be greater opportunity between, than within, classes, for cleavage or conflict, as in struggles over economic advantages or clashes in political loyalties.

Third, what difficulties beset the upwardly (or downwardly) mobile individual, and what strains does his mobility impose upon the group (such as his parents of one class) whom he leaves behind and upon the new group (such as his wife's parents of a different class) who must now absorb him?

Fourth, to the extent that answers can be found to these three sets of questions, what is the impact of the observed findings upon the society as a whole? If there are inequalities between classes, for example, what do these portend for the prosperity, the morality, or the stability of the overall structure of classes? What pressures for societal change are generated by differences, conflicts, or mobility between classes? (Riley, M.W. 1971. Social gerontology and the age stratification of society. *Gerontologist* 11:79. Reprinted by permission of The Gerontological Society of America. Emphasis in the original.)

In age stratification terms, the first question becomes: How does an individual's location within the age structure of a society influence his or her behavior and attitudes? We have already discussed in chapters on the biology and psychology of aging that age strata differ in physical and sensory capabilities, psychomotor performance, and probabilities of death. Psychologists of the life cycle often describe age strata in terms of their involvement in different developmental tasks. In addition, research shows that age strata differ in political and social attitudes, world outlook, style of life, organizational attachments, happiness and so on (Riley and Foner 1968). How do age stratification theorists explain these differences in behavior and attitudes among people of different age strata and the similarities among people within a stratum?

Riley (1971) suggests that two coordinates or dimensions useful for locating an individual in the age structure of a society are the *life course dimension* and the *historical dimension*. The first of these reflects chronological age, itself a rough indicator of biological, psychological, and social experience. This is only to say that individuals of the same age have much in common. They are alike in biological development as well as in the kinds of social roles they have experienced (worker, spouse, parent). The second dimension refers to the period of history in which a person lives. People born at the same time (a cohort) share a common history. Those born at different times have lived through a different historical period. Even when people born at different times share an historical event, they are likely to experience it differently. For example, persons born in 1920 and 1950 were likely to experience the Vietnam War quite differently. Riley uses the term *cohortcentric* to describe the view of the world (that is, the behavior and attitudes) that develops from a particular intersection of the life course and historical dimensions. People in the same place on the life course dimension (in the same age stratum) experience historical events similarly and, as a result, may come to see the world in a like fashion. The cohort-centricity of different age strata explains the different behaviors and attitudes associated with those age strata. More recently, Riley (1985) has described the *fallacy of cohortcentrism*—that is, the erroneous assumption that members of all cohorts will age in exactly the same fashion as members of our own cohort.

The second question becomes: How do individuals relate to one another within and between age strata? This question stimulates thinking about the nature of social relationships within age strata and the nature of intergenerational relations. From the age stratification perspective, within-age stratum solidarity and consciousness are predictable. People's similarity in age and cohort membership often signals mutuality of experiences, perceptions, and interests that may lead to integration or even to age-based groups and collective movements (Riley 1985). Yet, the continuous flow of cohorts in and out of age-stratum weakens identification with a particular stratum. As Foner (1975) points out, this is quite different from class strata, members of which share common experiences and often have a lifetime to reinforce identification with the group.

Relations among age strata reflect many factors, not the least of which is the distribution of power and wealth in a society. What about intergenerational relations within the family? Are they sequential or reciprocal? Foner (1969, cited in Riley 1971) asked parents of high school students what they would do with money unexpectedly received. Two percent said they would use it to help their aged parents; most indicated a willingness to use the money to help the children get started in life. Furthermore, she reports that the aged generation concurs with this decision. This suggests agreement among generations about the flow of material support—sequential, not reciprocal, with each generation attempting to aid the younger generation.

The third set of questions asks about age mobility. When aging is viewed as mobility through the age strata, it is revealed as a process that brings many of the same strains and stresses as does class mobility. Still, age mobility is different. In the first place, social mobility affects only a few; age mobility affects everyone. Although individuals age in different ways and at different rates, no one can achieve downward age mobility. As Mannheim (1952, 290) wrote, the "sociological phenomenon of generations is ultimately based on the biological rhythm of birth and death." Over time, a succession of waves of new individuals reach adulthood. Each wave, or cohort, is changed by *and* changes the prevailing culture. Mannheim described this as "fresh contact" (Kertzer 1983). Second, thus, because of its special relationship to historical events, each cohort experiences age mobility differently. For example, successive cohorts in our society in this century have increased longevity and formal education. Both these facts have dramatically changed how successive cohorts have aged.

Finally, the fourth set of questions reminds us that age stratification cannot be viewed in isolation. The system of age stratification in society influences and is influenced by the changing social–political–economic fabric of society. Sometimes, social changes may directly reflect "innovations" that emanate from one or more cohorts (Riley 1971). Thus, for example, the large proportion of "early" retirements from the labor force in recent cohorts of those aged fifty-five to sixty-five has already had enormous impact throughout the society— for example, on the financing of Social Security and other pension plans, on housing, and on leisure—and will continue to do so in the future. On the other hand, when many individuals in the same cohort are affected by social change in similar ways, the change in their collective lives can in turn produce further social change. That is, new patterns of aging are not only caused by social change; they also contribute to it (Riley 1985).

In Maoist China (1949–1976), three policies were implemented that are repeatedly cited as evidence for a decline in the status of older people in that country. First, a new marriage law, enacted in 1950, replaced absolute parental authority with reciprocity between parents and children. Second, the elimination of private property removed the parental control of family wealth as a power resource. Third, the state emphasized patriotism over filial piety; children were encouraged to expose family members who were ideologically against the state. In the 1970s, with the death of Mao, modernization in the form of economic development was emphasized in earnest. Although research on the impact on the aged of this intensive modernization is still ongoing, application of the modernization theory would seem to predict a further decline in the status of old people.

Peter Yin and Kwok Hung Lai (1983) have attempted to understand the changes in status experienced by the elderly in Maoist China within the context of the age stratification theory. In effect they ask: Did the aged lose status because they were old (*age effect*) or because of their life experiences (*cohort effect*)?

Yin and Lai argue for an explanation of the status of older people in China based on cohort effects. Their position is that older age groups suffered diminished status in Maoist China, mainly because of their life experience in the prerevolutionary era, when the previous government advocated capitalism and communists were in the role of revolutionaries. When the communists came to power, they feared that older adults could provide a major impetus to a revival of capitalism. In sum, these authors suggest that the position of the aged was diminished in Maoist China not as a function of their old age but rather as a result of generational conflict based on different life experiences.

The age stratification approach suggests a new way of viewing an increasing body of information on growing old and being old. The research literature on age stratification is still relatively scarce. Yet, it is clear the approach raises interesting and important questions. Only additional research efforts will determine its viability.

Political Economy of Aging

The political economy perspective on aging requires that we view the problems of aging in social structural rather than in individual terms. According to Estes, Swan, and Gerard (1984, 28), this perspective "starts with the proposition that the status and resources of the elderly and even the trajectory of the aging process itself are conditioned by one's location in the social structure and the economic and social factors that affect it." Clearly, the political economy perspective is not concerned with old age as a biological or psychological problem but rather as a problem for societies characterized by major inequalities in the distribution of power, income, and property. Implicit in this approach is the question of whether the logic of capitalism as a productive social system is reconcilable with the needs of elderly people.

Radical political economists of aging answer that capitalism is irreconcilable with meeting the needs of the elderly. Phillipson (1982) offers four arguments:

1. Whenever capitalism is in crisis—as in the 1930s and in the early 1980s—it attempts to solve its problems through cuts in the living standards of working people.

2. Capitalism has a distinct set of priorities, which almost always subordinates social and individual needs to the search for profits.

3. Because of the cyclical nature of the capitalist economies, elderly people often find themselves caught between their own need for better services and the steady decline of facilities within their neighborhood.

4. In capitalist economies, a ruling class still appropriates and controls the wealth produced by the working class.

Navarro (1984) has analyzed the health-care problems of older Americans, using a political economy approach. He concludes that the misery and impoverishment many elderly suffer today is a function of the dominance of the capitalist class over U.S. political, economic, and social institutions. From his view, defense of capitalist class interests has required shifting government resources from social and health expenditures, which benefit the majority of the U.S. population, to military expenditures, which benefit the few. Interestingly, Navarro remains optimistic enough to suggest that the interest-group mentality prevalent in the United States be replaced by an appreciation among the majority of Americans (whites, blacks, Latinos, females, the young, and the old) for their shared working-class status and hence for their collective power.

The political economy of aging is not a theory in the strictest sense. It is not presented in the form of a set of systematically organized statements. Rather, political economy is an orientation or perspective, which at this relatively early stage in its development may provide a useful guide for aging policy and research. Estes, Gerard, and Minkler (1984) employ the perspective to frame four important questions about aging policy. They believe that the answers to these questions speak to the heart of the relationship between this society and its aged constituents:

1. To what extent will aging interest groups ally themselves with a broader base and expand their concerns to encompass generic issues rather than those identified as aging issues only?

2. To what extent will state and local officials continue to accept the federal retrenchment and shift of governmental responsibility to state and local government?

3. Will the interests of the wealthy and the middle class continue to dominate public policy for the aging?

4. To what extent will the organizations serving the aging, as well as professionals and individuals, involve themselves in attempting to set the agenda for future public policy?

SUMMARY

Theories in social gerontology reviewed in this chapter were divided into two broad categories. One group of theories that attempts to conceptualize the adjustment of individuals to their own aging, while other theories deal with societal change and aging. Theories in the first category include the role, activity, disengagement, socio-environment, exchange, and symbolic interactionist theories. Those in the latter category include the subcultural, modernization, and age stratification theories, as well as the political economy perspective. None of the theories has been sufficiently tested to be completely rejected. Each acts as a guide to further research.

The earliest theory in social gerontology concentrated on adjustments to role change among the elderly. In general, this approach pointed out that role loss led to maladjustment. The activity theory states a positive relationship between activity and life satisfaction. Activity theorists argue that, although aging individuals face inevitable changes, many psychosocial needs remain the same. Thus, individuals able to maintain the activities of the middle years will be well satisfied with life in the later years. Several empirical tests of the theory show only social activity with friends to be related to life satisfaction in later life.

Standing in some contrast to the above approaches, disengagement theory characterizes old age as a time of mutual withdrawal between the aging individual and society. This mutual withdrawal is seen as functional for and desired by both aging individuals and the social system. Much critical discussion still surrounds the theory, although most research efforts are unable to provide empirical support for it.

Socioenvironmental theory is directed at acknowledging the effects of the social and physical environment on the activity patterns of aged individuals. Exchange theory attempts to explain the interaction patterns of the old in terms of the relationship between support given and received. When these are out of balance, injustice results, and life satisfaction declines. Symbolic interactionism emphasizes the power of aged individuals to socially construct their reality.

Rose (1965) offered the concept of an aged subculture to explain the impact of trends promoting the segregation of the old from the rest of society. The development of an aged subculture has both negative and positive consequences. The most positive of these includes the potential for the elderly forming a social action group.

Modernization theory describes the relationship between modernization and the changes in role and status of older people. Stated briefly, the theory holds that increasing modernization brings a decline in the status of the aged. Riley proposes an age stratification approach to understanding the aging process and old age. She advises that an approach similar to that used in the analysis of class stratification would be useful for shedding light on problems of growing old and being old.

Political economy is a new perspective that sees the aged and the aging process as conditioned by location in the social structure. The perspective questions whether the logic of our economic system is reconcilable with the needs of older people.

STUDY QUESTIONS

1. Discuss the role theory in relation to adjustment in old age. What are the major role changes individuals experience during the aging process according to this theory? What happens to sex role differentiation with aging?

2. Compare and contrast disengagement and activity theory.

3. Explain how Gubrium integrates the concepts of physical proximity and age-homogeneity into the socioenvironmental theory of aging. List and describe his resulting typology of social contexts.

4. Discuss exchange theory and explain how it can be applied to understand the support networks of older people.

5. Explain how the theory of symbolic interactionism can be used to provide a basis for understanding how older people perceive and assign meaning to things, events, and people in their lives.

6. Discuss the positive and negative consequences of development of an aged subculture.

7. Four aspects of modernization have been identified as salient to the conditions of older people in a society. List them and explain how each affects the status of the elderly.

8. Explain how questions of social stratification can be adapted to a conceptual framework of age stratification.

9. According to radical political economists of aging, is capitalism reconcilable with meeting the needs of the elderly? Why? How may the political economy perspective help frame future policy and research questions?

BIBLIOGRAPHY

Achenbaum, A., and Stearns, P. 1978. Old age and modernization. *Gerontologist* 18(3):307–312.

Amoss, P.T. 1984. Coastal Salish elders. In P.T. Amoss and S. Harrell (eds.), *Other ways of growing old*. Stanford, Calif.: Stanford University Press.

Atchley, R. 1971. Disengagement among professors. *Journal of Gerontology* 26:476–480.

Blumer, H. 1969. *Symbolic interactionism*. Englewood Cliffs, N.J.: Prentice-Hall.

Bultena, G., and Wood, V. 1969. The American retirement community: Bane or blessing? *Journal of Gerontology* 24:209–217.

Carp, F. 1969. Compound criteria in gerontological research. *Journal of Gerontology* 24:341–347.

Cavan, R., Burgess, E., Havighurst, R., and Goldhammer, H. 1949. *Personal adjustment in old age*. Chicago: Science Research Associates Inc.

Conner, K., Powers, E., and Bultena, G. 1979. Social interaction and life satisfaction: An empirical assessment of late-life patterns. *Journal of Gerontology* 34:116–121.

Cottrell, L. 1942. The adjustment of the individual to his age and sex roles. *American Sociological Review* 7:617–620.

Cowgill, D. 1974. Aging and modernization: A revision of the theory. In J. Gubrium (ed.), *Late life: Communities and environmental policy*. Springfield, Ill.: Charles C Thomas, Publisher.

Cowgill, D., and Holmes, L. 1972. *Aging and modernization*. New York: Appleton-Century-Crofts.

Crawford, M.P. 1971. Retirement and disengagement. *Human Relations* 24:255–278.

Cumming, E. 1963. Further thoughts on the theory of disengagement. *International Social Science Journal* 15(3):377–393.

Cumming, E., and Henry, W. 1961. *Growing old: The process of disengagement*. New York: Basic Books.

Dowd, J. 1984. Beneficence and the aged. *Journal of Gerontology* 39(1):102–108.

———. 1980. *Stratification among the aged: An analysis of power and dependence*. Monterey, Calif.: Brooks-Cole.

———. 1978. Aging as exchange: A test of the distributive justice proposition. *Pacific Sociological Review* 21:351–375.

———. 1975. Aging as exchange: A preface to theory. *Journal of Gerontology* 30 (September):584–594.

Emerson, R.M. 1976. Social exchange theory. In A. Inkeles, J. Coleman, and N. Smelser (eds.), *Annual review of sociology*, Vol. 2. Palo Alto, Calif.: Annual Reviews.

Estes, C.L., Gerard, L.E., and Minkler, M. 1984. Reassessing the future of aging policy and politics. In M. Minkler and C.L. Estes (eds.), *Readings in the political economy of aging*. Farmingdale, N.Y.: Baywood Publishing.

Estes, C.L., Swan, J.H., and Gerard, L.E. 1984. Dominant and competing paradigms in gerontology: Towards a political economy of aging. In M. Minkler and C.L. Estes (eds.), *Readings in the political economy of aging*. Farmingdale, N.Y.: Baywood Publishing.

Fischer, D. 1977. *Growing old in America*. New York: Oxford University Press.

Foner, A. 1975. Age in society: Structures and change. *American Behavioral Scientist* 19(2):289–312.

Gouldner, A.W. 1960. The norm of reciprocity. *American Sociological Review* 25(April):161–178.

Gubrium, J. 1973. *The myth of the golden years: A social-environmental theory of aging*. Springfield, Ill.: Charles C Thomas, Publisher.

———. 1975. *Living and dying at Murray Manor*. New York: St. Martin's Press, Inc.

Havighurst, R. 1968. Personality and patterns of aging. *Gerontologist* 8:20–23.

Hendricks, J., and Hendricks, C.D. 1986. *Aging in mass society: Myths and realities* (3d ed.). Boston: Little, Brown and Co.

Hochschild, A. 1975. Disengagement theory: A critique and proposal. *American Sociological Review* 40:553–569.

Homans, G. 1974. *Social behavior: Its elementary forms* (rev. ed.). New York: Harcourt, Brace and World.

———. 1958. Social behavior as exchange. *American Journal of Sociology* 63(May):597–606.

Kart, C.S., and Longino, C.F. 1987. The support systems of older people: A test of the exchange paradigm. *Journal of Aging Studies* 1(3):239–251.

Kertzer, D.I. 1983. Generation as a sociological problem. *Annual Review of Sociology* 9:125–149.

Knapp, M. 1977. The activity theory of aging: An examination in the English context. *Gerontologist* 17(6):553–559.

Lemon, B., Bengtson, V., and Peterson, J. 1972. Activity types and life satisfaction in a retirement community. *Journal of Gerontology* 27:511–523.

Longino, C.F. 1980. The retirement community. In F. Berghorn and D. Schafer (eds.), *Dynamics of aging: Original essays on the experience and process of growing old*. Boulder, Colo.: Westview Press.

Longino, C.F., and Kart, C.S. 1982. Explicating activity theory: a formal replication. *Journal of Gerontology* 17(6):713–722.

Longino, C.F., McClelland, K.A., and Peterson, W.A. 1980. The aged subculture hypothesis: Social integration, gerontophilia and self-conception. *Journal of Gerontology* 35(5):758–767.

Mannheim, K. 1952. The problem of generations. In *Essays on the sociology of knowledge*. New York: Oxford University Press.

Marshall, V. 1979. No exit: A symbolic interactionist perspective on aging. *International Journal of Aging and Human Development* 9:345–358.

Messer, M. 1967. The possibility of an age-concentrated environment becoming a normative system. *Gerontologist* 7:247–250.

Monge, R.H. 1975. Structure of the self-concept from adolescence through old age. *Experimental Aging Research* 1(2):281–291.

Navarro, V. 1984. The political economy of government cuts for the elderly. In M. Minkler and C.L. Estes (eds.), *Readings in the political economy of aging.* Farmingdale, N.Y.: Baywood Publishing.

Neugarten, B., Crotty, W., and Tobin, S. 1964. Personality types in an aged population. In B. Neugarten et al. (eds.), *Personality in middle and late life.* New York: Atherton Press.

Neugarten, B., Havighurst, R., and Tobin, S. 1961. The measurement of life satisfaction. *Journal of Gerontology* 16:134–143.

Palmore, E. 1968. The effects of aging on activities and attitudes. *Gerontologist* 8:259–263.

———. 1975. *The honorable elders: A cross-cultural analysis of aging in Japan.* Durham, N.C.: Duke University Press.

Palmore, E., and Manton, K. 1974. Modernization and status of the aged. *Journal of Gerontology* 29(2):205–210.

Palmore, E., and Whittington, F. 1971. Trends in the relative status of the aged. *Social Forces* 50:84–90.

Phillips, B. 1957. A role theory approach to adjustment in old age. *American Sociological Review* 22:212–217.

Phillipson, C. 1982. *Capitalism and the construction of old age.* London: Macmillan.

Reichard, S., Livson, F., and Peterson, P. 1962. *Aging and personality.* New York: John Wiley and Sons, Inc.

Riley, M.W. 1971. Social gerontology and the age stratification of society. *Gerontologist* 11:79–87.

———. 1977. Age strata in social systems. In R. Binstock and E. Shanas (eds.), *Handbook of aging and the social sciences.* New York: Van Nostrand Reinhold Co.

———. 1985. Age strata in social systems. In R. Binstock and E. Shanas (eds.), *Handbook of aging and the social sciences* (2nd ed.). New York: Van Nostrand Reinhold Co.

Riley, M.W., and Foner, A. 1968. *Aging and society: An inventory of research findings.* New York: Russell Sage Foundation.

Riley, M.W., Johnson, M., and Foner, A. 1972. *Aging and society: A sociology of age stratification.* New York: Russell Sage Foundation.

Rose, A. 1965. The subculture of the aging: A framework in social gerontology. In A.M. Rose and W.A. Peterson (eds.), *Older people and their social worlds.* Philadelphia: F.A. Davis Co.

Rosow, I. 1967. *Social integration of the aged.* New York: The Free Press.

Shanas, E. 1979. The family as a social support system in old age. *Gerontologist* 19:169–174.

Sinnott, J.D. 1977. Sex-role inconstancy, biology, and successful aging: A dialectical model. *Gerontologist* 17(5):459–463.

Spence, D.L. 1986. Some contributions of symbolic interaction to the study of growing old. In V.W. Marshall (ed.), *Later life: The social psychology of aging*. Beverly Hills, Calif.: Sage Publications.

Stoller, E.P., and Earl, L.L. 1983. Help with activities of everyday life: Sources of support for the noninstitutionalized elderly. *Gerontologist* 23(1):64–70.

Streib, G. 1965. Are the aged a minority group? In A. Gouldner and S.M. Miller (eds.), *Applied sociology*. New York: The Free Press.

Sussman, M. 1976. The family life of old people. In R. Binstock and E. Shanas (eds.), *Handbook of aging and the social sciences*. New York: Van Nostrand Reinhold Co.

Tallmer, M., and Kutner, B. 1970. Disengagement and morale. *Gerontologist* 10(Winter):317–320.

Thoits, P. 1982. Conceptual, methodological, and theoretical problems in studying social support as a buffer against life stress. *Journal of Health and Social Behavior* 23:145–159.

Ward, R.A. 1984. *The aging experience* (2nd ed.). New York: Harper and Row.

———. 1985. Informal networks and well-being in later life: A research agenda. *Gerontologist* 25:55–61.

Ward, R.A., Sherman, S., and Lagory, M. 1984. Subjective network assessments and subjective well being. *Journal of Gerontology* 39:93–101.

Weiss, R. 1969. The fund of sociability. *Transaction* 6:26–43.

Yin, P., and Lai, K.H. 1983. A reconceptualization of age stratification in China. *Journal of Gerontology* 38(5):608–613.

Youmans, E.G. 1967. Disengagement among older rural and urban men. In E.G. Youmans (ed.), *Older rural Americans*. Lexington, Ky.: University of Kentucky Press.

PART IV

THE AGED AND SOCIETY

CHAPTER 10

AGING AND FAMILY LIFE

CHAPTER 11

THE ECONOMICS OF AGING

CHAPTER 12

**WORK, RETIREMENT,
AND LEISURE**

CHAPTER 13

THE POLITICS OF AGING

CHAPTER 14

RELIGION AND AGING

CHAPTER 10

AGING AND FAMILY LIFE

The institution of the family is the one that is best known and that affects most people. Obviously, we feel the effects of other institutions—political, educational, and economic—but it is the family that touches us more deeply and continuously than any other. Families help regulate sexual activity and provide a context within which children are conceived and raised. Families afford individuals protection, intimacy, affection, and social identity (Federico 1979).

Among social scientists there is greater consensus about the functions of the family than about its organization or structure. For example, anthropologists have largely been unable to agree on a common definition of a family. This should not be surprising, since much of the literature of anthropology and family sociology highlights the wide variety of forms families can take. This becomes especially clear in comparing different cultures—their mate-selection procedures, child-rearing practices, and degree of interaction allowed among family members. Variation in family structure exists within societies as well. As we shall see, although more Americans today live in some form of nuclear family (husband and wife couple with children living in a common household) than in any other type of living arrangement, there is a wide array of family types in the United States.

There has been much discussion about the relationship between family structure and the role and status of aged people in a society. One form of family structure is often considered advantageous for the aged—the extended family. The term *extended family* is conventionally used to describe all those individuals one is related to through blood and marriage; yet, the term is also used to characterize three or more generations who share living arrangements. Premodern, or preindustrial societies, generally believed to be served by the extended form of family organization, are often offered as evidence of the

217

favored status of older people in extended family settings. In such societies, the aged are thought to be well integrated into family life, with family members living and working together harmoniously. This view is most likely an overly simplistic one: The premodern family should not be seen as a monolithic entity. First, if we reflect on the patterns of longevity in such societies, it is clear at once that there were too few people surviving to old age (as we define it) for families including three or more generations to be universal. Also, preindustrial societies evinced a wide variation in family organization; many, even those in which the extended family was evident, treated old people quite poorly. Sieroshevski (1901, quoted in Simmons 1945) has written of the Yakuts of Siberia as follows:

> The Yakuts treat their old relatives, who have grown stupid, very badly. Usually they try to take from them the remains of their property, if they have any; then constantly, in measure, as they become unprotected they treat them worse and worse. Even in houses relatively self-sufficient, I found such living skeletons, wrinkled, half-naked, or even entirely naked, hiding in corners, from where they crept out only when no strangers were present, to get warm by the fire, to pick up together with children bits of food thrown away, or to quarrel with them over the licking of the dish emptied of food. (Simmons, L., *The Role of the Aged in Primitive Society*, 197. New Haven, Conn.: Yale University Press, 1945.)

Simmons (1945, 1960), a student of aging in many different societies, argues that throughout human history the family has been the safest haven for the aged, even though the condition of the Yakut elderly shows otherwise. Simmons studied the position of the aged among seventy-one primitive peoples, and his data reveal that it was the organization of kinship relationships that primarily determined the destiny of aged people. In particular, opportunities for the aged to remain effective participants in society seemed to be related to their opportunities: (1) to marry younger mates, (2) to exercise managerial roles in the family, (3) to rely upon family care and support, and (4) to rely on the support of their sons-in-law. Important as kinship relationships were, however, they were not the only determinants of the position of the aged in these primitive societies. Cultural factors, including the principal means of economy, the permanency of residence, the constancy of food supply, the nature of the political system, and the establishment of property rights in land, crops, herds, goods, and women—in addition to the nature of the climate and physical environment—also affected the status and prestige of aged people.

What about the relationship between family structure and the position of aged people in modern societies such as our own?

OLD AGE AND THE AMERICAN
FAMILY: A LOOK BACKWARD

In the United States, the past—that is, the preindustrial and early industrial period from the country's beginnings up to the turn of the twentieth century—is often characterized as an idyllic time during which three or more generations of relatives lived harmoniously together on the family farm. Such extended families were thought to be led by the elders, those respected members of the family and community. As Hess and Waring (1978) remind us, however, this respect, along with the obligation to care for elders, often was based on their control of resources and was reinforced by religious tradition and normative sanction.

This picture of family life in an earlier time is often contrasted with that of contemporary family life, involving nuclear family units composed of husband and wife couples and their children. Conventional wisdom has it that these nuclear family units live apart from one another and that bureaucratic institutions perform many of the functions once fulfilled by the family, including care of the elderly sick. Moreover, younger people no longer give the parental generation the love and respect that traditionally has been its due. In fact, as Treas (1977) points out, many blame this family indifference for the social isolation and economic insecurity that confront many older people.

The major cause of this shift in family organization from the extended to the nuclear family is thought to be industrialization. Advocates of this view argue that extended families are advantageous in agrarian societies because all family members (including children and the elderly) contribute economically to the family. This is not the case in an industrial society, however, where children and the elderly are largely unemployable. Moreover, because they consume at a high rate, these dependent relatives are a burden rather than an advantage.

This unemployability of dependent relatives is seen as only one cause of the transformation of the extended family into the nuclear family in industrialized societies. With industrialization, the location of work shifted away from the home. Workers migrated to places where job opportunities existed. Purportedly, this geographical mobility strained kinship bonds and decreased the frequency and intimacy of contact among family members. In addition, some have argued that industrialization opened up opportunities for women to participate in work activities outside the home, thus diminishing the importance of some extended family functions.

With the passing of the extended family, it is believed that older people lost their economic role and became isolated from their children and relatives. Even the most noted sociologist adopted this view: Talcott Parsons (1942) wrote that with marriage and occupational independence of children comes "the depletion of [the] family until the older couple is finally left alone." Parsons contrasted this situation with that of other kinship systems (for example, extended families) "in which membership in a kinship unit is continuous throughout the life cycle."

Although the position of the aged in the family and in U.S. society certainly has undergone some historical change, not all share the above common perspective that a change in family structure from extended to nuclear is associated with decreased status and greater isolation for the elderly. For example, historical demographers now argue that the nuclear family has been viable throughout history and probably was the dominant type of family structure during the colonial period in the United States (Seward 1974).

As we shall see in more detail, it is *not at all likely* that the family evolved from an extended to a nuclear form. Rather, it has probably remained much the same. Gerontologist Clark Tibbitts (1968) has written that "it is now clear that the nuclear parent-child family has always been the modal family type in the United States and three-generation families have always been relatively rare."

Many family sociologists today have come to use the notion of a *modified extended family structure* to describe the interchange of visits and help between older parents and their children, which they believe to be more the rule than the exception (Troll 1971). From this view, they argue that the family—far from being irrelevant, as some contend—is becoming increasingly important as a place where older people can find support and interpersonal warmth as society becomes more technological and impersonal (Shanas 1979).

How do we account for the fictionalized (some would say idealized) version of the American extended family of the past? This is a difficult question. While arguing that this idealization of the past obscures its real character, Goode (1963) points out that "in each generation people write of a period *still* more remote, *their* grandparents' generation, when things really were much better." Perhaps, then, the answer lies in some universal belief that things were better in the past.

The general view in sociology has been that the nuclear family was founded in Western Europe and the United States and is a result of the urban-industrial revolution. As we have already indicated, the extended family is the form thought to have been prevalent prior to the urban-industrial revolution. Recently, however, this view has come into question. Much evidence now suggests that the nuclear family was the dominant form of family organization in the West during the preindustrial period as well.

Greenfield (1967) argues that the "small nuclear family was brought to the United States and Great Britain by its earliest settlers" and even suggests that the nuclear family helped produce the industrial revolution. Arensberg (1955) also believes that the nuclear family "came with (the) Yankees from England." Additional support for this belief is available. Stone (1967), in his study of the English aristocracy between 1558 and 1641, saw "little encouragement of younger sons to remain home, and daughters were almost invariably married off at an early age." Laslett and Harrison (1963) in their study of two seventeenth-century

English counties, Clayworth and Cogenhoe, found that the family was not extended; in most cases the "household did not ordinarily contain more generations than two, . . . living with in-laws or relatives was on the whole not to be expected." Laslett (1969) supported these conclusions in a later study of the composition of English households across three centuries.

Two more recent studies deserve mention. Back (1974) examined census records in England from 1574 to 1821 and found that only 6 percent of households contained three or more generations of family members. It is interesting that these extended households appeared to result almost always from a family tragedy of some sort, such as widowhood. Back concluded that there is no evidence that three-generation households were the preferred family pattern during the preindustrial period. Given the low percentage of extended families to begin with (6 percent), one would be hard pressed to argue that industrialization caused a decline in multigenerational households.

Apparently, England was not the only western society in which the nuclear family was the predominant form. Examining census records from 1847 to 1866 for a small community in Belgium, Van de Walle (1976) found that about two-thirds of the households were nuclear families; approximately 10 percent consisted of extended families, and 11 percent consisted of households in which more than one nuclear family lived together. Van de Walle observed nuclear families to be more lasting and suggested (in support of Back) that extended households were transitional patterns that resulted from family disruption.

What about the *American* past? Were extended families indigenous to the United States?

A number of recent studies of the American colonial family conclude that the extended structure was the exception rather than the rule. Demos (1965, 279), using family wills as a source, observed of the Plymouth colony that "there were no extended families at all in the sense of 'under the same roof', . . . married brothers and sisters never lived together in the same house," and "as soon as a man becomes betrothed, plans were made for the building, or purchase, of his own house." It was most unusual for married fathers with married sons to live together in an extended family group.

Greven (1966) describes the family structure in seventeenth-century Andover, Massachusetts. He distinguishes between the family of residence, which is nuclear, and the family of interaction or obligation, which he terms *modified extended*. Greven defines the modified extended family as a kinship group of two or more generations living within a single community in which the children continue to depend upon their parents after they have married and are no longer living under the same roof. Demos (1968, 44) supports this distinction in more recent studies of family structure in colonial New England. In Bristol, Rhode Island, "married adults normally lived with their own children and *apart* from all other relatives." Yet, a man's children, grown and established in their own households, were still very much a part of his social environment. As Demos (1978) points out, the details of intrafamilial relationships in colonial times remain somewhat obscure; although there is little reason to assume special closeness or harmony, the simple fact of the children's presence within the same community was important in its own right.

Kart and Engler (1985) reviewed wills probated in New York State between 1704 and 1799 in order to reconstruct the family relations of aged colonial Jews. Little evidence was found in the wills of explicit exchanges, or bargaining, between testators and their children, indicating, they argue, a relatively high degree of social and economic independence on the part of the younger generation. Kart and Engler speculate that by the eighteenth century encroaching forces of modernization (commercial trade and urbanization) were already reducing the amount of direct control parents had over offspring. And, especially because these colonial Jewish testators were not tied to the land, three of four were merchants, they were without the traditional power resources of land to withhold from children in exchange for service or provision of care (Kart and Engler 1985).

Has this revised picture of the early American family altered the view gerontologists have of the elderly during this period? Remember, it is generally believed that in early America the elderly were in a more favorable position with regard to family and society than they are today. Many associate this historically favorable position with the extended family and the subsequent loss of status and prestige with the change in family structure. The change in family structure (from extended to nuclear) appears to be more fiction than fact, but the change in the way Americans view the elderly is not.

The historian David H. Fischer has written about this changing American disposition toward the elderly. In the following summary of his writing, notice that Fischer does not associate the historical decline in the status of older people with a change in family structure, but rather with the kinds of cultural, demographic, and technological changes often associated with the modernization theory discussed in Chapter 9.

David Hackett Fischer (1977) lends support to the positive characterization of the position of the elderly in families of bygone days. At least, he argues, through its colonial phase, the United States was a gerontophilic place where being old conferred power and prestige. As Cotton Mather wrote in 1726, "the two qualities together, the ancient and the honorable." Seating arrangements in Massachusetts meetinghouses were determined by age rather than by wealth or status. Elders ran the churches. The aged occupied positions of community leadership; "grey champions" were turned to in crucial times. Names for persons in authority, like senator and alderman, were derived from words meaning old. Men tended to overstate rather than understate their age, and powdered wigs and long coats were used to give an older appearance.

Fischer believes that between 1770 and 1820 a revolution in age relations took place in the United States. This revolution, fueled by the ideology of liberty and equality, had the effect of dissolving the authority formerly vested in age. Fischer offers numerous manifestations of this revolution in age relations. By the later part of the eighteenth century, most New England town meetings had abandoned the practice of seating members on the basis of age. Northampton, Massachusetts, sold seats at auction rather than assigning them on the basis of age. Thus, the best seats went to the highest bidder, and rank and status in the meetinghouse thereafter rested upon wealth, without regard to age.

Mandatory retirement for public officials first appeared in America at the end of the eighteenth century. In 1777 the state of New York introduced compulsory retirement at age seventy for judges. New Hampshire followed suit in 1792, Connecticut in 1818. New York reduced the retirement age to sixty in 1821. These statutes angered former President John Adams, who wrote to Thomas Jefferson of his indignation: "I can never forgive New York, Connecticut, or Maine for turning out venerable men of sixty or seventy, when their judgment is often the best." Jefferson later responded, "It is reasonable we should drop off, and make room for another growth. When we have lived our generation out, we should not wish to encroach upon another" (Fischer 1977, 77). Jefferson, it seems, shared the revolutionary spirit in a way Adams could not.

Further evidence of a revolution in age relations between 1770 and 1820 in the United States included a shift in age preference, so that people began to pretend to be younger than they actually were; a shift in the age bias of dress, so that fashion flattered the young rather than the old; and a reduction in the frequency with which children were given the same names as their grandparents.

What caused this revolution? Fischer suggests that one key factor was the changing age composition of society. The number of aged was increasing, partly because more people were surviving to old age. Perhaps more important, however, is the fact that in the decade from 1800 to 1810 birth rates began to fall (and continued to do so for about 150 years); then the aged became a slowly increasing proportion of the population. At the same time that old age became more common, it also became more comtemptible: "Where the Puritans had made a cult of age, their posterity made a cult of youth instead" (Fischer 1977, 114). By 1847, Henry David Thoreau could write:

> Age is no better, hardly so well, qualified for an instructor as youth, for it has not profitted so much as it has lost. . . . Practically, the old have no very important advice to give the young, their experience has been so partial, and their lives have been such miserable failures, for private reasons, as they must believe; and it may be that they have some faith left which belies that experience, and they are only less young than they were. (Fischer 1977, 115–116)

The developing urbanization and industrialization of U.S. society accompanied demographic changes. The young, instead of waiting to inherit the family land, could move to the city and find work. Through the nineteenth and into the twentieth century, moving to the city became a strategy for leaving farming and parental control alike. Industrialization and urbanization contributed to changes in the character of generational relations. The young were no longer captive to a parental generation that controlled the family property and other economic resources.

THE FAMILY IN
CONTEMPORARY SOCIETY

Sussman (1976) has examined the structure of contemporary American families. The result is a taxonomy of American families, represented in Table 10-1. The statistics in this table are best "guesstimates" based on data collected in the mid-1970s from a wide array of largely governmental sources. These figures continue to provide guidelines for estimating the proportion of the adult population living in various family arrangements.

Approximately six in ten of all adults live in a nuclear family. This includes 37 percent living in the traditional "intact" U.S. family (nuclear family living with children) and 11 percent each of couples who have no children (or whose children no longer live at home) and couples who have remarried. Single-parent families represent about 12 percent of all adults, and approximately 19 percent of the U.S. adult population is single, widowed, separated, or divorced and living alone. Only 4 percent of adults live in an extended family household in which three or more generations share living arrangements.

Although some scholars view such data as evidence that the American family is not only nuclear but isolated as well, contrary arguments abound. Many contemporary family sociologists and gerontologists simply do not agree that the American nuclear family lives in isolation from its extended kin network.

Eugene Litwak (1965) was one of the first to question the isolation of the American nuclear family. In his studies, he found that most Americans function in *modified extended families* made up of numerous nuclear families that exhibit partial dependence on each other and exchange services. Lillian Troll (1971) supports this view and has made special reference to the position of the "post-parental" couple in this modified extended kin structure. In her view, the aged conjugal unit is not isolated.

Marvin Sussman has argued that the isolated nuclear family is a myth, and that there exists in modern urban–industrial societies "an extended kin system, highly integrated within a network of social relations and mutual assistance, that operates along historical kin lines and vertically over several generations" (1965, 179). According to Sussman, this extended kin network is the basic social system in U.S. urban society. More recently he has argued that the proliferation of services for the elderly has created new roles for kin as mediators between institutional bureaucracies and elderly relations. Children and relatives act as

---

TABLE 10-1   Family Type by Estimated Percentage Distribution, United States, 1976

Family Type	Estimated Percentage Distribution
Nuclear family—husband, wife, and offspring living in a common household ("intact")	37
Single career	18
Dual career	19
Nuclear dyad—husband and wife alone; childless, or no children living at home	11
Single career	4
Dual career	7
Nuclear family—husband, wife, and offspring living in a common household (remarried)	11
Single-parent family—one head, as a consequence of divorce, abandonment, or separation (with financial aid rarely coming from the second parent), and usually including preschool and/or school-age children	12
Career	8
Noncareer	4
Kin network—three-generation households or extended families in which members live in geographical proximity and operate within a reciprocal system of exchange of goods and services	4
Other single, widowed, separated, or divorced adults	19
Emerging experimental forms	6
Commune family—household of more than one monogamous couple with children, sharing common facilities, resources, and experiences; socialization of the child is a group activity. Household of adults and offspring—a "group marriage" known as one family in which all individuals are "married" to each other and all are "parents" to the children; usually develops a status system with leaders believed to have charisma.	
Unmarried parent and child family—usually mother and child, in which marriage is neither desired nor possible.	
Unmarried couple and child family—usually a common-law type of marriage with the child their biological issue or informally adopted.	
Total	100

Source: M. Sussman, "The Family Life of Old People," in R. Binstock and E. Shanas (eds.), *Handbook of Aging and the Social Sciences* (New York: Van Nostrand Reinhold, 1976), p. 230.

---

information sources for the elderly, informing them about housing, pensions, medical care, and other available options and entitlements. They also assist the aged in dealing with housing authorities, pension trustees, insurance companies, and hospitals (Sussman 1985).

PARENTS AND THEIR
ADULT CHILDREN

How do we know whether an old person is isolated or well-integrated into an extended kin network? To answer this question, many researchers have studied relationships between older people and their relatives. In particular, research has focused on relationships between older parents and their adult children. In a 1975 nationwide poll, Louis Harris and associates found that 81 percent of those sixty-five and over reported having children (NCOA 1976). According to Troll, Miller, and Atchley (1979), most older people who have no living children have never married. In this section we review some of the available research on aged parent–adult child relationships.

Residential Proximity. Almost all studies show that older people prefer to live near, but not with, their children. Shanas and associates (1968), in a study of old people in three industrial societies, found that 84 percent of those over sixty-five lived less than one hour away from one of their children. Most elderly wish to retain their independence as long as possible, sharing "intimacy, but at a distance" (Rosenmayr and Kockeis 1963). Reasons usually cited for preferring separate households include the desire to preserve independence and privacy and to avoid interference and potential conflict with children (Connidis 1983; Lopata 1980a).

Using data from nationwide surveys of the adult noninstitutionalized population of the United States, Okraku (1987) has offered evidence that since 1973 attitudes toward multigenerational residence has become more positive. The relationship between age and level of approval is inverse, however. Younger cohorts expressed more unconditional support for coresidence, whereas older cohorts expressed more conditional approval. Situations that include poor health or inadequate finances most often seem to necessitate living with a child.

Approximately one in eight elderly women and one in twenty-five elderly men live in a household headed by one of their children. More of these elderly people are likely to live with an unmarried child than with a married one, and more with a daughter (65 percent) than with a son (35 percent) (Troll, Miller, and Atchley 1979). These joint households are usually two-generational, not three. As we have already seen in Table 10-1, only about 4 percent of U.S. households are true three-generation families.

Interaction with Children. Most older parents and their adult children see each other quite often. The Harris Poll referred to earlier found that 55 percent of those surveyed who were sixty-five and over had seen one of their children within the last day or so; 26 percent had seen one of their children within the last week or two. These findings are consistent with those of other studies. In Shanas's study of older people in Denmark, England, and the United States, she reports that 84 percent of the American elderly with living children had seen at least one of their children within the previous week (Shanas et al. 1968).

A recent study of aged ethnics in Washington, D.C., and Baltimore, Maryland, revealed that 90.5 percent of the respondents had frequent to almost daily contact with their children (Gutman et al. 1979). There was some variation in contact with children among the ethnic groups: Greeks had the most frequent contact, almost twice as much as did aged Estonians. The nature of the contact was also different among ethnic groups. Hungarians had the highest percentage of those who had face-to-face contact with children, whereas the Lithuanians had the highest amount of phone contact with their children.

Distance may also be a strong determinant of frequency of contact with family for older people. In their study of elderly black residents in Cleveland, Ohio, Wolf and her colleagues (1983) report that those who had adult children in the neighborhood had contact with them daily. Those whose children lived an hour away reported significantly less contact.

Conventional wisdom supports an expectation of greater kinship ties and more frequent interaction across the generations in rural areas. Krout (1988) interviewed 600 individuals aged 65 and over residing in a continuum of community settings from farm areas to the central city of a large metropolis in western New York State. His findings suggest that the impact of rurality on the elderly parent's in-person contact with children has been overstated. Proximity was a far stronger predictor of in-person contact between elderly parents and their children. Krout (1988, 202) concludes that "people in rural areas do not have especially strong family ties or at least they are not evidenced by greater frequency of in-person contact nor are urban areas characterized by a lower level of intergenerational contact."

There appears to be some truth to the maxim that "a son's a son 'til he gets a wife, and a daughter's a daughter all her life." Research does show visitation to be more frequent along the female line. Husbands are more likely to be in touch with the wives' parents than their own, unless the wife mediates contact with the husband's parents (Reiss 1962; Adams 1971). According to Atkinson, Kivett, and Campbell (1986), familial linkages between generations that are female-based are predictive of greater exchange of help. From the point of view of these researchers, women are indeed the keepers of kin.

The order of frequency of interaction among New York Jewish families is with wife's mother, husband's mother, wife's father, and husband's father (Leichter and Mitchell 1967). In a recent study of three-generation Mexican-American families in San Antonio, Texas, respondents were asked how often they engaged in certain activities (for example, recreation outside the home, religious activities, telephone conversation) with each of their family members in the other two generations. All-female dyads showed higher levels of association than all-male and cross-sex dyads (Markides, Boldt, and Ray 1986).

Quality of Interaction. Many people believe that as parents age, the parent–child relationship undergoes a role reversal. The parent assumes the role of dependent, whereas the child takes on the supportive role of the parent. Certainly, this should not be expected; in fact, many gerontologists argue that it cannot work. Clark and Anderson write:

> A good relationship with children in old age depends, to large extent, on the graces and autonomy of the aged parent—in short on his ability to manage gracefully by himself. It would appear that in our culture there simply cannot be any happy role reversals between the generations, neither an increasing dependency of parent upon child nor a continuing reliance of child upon parent. The mores do not sanction it and children and parents resent it. The parent must remain strong and independent. If his personal resources fail, the conflicts arise. The child, on the other hand, must not threaten the security of the parent with request for monetary aid or other care when parental income has shrunk through retirement. The ideal situation is when both parent and child are functioning well. The parent does not depend on the child for nurturance or social interaction; these needs the parent can manage to fulfill by himself elsewhere. He does not limit the freedom of his child nor arouse the child's feelings of guilt. The child establishes an independent dwelling, sustains his own family, and achieves a measure of the hope the parents had entertained for him. Such an ideal situation, of course, is more likely to occur when the parent is still provided with a spouse and where a high socioeconomic status buttresses the parent and child" (Clark, M., and Anderson, B. *Culture and Aging,* 275–276. Springfield, Ill.: Charles C Thomas, Publisher, 1967).

One measure of the quality of intergenerational family relationships that has interested researchers involves the patterns of assistance that exist between parents and their adult children. In general, it appears that assistance flows both from adult children to their parents, and from the parents to their children, although Riley and Foner (1968) conclude that "the proportions of old people who give help to their children tend to exceed the proportions who receive help from their children."

Assistance takes many forms. It may involve carrying out nonessential, informal services that people often perform for each other when they live nearby—occasional shopping, carrying packages, or helping with household maintenance. Or it may involve providing highly organized, essential assistance such as regular babysitting or continued financial aid. Most studies of aging families focus on the elderly as stressors rather than as resources. Greenberg and Becker (1988) found that aging parents become an important resource when their adult children experience major life changes, most notably in coping with divorce or chemical dependency. Bankoff (1983) reports that supportive elderly parents play a crucial role for their widowed daughters. In fact, her analysis of questionnaire data from a nationwide sample of widows indicates that parents are the single most important source of support for still grieving widows and that such support is strongly related with the psychological well-being of recently widowed women.

The type of assistance offered (and received) varies by the sex of the parents and the children as well as by social class. Older men are more likely to assist their children with household maintenance and repairs, whereas elderly women help with child-rearing and domestic functions. According to Harris and Cole (1980), adult male children are likely to receive monetary aid and daughters to receive services from their parents. Mutual aid in lower-class families usually involves exchanges of services and shared living arrangements; the middle classes are more likely to provide direct financial assistance (Sussman and Burchinal 1962).

The two-way flow of support may persist until the onset of extreme frailty in the elderly parent or relative. Even then, rarely are the elderly dumped into institutions. The formal system of government and community agency programs plays only a minor role in providing for the elderly and is viewed by caregivers to the elderly as a last resort when the responsibilities become too complex to handle even with assistance (Stone, Cafferata and Sangl 1987). Families act as "case managers," facilitating contact between the elderly individual and the bureaucracy (Seltzer, Ivry and Litchfield 1987), and provide between 80 and 90 percent of medically related care, home nursing, personal care, household maintenance, transportation, and shopping (Day, 1985).

Estimates from the 1982 National Long-Term Care Survey and Informal Caregivers Survey indicate that in the United States approximately 2.2 million caregivers were providing unpaid assistance to 1.6 million noninstitutionalized disabled adults. Almost three out of four (73%) caregivers were either a spouse or a child. The majority (72%) were women, with adult daughters comprising 29 percent of all caregivers and wives constituting 23 percent of this population; husbands comprise 13 percent of caregivers, while nine percent were sons. The average age of the caregiver population was 57 years; 36 percent were 65 years or older.

Mathews (1987) reports that when older families include more than one living adult child, filial responsibility is shared. Interestingly, though, her study of 50 pairs of sisters who had at least one parent over the age of 75 found that members of the same family may not share perceptions of how responsibility is being divided. For example, only 52 percent of the pairs of sisters agreed on the way responsibility was divided in the family for giving emotional or moral support to an elderly parent. Data from this same study highlight the impact of employment status on the division of responsibility between sisters. Nonemployed sisters contributed relatively more tangible services than their employed sisters, especially when parents' health status was poorer. Such services included taking a parent to a medical appointment or handling daytime emergencies and care (Mathews et al. 1989).

Does the mutual assistance that appears to characterize intergenerational relations in U.S. families simply reflect feelings of obligation or a sense of duty, or do older parents and their adult children really like each other? In a wide array of studies across geographically disparate areas, older parents and their adult children report positive feelings for each other as well as considerable satisfaction with their relationships. Among aged ethnics living in the Washington, D.C., and Baltimore metropolitan areas, over 80 percent of each ethnic group indicated satisfaction with their family relationships. The highest proportion of "very satisfactory" relationships (85.8 percent) was reported by Polish in Baltimore, the lowest (65 percent) by Latvians (Gutman et al. 1979).

Lowenthal and associates (1975), reporting on a San Francisco sample, found that middle-aged parents felt good about their children. Bengtson and Black (1973) discovered high levels of regard reported by both older parents and their middle-aged children, although higher levels of sentiment are reported by the older parents. Older parents in a Boston study also rated their relationships with their adult children higher than their children did (Johnson and Bursk 1977). As might be expected, generations felt better about each other when the parents were in good health and financially independent (Johnson and Bursk 1977). In Cumming and Henry's (1961) Kansas City sample of healthy, independent-living people over age fifty, respondents were asked to whom they felt closest. In most cases, the answer was their child or children.

Many studies about the feelings parents and children have for each other suffer methodologically. Often they rely on self-reports, and they rarely involve both parents and children involved in the research. Nevertheless, researchers' reports show remarkable consistency in the positive feelings older parents and their adult children have for one another. Perhaps this should not be surprising. Similar findings are reported in studies of parent–child relationships across the life cycle (for example, high school students and their parents). And why not? After all, Troll and Bengtson (1978) have reminded us of the high degree of intergenerational continuity there is within the family. Reviewing the available literature on generations in the family, they found parent–child similarity strongest in religious and political affiliations but important also in sex roles and personality. Although social and historical forces affect people of different ages in different ways, there appears to be great similarity in values within families. These similarities may help explain why aged parents and adult children like each other—although not entirely. As studies seem to indicate, even when aged parents and their adult children disagree, they continue to see each other.

THE FAMILY LIFE CYCLE

Families change with time. The functions the family fulfills shift in importance just as family structure and patterns of interrelationships change. Where Duvall (1977) speaks of the "generational spiral" and Hess and Handel (1959) of "family themes," some family sociologists now use the notion of the *family life cycle* to characterize the changes families undergo. A well-known and frequently adopted staging of the family life cycle has been put forth by Duvall (1977):

Stage 1. Establishment (newly married, childless)

Stage 2. New parents (infant to three years)

Stage 3. Preschool family (child three to six years, possibly younger siblings)

Stage 4. School-age family (oldest child six to twelve years, possibly younger siblings)

Stage 5. Family with adolescent (oldest child thirteen to nineteen years, possibly younger siblings)

Stage 6. Family with young adult (oldest twenty, until first child leaves home)

Stage 7. Family as launching center (from departure of first child to that of last child)

Stage 8. Postparental family (after all children have left home)

It is important to recognize that this sequence of stages is an ideal representation of the life of a couple that marries, has children, and stays together through the course of the life cycle. Obviously, some people never marry, others marry and do not have children, and many who marry later divorce. Furthermore, any sequencing of stages downplays the variation in family life that can be produced by differences in the earlier life experiences of family members and by changing historical conditions (Cherlin 1983).

Family life cycles can overlap and, as a result, a family chain may go on. Children born into a family (sometimes referred to as their *family of orientation*) may later marry and begin their own families (their *family of procreation*). It is the adult child's family of procreation that produces the role of grandparent for the older parent.

Although in this chapter we are particularly interested in the last stage of the family life cycle, it should be understood that the stages themselves are not stagnant: Within each stage, significant changes in family structure and relationships may take place. For example, much literature suggests that the quality of the marriage relationship changes significantly in stage 2 with the onset of parenthood (for example, Rollins and Feldman 1970). In addition, as we shall see shortly, events that occur during the last stage—birth of a grandchild, retirement, death of a spouse, remarriage—may clearly change the character of the older person's family life.

The Postparental Family

Marital status is a simple, obvious criterion for distinguishing older people who are in families from those who are not. Table 10-2 shows the marital status distribution of older males and females in 1984. The marital distribution of men differs sharply from that of women in the three age groupings shown. In 1984, four of five men aged sixty-five to seventy-four years were married and living with their wives; only about one of eleven (9 percent) was widowed. Women sixty-five years and over are much more likely to be widowed than married. In 1984, 49 percent of women aged sixty-five to seventy-four years and 23

TABLE 10-2 Marital Status of Older Males and Females, 1984

	Age 55 to 64		Age 65 to 74		Age 75 Plus	
	Males	Females	Males	Females	Males	Females
Percent in category						
Single	5	4	5	5	4	6
Married-spouse present	83	66	80	49	67	23
Married-spouse absent	2	3	2	2	3	1
Widowed	4	17	9	39	24	67
Divorced	6	9	4	5	2	3

Source: U.S. Bureau of the Census, Current Population Survey, March 1984, unpublished.

percent of women aged seventy-five and over were married and living with their husbands; over one half of all elderly women were widowed (67 percent among those aged seventy-five and over). The changes in marital status since the end of World War II have been quite substantial, especially for men. The proportion of elderly men who are married has increased, and the proportions of single and widowed have fallen significantly.

Two important factors contribute to the sharply different marital distributions of men and women. The first is the much higher mortality rates of married men than for married women. As we have seen, men have higher mortality rates than women do. In addition, husbands are typically older than their wives by a few years. Siegel (1976) indicates that the expectation of life at age sixty-five of married women exceeds that of their husbands at age seventy by about nine years. Thus, not only do most married women outlive their husbands, but they tend to do so by many years.

A second factor accounting for the significantly higher proportion of widows than widowers is the higher remarriage rate of widowers. The marriage rate of elderly men is about seven times that of elderly women. The vast majority of these are remarriages (Siegel 1976). Societal norms are much more supportive of an elderly man marrying a younger woman than of the opposite. Men also have a demographic advantage in the marriage market. As Table 10-2 shows, in each age group, the proportion of older women who are unmarried is more than twice as great as the proportion of unmarried men (18 versus 49 percent among those sixty-five to seventy-four years, for example).

The Older Couple

Most elderly couples today have grown old together. The average couple has launched a family and can expect about fifteen years of living together after the departure of the last child. At the turn of the century, more than half of all marriages were interrupted by the death of one spouse, usually the husband, before the last child left home (Harris and Cole 1980). The increase in these

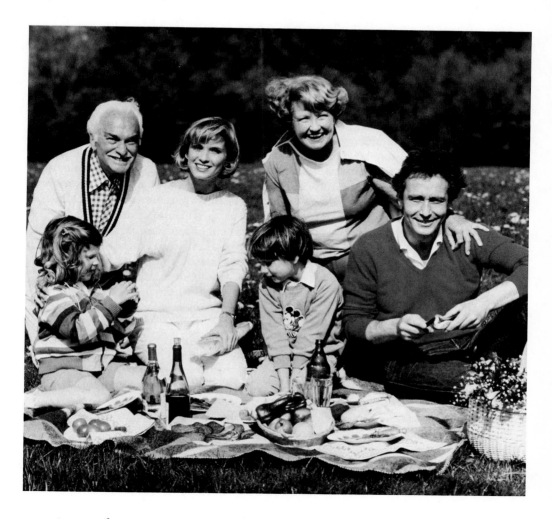

postparental years, sometimes referred to as the *empty nest period*, is due to increased life expectancies as well as to more closely spaced and smaller families.

Researchers have examined closely what happens after the launching of the children, yet consensus is difficult to achieve. Some studies show that marital satisfaction is as high or higher among older couples as it is among child-rearing couples, and that older couples report fewer marital problems (Riley and Foner 1968; Rollins and Feldman 1970). Several researchers have suggested that this pattern represents a "typical" marital life cycle in which satisfaction is high right after marriage, lower during the child-rearing years, and higher again during the postparental period (Rollins and Cannon 1974; Stinnett et al. 1972). Lowenthal and her colleagues (1975) found that most married couples look forward to the postparenting years. Many see the possibility for increased closeness and companionship. Stinnett, Collins, and Montgomery (1970) found the elderly couple to be happier, less lonely, and financially more stable than elderly single persons. Caregiving responsibilities may place a strain on some elderly marriages (Barusch 1988).

The marital relationship may not be a blessing for all older people, however. Marital disenchantment may surface during the latter stages of the family life cycle, resulting in reduced satisfaction with the relationship, loss of intimacy, and less sharing of activities (Pineo 1961). Clearly, for many couples, the marital relationship becomes subordinate during the child-rearing years and remains so after the children leave home. Atchley (1980) reports that every year nearly 10,000 older Americans are divorced. Divorce among older people has more than doubled since 1960 and divorce rates are currently higher among younger cohorts of adults (Uhlenberg and Myers 1981). Table 10-2 provides data to suggest that divorce is inclined to be more prevalent among future cohorts of older people; in 1984, men and women aged fifty-five to sixty-four years report being currently divorced at a rate higher than that for men and women aged sixty-five to seventy-four years.

Chiriboga (1982) points out that older persons appear particularly vulnerable to the divorce process. From a study of separated men and women living in the San Francisco–Oakland metropolitan area, he concludes that, relative to the young, older respondents were unhappier and reported fewer positive emotional experiences. Further, he notes that "their dealings with the social world appeared more tortured, there were more signs of personal discomfort, and their perceptions of the past and future reflected both greater pessimism and long-term dissatisfaction" (Chiriboga 1982, 113).

Cain (1982) argues that divorce among the elderly has been a hidden social phenomenon undistinguished from divorce among the young. She quotes one aged divorcee as follows:

> They lump us all together . . . . My daughter divorced at 33, and it was the pits for her, I well remember. But divorce for her was in no way the same as divorce for me . . . . She was heartbroken to be sure . . . but it was not the end of the world for her. She still had her children, a good job and a ton of divorced friends who "celebrated" the end of her marriage. When I was left at 64, the children were grown and scattered. I had no job, less than no confidence, and I did not know one woman my age who was similarly dumped. (pp. 89–90)

Deutscher (1964) found that, although the majority of older couples define the empty nest period favorably, some do experience serious problems. Women especially may find this to be a crucial time. A larger percentage of wives evaluated the postparental period both more favorably and more unfavorably than did husbands. The difficulties appear to center around three areas: (1) the advent of menopause and other disabilities associated with the aging process; (2) the final recognition and definition in retrospect of oneself as a "failure" in terms of either career or the child-raising process; and (3) the inability to fill the gap left in the family by the departure of the children.

Most elderly couples seem to adjust to retirement quite well. Research in this area focuses primarily on the changes in family role differentiation that occurs when a male retiree enters the wife's domain—the household. Some studies suggest that a large proportion of wives do not look forward to their husband's retirement (Donahue, Orbach, and Pollak 1960). Many wives resent the intrusion into the household of husbands who are home all day. They also express concern about having to live on reduced income. Heyman and Jeffers (1968) found a positive relationship between the length of a husband's retirement and the proportion of wives expressing negative attitudes toward their husband's retirement.

Kerckhoff (1966) observed social class differences in the effect of retirement on the redefinition of roles in the elderly household. Husbands' participation in domestic chores was welcomed by wives and seen as desirable by both spouses in upper- and middle-class households. Among working-class couples, however, both husbands and wives viewed increased participation in household chores by the husband as undesirable. Ballweg (1967) suggests that, although sharing domestic duties in general contributes to marital harmony among retirement couples, it does so especially when traditional sex-role task differentiation is continued. Thus, men may assume responsibility for "masculine" household tasks involving physical and mechanical skills, whereas women retain the more "feminine" tasks such as laundry and dusting. A recent study of couples married for fifty or more years seems to substantiate this finding (Sporakowski and Hughston 1978).

Widowhood

The majority of aged women are widows, and they outnumber widowers by a ratio of about five to one. Thus, it is not surprising that most of the research literature on widowhood deals with aged women. The few studies of widowers indicate that their main problems include loneliness and discomfort over self-maintenance. These studies have been principally concerned with the question of whether widowhood is harder on men or on women. Although widowers may be confronted with unfamiliar domestic and self-maintenance tasks, widowers also are more likely to belong to social organizations, to have more friends, to drive a car, and to have higher income than widows do (Atchley 1975; Crandall 1980). Adjustment to widowhood is especially problematic for men when they suffer several role losses within a short time span. As one would expect, the combination of loss of job, reduction of income, declining health, and loss of spouse can be traumatic.

In the United States the role of older widow is ambiguous. The term *widow* is useful for describing a marital status, but it is not at all useful for understanding how someone who occupies this status is expected to behave. In fact, there are no clear expectations for behavior in this role. Given the anomic situation in which older widows find themselves, it is no wonder that the great bulk of the research on widowhood highlights the negative personal consequences that accompany the change from spouse to widow. Statistics indicate that the widowed have higher rates of mortality, mental disorders, and suicide. It has generally been assumed that widowhood brings low morale (Atchley 1975). Shulman (1975) has reported that widows are more likely than single or married aged to describe the past as the happiest time of life and twice as likely to be depressed or lonely.

Helena Lopata, perhaps the foremost student of widowhood, believes that modern urban United States presents a unique cultural context for widowhood. Three factors appear to contribute to this uniqueness relative both to the historical past and to some other parts of the contemporary world:

1. The modern American nuclear family is expected to be socially and economically independent. Ties to the broader kinship network are there, but they are loose. In particular, ties to the male family line are weak.

2. Although the situation is beginning to change in the United States, it is still clearly the case that wives are economically dependent upon their husbands' sources of income.

3. U.S. society places extremely high importance on the marital relationship and on the development of strong mutual dependence between marital partners (Lopata 1980b).

Lopata (1973) has attempted to divide the widowhood experience into four stages: (1) official recognition of the event; (2) temporary disengagement or withdrawal from established lines of communication; (3) limbo; and (4) reengagement. The first stage typically begins with the funeral and includes the initial mourning period. *Grief work* is a term that describes the confrontation that must be made with the death of a spouse. This takes time and may involve a temporary withdrawal from previous social activities and responsibilities. Reengagement may begin with the question, "How and where do I go from here?"

Reengagement does not bring with it an end to the problems associated with widowhood: It may only be the beginning. The most serious problems widows must face are loneliness and a severe drop in income. Recently, Lopata (1978) has written of the failure of community resources to provide supports for widows who are trying to rebuild their lives and who have difficulty dealing with their problems.

Despite our understanding of the trauma of widowhood and of the adjustments it necessitates for many aged women, we must be careful not to overstate its impact. Some women downgrade the wife role, have less satisfying relationships with their husbands, and are in marriages that are less couple-oriented than more successful marriages are. This configuration of attitudes may reduce the impact of widowhood.

It is also the case that the lower morale experienced by widows may come not from widowhood but from changes brought about as a result of widowhood. Morgan (1976) has looked at the relationship between widowhood and morale while controlling for some accompaniments of widowhood, such as loss of income and loss of self-image. He found that, when these things were held constant, the morale scores of widowed women were not different from those of their nonwidowed counterparts.

Remarriage

Remarriage may be a desirable alternative for many divorced or widowed aged people. Whether or not it is a realistic alternative is another matter. In 1975, only 1 percent of the brides and 2 percent of the grooms in the United States were sixty-five years old and over (Glick 1979). The 1970 Census reports about 15 percent of older men and 6 percent of older women as remarried. This situation is not likely to change dramatically in the near future. As Treas and VanHilst (1976) point out, our culture offers little impetus to marry in the later years. The reasons for marriage in the United States today are not pertinent to the single aged: premarital pregnancy or the desire for children, escape from parental domination, social validation of adult heterosexuality, and pressure for conformity.

Aged marriages appear to be successful. Treas and VanHilst (1976) found that remarriages of the aged were most successful when based upon mutual affection and financial security. Children's approval seemed to contribute to the success of the marriages. Vinick (1978) studied remarriage in a small sample of Massachusetts elderly. Most remarriages were formed on the basis of companionship. Many in the sample used the statement, "It just turned into something," to describe the courtship. The desire for care was also important to the men; the personal qualities of the mate were important to the women. Those who were unhappy with their remarriages felt forced into the marriage because of external circumstances, such as financial need. For men, marital satisfaction was positively correlated with their past attitudes toward remarriage and their mental and physical health. For women, marital satisfaction was associated with the attitudes of peers, the quality of housing, and financial position.

Grandparenting

Grandparenting has become an event of middle-age. Early marriage, earlier childbearing, and longer life expectancy are producing grandparents in their forties (Troll, Miller, and Atchley 1979). The rocking-chair image of grandparents seems to be disappearing. Grandparents still work and remain quite active. Moreover, as Troll and her associates point out, many find their loyalties split between helping to care for their grandchildren and helping to care for their aged parents.

In 1970, 95 percent of all ten year olds had one living grandparent, 75 percent had at least two, and 71 percent had four living grandparents (Harris and Cole 1980). About 75 percent of the elderly in the United States have living grandchildren (Troll, Miller, and Atchley 1979). The Harris poll referred to earlier in this chapter reports that nearly one-half of all American grandparents see a grandchild approximately every day.

The high rates of divorce and remarriage in the United States have provided dramatic changes in the kinship networks of grandparents. Expanding networks are much more common among paternal grandmothers; they are much more likely to retain relationships with former daughters-in-law than are maternal grandmothers with former sons-in-law (Johnson and Barer 1987). But the expansion may be considerably broader. From the grandmothers' perspective, the relatives of children's divorces include former children-in-law, their parents and children, and even their new spouses and their relatives. With the remarriage of children, potential relatives include new children-in-law, their parents and children and even their former spouses and relatives (Johnson and Barer 1987). This "stretching out" of kinship networks can force role changes for many grandparents; some may even have to employ several different styles of grandparenting.

The grandparent role has different meanings for different people, and often the meaning of the role is reflected in the style of grandparenting. Neugarten and Weinstein (1964) have classified the different styles of grandparenting into five categories:

1. The *formal* grandparent likes to provide special treats and indulgences for the grandchild but maintains clearly demarcated lines between parenting and grandparenting. This grandparent leaves parenting strictly to the parents, maintaining constant interest in the grandchild but offering no advice.

2. The *fun seeker* maintains a playful and informal relationship with the grandchild, with the emphasis on mutual satisfaction.

3. The *surrogate parent* role is played by grandmothers whose daughters work and who assume responsibility for taking care of the child during the day.

4. The *reservoir of family wisdom* refers mainly to grandparents who possess special skills or resources and who expect young parents to maintain a subordinate position.

5. The *distant figure* is the grandparent who has contact with the grandchildren only on holidays and special occasions but otherwise remains distant and remote from the grandchild's life.

The styles of grandparenting are related to age. *Fun seekers* and *distant figures* are usually younger, whereas *formal* grandparents are more typically older.

McCready (1985) has used national survey data gathered between 1972 and 1984 to determine whether or not ethnicity can usefully explain variation in the styles of grandparenting that are adopted. Although not every older person in these national surveys is an actual grandparent, the respondents represent a "grandparent cohort" of people of like age and experience. The ethnic groups represented were English, Scandinavian, German, Irish, Italian, and Polish. Characteristics of children were grouped in a fashion that approximated the five styles of grandparenting described above, though the *formal* and *distant* styles were combined because there was no measure of contact frequency upon which to base distance (McCready 1985).

Generally, males were more likely to exhibit attitudes and responses linked to the formal/distant style of grandparenting, whereas the women emphasized the more informal and affect-oriented styles of behavior (McCready 1985). Scandinavians, Irish, and the Italians (grandmothers and grandfathers alike) were above the mean on scores of the formal/distant and surrogate styles; English and Italian grandmothers were the only groups to score above the mean on measures representing the reservoir-of-wisdom style of grandparenting. German grandfathers scored high on the formal/distant and surrogate styles, though German grandmothers only scored positively on the latter. Almost uniformly, representatives of the ethnic groups in this study scored low or negatively on indicators of the fun-seeking style. McCready (1985, 57) suggests that "the affective dimensions of the grandparent–grandchild relationship are not as prized by these respondents as the more behavioral and 'correct' dimensions of children's behavior." Clearly the cultural diversity that exists within grandparent populations in the United States reveals itself in diverse styles of grandparent–grandchild interaction.

Recently, some attention has begun to focus on the growing number of greatgrandparents in the United States. Employing data from a small sample, Doka and Mertz (1988) identified two basic styles of greatgrandparenting: remote and close. In the *remote* style, greatgrandparents had limited and ritualistic contact with their greatgrandchildren. Typically, this occurred on family and holiday occasions. Those who adopted a *close* style had frequent and regular contact with their greatgrandchildren, often babysat for them, and took them on trips or shopping. As Doka and Mertz conclude, there are many similarities between grandparenthood and great-grandparenthood, but clearly more research is needed to gain a fuller perspective on the dynamics of four, and even five, generation families.

What do grandchildren think of their grandparents? Children often develop attitudes toward their grandparents (and perhaps to the aged in general) that are consistent with the attitudes of their parents. Some research suggests that children observe how their parents treat their grandparents, and then treat their parents similarly when they become old.

The type of grandparent a child prefers appears strongly related to the age of the child. Kahana and Kahana (1970) found that younger children (preschool age) favored indulgent grandparents who gave them gifts; older children wanted grandparents to be active and fun-sharing. Robertson (1976) found that grandchildren between the ages of sixteen and twenty-six had extremely favorable attitudes toward their grandparents; 92 percent of them indicated that they would miss not having grandparents. The most desirable qualities that these grandchildren wanted in a grandparent were intelligence, love, gentleness, understanding, sense of humor, ability to communicate, and industriousness. It appears that, although the role of grandparent is not meaningful to all older people, most grandchildren seem to have strong affection toward their grandparents.

SUMMARY

The common perspective that family structure has changed in the United States from the extended to the nuclear type has come under serious question. Historical demographers now argue that the nuclear family probably was the dominant type of family structure during the U.S. colonial period and has since been the modal family type in the United States.

In its colonial phase the United States had a gerontophilic society, where being old conferred power and prestige. Cultural, demographic, and technological changes have brought a loss of status to older people.

Family sociologists and gerontologists use the notion of a modified extended family to describe the place of the elderly in the contemporary U.S. kin network. There is little evidence that older people are isolated from their families. Most older people live near, but not with, their children and interact with them frequently. Assistance in the form of goods, services, and financial aid flows both from adult children to their parents, and from the parents to their children.

The marital distribution of elderly men differs sharply from that of elderly women. Most elderly men are married, whereas over half of all elderly women are widowed. Most older couples are satisfied with their marriages and have adjusted to retirement.

Widowhood is a more difficult adjustment. The widowed have high rates of mortality, mental disorders, and suicide. The most serious problems that widows face are loneliness and a drop in income. Few elderly get the opportunity to remarry, although there is a demographic advantage to men, who are a relatively scarce resource. Aged marriages do seem to be successful.

Many, but not all, grandparents find grandparenting a significant role to play. There is significant diversity in grandparenting styles in the United States today. Most grandchildren seem to have strong affection for their grandparents.

STUDY QUESTIONS

1. Discuss the contrasting views social historians have of the U.S. family of bygone days.

2. Define *modified extended family*. How does such a family differ from the extended and nuclear family?

3. Discuss Fischer's notion of a "revolution in age relations" that occurred in the

United States between 1770 and 1820. What are its implications for the position of the elderly in families?

4. In relation to frequency and quality of interaction, discuss the relationship between aging parents and adult children in the contemporary U.S. family.

5. Explain what is meant by the empty-nest period. What are the positive and negative implications for the older couple experiencing the period of the family life cycle?

6. Helena Lopata divided widowhood into four stages. List and explain each of these stages.

7. Neugarten and Weinstein have classified the different stages of grandparenting into five categories. List and explain each of these stages.

BIBLIOGRAPHY

Adams, B. 1971. Isolation, function and beyond: American kinship in the 1960s. In C. Broderick (ed.), *A decade of family research and action.* Minneapolis: Council on Family Relations.

Arensberg, C. 1955. American communities. *American Anthropologist* 57:1143–1162.

Atchley, R. 1975. Dimensions of widowhood in later life. *Gerontologist* 13(2):176–178.

———. 1980. *Social forces in later life* (3d ed.). Belmont, Calif.: Wadsworth Publishing Co., Inc.

Atkinson, M.P., Kivett, V.R., and Campbell, R.T. 1986. Intergenerational solidarity: An examination of a theoretical model. *Journal of Gerontology* 41(3):408–416.

Back, K. 1974. The three-generation household in preindustrial society: Norm or expedient. Paper presented at the meeting of the Gerontological Society, Portland, Oregon, October 1974.

Ballweg, J. 1967. Resolution of conjugal role adjustment after retirement. *Journal of Marriage and the Family* 299:277–281.

Bankoff, E. 1983. Aged parents and their widowed daughters: A support relationship. *Journal of Gerontology* 38(2):226–230.

Barusch, A.S. 1988. Problems and coping strategies of elderly spouse caregivers. *Gerontologist* 28(5):677–685.

Bengtson, V., and Black, K. 1973. Intergenerational relations and continuities in socialization. In P. Baltes and K. Schaie (eds.), *Life-span development psychology.* New York: Academic Press, Inc.

Cain, B. 1982. Plight of the gray divorcee. *New York Times Magazine* December 19:89–90, 92, 94.

Cherlin, A. 1983. A sense of history: Recent research on aging and the family. In M.W. Riley, B.B. Hess, and K. Bond (eds.), *Aging in society: Selected reviews of recent research.* Hillsdale, N.J.: Lawrence Erlbaum Associates.

Chiriboga, D. 1982. Adaptation to marital separation in later and earlier life. *Journal of Gerontology* 37(1):109–114.

Clark, M., and Anderson, B. 1967. *Culture and aging.* Springfield, Ill.: Charles C Thomas, Publisher.

Connidis, I. 1983. Living arrangement choices of older residents. *Canadian Journal of Sociology* 8:359–375.

Crandall, R. 1980. *Gerontology: A behavioral science approach.* Reading, Mass.: Addison-Wesley Publishing Co., Inc.

Cumming, E., and Henry, W. 1961. *Growing old.* New York: Basic Books.

Day, A.T. 1985. *Who cares? Demographic trends challenge family care for the elderly.* Number 9, Population Trends and Public Policy. Washington, D.C.: Population Reference Bureau, Inc.

Demos, J. 1965. Notes on life in Plymouth Colony. *William and Mary Quarterly,* (Third Series) 22:264–286.

———. 1968. Families in colonial Bristol, Rhode Island: An exercise in historical demography. *William and Mary Quarterly* (Third Series) 25:40–57.

———. 1978. Old age in early New England. *American Journal of Sociology* 84(Supplement):S248–287.

Deutscher, I. 1964. The quality of postparental life. *Journal of Marriage and the Family* 26(1):52–59.

Doka, K.J. and Mertz, M.E. 1988. The meaning and significance of great-grandparenthood. *Gerontologist* 28(2):192–197.

Donahue, W., Orbach, H., and Pollak, O. 1960. Retirement: The emerging social pattern. In C. Tibbitts (ed.), *Handbook of social gerontology.* Chicago: University of Chicago Press.

Duvall, E.M. 1977. *Marriage and family development* (5th ed.). Philadelphia: J.B. Lippincott Co.

Federico, R. 1979. *Sociology* (2nd ed.). Reading, Mass.: Addison-Wesley Publishing Co., Inc.

Fischer, D. 1977. *Growing old in America.* New York: Oxford University Press.

Glick, P. 1979. The future marital status and living arrangements of the elderly. *Gerontologist* 19:301–309.

Goode, W. 1963. *World revolution and family patterns.* New York: The Free Press.

Greenberg, J.S., and Becker, M. 1988. Aging parents as family resources. *Gerontologist* 28(6):786–791.

Greenfield, S. 1967. Industrialization and the family in sociological theory. *American Journal of Sociology* 67:312–322.

Greven, P. 1966. Family structure in seventeenth century. Andover, Mass. *William and Mary Quarterly* (Third Series)23:234–356.

Gutman, D., et al. 1979. *Informal and formal support systems and their effect on the lives of the elderly in selected ethnic groups.* Washington, D.C.: The Catholic University of America.

Harris, D., and Cole, W. 1980. *Sociology of aging.* Boston: Houghton Mifflin Co.

Hess, B., and Waring, J. 1978. Changing patterns of aging and family bonds in later life. *The Family Coordinator* 27(4):304–314.

Hess, R., and Handel, G. 1959. *Family worlds.* Chicago, University of Chicago Press.

Heyman, D., and Jeffers, F. 1968. Wives and retirement: A pilot study. *Journal of Gerontology* 23:488–496.

Johnson, C.L., and Barer, B.M. 1987. Marital instability and the changing kinship networks of grandparents. *Gerontologist* 27(3):330–335.

Johnson, E., and Bursk, B. 1977. Relationships between the elderly and their adult children. *Gerontologist* 17:90–96.

Kahana, B., and Kahana, E. 1970. Grandparenthood from the perspective of the developing grandchild. *Developmental Psychology* 3(1):98–105.

Kart, C., and Engler, C. 1985. Family relations of aged colonial Jews: A testamentary analysis. *Ageing and Society* 5:289–304.

Kerckhoff, A. 1966. Family patterns and morale in retirement. In I. Simpson and J. McKinney (eds.), *Social aspects of aging.* Durham, N.C.: Duke University Press.

Krout, J. 1988. Rural versus urban differences in elderly parents' contact with their children. *Gerontologist* 28(2):198–203.

Laslett, P. 1969. Size and structure of the household in England over three centuries. *Population Studies* 23:199–224.

Laslett, P., and Harrison, W. 1963. Clayworth and Cogenhoe. In H. Bell and R. Ollard (eds.), *Historical essays, 1660–1750.* London: Adam and Charles Black.

Leichter, H., and Mitchell, W. 1967. *Kinship and casework.* New York: Russell Sage Foundation.

Litwak, E. 1965. Extended kin relations in an industrial democratic society. In E. Shanas and G.F. Streib (eds.), *Social structure and the family.* Englewood Cliffs, N.J.: Prentice-Hall.

Lopata, H. 1973. *Widowhood in an American city.* Cambridge: Schenkman Publishing Co.

———. 1978. The absence of community resources in support systems of urban widows. *Family Coordinator* 27(4):383–388.

———. 1980a. The widowed family member. In N. Datan and N. Lohmann (ed.), *Transitions of aging.* New York: Academic Press.

———. 1980b. Widows and widowers. In H. Cox (ed.), *Aging* (2nd ed.). Guilford, Conn.: Dushkin Publishing Group, Inc.

Lowenthal, M., Thurnher, M., and Chiriboga, D. 1975. *Four stages of life.* San Francisco: Jossey-Bass, Inc., Publishers.

Markides, K.S., Boldt, J.S., and Ray, L.A. 1986. Sources of helping and intergenerational solidarity: A three-generations study of Mexican Americans. *Journal of Gerontology* 41(4):506–511.

Mathews, S.H. 1987. Provision of care to old parents. *Research on Aging* 9(1):45–60.

Mathews, S.H., Werkner, J.E., and Delaney, P.J. 1989. Relative contributions of help by employed and nonemployed sisters to their elderly parents. *Journal of Gerontology* 44(1):S36–44.

McCready, W.C. 1985. Styles of grandparenting among white ethnics. In V.L. Bengtson, and J.F. Robertson (eds.), *Grandparenthood.* Beverly Hills, Calif.: Sage Publications.

Morgan, L. 1976. A reexamination of widowhood and morale. *Journal of Gerontology* 31(6):687–695.

National Council on the Aging. 1976. *The myth and reality of aging in America.* Washington, D.C.: NCOA.

Neugarten, B., and Weinstein, K. 1964. The changing American grandparent. *Journal of Marriage and Family* 26(2):199–204.

Okraku, I.O. 1987. Age and attitudes toward multigenerational residence, 1973 and 1983. *Journal of Gerontology* 42(3):280–287.

Parsons, T. 1942. Age and sex in the social structure of the U.S. *American Sociological Review* 7:604–616.

Pineo, P. 1961. Disenchantment in the later years of marriage. *Marriage and Family Living* 23(1):3–11.

Reiss, P. 1962. Extended kinship system: Correlates of and attitudes on frequency of interaction. *Marriage and Family Living* 24:333–339.

Riley, M.W., and Foner, A. 1968. *Aging and society,* Vol. I. New York: Russell Sage Foundation.

Robertson, J. 1976. Significance of grandparents: Perception of young adult children. *Gerontologist* 16(2):137–140.

Rollins, B., and Cannon, K. 1974. Marital satisfaction over the family life cycle. *Journal of Marriage and Family* 36:271–282.

Rollins, B., and Feldman, H. 1970. Marital satisfaction over the family life cycle. 32(1):20–28.

Rosenmayr, L., and Kockeis, E. 1963. Propositions for a sociological theory of aging and the family. *International Social Science Journal* 15:410–426.

Seward, R. 1974. Family size in the U.S.: An exploratory study of trends. *Kansas Journal of Sociology* 10:119–136.

Seltzer, M.M., Ivry, J., and Litchfield, L.C. 1987. Family members as case managers: Partnership between the formal and informal support networks. *Gerontologist* 27(6):722–728.

Shanas, E. 1979. Social myth as hypothesis: The case of the family relations of old people. *Gerontologist* 19(1):3–9.

Shanas, E., Townsend, P., Wedderburn, D., Friis, H., Milhhoj, P., and Stehouver, J. 1968. *Old people in three industrial societies.* New York: Atherton Press.

Shulman, N. 1975. Life-cycle variations in patterns of close relationships. *Journal of Marriage and Family* 37(4):813–821.

Siegel, J. 1976. *Demographic aspects of aging and the older population in the United States.* Current Population Reports, Special Studies Series P-23, No. 59. Washington, D.C.: U.S. Department of Commerce, Bureau of the Census.

Simmons, L. 1945. *The role of the aged in primitive society.* New Haven, Conn.: Yale University Press.

———. 1960. Aging in preindustrial societies. In C. Tibbitts (ed.), *Handbook of social gerontology.* Chicago: University of Chicago Press.

Sporakowski, M., and Hughston, G. 1978. Prescriptions for happy marriages: Adjustment and satisfaction of couples married for 50 years or more. *Family Coordinator* 27(4):321–327.

Stinnett, N., Carter, L., and Montgomery, J. 1972. Older persons' perceptions of their marriages. *Journal of Marriage and Family* 34:665–670.

Stinnett, N., Collins, J., and Montgomery, J. 1970. Marital need satisfaction of older husbands and wives. *Journal of Marriage and Family* 32:428–434.

Stone, L. 1967. *The crisis of the aristocracy, 1558–1641.* New York: Oxford University Press.

Stone, R., Cafferata, G.L., and Sangl, J. 1987. Caregivers of the frail elderly: A national profile. *Gerontologist* 27(5):616–626.

Sussman, M. 1965. Relationships of adult children with their parents in the U.S. In E. Shanas and G.F. Streib (eds.), *Social structure and the family.* Englewood Cliffs, N.J.: Prentice-Hall.

———. 1976. The family life of old people. In R. Binstock and E. Shanas (eds.), *Handbook of aging and the social sciences.* New York: Van Nostrand Reinhold Co.

———. 1985. The family life of old people. In R. Binstock and E. Shanas (eds.), *Handbook of aging and the social sciences* (2nd ed.). New York: Van Nostrand Reinhold Co.

Sussman, M., and Burchinal, L. 1962. Parental aid to married children: Implications for family functioning. *Marriage and Family Living* 24:32–332.

Tibbitts, C. 1968. Some social aspects of gerontology. *Gerontologist* 8(2):131–133.

Treas, J. 1977. Family support systems for the aged: Some social and demographic considerations. *Gerontologist* 17(6):486–491.

Treas, J., and VanHilst, A. 1976. Marriage and remarriage rates among older Americans. *Gerontologist* 16:132–136.

Troll, L. 1971. The family of later life: A decade review. *Journal of Marriage and the Family* 33:263–290.

Troll, L., and Bengtson, V. 1978. Generations in the family. In W.R. Burr, R. Hill, F.I. Nye, and I.L. Reiss (eds.), *Contemporary theories about the family*, Vol. I. New York: The Free Press.

Troll, L., Miller, S., and Atchley, R. 1979. *Families in later life.* Belmont, Calif.: Wadsworth Publishing Co., Inc.

Uhlenberg, P., and Myers, M.A. 1981. Divorce and the elderly. *The Gerontologist* 21:276–282.

Van de Walle, E. 1976. Household dynamics in a Belgian village, 1874–1866. *Family History* 1(1):80–94.

Vinick, B. 1978. Remarriage in old age. *Family Coordinator* 27(4):359–364.

Wolf, J.H., Breslau, N., Ford, A., Ziegler, H., and Ward, A. 1983. Distance and contacts: Interactions of Black urban elderly adults with family and friends. *Journal of Gerontology* 38(4):465–471.

CHAPTER 11

THE ECONOMICS OF AGING

Mrs. Mary Fremont is a seventy-seven-year-old black woman who has lived alone for twenty years. She rents an apartment in the inner city of a major metropolitan area in the upper Midwest. Her yearly income in 1985, which she received from the federally administered Supplemental Security Income (SSI) program, was $2,016 or about the average for all aged recipients of SSI in 1985. The actual poverty threshold for an aged individual in 1985 was $5,156.

The Evans's are recent migrants to a retirement community in the Southwest. They are white, middle class, and college educated. Mr. Evans worked in an executive capacity for a large corporation in the East. His approximate current retirement income is $26,000 and includes income from Social Security, a private pension, and other assets. The Evans's income is four times the 1985 poverty threshold level for an aged couple.

Mrs. Fremont fits the stereotype of an aged person living on what appears to be inadequate income. Certainly, most readers must be wondering how anybody in the United States today (or even in 1985) could get by on $2,000 in yearly income. What about the Evans's? It is difficult to think about them as being disadvantaged. Which case example best represents the economic situation of the elderly? A nationwide survey of adults between the ages of eighteen and sixty-four found 63 percent of them expressing the view that not having enough money to live on was a "very serious" problem for most people over sixty-five years of age (NCOA 1975). Interestingly, this same survey found only 15 percent of those over sixty-five themselves indicating that lack of money was a very serious problem.

How do we account for this discrepancy? Is economic deprivation among the elderly a myth? Or, are the elderly just kidding themselves about their financial situation? This chapter attempts to answer these and other important

246

questions. We begin by describing the economic status of the elderly and then investigating the adequacy of their financial resources in relation to their needs.

THE ECONOMIC STATUS
OF THE ELDERLY

The importance of one's economic status in old age cannot be exaggerated. The presence (or absence) of financial resources will have considerable impact on an individual's capacity to adjust to aging. Income will affect whether or not a retiree's values and preferences can be realized (Irelan and Bond 1976). The older person with adequate financial resources can maintain some degree of control over his or her life, including making decisions about which leisure activities to pursue, how much to travel, what kind of diet to maintain, and the amount of preventive medical care to seek. Older people without money can do none of these things.

Money Income of the Aged

Older Americans receive direct money income from a variety of sources. Some have earnings, either salaries or wages or self-employment income; most have a retirement pension (including Social Security) of one kind or another. Direct money income can also come from welfare payments, dividends, interest, rents, alimony, unemployment, veterans' and workmen's compensation payments, and gifts from others.

Figure 11-1 shows the sources of money income for the elderly. Clearly, Social Security is the major source (39 percent), although earnings (16 percent) and asset income (28 percent) contribute to the income position of many elderly. Not all elderly individuals receive income from all the sources identified in the figure. Table 11-1 describes the proportion of the elderly receiving income from a diverse list of income sources for 1962 and 1984. In 1984, 91 percent of the elderly received some income from Social Security. Married elderly people were more likely to receive income from wages, assets, private pensions, and government pensions than were the single aged. A higher proportion of unmarried aged received income from public assistance than did the married aged.

The accessibility of some income sources for the elderly has changed since the early 1960s. This is the result of broadened coverage of Social Security benefits and the rising impact of private pensions. For example, in 1962 only 69 percent of the aged were receiving income from Social Security. In addition, the proportion of the aged with private pension income rose from 9 percent in 1962 to 24 percent in 1984 (Yeas and Grad, 1987).

The accessibility of income sources for the elderly is likely to continue to change in the future. In particular, the impact of private pensions, and especially

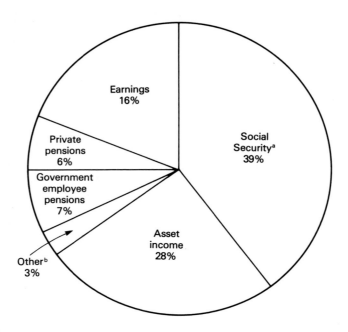

^a Includes railroad retirement (1%).
^b Includes public assistance (1%).

FIGURE 11-1   1984 sources of aged income. *Source: Yeas and Grad (1987, Table 4).* Note: Percentages have been rounded off to the nearest whole number.

individual retirement accounts (IRAs), is expected to alter the configuration of sources from which the elderly derive income. In 1981, the great majority of Americans became eligible to open IRAs. According to the Internal Revenue Service, almost 12 million tax returns for 1982 listed this deduction. The Tax Reform Act of 1986 placed significant limitations on the use of IRAs, although individuals not covered by company retirement plans remain eligible to take a tax deduction of up to $2,000 annually for a deposit in an individual retirement account. Individuals can begin withdrawing on these funds on reaching the age of fifty-nine and a half years or older, when their incomes are expected to be lower than during their peak working years.

Just how much income do the elderly have? Table 11-2 shows the total money income of persons sixty-five and over, by sex, in 1986. Most elderly persons had incomes under $10,000. This is the case for 43 percent of the men; 65 percent of the women had incomes under $8,500. The median income of aged women is $6,425; that of the men is $11,544. This constitutes an income ratio of 55.7 percent. Fifteen percent of aged men and 5 percent of aged women had incomes of $25,000 or more in 1986.

TABLE 11-1   Percentage of Aged Units with Income from Various Sources, 1962 and 1984

Source	1962	1984
Earnings	36	21
Social Security	69	91
Government employee pensions	5	14
Private pensions or annuities	9	24
Income from assets	54	68

Source: Yeas and Grad (1987, Table 1).

Another way to describe the income picture for the aged is in terms of family data. After all, many of the people whose incomes are reflected in Table 11-2 are married to someone with additional income. Table 11-3 provides the median incomes of all families in the United States in 1986, including the median income for families in which the head of household is aged sixty-five or over (hereafter referred to as *aged families*). The income of aged families is substantially higher than the income received by unrelated individuals, although it is still considerably below that of all families in the United States. The median income of aged families in the United States in 1986 was $19,932, $9,526 less than the median for all families.

TABLE 11-2   Total Money Income of Persons Aged Sixty-five and Over, by Sex, 1986

Total Money Income*	Men (%)†	Women (%)†
Less than $2,000	2.7	5.8
$2,000–3,999	4.7	17.0
$4,000–5,999	11.9	24.4
$6,000–8,499	16.5	18.1
$8,500–9,999	7.6	6.6
$10,000–14,999	22.4	12.9
$15,000–19,999	12.8	7.0
$20,000–24,999	7.0	3.4
$25,000–29,999	4.7	1.9
$30,000–34,999	2.5	1.0
$35,000–49,999	4.0	1.3
$50,000 and over	3.7	0.7
Total	100.0	100.1

* Includes salaries and wages; self-employment income; social insurance benefits; welfare payments; dividends, interest, and rents; pensions, alimony, and contributions from others; and unemployment, veterans', and workmen's compensation payments.

† Median income: men, $11,544; women, $6,425.

Source: U.S. Department of Commerce, Bureau of the Census, *Money income and poverty status of families and persons in the United States: 1986*, CPR, Series P-60, No. 157 (Washington, D.C.: U.S. Government Printing Office, 1987).

TABLE 11-3   Median Total Money Income by Age of Head of Family, 1986

	Median Income ($)
Families	
All ages	29,458
Head 65 years and over	19,932
Unrelated individuals	
All ages	12,116
65 years and over	7,731

Source: U.S. Department of Commerce, Bureau of the Census, *Money income and poverty status of families and persons in the United States: 1986,* CPR, Series P-60, No. 157 (Washington, D.C.: U.S. Government Printing Office, 1987).

Since 1965 the median income of aged families has increased almost six times from $3,514 to $19,932. The relative income position of the aged also has improved over this time period. For example, the ratio of median income of aged families to the median income of all families rose from 49.3 percent in 1965 to 56.9 percent in 1977 to 67.7 percent in 1986. This improvement in relative income status suggests that elderly families have enjoyed growth rates in income above the national average.

In describing the characteristics of an entire population, summary statistics, like those presented here, are frequently used. These measures represent statistical generalizations. It is important to recognize that the aged are a heterogeneous group, and there is wide variation in income among them. We have already seen how income varies along the lines of sex and family status. The most obvious other factors associated with income variation among the elderly are retirement status, age of the elderly, and race. The latter is discussed in great detail in Chapter 15, "The Minority Aged."

Not all older people are retired. In 1980, 20.1 percent of aged men and 8.0 percent of aged women were working. The income advantage to aged families with the head of household working is substantial. In 1986, aged families with the head working full-time, year-round had a median income of $39,434; the comparable figure for unrelated aged individuals was $19,122. Aged families with a head of household working full-time, year-round had median income almost twice that of all aged families.

The elderly are not age-homogeneous. Chapter 3 ("The Demography of Aging") distinguished between the "young-old" and the very old, or "old-old." Most data on the income of the aged groups all persons sixty-five and over together. Only recently has some income data distinguishing age groups among the elderly become available. Table 11-4 shows the decline in median income of aged family units, with the increasing age of the head of household.

Aged family units in which the head of household is eighty-five years or more have total money income that is about 55 percent of that for families headed by an individual sixty-five to sixty-nine years. Some of this income differential may be a function of current work experience, with the youngest elderly more likely to be participating in the labor force (even if only part-time). In addition, many of the old-old began their work careers before Social Security and private pension plans became commonplace.

Assets and In-Kind Income

Approximately twenty-five percent of all income to the elderly in this country comes from financial assets. These assets—sometimes referred to as *liquid assets* because of their easy conversion to goods, services, or money—generally take the form of bank deposits and corporate stocks and bonds. This income is not distributed equitably across the elderly population. In fact, about one-quarter of all elderly couples and over 40 percent of unrelated individuals had no financial assets in 1967 (Murray 1972); by 1975 about one-third of married couples and 60 percent of unrelated individuals had less than $15,000 in financial assets. This hardly constitutes a significant income supplement. Depending on the form of investment, even $15,000 will likely yield no more than about $1,500 per year in income. According to Riley and Foner (1968), assets tend to be correlated with income: Those families with the highest incomes are most likely to have substantial assets; those with the lowest incomes are least likely to have any assets.

Some assets have less liquidity because they require more time to convert to money. These *nonliquid assets* include equity in housing or a business and things such as automobiles. Homes are the most common asset (liquid or nonliquid) of older people. About 80 percent of elderly households reside in a privately owned home. Four-fifths of these homeowners own their homes free of any mortgage. This might suggest to some that older people need less

---

TABLE 11-4   Money Income of Aged Family Units, by Age of Unit Head, 1983

Age of Unit Head	Median Income ($)	Ratio to Median Income for All Aged Family Units
65–69	12,980	1.27
70–74	10,330	1.01
75–79	9,020	.89
80–84	8,210	.81
85 and over	7,110	.70
All, 65 and over	10,190	

Source: Radner, D.B. 1986. *Changes in the money income of the aged and nonaged, 1967–1983.* Studies in Income Distribution, No. 14, Social Security Administration, U.S. Government Printing Office.

income because they have no mortgage payments and have considerable equity tied up in a home. This may not be the case, however. Atchley (1977), contending that home ownership really does not reduce income requirements for aged persons, suggests that home ownership reduces income needs by less than $500 per year.

Just how much equity do the elderly have in their homes? Using data from the Survey of Income and Program Participation, Schulz (1988) reports that while 27 percent of elderly households in 1984 had no home equity, 53 percent had home equity of $40,000 or more. Until very recently, however, this equity was not available to the aged homeowner for day-to-day living expenses. Since January 1, 1979, the Federal Home Loan Bank Board has allowed federally chartered savings and loan associations to offer *reverse annuity mortgages*. Under this mortgage, a homeowner may sell some equity in the house, receiving in return a fixed monthly sum based on a percentage of the current market value of the house (Schulz 1988). This is similar to a plan that has existed in France for many years. In France, a homeowner can negotiate a home annuity plan, called a *viager* arrangement (the word literally means "for life"), with a buyer. The buyer pays an agreed-upon down payment and a monthly payment to the owner for the rest of the owner's life in return for the property at death (Schulz 1988). Over 400,000 of these annuity plans are thought to exist in France, but there is currently no data available on the number of such mortgages written in the United States.

The elderly receive indirect or in-kind income in the form of goods and services, which they obtain free or at reduced cost. According to the U.S. House Select Committee on Aging (1979), there are forty-three major federal programs benefiting the elderly over and above those providing direct income. Nevertheless, it is difficult to say how much in income these programs are worth today to the aged. Information on the value of comparable services available in the marketplace is sometimes difficult to obtain. In addition, the value recipients may place on in-kind services may differ sharply from the market value (Schmundt, Smolensky, and Stiefel 1975).

There are numerous programs aimed at providing housing to older people below the cost for similar housing on the open market. Under its various assistance programs the federal government houses nearly 1.5 million older persons in 1.25 million units (Lawton 1985). These programs are discussed in detail in Chapter 16, "Living Environments of the Elderly."

The food stamp program is another visible source of indirect income to those elderly who are eligible to participate (there are income and asset tests). Perhaps the largest government program providing indirect income to the elderly is Medicare, federal health insurance for the aged, established in 1965. Smeeding (1982) estimates that in 1980 the total market value of the major housing, food, and medical care benefits for both the aged and nonaged was $72.5 billion. The Social Security Administration reports that 85 percent of the aged receive *none* of the benefits from these services; only six percent of low-income aged received food stamps benefits in 1984, while four percent received public housing benefits (Social Security Administration 1986).

Taxes and Inflation

When we reported above that the median income of aged families in the United States in 1986 was $19,932, we were giving a pretax figure. Almost all income data, especially that published by the Social Security Administration and U.S. Census Bureau, is gross income or income before taxes. The scarcity of after-tax data makes it difficult to analyze the impact of taxation on the elderly and to determine whether, relative to the other age groups, they are advantaged or disadvantaged by tax laws.

Since 1984, up to one-half of Social Security benefits received by taxpayers whose incomes exceed certain base amounts are included in taxable income. The base amount is $25,000 for a single taxpayer, $32,000 for a married couple filing a joint return, and zero for married persons filing separate returns. The Tax Reform Act of 1986 increased the personal tax exemption to $1,900 for all individuals and allowed an additional deduction of $600 for an aged couple and $750 for a single person who is sixty-five years or older. Persons age fifty-five years and over are permitted to exclude from federal taxation up to $125,000 resulting from the sale of a personal residence. Property tax reductions are now granted to the elderly in virtually every state. The latter points would seem to be of more help to the higher income elderly—those who are more likely to itemize deductions on federal income tax returns and who are more likely to be property owners.

Inflation has been called a hidden tax, which can have disastrous impact on the economic situation of people of all ages. There is some controversy surrounding the analysis of the impact of inflation on the incomes of the aged. The economist Arthur Okun (1970) concludes that the "retired aged are the only major specific demographic group of Americans that I can confidently identify as income losers." Theodore Torda (1972) does not find support for the thesis that the elderly suffer greater losses as a result of inflation. Torda observed that the cost of living to aged retirees rose by about 2 percent more than it did for urban wage earners from 1960 to 1972. He believes this was more than offset by the indirect income received by the elderly through the introduction of Medicare in 1966.

Schulz (1988) lists five principal ways older people can be affected adversely by unanticipated inflation:

1. Assets that do not adjust with inflation depreciate in value.
2. Income sources may not adjust to inflation, reducing real income.
3. For employed people, adjustments in earnings may lag behind inflation, reducing real wages.

4. The tax burden may rise because the tax brackets are defined in money rather than real terms.

5. Elderly persons may allocate their budget differently from others (for example, more for food, housing, and transportation). Because indexes used to measure and adjust various sources of income may not correctly reflect aged buying patterns, the aged may not be fully compensated for increased prices.

The last two points deserve additional discussion. We should be mindful of the fact that many aged will not pay income taxes because their incomes are low. All but the highest income recipients of Social Security will be exempt from federal taxes as well. In the past, those who paid federal income taxes faced a problem: Some compensation received as protection from inflation was taxed away, moreover, at progressively higher rates (Schulz 1988). Starting in 1985, tax brackets were indexed to take inflation into account. The Tax Reform Act of 1986 simultaneously reduced the number of tax brackets and the progressivity in the federal tax structure. These actions have eliminated the problem.

Clearly, persons living primarily on fixed incomes or on pensions are hurt the most by the rising prices that accompany inflation. Historically, this has been the case for the elderly. Recent developments have changed this situation, though. The Social Security program, the major source of retirement income, now adjusts benefits automatically based on the rate of inflation; for 1984, for example, recipients of Social Security received a 3.5 percent increase consistent with the lower rate of inflation for that year. The Social Security Amendments of 1983 have affected cost-of-living adjustments (COLA) to Social Security benefits in two ways. First, the July 1983 COLA was delayed until January 1984, with all future automatic adjustments being effective on a calendar year basis. Second, if Social Security trust fund assets decline relative to the outflow of funds, then future automatic COLAs will be pegged to the lesser of increases in prices (measured by the Consumer Price Index) or to increases in wages.

Several in-kind income sources such as the food stamp program also peg their benefits to the rate of inflation. Some private pension benefits are also adjusted automatically as the cost of living increases. All this suggests that many elderly are in an advantaged position relative to other age groups—a major portion of their direct and indirect money income keeps pace with the rate of inflation.

THE ADEQUACY OF AGED INCOME

It is one thing to describe how much income the elderly have, quite another to say what they do with their income and whether or not it is adequate for their needs. We now attempt the latter below.

Like Americans of all ages, the aged are consumers of a vast array of goods and services. In 1970 older persons spent about $60 billion, or over 10 percent of the national total. This figure was consistent with the proportion of the United States population made up by older people in 1970, 10 percent. It is likely that, as the elderly population increases (and their incomes increase), so will the proportion of all goods and services they account for in purchases. On this basis, we would estimate personal expenditures of the aged in 1984 at about $260 billion, or little more than 11 percent of total personal consumption expenditures in the United States in 1984.

How do older Americans spend their income? Table 11-5 compares the annual expenditures of urban households with a head sixty-five years of age or older with all urban households. Older household units spend proportionately more of their income on housing, food, and health care, and less on transportation, clothing and, as might be expected, contributions to retirement pensions. The proportion spent on life insurance and other miscellaneous expenditures is about the same for both groups.

Herman Brotman (1978), former assistant to the Commissioner on Aging, recognized the pattern of expenditures among the elderly as being similar to the pattern of expenditures among low-income groups in general. Still, we must ask, is "low-income" an adequate income?

The most frequently used measure of income adequacy is the poverty index developed in the early 1960s by the Social Security Administration, based on the amount of money needed to purchase a *minimum adequate diet* as determined by the Department of Agriculture. The index has been described as follows:

The food budget is the lowest that could be devised to supply all essential

TABLE 11-5   Annual Expenditures of Urban Consumer Units, by Age of Householder, 1982–83

	All Consumer Units (%)	Age of Householder 65 Years and Over (%)
Housing	30.6	33.4
Food	16.6	18.5
Transportation	19.6	16.0
Health care	4.4	9.9
Clothing	5.5	4.2
Retirement pension, Social Security contributions	7.2	2.0
Life insurance	1.4	1.2
Other (entertainment, personal care, education, miscellaneous expenditures)	13.2	13.7
	100.0	100.0
Total expenditures	$18,892	$12,346

Source: U.S. Bureau of the Census (1985, Table 739).

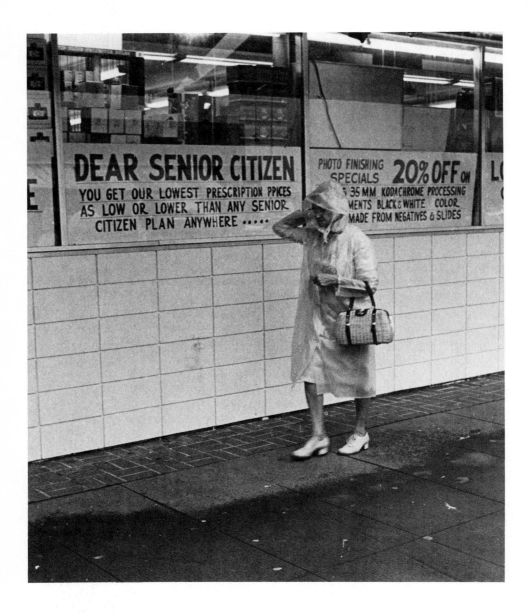

nutrients using food readily purchasable in the U.S. market (with customary regional variations). The poverty line is then calculated at three times the food budget (slightly smaller proportions for one- and two-person families) on the assumption—derived from studies of consumers—that a family that has spent a larger proportion of its income on food will be living at a very inadequate level. The food budgets and the derivative poverty income cutoff points are estimated in detail for families of differing size and composition (62 separate family types) with a farm/nonfarm differential for each type. This variation of the poverty measure in relation to family size and age of members is its most important distinguishing characteristic. (U.S. House Committee on Ways and Means 1967)

In 1986, the poverty index level for a two-person family with an aged head was approximately $6,630; the comparable level for a single person was about $4,255.

Table 11-6 shows that in general poverty has been declining among older people during the period from 1959 to 1986, although about one in eight older persons is still "officially" impoverished. Poverty varies among subgroups of the elderly. Aged whites are less likely to live in poverty than is anyone in the total United States population, with 10.7 percent living below the poverty level; however, 31 percent of aged nonwhites are living in poverty.

Critics of the poverty index argue that it is set too low. Remember that the index is calculated at three times the minimum adequate food budget, with different food budgets constructed for different types of families. The following characteristics are used in combination to develop indices for family units:

1. Age of head over or under age sixty-five

2. Size of family (two to seven or more)

3. Farm and nonfarm

4. Male and female head of household

5. Number of related children under age eighteen

6. "Unrelated" family units

The 3:1 ratio was set as a result of surveys made in 1955 and in 1960 to 1961 of the ratio of food consumption to other expenditures for *all* families in the

TABLE 11-6   Poverty Rates: 1959, 1968, 1977, 1982, 1986

	1959 (%)	1968 (%)	1977 (%)	1982 (%)	1986 (%)
Total population	22	13	12	15	13.6
Total aged population	35	25	14	15	12.4
Whites	33	23	12	12	10.7
Nonwhites	61	47	35	38	31.0

Source: Based on data in U.S. Bureau of the Census, *Consumer income*, CPR, Series P-60, No. 116 (Washington, D.C.: U.S. Government Printing Office, 1978); U.S. Department of Commerce, Bureau of the Census, *Money income and poverty status of families and persons in the United States: 1982*, CPR, Series P-60, No. 140 (Washington, D.C.: U.S. Government Printing Office, 1983; and U.S. Department of Commerce, Bureau of the Census, *Money income and poverty status of families and persons in the United States: 1986*, CPR, Series P-60, No. 157 (Washington, D.C.: U.S. Government Printing Office, 1987).

United States. A congressional report indicates that based on Consumer Expenditure Surveys of 1972 to 1973, the current ratio likely exceeds 5:1 (Poverty Studies Task Force 1976). In testimony before the U.S. House Select Committee on Aging, one student of aging in the United States suggested that shifting to more realistic levels of what constitutes poverty would more than double the number of aged poor, so that the number of either poor or near poor would include approximately 40 percent of the aged (Orshansky 1978). Orshansky (1978) also points out that the index is not applied to the "hidden poor"— those who are institutionalized or living with relatives. Thus, even the current figures on poverty status exclude millions of aged who are unable to live independently. According to Chen (1985), one in four of the aged had incomes at or below 125 percent of the poverty level measure in 1981. Had this near-poverty benchmark been employed, the number of aged persons defined as impoverished would have risen from 3.9 million to 6.4 million, an increase of 64 percent.

There is another criticism of the poverty index, one that argues poverty statistics are artificially high because the value of in-kind or noncash transfers are not included as income. In 1980, government expenditures for noncash transfer programs such as food stamps, Medicare, and Medicaid was over $72 billion (U.S. Bureau of the Census 1982). Should this money be included as income for the purpose of measuring poverty? If the answer is yes, then by definition many people will have additional income, and the poverty rate will decline.

Table 11-7 shows the poverty rates for all persons and those sixty-five years of age and older employing three different methods developed by the U.S. Bureau of the Census (1982) for valuing in-kind and noncash transfers: market value, recipient value, and poverty budget share value. *Market value* is equal to the purchase price in the private market of the goods and services received by the recipient. The *recipient value* is the amount of cash that would make the recipient just as well off as the in-kind transfer. It reflects the recipient's own

TABLE 11-7   Poverty Rate by Age, Using Alternative Methods of Valuing Noncash Benefits: 1984

	Current Poverty Definition (%)	Valuing Food and Housing Only			Valuing Food, Housing, and All Medical Benefits		
		Market Value (%)	Recipient Value (%)	Poverty Budget Share Value (%)	Market Value (%)	Recipient Value (%)	Poverty Budget Share Value (%)
All persons	14.4	12.9	13.2	13.0	9.7	12.2	12.1
65 years and over	12.4	10.5	10.8	10.5	2.6	7.3	7.6

Source: U.S. Bureau of the Census (1985, Table 774).

valuation of the benefit. The *poverty budget share value* limits the value of food, housing, or medical benefit transfers to the proportions spent on these items by persons at or near the poverty line from 1960 to 1961 when in-kind transfers were minimal. Remember also that the household consumption surveys of 1960 to 1961 are the continuing basis for the assumption in the poverty index that food represents one-third of household expenditures for the poor. According to the table, the market value approach has the effect of reducing poverty the most. Under the market valuation approach for food, housing, and medical benefits, the poverty rate for all persons in the United States would be under 10 percent (9.7 percent), and poverty would be near nonexistent for the aged (2.6 percent).

A second measure of the adequacy of aged income is the *Retired Couple's Budget* of the U.S. Bureau of Labor Statistics. The retired couple is defined as a husband aged sixty-five or over and his wife. They live independently and are assumed to be in good health. Actually, the Bureau of Labor Statistics provides three different budgets for aged couples reflecting different standards of living: lower, intermediate, and higher. Table 11-8 presents the monthly budget for a retired couple for the three different levels as it was set in the autumn of 1981. Budget items pertain to urban families only and have been updated based on changes in the Consumer Price Index. For the fall of 1981 (the last year for which the index is available), the budget for a retired couple living in an urban area was set at approximately $7,226 (lower level), $10,226 (intermediate level), and $15,078 (higher level).

One problem with the Retired Couple's Budget is that little explanation is given for why one of the three standards should be used over the other two. All those who are "officially" poor in terms of the poverty index are still so under terms of the Retired Couple's Budget. But, what of those who have incomes above the poverty level but below the budget level? Chen (1985) has

TABLE 11-8   Monthly Budget for a Retired Couple, Urban United States, Autumn, 1981

	Lower		Intermediate		Higher	
	$	%	$	%	$	%
Food	182	30	242	28	304	24
Housing	198	33	283	33	442	35
Transportation	46	8	89	10	163	13
Clothing and personal care	37	6	58	7	88	7
Medical care	90	15	91	11	92	7
Other family consumption	23	4	38	4	75	6
Other cost	26	4	51	6	93	7
Totals	602	100	852	99	1257	99

Source: U.S. Bureau of the Census. 1982. *Statistical Abstract of the United States, 1982–83* (Table 763, p. 465). Washington, D.C.: U.S. Government Printing Office.

calculated that in 1985 18 percent of retired couples had incomes below the lower budget and 35 percent had incomes below the intermediate budget. Whether such persons are officially deemed poor or not may be a moot issue. Clearly, many of these elderly have substantial economic difficulties that are likely to manifest themselves in poor nutrition, neglect of medical needs, inadequate housing, and the like.

THE SOCIAL SECURITY SYSTEM

Nine of ten U.S. workers are covered and over 90 percent of the elderly receive some income support through a public retirement pension system administered by the federal government and colloquially referred to as Social Security. Despite recent public attention to the problems involved in financing this system, few people are really familiar with its principles and provisions. In this section we discuss Social Security, focusing primarily on pension benefits and selected special issues such as the needed reform of provisions related to women. Several related programs, including Supplemental Security Income (SSI), will be reviewed.

Background

The notion of an old age pension received as a right by a person who had led a productive life was not seriously discussed until the end of the nineteenth century (Bromley 1974). Even then, the prevailing opinion was that an individual was solely responsible for making financial provision for himself or herself in old age. Such provision would come out of a lifetime's earnings, through either savings or insurance. Individuals unable to provide for themselves were subject to "poor laws" and the scarce resources of private charities (see Chapter 16, "Institutionalization," especially the section on the history of old-age institutions).

By 1889 a system of social insurance had been created in Germany that included a pension scheme. For the first time the aged were given a measure of economic security as a right rather than as a charity. In Denmark, state support for needy old people was introduced in 1891. Pension rights were introduced in Great Britain in 1908 for people over the age of seventy who had been in regular employment but had little or no income.

During the early part of this century and into the 1920s continuing attempts were made in the United States to define pensions as a right of aged Americans. These attempts met with limited success. Several states enacted old-age pension legislation, and reform groups such as the American Association of Old Age Security began to appear. The Great Depression, with its devastating economic impact on the lives of many Americans, helped create conditions that would ultimately allow the enactment of federal legislation promoting the pension rights of the aged and guaranteeing unemployment insurance.

Unemployment during the Great Depression was more than 25 percent among the elderly. Bank failures and the declining value of estates exhausted the financial resources of millions, including even those among the more prosperous middle and upper-middle classes. In 1932 the American Federation of Labor reversed its previous position and endorsed unemployment insurance and old-age assistance at the state and federal levels.

Utopian schemes were prevalent during this period. In 1933 Upton Sinclair put forth a twelve-point EPIC ("end poverty in California") plan to make people self-supporting and to grant a $50 a month old-age pension to all needy persons who had resided in California for at least three years. Sinclair won the Democratic nomination for governor but was soundly defeated as his opponents insisted EPIC actually meant "end property, introduce communism" in California (Fischer 1977).

The so-called "ham and eggs" movement, also based in California, proposed a weekly pension be given to everyone who was fifty years of age or over and out of work. The pension, initially proposed to be "twenty-five dollars every Tuesday" and later improved to "thirty dollars every Thursday," would be in the form of stamped scrip, which would expire at a given date. Not only would the economic situation of the older unemployed be enhanced by this scheme, but also the economy would be invigorated by increased circulation of money (Fischer 1977).

Perhaps the most popular of these utopian schemes was that put forth by Dr. Francis Townsend of Long Beach, California. The essence of the Townsend plan was that all Americans over sixty receive a monthly sum of $200 on the condition that they spent their pension within thirty days; a 2 percent tax on all business transactions was to pay for the plan (Achenbaum 1978). By 1936 Townsend claimed a national following of over 5 million and at least sixty U.S. representatives sympathetic to his measure (Putnam 1970).

Clearly the idea of an old-age pension had achieved legitimacy. The institutional structure needed to implement this idea was the Social Security Act of 1935. With its passage, the United States became one of the last industrial nations to establish a federal old-age pension program.

Principles

The influence of this piece of legislation on the whole question of retirement and pension in the United States is difficult to overestimate (Calhoun 1978). As one historian of old age in America has pointed out, the Social Security Act of 1935 (1) established the principle of a guaranteed "floor" income as a right bought by contributions over the course of a working life, (2) gave added impetus to demands for the extension of private pension coverage, (3) provided a standard age by which retirement could be defined, and (4) signaled a new era in financial arrangements for life after retirement (Calhoun 1978).

Still, it is important to remember that this legislation was very much a political document, which reflected divergent views prominent at the time. Should a program be aimed at preventing or relieving economic destitution? Should a straight government pension be provided or a contributing insurance system for wage earners? What of England's plan, which included both insurance *and* old-age assistance? Should there be a single federal system or an aggregate of state plans? Should the plan be voluntary or compulsory, universal or selective (Achenbaum 1978)?

Schulz (1988) outlines seven principles inherent in the Social Security legislation accepted by President Roosevelt and the Congress. Some of these principles clearly reflect a consensus or compromise position on questions raised here above.

1. For the designated groups, participation was compulsory.

2. Social Security was set up as an earnings-related system.

3. Social adequacy was taken into account in the determination of benefits for recipients. Weighted benefits favored workers with lower earnings.

4. Social Security was not intended to be the sole means of economic protection; it was only to provide a floor of protection.

5. Funds for operating the program were to come from earmarked taxes, called *contributions,* and employer contributions.

6. Workers were to earn their benefits through participation in the program; there was to be no means test.

7. A retirement test was established; pension benefits were withheld if an eligible person worked and earned above a specified amount.

Pension Benefits

The Social Security Act of 1935 established a federal old-age pension program (OAI) and a federal-state system of unemployment insurance. The original legislation, weak by comparison with other western nations, has been strengthened and expanded since 1939, when survivors' and dependents' benefits were added (OASI). Disability insurance (OASDI) was added in 1956, Medicare (OASDHI) in 1965. Changes legislated in 1972 included the automatic adjustment of benefits for inflation (begun in 1975) and the establishment of Supplemental Security Income (SSI) to replace aid to the indigent, blind, and disabled. Important changes were made again in the Social Security Amendments of 1983.

In 1948 only 13 percent of all persons aged sixty-five years and over were receiving Social Security payments. Since 1950, however, additional groups of workers have been brought into the system: certain farm and domestic workers (1950), the self-employed (1954), members of the uniformed services (1956), Americans employed by foreign governments (1960), physicians (1965), and ministers (1967). In 1974, the railroad retirement program was integrated into the Social Security system. As of January 1984 the following new groups have been covered under Social Security: (1) newly hired federal employees including executive, legislative, and judicial branch employees; (2) current employees of the legislative branch who are not participating in the Civil Service Retirement System; (3) all members of Congress, the president, the vice president, federal judges, and most executive-level political appointees; and (4) current and future employees of private, tax-exempt nonprofit organizations. Currently, nine of ten workers in this country are covered by Social Security.

Social Security eligibility is related to work rather than to need. An individual (and his or her dependents and survivors) is eligible if he or she has worked in employment that is covered and has worked long enough to have acquired "insured status." Most workers in jobs not covered are aware of this and are often covered by another retirement system. Insurance status is acquired by earning a minimum amount during a specified number of calendar quarters in jobs covered by Social Security. In 1988 a person was credited with a quarter of coverage for each $470 earned during the year, with a maximum of four quarters of coverage in a given year. A person who reached age sixty-two in 1983 needed thirty-seven quarters to achieve minimum eligibility for retirement benefits; a person who reaches age sixty-two in 1991 or later will need at least forty quarters of coverage for eligibility, or about ten years of covered employment.

Benefits are financed by payroll taxes paid by both employees and employers on income up to a certain level. In 1988 this tax is 15.02 percent (7.51 percent withheld from employees) applied to a base level of earnings, which (since 1974) rises automatically as average earnings rise. This is scheduled to increase to 15.30 percent in 1990. The self-employed can expect to pay this same rate of 15.30 percent in 1990.

Some have argued that this payroll tax is regressive. That is, since only income up to a certain level is subject to taxation, those with higher incomes pay a lower proportion of their income into the Social Security tax fund. For example, an individual earning $15,000 a year pays 7.51 percent or $1,126.50 to Social Security, but someone earning $100,000 a year pays approximately $3,380 (7.51 percent of the first $45,000), or about 3.4 percent of his or her total income. Thus, the tax contribution is a heavier burden for the lower-income worker, although such workers do receive *proportionately* higher benefits when they retire (see discussion of pension replacement rates, below). It is also likely (perhaps even *more* likely for the lower income worker) that the employer's share of tax contribution is borne by employees in lower wages and reduced benefits.

Benefits are paid to persons who have worked for a minimum period of time on a covered job. The minimum benefit of $2,556 in 1988 is provided workers (and survivors) who retire at age sixty-five and who would otherwise be eligible for very low benefits. Maximum benefits are limited by a ceiling placed on earnings on which the worker had made contributions. The benefit formula is neglected in favor of persons with a history of low earnings, on the assumption that they have a smaller margin for reduction in income (Yeas and Grad 1987).

A covered worker who had always earned the federal minimum wage and who claimed benefits at age sixty-five in January 1987 would have received a monthly benefit of $391. One who had always had earnings equal to average wages in covered employment would have received $593. Finally, a covered worker who always had wages at or above the maximum amount subject to Social Security taxes and who claimed benefits at age sixty-five in January 1987 would have received a monthly benefit of $789 (Social Security Administration 1987). The average monthly benefit actually paid to a retired worker in January 1987 was $5,868 a year, or $489 a month.

This relatively low average benefit level reflects the fact that over one-half of current Social Security recipients *do not* receive full benefits. This is in part due to the popularity of the early retirement option. Early retirement benefits may be paid to people who retire at ages sixty-two to sixty-four. These benefits are reduced to take into account the longer period over which they will be paid.

Delayed benefit credits (sometimes referred to as the *delayed retirement credit* or DRC) are also available. Up until 1979, benefits were increased 1 percent for each year after 1970 in which the worker between sixty-five and seventy-two did not receive any benefits. Starting with those reaching sixty-two in 1979, an additional 3 percent will be added to benefits for each year between age sixty-five and seventy-two that benefits are not received. The 1983 amendments to Social Security have increased the DRC payable to workers who delay retirement past the full-benefit retirement age and up to age seventy. DRCs will increase an additional 0.5 percent every other year until reaching 8 percent per year for workers aged sixty-two after 2004.

The Retirement Test

The Social Security Administration employs a "retirement test" to determine whether or not a person otherwise eligible for retirement benefits is considered retired. Unless a person can be considered substantially retired, benefits are not payable. Essentially, the retirement test acts to reduce benefits paid persons under age seventy who earn more than a certain amount. For example, a sixty-seven-year-old woman could earn up to $8,440 in 1988 ($703 monthly) *without* any reduction in her Social Security benefits. Benefits are reduced $1 for every $2 earned above the exempt amount. Prior to 1977 the retirement test involved both an annual and a monthly test. Benefits were payable in any month any individual earned wages of less than $200 regardless of total earnings in the year. In 1977 the monthly exemption test was eliminated, except for the first year of retirement; now, only an annual test applies.

Beginning in 1990, the retirement test "tax" will decrease from $1 for each $2 of earnings to $1 for each $3 of excess earnings for individuals who attain full-benefit retirement age. The full-benefit retirement age, currently age sixty-five, will gradually increase to age sixty-six in the year 2009 and to sixty-seven in 2027, according to the 1983 amendments of the Social Security system.

It is difficult to estimate how many people are affected by the retirement test. A Special Committee on Aging estimate of 1.5 million was made in 1975. Much controversy surrounds discussion of the test as evidenced by persistent congressional attempts to repeal or drastically modify it. Critics argue that the retirement test acts as a work-disincentive plan in that earnings above the exempt amount are, in effect, taxed at a 50 percent rate. Others suggest that the test itself is a form of age discrimination because persons seventy and older are not required to meet it. Proponents of the test point out that liberalization or even elimination of the retirement test would be very costly and would ultimately help only a small number of aged who are least in need. Complete elimination of the test is estimated to cost $6 or $7 billion in the first year (National Commission on Social Security 1981).

Social Security Replacement Rates

Social Security has had enormous impact on reversing the extent of poverty among the aged. In 1966, 60 percent of Social Security benefits went to people whose income otherwise would have been below the poverty line, and 90 percent of these were lifted from poverty by virtue of the Social Security payments (Hollister 1974). This has led at least one economist to characterize Social Security as the most successful social program in the history of the country (Hollister 1974). Still, many are uncomfortable with the program and especially with what is perceived to be an inadequate replacement of preretirement income. Is this perception accurate? An answer requires evaluation of Social Security replacement rates.

In 1967, a U.S. House Ways and Means Committee report specified that the retirement benefit of a man aged sixty-five and his wife should represent at least 50 percent of his average wages under the Social Security system. Some have argued that, even assuming reduced expenses and lower taxes, 50 percent of wages is not enough. Munnell (1977) and Schulz and his colleagues (1974) seem to agree that 65 to 80 percent of preretirement earnings is required by retirees. Schulz proposes that Social Security provide most of this—inflation protection benefits equal to at least 55 percent of preretirement average earnings. We must remember that Social Security is only one source of income for most of the elderly; many are able to supplement this income. Private pensions, wages, asset income, intrafamily aid, and even welfare and SSI benefits for the poorest of the elderly all provide help to individuals attempting to maintain a preretirement standard of living.

Munnell (1977) has evaluated the replacement rate structure of Social Security benefits in 1975 and finds it to be quite progressive: As the earnings record of a worker rises, the Social Security replacement rate falls. The proportion of income replaced for the worker with a history of low earnings ranges from 99.4 percent for the worker who retires at age sixty-five and whose spouse is also sixty-five or over, to 53 percent for a worker who retires at age sixty-two without a spouse or whose spouse is under age sixty-two. Among those with maximum earnings in 1975, this range is from 49.5 percent to 26.4 percent. The range of replacement rates among those with median earnings (69.3 to 36.9 percent) is high when compared with actual Social Security recipients studied by the Social Security Administration. Fox (1982) calculated the median after-tax replacement rates for Social Security recipients first receiving benefits between 1968 to 1976 to be 55 percent for couples, 52 percent for nonmarried women, and 46 percent for nonmarried men. Even when private and government pension income is taken into account, replacement rates fall well below a level necessary for many to maintain living standards in retirement.

Several authors have examined the adequacy of replacement rates in the United States in relation to those that exist in other countries. Horlick (1970) found that the average retired couple in the United States enjoys an intermediate replacement rate among the thirteen industrialized nations he studied. Five were significantly higher, three were about the same, two were slightly lower, and two were significantly lower. For example, Austria has a pension formula based on average earnings over the last seven years of coverage (changing to ten years from 1987). It is also time related, providing about 57 percent of earnings after thirty years of labor and increasing to 79.5 percent after forty-five years (U.S. Department of Health and Human Services 1986). In practice, a man who retired in 1986 after thirty-five years of working received about 65 percent of his average earnings in the seven years before retirement, aside from other benefits. One difficulty involved in making these international comparisons has to do with the varied systems that exist among nations. Schulz and his colleagues (1974) point out that many nations (for example, Australia, Finland, Ireland, Israel, the Netherlands, and New Zealand) have flat-rate systems, whereas others (for example, Sweden, Canada, and Great Britain) have double-decker systems. Such systems, including a flat pension benefit supplemented by an earnings-related pension program, provide higher replacement for low-wage workers and increased benefits for middle and high wage workers (Schulz et al. 1974). For example, aged Canadians receive a universal pension earned at a rate of one-fortieth of the maximum pension for each year of residence in Canada after age eighteen, up to a maximum of forty years and with a minimum of ten. In addition, earnings-related pensions are provided replacing approximately 25 percent of average earnings (U.S. Department of Health and Human Services 1986).

Women and Social Security

In recent years, a question has emerged about the equity of Social Security Coverage for certain groups, especially women. It is generally believed that women are at a disadvantage under the Social Security system. Flowers (1977), pointing out that most of the provisions of the law pertaining to women have been in effect for about forty years, asks "why significant controversy has developed only fairly recently." In answer, she notes that the women's liberation movement has heightened interest in all aspects of the treatment of women in U.S. society and that the Social Security benefit structure reflects a pattern of family life that is no longer typical in the United States.

In 1939 the Social Security Act was amended to provide additional protection for the wives, widows, and children of workers covered by the program. These amendments were based on two important presumptions generally accepted at the time: first, that a man is solely responsible for the support of his wife and children; and, second, that the overwhelming majority of married women *do not* work (U.S. Senate Special Committee on Aging 1975). Several important social trends have played havoc with these presumptions. Not the least of these is the dramatic increase of women, and particularly married women, in the labor force. In 1984, over 53 percent of all married women were working. Most of these women make a significant economic contribution to the standard of living of the family.

Just how are women disadvantaged by the Social Security system?

1. Benefits tend to be lower for women than for men. The average monthly benefit for a woman retiree was 76 percent of that of a retired man in December 1986 ($420 versus $550). Social Security benefits depend to a great extent on average earnings and length of participation in the labor force. Many women have marginal work careers with low earnings; in addition, many women earn substantially less than their equally skilled male counterparts. Finally, increasing numbers of married women divide their lives so as to spend a part as homemakers and another part in the paid labor force. This reduces their length of participation in covered employment.

2. Because homemaking yields no credit as work, a homemaker is fully dependent on her husband's benefits. It is generally recognized that work performed in the home by homemakers accounts for a very large amount of all unpaid work. Morgan, Sirageldin, and Baerwaldt (1966) have estimated that inclusion of unpaid work in the national accounts would increase the gross national product (GNP) by about 38 percent. Gauger (1973) estimates the contribution of household work alone to be an additional 26 percent of GNP. There is no consensus on an approach to placing a value on household work. One approach, the market cost approach, assumes that the wage rate for tasks performed in the marketplace can be applied to the same work performed *outside* the marketplace. Application of this

approach placed the average 1972 value of a housewife at $4,705 with wide variation by age (U.S. Senate Special Committee on Aging 1975). Treating household work as covered employment would give women Social Security work credit, leave them no longer fully dependent upon a husband's benefits, and increase the average monthly benefit for women. Homemaker credits are now used in several countries. In the United Kingdom, for example, voluntary contributions to the social security system are permitted by all the nonemployed, including homemakers (U.S. Department of Health and Human Services 1986).

3. Women who are divorced before ten years of marriage are *not* entitled to any of their husband's benefits.

4. Retired women workers are at a benefit disadvantage to widows with survivor's benefits. The average monthly benefit for a retired women is 94 percent of that for a woman receiving survivor benefits in December 1986 ($420 versus $445).

The Social Security Amendments of 1983 improved the benefit status of women in the Social Security system in several important ways. Two are identified here. First, Social Security benefits will no longer be terminated for surviving divorced spouses and disabled widows and widowers who remarry after entitlement to benefits. Previously, remarriage would result in termination. Second, effective January 1, 1985, a divorced spouse aged sixty-two or over who has been divorced for at least two years may receive benefits based on the earnings of a former spouse who is eligible for retirement benefits, regardless of whether the former spouse has applied for benefits or has benefits withheld under the earnings test. In the past, the divorced spouse could not qualify until the former spouse had filed an application.

Supplementary Security Income

The Social Security Act of 1935 included a mandate for the establishment of a separate program of old-age assistance under which benefits (coming mostly from federal funds) would be distributed to needy aged people and administered by the states. Similar programs for the blind and disabled were established in the 1935 act and subsequent amendments. Under the Social Security Amendments of 1972, a new federal program of Supplemental Security Income (SSI) for the aged, blind, and disabled replaced the former state-operated welfare programs. When the SSI program began making payments in January 1974, 3.2 million recipients were on the rolls. By the end of 1987, this figure had increased to 4.3 million, nearly half of whom were sixty-five years or older.

The SSI program was envisioned as a basic national income maintenance system for the aged, blind, and disabled (U.S. Senate Committee on Finance 1977). It was intended to present minimal barriers to eligibility by having few requirements other than lack of income. Yet, as its title indicates, the program was expected to supplement the Social Security program primarily by providing income support to those not covered by Social Security.

Since SSI is an assistance program, applicants must prove need by meeting an "assets test." As of January 1, 1989, assets may not exceed $2,000 for an individual and $3,000 for a couple. Excluded from the assets test are the value of a home (up to a certain market value), household goods, personal effects, an automobile with a market value under $4,500, and a life insurance policy with a face value of less than $1,500. In addition, $1,500 each may be set aside for the burial of the recipient and a spouse (Kahn 1987). In December, 1987, Federal SSI payments were $340.00 a month for an individual and $510 a month for a couple. Many states provide an additional supplement to the federal benefit.

Critics of SSI argue that although the program is targeted at the right population—the aged poor—eligibility requirements limit people's ability to lift themselves from poverty status. People who save by reducing expenses find these savings treated as income by SSI and often lose benefits (Estes 1979). A case report illustrates this problem:

> A seventy-two-year-old woman in Iowa lost her SSI benefits entirely because the rent she doesn't pay is more than the rent she does pay. This woman rents a trailer from her son for $60 a month and pays $25 a month for the space rental. In addition, her normal expenses include $25 for utilities and $24 for $56 worth of food stamps. The secretary of HEW determined that her son could rent the trailer to someone else for $150 a month. The woman was assessed $90 in "income" for rent she did not pay even though she was paying $85 a month in rent, almost 50 percent of her total cash income. Since her so-called "income," plus her Social Security benefits, put her over the income limit for SSI she has had to live on her $120 a month Social Security check. (National Senior Citizens Law Center, quoted in Estes 1979)

Another major concern has arisen because of the low participation level of eligible persons in the SSI program. The Social Security Administration estimates that about one in three eligible aged persons do not participate in the program. Drazaga, Upp, and Reno (1982) offer two reasons for the levels of participation in SSI: lack of knowledge about the program and stigma. Their study found that 45 percent of nonparticipants had never heard of the SSI program. And, even among the many who did know of SSI, some indicated a reluctance to become involved in a means-tested program.

The Future of Social Security

The most crucial questions about the future of the Social Security system concern its financial status. Current and future retirees (current contributors) want to know if the system is solvent or whether it will go bankrupt and deprive millions of a retirement pension they have counted on. The latter appears highly unlikely. As Dorcas R. Hardy (1987, 5), Commissioner of Social Security has written, "Social Security and justice are inextricably linked." According to Hardy, the system is sound, has a significant Trust Fund reserve which is expected to grow significantly out into the next century (see below), and is not likely to face another financial crunch until about the year 2040.

During the early years of Social Security, more revenue was collected from contributions than was paid in benefits, and a trust fund was developed. By 1976 this situation had changed. Boskin (1977) estimates that Social Security was paying out $4.3 billion more in 1976 than it was taking in. At that rate the trust fund would likely have run out during the mid-1980s. Significant amendments were made in the Social Security system in 1977. Many, including then President Carter, believed these changes provided a long-term financial solution for the system's problems. By 1982 economic conditions again made the financial status of the system appear vulnerable. On January 20, 1983, the National Commission on Social Security Reform (NCSSR) presented its recommendations. Passed with almost unprecedented speed after bipartisan effort, Public Law 98-21 was signed into law by President Reagan on April 20, 1983. This law represents the Social Security Amendments of 1983 and is substantially in line with the NCSSR recommendations. A number of the changes brought about by these amendments have already been noted in the discussion above. In signing the bill into law, the President stated

> This bill demonstrates for all times our Nation's ironclad commitment to Social Security. It assures the elderly that America will always keep the promises made in troubled times a half a century ago. It assures those who are still working that they, too, have a pact with the future. From this day forward, they have our pledge that they will get their fair share of benefits when they retire. Our elderly need no longer fear that the checks they depend on will be stopped or reduced. These amendments protect them. Americans of middle age need no longer worry whether their career-long investment will pay off. These amendments guarantee it. And younger people can feel confident that Social Security will still be around when they need it to cushion their retirement.

For approximately the next forty years or so, under current economic forecasts, the combined Social Security Trust Fund is expected to continually have excesses of income over outgo, creating a buildup that will peak in 2030 at about $12.5 trillion (Hambor 1987). The 1987 excess of income over outgo was estimated at $21.1 billion and increased the total in the Trust Fund to $60.1 billion. Can sour economic conditions again place the Social Security system in jeopardy? Perhaps, but Social Security is a vital program and, most important, it is guaranteed by the taxing power of the federal government of the United States of America.

PRIVATE PENSIONS

By 1984 about 40 million (49 percent) wage and salary workers in private industry were covered by private pension plans of one sort or another. This represents significant growth over the last forty years or so. In 1940, only about 12 percent of the labor force was covered by private pensions. In 1982, only 23 percent of all those aged sixty-five and over received money income from private pensions or annuities. Table 11-9 shows which U.S. workers were *not* covered by pension plans in 1979 (President's Commission on Pension Policy 1981). Almost 50 million workers did not participate in a private pension plan in 1979. According to Schulz (1988), the two key factors are union status and firm size: Almost all workers without pension coverage are nonunion and work for firms with a relatively small number of employees.

Private pensions were first introduced into U.S. industry by the railroad and express companies. The first plan, established by the American Express Company in 1875, was financed solely by the employer. The first plan supported jointly by employee and employer contributions was inaugurated by the Baltimore and Ohio Railroad Company in 1880. The railroad industry was the first to adopt pension plans rather widely; by World War I over half of all railroad employees were covered by such plans, and by the late 1920s the proportion covered had risen to four-fifths (Institute of Life Insurance 1975).

TABLE 11-9   Workers Not Covered by Pension Plans in 1979

In 1979, 49.4 million workers were not covered by a pension plan:

Sex:	54% of these were *men*; 46% were *women*
Hours Worked:	71% of these worked *full time*; 29% *part time*
Age:	68% were *over age 25* and 51% of noncovered were over 25 and had one or more years of service with their employer
Sector:	8.2 million were employed in the *public sector*
	38.1 million were wage and salary workers in the *private sector*

Of private sector noncovered wage and salary workers:

Industry:	78% worked in *three main industries:*
	• 32% in trade
	• 28% in service
	• 18% in manufacturing
Earnings:	30% earned less than $5,000 in 1978
	36% earned between $5,000 and $10,000 in 1978
	19% earned between $10,000 and $15,000 in 1978
	15% earned over $15,000 in 1978
Firm Size:	79% were in firms with fewer than 100 employees
	8% were in firms with 500 or more employees
Union Status:	About 90% were not members of unions

Source: Based on President's Commission on Pension Policy (1981, Chart 6).

Labor unions played an important part in the expansion of pension coverage. Many unions developed their own plans in industries that provided no company coverage. The first trade union plan was that of the Granite Cutters in 1905. Two years later, the first of the larger international unions, the International Typographic Union, adopted a formal pension plan for its members. By 1930 about 20 percent of all trade union members in the United States and Canada were covered by a union pension plan (Institute of Life Insurance 1975).

Economic conditions during the 1930s reduced the growth of the private pension movement. The passage of the Social Security Act of 1935 did help create a climate in which the idea of pension planning would continue to flower. Schulz (1988) attributes the tremendous growth in private pension coverage since 1940 to a variety of reasons. These include (1) the continued industrialization of the U.S. economy, (2) wage freezes during World War II and the Korean War that encouraged fringe benefit growth in lieu of wages, (3) inducements offered by the federal government such as the Revenue Act of 1942, which made employer contributions to qualified pension plans tax deductible, (4) a favorable decision by the Supreme Court in 1949 that pensions were a proper issue for collective bargaining, and (5) the development of multiemployer pension plans.

In 1974 Congress passed the Employee Retirement Income Security Act (ERISA). This legislation established minimum standards for pension programs and strengthened the regulation and supervision of such programs. Prior to this, the policing function was left primarily in the hands of participants. Unfortunately, this had tragic consequences in many cases. Workers lost pension benefits as a result of company bankruptcies, plant closures, and unemployment. In addition, financial irregularities, including mismanagement of funds, left many new retirees with nothing despite a lifetime of paying into the company's pension fund. One report, based on examination of data from the Social Security Administration's Retirement History Study, found that 45 percent of recent retirees were covered by a pension on their longest or most recent job. Amazingly, 28 percent of men covered and 45 percent of women covered never received a benefit (Thompson 1978).

The major provisions of ERISA as passed in 1974 are as follows (Skolnick 1974):

1. A company must permit an employee to participate in a pension plan if he or she has reached the age of twenty-five and has worked for the employer for one year.

2. Vesting is the nonforfeitable right of an individual to receive a future pension based on his or her earned credits even if the person leaves the job before retirement age. All private pension plans must now vest benefits according to one of the three ways:

    a. Twenty-five percent of pension benefits would be vested after five years with the company, increasing to 100 percent after fifteen years of service.

    b. One hundred percent pension benefits would be vested after ten years of service.

    c. Fifty percent of pension benefits would be vested after ten years of service when age and years of service total forty-five years, followed in five years by 100 percent vesting (all employees must be 50 percent vested after ten years and fully vested after fifteen years of service).

3. Plan termination insurance is established up to a certain level for employees whose plans terminate with insufficient funds.

4. Individual retirement accounts (IRAs) may be established by workers without private or public employee pension coverage. There are limits on the annual investment allowed.

5. Employees may transfer vested pension rights (portability) on a tax-free basis from one employer to another or to an IRA.

ERISA contains quite specific reporting and disclosure requirements for private pension plans. In addition, amendments have been made since 1974. For example, ERISA now mandates that all pension plans subject to its provisions provide workers with a *joint and survivor option* at the time of retirement. If chosen, this option provides income to the surviving spouse in an amount equal to some percentage of the income payable during the time the employee and spouse were alive. In the absence of such a provision, the surviving spouse often loses his or her interest in the pension benefit.

ERISA has not solved all the pension problems of individuals or their employers. Special concerns remain for women who, because of their home and family responsibilities, are likely to accumulate far fewer private pension credits than men. A U.S. Department of Justice Task Force on Sex Discrimination (cited in Schulz 1988) identified some specific problem areas for women:

1. Workers under age twenty-five may be excluded from coverage, although the twenty to twenty-four age group has the highest female participation rate.

2. Coverage was not required for part-time employees.

3. "Breaks in service" by women were likely to exceed current allowable limits.

4. Vesting requirements were too long (most companies allow vesting of 100 percent of accrued benefits after ten years of service).

5. Vested rights, if acquired through service early in an employee's working life, might be worth little at retirement as they are not adjusted upward to compensate for inflation or a higher level of real benefits.

The following legislative provisions of the Retirement Equity Act of 1984 and the 1986 Tax Reform Act were passed as part of an effort to address those aspects of ERISA that did not provide full private pension protection for women:

1. The age before which years of service can be excluded for vesting purposes is 18.

2. The minimum age for plan participation for most workers is 21 (with one year of service).

3. "Break in service" rules are liberalized.

4. One hundred percent vesting is specified after five years of service.

5. Pension plans are required to provide automatic joint and survivor protection to participants with vested benefits.

6. Pension beneficiary decisions and changes must have direct consent of spouses.

Private pensions have generally been designed as supplements to Social Security. Thus, it is no surprise that average benefits are quite low. Schulz, Leavitt, and Kelly (1979) studied 977 pension plans identified by the Bureau of Labor Statistics as providing determinable benefits. They estimated that the median annual benefit for a male earner after thirty years of pension service was $2,720; a comparable female would receive $2,046. This constitutes a pre-retirement income replacement ratio of 22 percent for men and 28 percent for women. Replacement ratios varied widely by industry, type, and size of plan.

A more recent study of pension benefit levels in 1979 by the same authors (Schulz, Leavitt, Kelly, and Strate 1982) found slight increases in these replacement rates. Median private pension replacement rates for workers with thirty years of service and average earnings were 27 percent for men and 34 percent for women. The rates varied from a low of 23 percent for men and women in the service industry to a high of 35 percent for women in manufacturing.

Such low replacement ratios are inadequate for the great majority of retirees. Benefit levels may improve as these plans mature; most private pension plans are *not* on a pay-as-you-go basis (as is Social Security), but are funded. Yet in many plans benefit levels are subject to collective bargaining agreements. Kassachau (1976) points out that unions are often dominated by younger workers, making retirees and their needs relatively unimportant. Retired persons who are "double dippers"—drawing both private pension and Social Security retirement benefits—are considerably better off. Unfortunately, they represent a minority of retirees who tend to have been concentrated in high-earning jobs and industries.

The United States is likely to continue to have a mixture of public and private pension systems. We have already discussed some of the advantages of Social Security including almost-universal coverage, cost-of-living adjustment, and financing backed by the federal government. In addition, administrative costs are quite low. In 1987 administrative costs for Social Security amounted to 1.2 percent of contributions. Private pensions provide greater flexibility for different worker groups as well as the potential for investing pension funds in the national economy. Some disadvantages of private pensions include higher administrative costs, a general absence of indexing to protect retirees against inflation, and the difficulty involved in achieving portability, among others mentioned above.

Robert Butler (1975) has suggested what seems to be an ideal pension system based on current standards of living: universal coverage, immediate 100 percent vesting, portability, full insurance including survivors' benefits, and two benefit escalators—one tied to the cost of living and another tied to the nation's economic growth. Historian David Fischer (1977) believes that instead of supporting the aged with pensions at the end of life, it would be cheaper and easier to give each American a grant of capital at the beginning of life. He proposes that every American receive at birth a "national inheritance gift" in the amount of $4,400. The gift would be surrounded by restrictions. It would have to be invested in a savings account or government security and could not be spent, loaned, borrowed, or employed as collateral in any way. The money would not be taxed and would be left to earn interest until the infant who originally received it reached the age of sixty-five. At 6 percent annual interest over sixty-five years, the original $4,400 would grow to $200,000. The average aged couple would have nontaxable income of more than $25,000 a year. On their death, the money would return to the United States Treasury. According to Fischer, supporting such a program would cost less than current government expenditures for the aged and might actually reduce inflation because the plan would be funded before the money was spent (this is the opposite of deficit spending). The likelihood of either of these proposals receiving serious consideration in the near future, though, is quite small.

SUMMARY

The major sources of income for the elderly are Social Security, earnings, and asset income. A considerable proportion of the elderly receive in-kind income in the form of goods and services they obtain free or at reduced expenditure. Examples include housing, health care, and food stamps. It is difficult to estimate how much in income these programs are worth to the aged. Since the mid-1960s, the median income of elderly has increased more than two and one-half times. In 1986, the median income of families with an aged head was $19,932. Retirement status, age, and race are factors associated with income variation among the elderly. Tax advantages received by the elderly would seem to be of more help to property owners and those with higher incomes. Inflation has adverse implications for all people, although Social Security benefits, some private pensions, and in-kind programs such as food stamps are now indexed to the rate of inflation. This gives the aged an advantage relative to other age groups.

The elderly show a pattern of expenditures quite like that of other low-income groups. Poverty has been declining among the elderly, although 12.4 percent of older persons are considered to be officially poor. Poverty varies among subgroups of the elderly; 31 percent of aged nonwhites were officially poor in 1986. Orshansky argues that the government's poverty index is set too low and is not applied to those aged who are institutionalized or living with relatives. Adjusting the poverty index and applying it to these hidden poor might show as many as 40 percent of the aged to be living in poverty.

The Social Security Act of 1935 signaled a new era in financial arrangements for life after retirement. Nine out of ten workers are covered, and over 90 percent of the elderly receive some income from Social Security. Social Security is an earnings-based program; for the designated groups, participation is compulsory. Retirement is defined through a "retirement test" that withholds pension benefits if earnings are above a specified amount. Average benefits are relatively low as a result of the popularity of the early retirement option. Early retirement benefits (to those who retire at ages sixty-two to sixty-four) are reduced because of the longer period over which they will be paid. It is generally believed women are disadvantaged by the Social Security system, although, as a proportion of the total of all benefits, the amount paid on the earnings of women is slightly greater than that paid on the earnings of men. At least for now, the Social Security Amendments of 1983 appear to have laid to rest fears about the financial status of the Social Security system.

Private pension plans have generally been designed as supplements to Social Security. About 49 percent of U.S. workers are covered by one sort of private pension plan or another. In 1974, the Congress passed important legislation establishing minimum standards for these plans. Previously, the policing of private pension programs was irregular and ineffectual.

STUDY QUESTIONS

1. Discuss the economic position of American elderly with regard to variation by sex, marital status, age, race, and retirement status.

2. List and explain the various forms of indirect or in-kind income available to the elderly through federal programs.

3. Explain some of the ways in which inflation can have a detrimental impact on the economic situation of the elderly.

4. Discuss the *poverty index* and explain how it is used to determine the adequacy of elderly income. What are the problems inherent in using this measure of income adequacy?

5. With the passage of the Social Security Act of 1935, the United States became one of the last industrialized nations to execute a federal old-age pension program. Discuss the principles behind this legislation.

6. Explain why the Social Security payroll tax schedule is considered by many to be regressive.

7. Discuss the advantages and disadvantages women experience with respect to Social Security benefits.

8. Explain why ERISA was deemed a necessary piece of legislation. What are some of the major provisions of this act? Which provisions were thought to disadvantage women? How were these remedied?

BIBLIOGRAPHY

Achenbaum, W.A. 1978. *Old age in the new land.* Baltimore: The John Hopkins University Press.

Atchley, R. 1977. *Social forces in later life* (2nd ed.). Belmont, Calif.: Wadsworth Publishing Co., Inc.

Boskin, M. 1977. *The crisis in social security: Problems and prospects.* San Francisco: Institute for Contemporary Studies.

Bromley, D. 1974. *The psychology of human ageing.* Middlesex, England: Penguin Books.

Brotman, H. 1978. The aging of America: A demographic profile. *National Journal* October 7: 1622–1627.

Butler, R. 1975. *Why survive?: Being old in America.* New York: Harper and Row.

Calhoun, R. 1978. *In search of the new old.* New York: Elsevier Scientific Publishing Co.

Carp, F. 1976. Housing and the living environments of older people. In R. Binstock and E. Shanas (eds.), *Handbook of aging and the social sciencies.* New York: Van Nostrand Reinhold Co.

Chen, Y.P. 1985. Economic status of the aging. In R. Binstock and E. Shanas (eds.), *Handbook of aging and the social sciences* (2nd ed.). New York: Van Nostrand Reinhold Co.

Clark, R., Kreps, J., and Spengler, J. 1978. Economics of aging: A survey. *Journal of Economic Literature* 41:919–962.

Drazaga, L., Upp, M., and Reno, V. 1982. Low-income aged: Eligibility and participation in SSI. *Social Security Bulletin* 45(May):28–35.

Estes, C. 1979. *The aging enterprise.* San Francisco: Jossey-Bass, Inc., Publishers.

Fischer, D. 1977. *Growing old in America.* New York: Oxford University Press.

Flowers, M. 1977. *Women and social security: An institutional dilemma.* Washington, D.C.: American Enterprise Institute for Public Policy Research.

Fox, A. 1982. Earnings replacement rates and total income: Findings from the Retirement History Study. *Social Security Bulletin* 45(October):3–24.

Gauger, W. 1973. Household work: Can we add it to the GNP? *Journal of Home Economics* (October):12–15.

Grad, S. 1984. *Income of the population 55 and over, 1982.* Washington, D.C.: U.S. Department of Health and Human Services, Social Security Administration.

Hambor, J.C. 1987. Economic policy, intergenerational equity, and the Social Security Trust Fund buildup. *Social Security Bulletin* 50(10):13–18.

Hardy, D.R. 1987. The future of Social Security. *Social Security Bulletin* 50(8):5–7.

Hollister, R. 1974. Social mythology and reform: Income maintenance for the aged. *Annals of the American Academy of Political and Social Sciences* 415:19–40.

Horlick, M. 1970. The earnings replacement rate of old-age benefits: An international comparison. *Social Security Bulletin* (March):3–16.

Institute of Life Insurance. 1975. *Pension facts.* New York: Institute of Life Insurance.

Irelan, L., and Bond, K. 1976. Retirees of the 1970s. In C. Kart and B. Manard (eds.), *Aging in America: Readings in social gerontology.* Sherman Oaks, Calif.: Alfred Publishing Co.

Kahn, A.L. 1987. Program and demographic characteristics of Supplemental Security Income recipients, December 1985. *Social Security Bulletin* 50(5):23–57.

Kassachau, P. 1976. Retirement and the social system. *Industrial Gerontology* 3:11–24.

Lawton, M.P. 1985. Housing and living environments of older people. In R. Binstock and E. Shanas (eds.), *Handbook of aging and the social sciencies* (2nd ed.). (New York: Van Nostrand Reinhold.

Morgan, J., Sirageldin, I., and Baerwaldt, N. 1966. *Productive Americans: A study of how individuals contribute to economic progress.* Ann Arbor: Institute for Social Research, University of Michigan.

Munnell, A. 1977. *The future of Social Security.* Washington, D.C.: The Brookings Institution.

Murray, J. 1972. Homeownership and financial assets: Findings from the 1968 Survey of the Aged. *Social Security Bulletin* 35:3–23.

National Commission on Social Security. 1981. *Social Security in America's future.* Report of the Commission to the President. Washington, D.C.: The Commission.

National Council on Aging. 1975. *The myth and reality of aging in America.* Washington, D.C.: National Council on Aging.

Okun, A. 1970. Inflation: The problems and prospects before us. In A. Okun, H.M. Fowler, and M. Gilbert (eds.), *Inflation.* New York: New York University Press.

Orshansky, M. 1978. Testimony in U.S. House Select Committee on Aging. *Poverty among America's aged.* Washington, D.C.: U.S. Government Printing Office.

Poverty Studies Task Force. 1976. *The measure of poverty.* Washington, D.C.: U.S. Department of Health, Education, and Welfare.

President's Commission on Pension Policy. 1981. *Coming of age: Toward a national retirement income policy.* Washington, D.C.: The Commission.

Putnam, J.K. 1970. *Old-age politics in California: From Richardson to Reagan.* Stanford, Calif.: Stanford University Press.

Riley, M.W., and Foner, A. 1968. *Aging and society: An inventory of research findings.* New York: Russell Sage Foundation.

Schmundt, M., Smolensky, E., and Stiefel, L. 1975. The evaluation of recipients of in-kind transfers. In I. Laurie (ed.), *Integrating income maintenance programs.* New York: Academic Press, Inc.

Schulz, J. 1988. *The economics of aging* (4th ed.). Dover, Mass. Auburn House Publishing Co., Inc.

Schulz, J., Carrin, G., Krupp, H., Peschke, M., Sclar, E. and Van Steenberge, J. 1974. *Providing adequate retirement income—Pension reform in the U.S. and abroad.* Hanover, N.H.: New England Press.

Schulz, J., Leavitt, T., and Kelly, L. 1979. Private pensions fall far short of preretirement income levels. *Monthly Labor Review* 102 (February):28–32.

Schulz, J., Leavitt, T., Kelly, L., and Strate, J. 1982. *Private pension benefits in the 1970s.* Bryn Mawr, Pa.: McCahan Foundation for Research in Economic Security.

Skolnick, A. 1974. Pension reform legislation of 1974. *Social Security Bulletin* 37(12):35–42.

Smeeding, T. 1982. *Alternate methods for valuing selected in-kind transfer benefits and measuring their effects on poverty.* Technical paper 50. Washington, D.C.: U.S. Bureau of the Census.

Social Security Administration. 1986. *Income and resources of the population 65 and over.* Washington, D.C.: U.S. Government Printing Office.

———. 1987. Fast facts and figures about Social Security. *Social Security Bulletin* 50(5):5–22.

Thompson, G. 1978. Pension coverage and benefits, 1972: Findings from the Retirement History Study. *Social Security Bulletin* 41:3–17.

Torda, T. 1972. The impact of inflation on the elderly. *Federal Reserve Bank Cleveland Economic Review.* (October/November):3–19.

U.S. Bureau of the Census. 1982. *Alternative methods for valuing selected in-kind benefits and measuring their effect on poverty.* Technical paper No. 50. Washington, D.C.: U.S. Government Printing Office.

———. 1985. *Statistical abstract of the United States: 1986.* Washington, D.C.: U.S. Government Printing Office.

U.S. Department of Health and Human Services. 1986. *Social Security programs throughout the world—1985.* Research report #60. Washington, D.C.: U.S. Government Printing Office.

U.S. House Committee on Ways and Means. 1967. *President's proposals for revision in the Social Security system: Hearings Part I.* Washington, D.C.: U.S. Government Printing Office.

U.S. House Select Committee on Aging. 1979. *Federal responsibility to the elderly.* Washington, D.C.: U.S. Government Printing Office.

U.S. Senate Committee on Finance. 1977. *The Supplementary Security Income Program.* Washington, D.C.: U.S. Government Printing Office.

U.S. Senate Special Committee on Aging. 1975. *Women and Social Security: Adapting to a new era.* Washington, D.C.: U.S. Government Printing Office.

Yeas, M.A., and Grad, S. 1987. Income of retirement-aged persons in the United States. *Social Security Bulletin* 50(7):5–14.

CHAPTER 12

WORK, RETIREMENT, AND LEISURE

Jacob Jensen[1] (a fictitious name) had been a happy, successful man. Thirty-seven years ago he had begun as a stock boy, and today he was the number two man in the company. A fine family, plenty of money, good health, and respect in the community reflected this success. Yet, as he approached age sixty, he was given a a stark choice by the board chairman: retire or be transferred. Jensen had never given thought to retirement, because it seemed there would always be time to prepare for such a distant event. Jensen found himself in great psychological pain. A psychiatrist, later writing his case history, described him as depressed, suicidal, and highly susceptible to a debilitating physical illness such as a stroke.

Jimmy Kilpatrick[2] is another story. He worked in a factory in Detroit touching up paint on new Cadillacs. According to Mr. Kilpatrick, he had been working since he was ten years old—and it was time to rest. At the age of fifty-one, he took that rest and retired from the assembly line at Cadillac. His monthly pension is $634, and the mortgage payment on the house he bought fifteen years ago is only $127 a month. His children are grown and self-supporting, and his wife is considering going back to work. Kilpatrick says that if money gets a little short, "I'm not bragging, but I'm pretty good with paints."

Explaining the different responses of these two individuals toward retirement is not simple. Nevertheless, in many respects, both cases represent the American experience with retirement. Mr. Jensen represents the situation of

---

[1] From Rosenfeld, A. 1978. "The Willy Loman Complex," in Gross, R., Gross, B., and Seidman, S. (eds.), *The New Old: Struggling for Decent Aging.* Garden City, N.Y.: Anchor Books.

[2] From Flint, J. 1977. Early retirement is growing in the U.S., *New York Times,* July 10.

being at the top of his profession one day and then, the next, because of a fixed retirement policy, anticipating himself outside the arenas of achievement and competition. Mr. Kilpatrick, on the other hand, represents what has become a significant trend in the work style of Americans—early retirement. Growing numbers of workers have an opportunity to retire early, and many are taking it.

Most Americans, men and women, in the labor force or about to enter it, will face retirement, which itself is a radical transformation from the past. What we know about changes in survivorship rates alone should support this fact. Retirement requires longevity; if people do not live long enough to work and still have years left over, there can be no retirement. According to the gerontologist Robert Atchley (1976), three additional conditions are necessary for the emergence of retirement as a social institution. These include the following:

1. An economy that produces enough surplus to support adults who do not hold jobs.

2. The presence of mechanisms, such as pensions or Social Security, to divert part of the surplus to support retired people.

3. The acceptance in a society of the idea that people can live in dignity as older adults without working at a job.

Other factors have contributed to the appearance of retirement in the United States. These include the decline of agriculture as a provider of jobs to U.S. workers and the increasing importance of formal education as an asset valued over experience (Achenbaum 1978).

Still, the United States has been described by many as a work-oriented society where who you are is determined by what you do. The pollster Daniel Yankelovich (1974), on the basis of survey studies, has written that the majority of Americans in the mid-1960s associated four ideas with work: (1) To be a man in our society means being a good provider for his family; (2) work earns one freedom and independence; (3) hard work leads to success; and (4) a man's worth is reflected in the act of working.

Various national groups make competing claims about who works hardest, but there may be no people for whom work means more than it does among Americans. Ethel Shanas (1968) found, in a comparison of men aged sixty-five and over living in Denmark, Britain, and the United States, that, although aged Americans were as likely to retire as were aged citizens of the other two countries, retired Americans were much more likely to say that they missed some aspect of their work. Interestingly, although they did not miss the work itself, they missed the sense of feeling useful that their jobs had provided, the people they had met at work, and the money they had earned—more than the Danes or British did.

Why do we attach this special importance to work? The eminent German sociologist Max Weber offered one explanation, which is rooted in the religious ideals of Calvin and his followers. Calvin, following Luther, believed that man (and, no doubt, woman as well) had a calling to God in this world, and that this calling included one's work. Whatever that work was, it was a person's duty to do the best he could in order to please God. Calvin added the notion of predestination to the Lutheran theology. According to Calvin, God had already decided on the future course of man- and womankind, including who would be saved and who would be damned. Thus, although one could still have a calling to God, following it no longer necessarily meant salvation.

Rather than simply accepting their fate, Calvinists sought signs of God's determination for them. Success in earthly endeavors became an indication of God's favor. Hard work (and the financial success it often brought) meant being in God's good graces, unlike the perspective of early Christianity, when hard work reflected condemnation related to original sin.

Historically, the religious context for work eroded, although, despite this secularization process, work still remained "the stuff of life." The Protestant ethic became the work ethic. Some argue that this work ethic has become increasingly outmoded in the twentieth century. Calhoun (1978) believes that technological progress, population growth, the accompanying contraction of manpower needs relative to availability, and increasing ability to control the business cycle have caused a devaluation of the work ethic.

Streib and Schneider (1971) suggest that it is an oversimplification to call American society work oriented. They point out that, given the enormous range of jobs in the United States (from cab driver to Supreme Court Justice) and the difficult skills required to carry out these jobs, there may not be enough equivalent meaning among jobs to speak of a common meaning attached to work. Simpson, Back, and McKinney (1966) found that the type of job had a strong impact on a person's commitment to the identification with the job. Upper white-collar job holders (for example, executives, professionals) were oriented toward autonomy and self-expression in their jobs, whereas semi-skilled workers were oriented toward job security and income. Another early study along these lines found very few steelworkers or coal miners viewing their jobs as sources of meaningful life experiences (Friedmann and Havighurst 1954). Williams and Wirths (1965), in their study of Kansas City adults, found that the world of work was the central element in the life-style of only 15 percent of their cases.

Much work in the United States *is* highly routinized, boring, exhausting, and unsatisfying. Mike Lefevre, a steel mill worker, talked to Studs Terkel about his "alienation" from work:

> It's hard to take pride in a bridge you're never gonna cross, in a door you're never gonna open. You're mass-producing things and you never see the end result of it. . . . In a steel mill, forget it. You don't see where nothing goes. . . . My attitude is that I don't get excited about my job. I do my work, but I don't say whoopee-doo. The day I get excited about my job is the day I go to

a head shrinker. How are you gonna get excited when you're tired and want to sit down. (Terkel, S. *Working: People Talk About What They Do All Day and How They Feel About What They Do.* New York: Random House, Inc., 1972.)

Karl Marx saw the potential for alienation from work in industrial societies. According to Marx, work constitutes man's most important activity—in fact, he calls it "life activity." Marx said that work is "creative" and that through it people create their world, and as a consequence, create themselves. The Swedish sociologist Joachim Israel (1971) summarizes the conditions under which work is truly creative:

1. Work must be freely chosen.
2. It must allow an expression of capabilities.
3. It must allow an individual to express his or her social nature.
4. It should be *more* than a means for maintaining subsistence.

For Marx, any other kind of work is "forced" and alienating. Alienating work produces estrangement from one's labor and, perhaps more important, from one's self and the social world. "What is true of man's relationship to his work, to the product of his work and to himself, is also true of his relationship to other men" (Marx, in Israel 1971).

One does not have to be a Marxist to recognize that many workers, old and young, are doing "forced labor." Yet the relationship between people and their jobs is a complicated one. How people feel about their job (and themselves) and how central their work is to their life-style will strongly affect how they view the prospect of retirement. These factors may also determine how prepared a person is to deal with the demands of retirement. In the next section we survey the complicated and changing relationships between aging and work, retirement and leisure. We begin by describing the status of elderly Americans in the labor force and how this status has changed in the twentieth century.

THE OLDER WORKER

Older people have always worked. In fact, it was not until sometime between 1930 and 1940 that the rate of labor force participation by elderly American males dipped below 50 percent. This rate has continued to decline and, as Table 12-1 shows, by 1980 about one-fifth (19.0 percent) of all aged males were in the labor force. Among males aged fifty-five to sixty-four years (those approaching "normal" retirement age), labor force participation rates have declined during the twentieth century and are quite in line with overall employment trends among males. By 1950, 86.4 percent of all males sixteen years of age and over were in the labor force; this figure had dropped to 77.0 percent

TABLE 12-1   Civilian Labor Force and Participation Rates by Sex and Age: U.S., 1950–1995

	Males		Females	
	55–64 Years	65+ Years	55–64 Years	65+ Years
1950	86.9	45.8	27.0	9.7
1960	86.8	33.1	37.2	10.8
1970	83.0	26.8	43.0	9.7
1980	72.1	19.0	41.3	8.1
1990	65.5	14.9	41.5	7.4
1995	64.5	13.3	42.5	7.0

Source: U.S. Bureau of the Census, "Demographic Aspects of Aging and the Older Population in the U.S.," *Current population reports,* Special Studies, Series P-23, No. 59, Table 6-5, May, 1976; and U.S. Bureau of the Census, 1987, Table 660.

by 1980. The comparable figures for males aged fifty-five to sixty-four years were 86.9 percent and 72.1 percent.

The percentage of women aged sixty-five years and over employed outside the home has not exceeded 11 percent in this century. Table 12-1 shows the narrow range within which the labor force participation rate of older females has fluctuated since 1950. This is despite the fact that the proportion of gainfully employed women of all ages has increased dramatically in the first three-quarters of the twentieth century. About 18 percent of all women were employed in 1890; this figure has risen to over 50 percent in the 1980s. The labor force experience of women aged fifty-five to sixty-four reflects this phenomenon. Since 1950, labor force participation rates for this group have increased from 27.0 to 41.3 percent in 1980, although the rate peaked in 1970 (43 percent) and has shown minimal decline since.

Nonwhites (old and young) have had labor force experiences similar to those described above (see Table 12-2). The labor force participation rates of all nonwhite males has declined somewhat, whereas that of elderly nonwhite males has fallen dramatically in this century. Almost 85 percent of aged black males were employed in 1900 (Achenbaum 1978), 40 percent in 1955, 20.9 percent in 1975, and 14.7 percent in 1984. Aged black females have always had higher rates of employment than their white counterparts have had, although the difference in rates has narrowed. By 1984, only 8.2 percent of aged black females were employed—a modest decline from the recent peak of 12.9 percent in 1965, though a more significant percentage decline from the employment rate of 16.5 percent in 1950.

Rose C. Gibson (1987) reminds us that despite the formal definition of retirement employed by the United States Bureau of the Census and other governmental agencies, for many older blacks, the line between working or being retired is not so clear. Work in low status jobs is a necessity for many aged blacks and this continues a disadvantaged work pattern from youth through old age. As Gibson (1987, 691) describes it, "this sameness of sporadic work patterns over the life course . . . may create for older blacks a certain ambiguity between work and retirement which, in turn, may affect the ways in which blacks define retirement." Using data from the National Survey of Black Americans, Gibson identified four factors which in combination contribute to many older blacks thinking about themselves as being in an "unretired-retired" status: (1) an indistinct line between work in youth and work in old age; (2) the receipt of income from other than private pension sources; (3) the knowledge that one must work during old age; and (4) the benefits of defining oneself as sick or disabled rather than retired.

What kind of work do older workers do? Historically, farming was the occupation in which most elderly men found work; it was a lifelong occupation. Retirement on a farm was rare. An older worker physically unable to perform some duties could assume other less demanding though equally important chores. This was especially true for white farmers. A greater proportion of blacks than whites were in farming, but whites were much more likely to be owners or managers. Thus, they were in a position to remain in charge of planning and overseeing farm activities when they themselves were no longer able to carry out more physically taxing farm duties.

Obviously farming has diminished in importance as a source of jobs, and not just for older men but for younger men as well. Still, older workers are more likely to be found in farming than is the total population of employed persons. As can be seen from Table 12-3, elderly male workers are almost three times more likely to be found in farm work than are all male workers (11.3 percent versus 4.3 percent), and elderly females in the labor force are about twice as likely to be in farm work as are female workers of all ages (1.8 percent versus 1.0 percent).

TABLE 12-2   Labor Force Participation Rates for Nonwhites 65 Years of Age and Older, By Sex: United States, Selected Years 1950–1984

	Males	Females
1950	45.5	16.5
1955	40.0	12.1
1960	31.2	12.8
1965	27.9	12.9
1970	27.4	12.2
1975	20.9	10.5
1984	14.7	8.2

Source: U.S. Bureau of the Census, "Demographic Aspects of Aging and the Older Population in the U.S.," *Current population reports*, Special Studies, Series P-23, No. 59, Table 6-5, May, 1976; U.S. Senate Special Committee on Aging (in conjunction with AARP, the Federal Council on the Aging, and the Administration on Aging), *Aging America: Trends and projections, 1985–86 Edition*. Washington, D.C.: U.S. Government Printing Office.

TABLE 12-3   Occupational Distribution of Employed Persons: The Total Population and the Elderly Population, 1980

	Total Population		Population 65 +	
	Male (%) (56,004,690)	Female (%) (41,634,665)	Male (%) (1,875,253)	Female (%) (1,172,711)
White-collar	42.6	67.0	46.4	58.3
Managers and administrators	12.6	7.4	13.1	6.9
Professional and technical	11.0	14.1	11.3	11.1
Sales	9.1	11.2	14.2	15.0
Clerical and kindred	9.9	34.3	7.8	25.3
Blue-collar	43.9	14.0	26.7	10.9
Craftsmen and kindred	20.7	2.3	13.1	2.5
Operatives (except transport)	9.7	8.8	5.0	6.5
Transport equipment workers	7.2	0.8	4.7	0.4
Helpers and laborers	6.3	2.1	3.9	1.5
Farm	4.3	1.0	11.3	1.8
Farm operators and managers	2.1	0.3	8.0	1.0
Other farm occupations	2.2	0.7	3.3	0.8
Service	9.2	17.9	15.0	29.0
Private household	—	1.4	0.2	7.4
Protective service occupations (e.g., police officer, firefighter)	2.3	0.4	4.0	0.4
Other service (e.g., health and personal service)	6.9	16.1	10.8	21.2

Source: U.S. Bureau of the Census, *Detailed population characteristics. United States summary: 1980*, Table 280.

Older workers are less likely than all workers to have blue-collar jobs. Many of these jobs are in industries where mandatory retirement has been the rule and where pension plans are prevalent. Moreover, many blue-collar jobs are physically arduous—truck driving and construction work, for example.

Many older workers are self-employed or work for small businesses. These include accountants, lawyers, and tavern keepers, who simply continue at the same work beyond normal retirement age. Sales and clerical work offer part-time employment and are thus amenable to elderly individuals' attempting to supplement retirement income; over 40 percent (40.3 percent) of all elderly female workers were employed in these categories in 1980.

Elderly workers are more likely than all other workers to be found in service jobs: gardeners, seamstresses, practical nurses, washroom attendants, night watchmen, ticket takers, and domestics, for example. The 1980 Census reports relatively large proportions of elderly people in each of these occupations. A recent *New York Times* article (Collins 1987) reports that the child-care industry has begun to turn to older Americans to help care for the nation's preschool children. While McDonald's, the giant fast food firm, gains attention for its recent television advertising campaign involving older adult employees, the largest national chain of child-care centers, Kinder-Care Inc., estimates that about 10 to 12 percent of the company's 16,400 workers are over the age of fifty-five. It is recruiting more older workers through community groups and local and national organizations for the elderly.

Through the course of this century, increased longevity and changing social and work patterns have contributed to changes in the time people devote to life activities such as education, work, and retirement. Compared to the population of 1900 (see Figure 12-1), children today are spending more time in school, both men and women spend more time in work, and older people are spending more time in retirement (U.S. Senate Special Committee on Aging 1985).

On the average, males spent five more years in the labor force in 1980 than in 1900. Nonetheless, a smaller proportion of their lives was spent working, 55 percent, than in 1900 when males spent 69 percent of their lives working. Since 1900, the average number of years women spent in the labor force increased from 6.3 to 27.5 years and from 13 to 36 percent of average life expectancy.

The portion of life spent in retirement also has increased substantially since the beginning of the century. In 1900, average life expectancy for males was forty-six or forty-seven years and only 1.2 years or about 3 percent of that was spent in retirement. By 1980, the average male spent almost fourteen of his seventy years in retirement (20 percent). Thus, although average life expectancy increased by 50 percent since 1900, average years in retirement increased by eleven times.

Although the twentieth century has brought with it increased life expectancy, increased work life expectancy, and an increased expectation of retirement, as we have already noted, it has also brought significant decline in labor force participation rates among older men. How do we explain the declining employment level of older persons? What factors have become important in setting that employment level?

Several explanations for the decline in labor force participation of older men have been put forth. A growing number of studies identify health status and the development of pension systems (including Social Security) as the most significant factors influencing the labor supply of older workers. Research also shows changes in the population age structure, changes in labor force composition, and age discrimination in employment to be contributors to the declining employment rates of older workers. Each factor deserves some attention.

Health Status

One interpretation of the decline in labor force participation of older persons has to do with the decline in death rates during this same period. This interpretation assumes that, compared with today's elderly, those in the past were

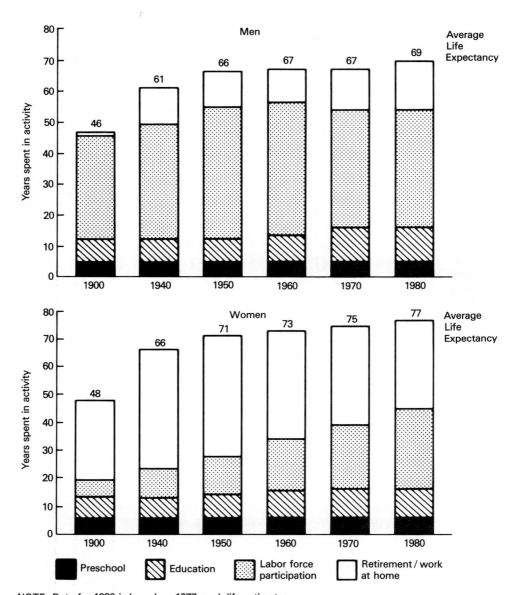

NOTE: Data for 1980 is based on 1977 work life estimates.

FIGURE 12-1   Lifecycle distribution of education, labor force participation, retirement and work in the home: 1900–1980. *Source: Median School Years Completed, Bicentennial Edition: Historical Statistics of the United States: Work Sharing Issues, Policy Options and Prospects, Upjohn Institute for Employment Research, 1981, Bureau of Labor Statistics Bulletin 1982.* Life expectancy from U.S. Bureau of the Census.

healthier and thus more able to work. This assumption is based on recognition of the increasing numbers of chronically ill and physically debilitated people who today survive well into old age.

This proposition is difficult if not impossible to test empirically. Although life expectancy has increased dramatically and mortality rates are down significantly since 1900, we really do not know whether the elderly are healthier or less healthy now than in the past. The National Health Survey, which reports on the health status of Americans, was not initiated in the United States until 1956 and is plagued by methodological problems. For example, it is difficult to obtain accurate information on the health of older people (or people of any age, for that matter), who vary considerably in their ability to describe symptoms and in the symptoms to which they give attention. Misattribution of illness symptoms is a problem among the elderly (Kart 1981), as is underreporting of illness. And, as one prominent medical sociologist (Mechanic 1968, 230) has pointed out, "Information obtained from respondents tends to be highly discrepant from information obtained from clinical evaluations of the same populations." Finally, the survey counts as illnesses only those conditions for which there is restriction of usual activities, bed disability, work loss, the seeking of medical advice, or the taking of medicines (U.S. National Center for Health Statistics 1964). Thus, changes over time and differences among the elderly in the reported incidence of illness may actually reflect variations in access to medical information and care or willingness to take a day off from work.

Despite the methodological difficulties involved in determining the health status of the current elderly population as compared with past elderly populations, a body of literature shows poor health to be a correlate of retirement. The 1968 Survey of Newly Entitled Beneficiaries (SNEB) conducted by the Social Security Administration found that 44 percent of wage and salaried male workers gave health problems as the main reason for leaving their last job (Bixby 1976), although this influence declined with age; 57 percent of men aged sixty-two give this reason, and only 23 percent of those aged sixty-five did so. Data from the Social Security Administration's 1969 Retirement History Study, comprising 11,153 members of the birth cohort from 1905 to 1911, indicated that a health problem was a primary generator of early retirement for men (Schwab 1974) and women (Sherman 1974).

Parnes and his colleagues (1975), reporting on results from the National Longitudinal Study (NLS) of older men, found that men who reported health problems in 1966 were twice as likely to have retired between 1966 and 1971 as men who were free of health impairments. This study is particularly important because it reflects a *causal* sequence of events: Health problems lead to retirement. Other studies are open to the charge that respondents cite health as a reason for retirement because they deem it to be a socially acceptable response. Kingson used this data set in studying men who retired before age sixty-two between 1966 and 1975. (U.S. Senate Select Committee on Aging

1981). He found the labor force withdrawal of these very early retirees to be involuntary; 80 percent of the black and 66 percent of the white very early retirees did so involuntarily. Of these early withdrawees, 87 percent claimed disability or poor health. The legitimacy of reported health problems is sometimes questioned. Reporting a health problem provides a socially acceptable reason for leaving work; thus, it was important for Kingson to determine the validity of such claims. One such test involves looking to the mortality rates of those claiming poor health as a reason for retirement and comparing the rates with those healthy retirees. As Kingson notes, unfortunately for these early retirees, their claims of ill health were validated by their deaths. For example, by 1975, among white early retirees, the unhealthy group had died at a rate (42 percent) almost three times that of the healthy group (15 percent).

Not only do early retirees leave work voluntarily as a result of health problems, but, according to Kingson (1981), the research also shows these men to be among the most financially vulnerable retirees. One study of newly eligible beneficiaries for Social Security found that only one in four of all nonworking men entitled to Social Security benefits at age sixty-two retired voluntarily and had pension income in addition to Social Security; 45 percent had no pensions and did not want to retire when they had to leave their jobs. It seems that early retirees can be divided into two groups; there are those who leave work voluntarily—retirees in good health and with adequate pension income—and those—more numerous—with opposite characteristics.

Changing Retirement Policies

In 1980 almost 90 percent of all persons over the age of sixty-five received money from one retirement program or another. This is a different picture from that in 1935, when Congress passed the Social Security Act. The increasing number of people eligible for Social Security benefits, the rising payment level of the benefits, and the growth of other public and private pension plans not only have provided security to many people in old age but also have permitted many older people financially to afford retirement.

Data from the Retirement History Survey show that eligibility for Social Security benefits reduced the probability of working 15 to 20 percentage points (Quinn 1975). Barfield and Morgan (1969) and Barfield (1970) found pension income to be significantly related to retirement among a sample of auto workers. A threshold effect appeared to operate at $4,000 retirement income in 1967 and $5,000 in 1969. Parnes and his colleagues (1975) found a similar threshold effect among respondents in the National Longitudinal Survey. Sixty-five percent of those with an expected monthly income of $300 or more expected to retire early, but only 47 percent of those with monthly benefits below $300 expected an early retirement.

The availability of early retirement benefits built into Social Security and other public and private pension programs has obviously contributed to the decline in old-age work participation rates. In 1956 the Social Security Act was amended to allow women workers to receive reduced benefits for early retirement between the ages of sixty-two and sixty-four. This amendment was extended to men in 1961. According to the Social Security Administration, a majority of the men awarded initial retirement benefits each year since 1962 have received reduced benefits (Schulz 1976).

In addition, mandatory retirement policies have historically been tied to many pension plans. One might argue that even the Social Security Administration's retirement test exemplifies a form of compulsory retirement. The retirement test, by reducing or eliminating benefit payments if a potential recipient earns above an earnings exemption ceiling, thus effectively discourages some workers from staying in the labor force. The estimated earnings exemption ceiling in 1987 is $6,000 for retirees under age sixty-five and $8,160 for those sixty-five years or over. Benefits are reduced $1 for every $2 earned above the exempt amount.

Bowen and Finegan (1969) have estimated that compulsory retirement policies reduced the labor force participation rate of older males approximately 5 percent between 1948 and 1965. Reno (1976) reports that only 1 percent of the SNEB men aged sixty-two and 7 percent aged sixty-three to sixty-four gave mandatory retirement as the most important reason for leaving their last job, whereas 36 percent of those sixty-five year olds gave this reason.

Changing Age Structure

Another explanation for the appreciable change in the occupational status of the elderly lies in the aging of the elderly population itself. Because work force participation rates for men tend to decline with age, the mere presence of more and more people living past the age of sixty-five, and especially past seventy-five, may reduce the proportion of the elderly population that is employed. Table 12-4 shows the impact of a changing age structure among the elderly on the proportion of old people in the labor force. Following Sheldon (1958), the table presents the results of a calculation of the labor force participation rate that could have been expected in 1970 for men sixty-five years and over had the age distribution for the group been identical with that of 1890, and had the age-related labor force participation rates observed in 1970 been obtained. The table shows 24.8 percent of the 1970 elderly population to be in the labor force; it also shows that we could have expected 26.6 percent of this population to be at work had the age composition of the elderly *not* changed between 1890 and 1970. This resulted in approximately 150,000 fewer people in the 1970 labor force.

Changes in the *overall* age structure must also be assessed for possible impact on the labor force participation rates of the elderly. After all, if the working population has increased or decreased as a proportion of the total population, then work opportunities for the elderly may be likewise affected.

TABLE 12-4 Observed and Expected Male Labor Force 65 Years Old and Over, 1970

Age	Total, 1890[a]		Observed, 1970				Expected, 1970[b]		
			Total		Labor force		Total	Labor force	
	Number	Percent	Number	Percent	Number	Percent	Total	Number	Percent
Total	1,233,719	100.0	8,437,630	100.0	2,092,496	24.8	8,437,630	2,245,650	26.6
65–69 yrs	525,627	42.6	3,113,144	36.9	1,213,000	39.0	3,594,430	1,401,828	39.0
70–74 yrs	363,642	29.5	2,319,748	27.5	520,059	22.4	2,489,101	557,559	22.4
75–79 yrs	199,093	16.1	1,585,351	18.8	224,654	14.2	1,358,458	192,901	14.2
80–84 yrs	97,862	7.9	877,139	10.4	79,388	9.1	666,573	60,658	9.1
85 yrs and over	47,495	3.8	542,248	6.4	55,395	10.2	320,630	32,704	10.2

[a] Data on 1890 taken from Table C-6 in H. Sheldon, *The Older Population of the United States*. New York: John Wiley & Sons, 1958; reprinted by permission of the Social Science Research Council, 605 Third Avenue, New York. Data on 1970 taken from Table 215, "Employment Status by Race, Sex and Age," in the *1970 Census of Population, Characteristics of the Population, U.S. Summary*.

[b] Computed on the basis of the observed age-specific labor force participation rates of 1970 and the percentage age distribution of 1890.

Table 12-5 presents data on changes in the working population between 1890 and 1970. Following procedures used by Sheldon (1958), the population of working age was defined as that between the ages twenty and sixty-four. Any definition of the working population in terms of chronological age is crude; it fails to allow for those (in this case) between twenty and sixty-four who do not work and for those under twenty and over sixty-five who do. Despite limitations, such a device is used because large differences in the proportion of the total contributed by the population of working age do reflect in a general way the need for manpower (Sheldon 1958, 174). When the proportion of those aged twenty to sixty-four drops, there may be an insufficient workforce to support the economy; increases in the proportion of those of working age may indicate an overavailability of workers. In the former situation, older workers are needed to help support the economy; the latter situation is a depressant on work opportunities for the aging.

As can be seen in Table 12-5, there was an increase between 1890 and 1970 in the size of the working-age population and in the proportion of the total population made up by those of working age (49.9 percent versus 52.5 percent). In addition, if the proportion of the total population made up by those twenty to sixty-four years in 1890 had remained the same in 1970, the population of working age would have been reduced by almost 5 million. This number is sufficiently large to suggest that the intensity of need for manpower was greater in 1890 than in 1970. If this is so, we can assume that the decline in labor force participation rates among the elderly is, in some part, attributable to a decline in need for manpower.

TABLE 12-5   Observed and expected "working population" by sex: 1970

Year	Population (all ages)	Total Observed Working Population (20–64 yr)		Expected Working Population (20–64 yr)	
		Number	Percent	Number	Percent
1890	62,622,250	31,243,034	49.9	—	—
1970	203,211,926	106,176,024	52.2	101,402,740	49.9
		Males			
1890	32,067,880	16,191,913	50.5	—	—
1970	98,912,192	47,733,630	48.3	49,950,656	50.5
		Females			
1890	30,554,370	15,051,121	49.3	—	—
1970	104,299,734	54,818,119	52.6	51,419,766	49.3

Source: U.S. Bureau of the Census. *Historical Statistics of the United States, Colonial Times to 1970*, Pt. I. Series A119–134, 1975.

This assumption is weakened, however, by data presented in Table 12-5 on changes in the age structure by sex. For males, the proportion of the total population in the working years declined between 1890 and 1970 from 50.5 to 48.3 percent. If the proportion had remained the same during this period, over 2 million *more* men would have been in the population of working age in 1970. This decline in the working population should have provided job opportunities for older male workers.

Women show a different pattern. The proportion of the total female population in the working years increased between 1890 and 1970 from 49.3 to 52.6 percent. If the 1890 proportion had held constant in 1970, the female population of working age would have been reduced by more than 3 million. It seems likely that this situation acted to constrain older female labor force participation rates.

Changing Occupational Structure

Two theories related to changes in the composition of the labor force often surface as explanations for the changes in the work status of elderly people during the past seventy-five years. The first is the argument that changing technology places older persons at a disadvantage. Occupational skills may become outmoded with technological innovation, and emphasis on assembly-line production may place a greater premium on speed and physical stamina than on work experience.

At first glance the theory may seem credible, though evidence in support of it is difficult to obtain. Technological change that makes work skills obsolescent should do so for all workers in an occupational category—not just the old. Moreover, older workers may be in a stronger position to hang on in such situations through recognition of seniority. Work careers sometimes involve shifts from one occupational group to another. Managers and administrators often are recruited from clerical and sales personnel, foremen from operatives. Typically, such a career pattern might tend to favor an older worker under conditions of changing technology. Additionally, in occupations where opportunities are undergoing contraction (because of technological change or otherwise), the greatest impact often is felt by young workers attempting to enter the occupation. Frequently, this is seen in the way craft unions regulate apprenticeship when demand for a particular skill is declining.

We should not forget that, while new technology makes some job skills unnecessary, it also prolongs working lives. Machines and automation often reduce the physical burdens and stress associated with industrial jobs (Achenbaum 1978). Bowen and Finegan (1969) have suggested that the reduction in the work week, itself often associated with mechanization in the labor force, may have *offset* the decline in elderly men's labor force participation rates by as much as 3.5 percent between 1948 and 1965.

One place where older workers may have had special difficulty in the face of mechanization is in rural areas. Historically, rates of employment among older men have declined more in rural than in urban places (Long 1958). In rural areas, nonfarm employment opportunities for older people are minimal, and it seems likely that elderly men who followed the migration to urban areas did not do well. How much the population migration from rural to urban areas contributed to declining labor force opportunities for older workers is difficult to discern, although it appears less than might have been expected. On the basis of his labor force analysis, Long (1958) concluded that the effect of population migration between 1890 and 1950 on the elderly male labor force rate was "relatively little." According to one study, rural to urban migration accounted for about a 3 percent decline in elderly male workers between 1948 and 1965 (Bowen and Finegan 1969).

A second theory regarding changes in labor force composition is that decline in the importance of farming as a source of jobs has had a depressing effect on the employment of older people. In 1890 almost 61 percent of all employed aged men were farmers; by 1980, the figure was 11.3 percent. Yet, older workers were not the only ones affected by the twentieth-century revolution in agriculture. The increased technology and science in farming, the consolidation of small farms, and the development of multinational agribusiness had significant impact on farming employment for people of all ages. In 1900 about 36 percent of all those in the labor force were employed in agriculture, compared with about 4.3 percent in 1980.

These changes have affected younger and older men differently. Rapid expansion of the nonfarming components of the labor force has been a source of opportunities for younger workers; no concomitant compensatory expansion of opportunities has occurred for older workers. Further, occupational longevity is greater for farmers than for other workers: "age grading" is less relevant in agriculture. Retirement on the farm does not have the same meaning it does in other industries. The decline in the number of persons engaged in farming has been large enough to affect appreciably the labor force participation rates of older men. In 1910, over 12 million workers were engaged in farming; by 1980 this figure had dropped to about 2.8 million.

Age Discrimination in Employment

No one really knows the extent of age discrimination in employment that exists in U.S. society, although it is considered pervasive and in recent years has drawn increasing attention. A 1964 Department of Labor study reported that over 1 million man-years of productive output are lost each year in the United States because of age discrimination. In 1967 the Congress passed the Age Discrimination Employment Act (ADEA) and amended it in 1974, 1978, and 1986. The federal law prohibits the following:

1. Discrimination in the hiring of an employee on the basis of age
2. Discrimination in discharging a person on the basis of age

3. Discrimination in pay and other privileges and conditions of employment because of age

4. Instructions to an employment agency not to refer a person to a job because of age or to only certain kinds of jobs

5. Placement of any advertisement that shows preferences based on age or which specifies an age bracket

Currently, all employers with more than twenty employees are subject to the provisions of ADEA, as well as employment agencies, labor organizations, and states and their agencies and subdivisions. With the 1986 amendments, virtually all employees aged forty or older are protected. Exceptions include firefighters, law enforcement officers, and tenured faculty at institutions of higher learning, who until December 31, 1993, may be discharged on the basis of age at age seventy or older.

One study of employed aerospace workers aged forty-five and over reported that *half* of them had at least one personal experience with discrimination in employment because of their age (Kasschau 1976). Many workers suffer from age discrimination but do not identify it as such; others may be unaware of their protection under ADEA.

Instances of age discrimination in employment can be difficult to identify. For workers not covered by federal law, states may vary in the protection they offer an older worker. According to one report, although state laws generally are not as broad as the federal ADEA, many states do offer better protection to public than private employees (Goldberg 1978). This same report found only four states having coverage equal to or better than federal laws.

Because the ADEA covers all employees aged forty or older, discrimination based on age is not as clear-cut or obvious as race or sex discrimination (where unchanging characteristics are involved). When race or sex discrimination is proven, it usually affects the protected group as a whole. Age discrimination, on the other hand, may be directed at a subgroup of the protected class. For example, in one case brought before the U.S. Court of Appeals in Denver in 1980 (*Equal Employment Opportunity Commission v. Sandia Corporation*), the trial court found that in the company's layoff decisions a pattern and practice of age discrimination began to appear for employees aged fifty-two, and the inference that age was a factor became stronger after age fifty-five, increasing up to age fifty-eight, where it remained a steady influence in decisions until age sixty-four.

RETIREMENT

Retirement as a mass phenomenon is a modern industrial creation. People certainly retired in preindustrial times, but only if they could generate income by performing some productive function or if they owned enough property to provide income. People who stopped working because they were too old or sick led a difficult life. They were "dead weight"—often treated, at least figuratively, like the Eskimo grandmother who, when she could no longer function, was abandoned or walled up in an igloo to await death (Donahue, Orbach, and Pollak 1960).

Richard Calhoun (1978) points out that in the sense of giving up "business or occupation in order to enjoy more leisure or freedom" the *Oxford English Dictionary's* first example of retirement comes from a 1667 entry in Samuel Pepys's diary. The example makes clear, through reference to pensions and "competences," that retirement was a status available only to the nobility or mercantile elites. Working people of the day did not retire. Generally they did not have access to pensions. Also, "busy hands are happy hands"; retirement was not valued.

In the U.S. context, the historian Achenbaum (1978) tells us that the word retirement, meaning stopping work at some prescribed age, was literally absent from pre–Civil War vocabulary. People retired, but as in "retiring" from winter storms to the warmth of a family circle. Webster, in the first edition of *An America Dictionary* (1828), defined retirement as "1. the art of withdrawing from company or from public notice or station; 2. the state of being withdrawn; 3. private abode; 4. private way of life." Obviously, old age was no prerequisite to retirement; anyone might retire. By the 1880 edition, however, a new meaning was attributed to the verb *to retire:* "to cause to retire, specifically to designate as no longer qualified for active service, as to retire a military or naval officer." The reference to naval officer is interesting. According to Achenbaum, the first federal retirement measure became law in December 1861 when Congress passed an act requiring any naval officer below the rank of vice admiral who was aged sixty-two or older to resign his commission; the retirement age for naval officers was raised to sixty-four in 1916. Also noteworthy in the 1880 definition is the implicitly negative attitude toward old age. People were retired when they were no longer qualified for employment because of age.

From the midnineteenth to the midtwentieth century, retirement policies became more prevalent in both public and private sectors. During this period, much debate surrounded issues of a standard age for defining superannuation (retirement), mandatory versus voluntary retirement, and the adequacy of pension income. Debaters differed on the advantages and disadvantages of various retirement policies to the older worker and the national economy. Business, for example, regarded the issue of adequacy of pension as the price of management gaining prerogative over setting retirement age. Such power was essential for manipulating the size of the labor pool during business up- or downturns. Organized labor, on the other hand, viewed pension adequacy as a bread and butter issue—a right of every worker. Academicians and social reformers saw pension reform as extraneous, an issue used to exclude older workers from the labor force and deny them the freedom to work as long as they are able and desirous of doing so (Calhoun 1978).

Many older workers saw retirement as a threat. They recognized that retirement (particularly forced retirement) might create an economically disadvantaged situation. Some believed the myth that death comes at retirement. Others believed in work as the American way of life.

In 1949 novelist James Michener published a short story in *Nation's Business* that he believed reflected the attitude of Americans toward retirement. John Bassett was the head accountant at J.C. Gower and Company. The story involved his last day of work at the firm, which was forcing Mr. Bassett into retirement. He plotted revenge, but his employer—concerned about the impact of the forced retirement on Bassett and aware of the accountant's work record— waived the company's sixty-five-and-out rule. Bassett stayed on the job, though at half pay. Mr. Gower also gave the employee a set of woodworking tools in an effort to increase the accountant's avocations. Mr. Bassett gave the tools to his grandson and in doing so summed up the attitude that Michener believed to be prevalent among U.S. workers: "Such substitutions for paid employment are for kids; what a man needs is a job."

Nevertheless, by the 1960s something had changed. Retirement was becoming an accepted part of the life cycle for a greater proportion of the population. Ash (1966) studied the attitudes toward retirement among steelworkers. He found that in 1951 retirement was justified only if an individual was physically unable to continue working. By 1960, however, retirement was justified as reward for a lifetime of work. The gerontologist Robert Atchley (1974) also found that retirement had become an overwhelmingly favorable concept. In his research he discovered that people saw retirement as an active, hopeful, meaningful, healthy, relaxed, and independent time.

Even early retirement became acceptable. Apparently, when workers are provided adequate income for retirement before age sixty-five, even to age fifty, there is little resistance to retirement. Whereas in the immediate postwar environment unions debated whether or not to set the retirement age at sixty-five, by the 1960s thirty-years-service-and-out by age fifty-five was not atypical of union demands. The United Auto Workers' (UAW) 1965 plan had the effect of reducing retirement age to sixty. Under the plan, an auto worker aged sixty with thirty years of service retired on a monthly pension plus a supplement until such time as the worker qualified for full Social Security benefits. Currently, 30 percent of those eligible under the UAW's thirty-and-out plan are retiring. General Motors reports that the average age at retirement has come down steadily, to fifty-eight in 1975. In 1976, only 2 percent of that company's hourly rate employees retired at the mandatory age.

Ekerdt, Vinick, and Bosse (1989) provide formal support for the view that retirement—early or otherwise—has been institutionalized as an anticipated and orderly event in the life course. These researchers found that 66 percent of workers participating in the Veterans Administration's Normative Aging Study accurately predicted their eventual date of retirement within plus or minus one year; 40 percent were exact to within three months.

Mandatory Retirement[3]

Some attribute the choice of age sixty-five as the age for retirement to the Old Age and Survivors Pension Act that Otto Von Bismarck pushed through as the first chancellor of the German Empire in 1889. One unverifiable account of how this came to be suggests that Bismarck's actuaries recommended sixty-five as a safe age because life expectancy at birth during the 1880s was about forty-five years and few people could be expected to reach age sixty-five. The English, playing it even safer, passed similar legislation in 1908 using seventy as a retirement age (they later reduced it to sixty-five). The United States followed in 1935 with its own Social Security program. Wilbur Cohen (1957), former Secretary of Health, Education, and Welfare, and one of the staff members who helped draft the 1935 legislation, wrote that the choice of age sixty-five as a boundary line for providing old age assistance had no scientific, social, or gerontological basis. There was simply a general political concensus that sixty-five was an acceptable age.

Although the original Social Security Act of 1935 was not involved in establishing a compulsory retirement age, the choice of age sixty-five seems to have carried over from Social Security to mandatory retirement policies. As we have already pointed out, recent amendments to the Age Discrimination Employment Act (ADEA) have, for the most part, eliminated sixty-five as the age for mandatory retirement. The Act protects individuals from employment discrimination who are aged forty and older.

It is difficult to say who has been affected by mandatory retirement policies. A 1961 Cornell University sample survey (Slavick 1966) of industrial firms in the United States with fifty or more employees found that most establishments had flexible retirement policies. Almost 95 percent of firms without pension plans, almost 70 percent of those with profit-sharing, and 60 percent of those with formal pension plans had flexible retirement policies. The Brandeis economist James Schulz (1976) has pointed out the relationship between flexible retirement rules and establishment size that was evident in this survey. For example, 68 percent of the firms with fifty to ninety-nine employees had flexible rules, yet only 30 percent of those with 500 or more employees had such rules. Thus, it is possible that relatively few firms have had mandatory retirement rules, while at the same time many workers have been subject to such policies.

A 1972 survey of the largest state and local government retirement systems covering about 70 percent of all employees enrolled in such systems showed that most had a mandatory retirement age; for two-thirds of the plans retirement age was set at age seventy or later. James Schulz has developed the tabulations of responses from this survey, which shows the incidence of mandatory retirement. Although 54 percent of male retirees were subject to mandatory

---

[3] This section relies heavily on the August 1977 report by the Select Committee on Aging, *Mandatory Retirement: The Social and Human Cost of Enforced Idleness.* Washington, D.C.: USGPO.

retirement rules, only 7 percent of the total cohort of retired workers were able and willing to work but unable to find a new job. This small proportion of workers affected by mandatory retirement policies supports data on this issue provided by some of America's largest corporations.

Why the fuss over mandatory retirement practices in light of how relatively few workers are forced out of work because of them? One reason may have to do with the adverse effects mandatory retirement has had on many retirees. Robert Butler (1975) describes these effects as the "retirement syndrome." Although not all retirees develop these characteristics, many formerly healthy workers do develop headaches, irritability, nervousness, lethargy, and the like in connection with retirement. Susan Haynes of the National Heart, Lung, and Blood Institute found that the mortality rate of workers who were in good health when mandatorily retired at age sixty-five was 30 percent higher than expected three and four years following retirement.

A second reason for concern over mandatory retirement may have to do with the traditional arguments made for and against mandatory retirement. These are often based on misconceptions and myths associated with the aging process and the employment of older people. Many studies indicate that older workers produce a quality of work as good or better than that of younger workers. As has already been pointed out in Chapter 7, "Psychological Aspects of Aging," there is no reason to expect a decline in intellectual capacities with age and every reason to assume that older workers in good health are capable of learning new skills when circumstances require it.

The argument that the mandatory retirement of older workers opens needed jobs for the young may be especially appealing to some. Yet no study can be cited that demonstrates that the termination of an older worker because of mandatory retirement directly caused the hiring of young workers. Given the high rate of early retirement and the small proportion of retirees who would have continued working without mandatory retirement, it does not appear that the elimination of mandatory retirement policies would have any substantial impact on the labor supply or the unemployment rate.

Adjustment to Retirement

Adjustment to retirement can be difficult for many people, although most studies show a majority of people adjust reasonably well. Finances, health, physical mobility, social involvement, and the specific circumstances of the retirement appear to top the list of factors researchers have identified as affecting adjustment to retirement. For example, Beck (1982) has identified poor health, lower income, and retirement earlier than expected as main determinants of a negative evaluation of retirement. Boaz (1987) implies some anxiety about retirement in her study of work as a response on the part of retirees to low and decreasing real retirement income. Findings from this research suggest that work during retirement among men *and* women "is a response to low or moderate levels of nonwage income at the beginning of retirement and, for

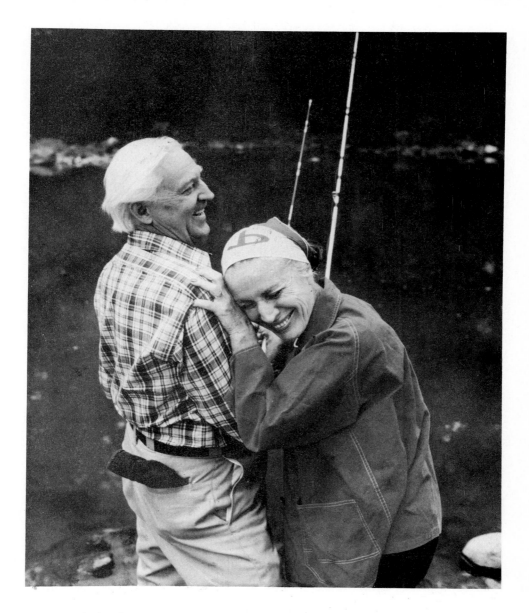

men, work is also a response to a decrease in the real value of such income during retirement'' (p. 437). Fillenbaum and her colleagues (1985) found few consequences of retirement, however. Blacks and men at poverty level were minimally affected by retirement, perhaps as a result of government-provided income supports.

Evans, Ekerdt, and Bosse (1985) used data from 816 male workers participating in the Normative Aging Study of the Veterans Administration in Boston to investigate the preretirement socialization process. These researchers found a strong linear relationship between proximity to retirement and informal pre-retirement involvement (measured by how often the preretiree had talked with his wife, his relatives, his close friends, or people on the job or had read articles about retirement). This finding indicates that an anticipatory self-socialization to retirement was underway at least fifteen years prior to the retirement itself. In addition, other factors such as attitudes toward retirement, job characteristics, and personal resources (especially the existence of an already-retired good friend) were of relevance in explaining variation in preretirement involvement.

Attitudes toward retirement may directly determine adjustment. A recent study of college professors showed that about three-quarters of them looked forward to retirement; one-fourth did not have a positive attitude. A professor of the biological sciences held this negative view:

> The problem I see about retirement is the failure of our society to appreciate the worth of all the education experience, teaching quality, and knowhow packed into an academic. One can be a professor one minute, then a park bench occupant the next, and yet I am constantly reading about inadequately informed congressmen, schools with teaching deficits, etc. The concept of the golden years of travel, etc., is based largely on romantic novels and the cinemas. The greatest tragedy of retirement is the lack of imagination of our institutions including universities to develop a plan whereby individuals' worth and self-esteem can be maintained in a meaningful way. (Patton, C. 1977. Early retirement in academia: Making the decision. *Gerontologist* 17(4):350. Reprinted by permission of The Gerontological Society of America.)

The feelings of worth and self-esteem referred to by this professor may be at the core of discussions about adjusting to retirement. Miller (1965) has taken the position that retirement brings with it an identity crisis. He argues that retirement is basically degrading because it implies that the individual is no longer able to carry out the work role. This is especially problematic, Miller says, because occupational identity is so much a part of a person's life. It affects how all the other roles (spouse, parent, friend, and so on) are played. Leisure roles cannot replace work as a source of self-respect and identity because society does not support them in the same way it supports work roles. According to Miller, leisure is not sufficient replacement for work as a source of worth and self-esteem. The crisis comes because the individual's former claims to prestige and status are negated by retirement, and no replacement sources of prestige and status are available. This embarrasses the individual and causes withdrawal from social life.

In response to Miller's "identity crisis theory," the gerontologist Robert Atchley (1971) put forth an "identity continuity theory" of adjustment to retirement. Atchley points out that few people rest their entire identity on a single role. Rather, most people have several roles in which to base identity. The probability that retirement will lead to identity crisis or breakdown is slim because other roles (for example, parent, grandparent, or spouse) are maintained well into old age. Also, retired workers will likely continue to identify with their occupation even though they no longer play the role. Thus, the retired professor will continue to see himself or herself as a professor beyond the retirement age. Furthermore, Atchley argues that people *can* gain self-respect from leisure pursuits in retirement, especially if they have sufficient financial resources available and a cohort of retired friends who accept full-time leisure as a legitimate enterprise. A final point of identity continuity theory is that many people develop skills during the course of their occupational careers that are quite useful in retirement and do provide a degree of identity continuity. Skill in interpersonal interaction developed in careers in sales or teaching, for example, may serve a person well in leisure activities and at the same time facilitate a sense of continuity in their life.

Although it does not appear to be a typical pattern, some people, especially those forced to retire, do undergo the identity crisis described by Miller. The "retirement syndrome" Butler referred to may reflect this identity crisis. Ellison (1968) suggests that this crisis can be an important precipitating factor in the adoption of the sick role. Having come to define illness as a more legitimate role to occupy than being retired, retirees may become "sick" (that is, behave as if they were ill). It may be easier in our society to say you have retired because of poor health than to explain that the employer no longer considers you competent to do a job.

A more typical pattern of adjustment in retirement involves those whose experiences fit the continuity perspective. Snow and Havighurst (1977) studied the careers after age sixty of administrators in American higher education. One life-style pattern that they identified, the *maintainers,* were able to hold onto their professional activities successfully even after formal retirement, pursuing part-time assignments and filling time with other activities. Interestingly, the maintainers were contrasted with another group, the *transformers.* The transformers changed their life-styles with retirement, reduced their professional activities (by choice), and created a new pattern of living that often emphasized nonprofessional areas of activity (such as hobbies, arts and crafts, or travel). As one transformer put it:

> My post-retirement activity represents a relatively sharp change of the content of my experience. At the time of my full retirement, I was confronted by a series of invitations and opportunities to engage in continued professional work in various cities and as far away as Taiwan. On reflection, my wife and I decided to reject all of them. I had had more than enough of riding in airplanes and living in hotels and we wished to stay here among our good friends. This would give me opportunity to activate a long smouldering interest in painting. The painting now claims my primary interest and labor, and I have become President of our local Art League. I keep some professional work going in education but really, I have opened up a new career which beckons me on to achievement and a new kind of fulfillment. (Snow, R., and Havighurst, R. 1977. Life-style types and patterns of retirement of educators. *Gerontologist* 17(6):548. Reprinted by permission of The Gerontological Society of America.)

Still, even this transformer maintains continuity by keeping "some professional work going in education."

More recently, Mutran and Reitzes (1981) have added to this discussion of "identity crisis" versus "identity continuity" through their secondary analysis of the 1974 national survey data collected by the National Council on Aging. In particular, they were interested in the way retirement (and a series of background variables) affects participation in community activities, visits with friends, self-identity, and feelings of well-being among men aged fifty-five and older in the survey. These researchers found that retirement is not directly associated with visiting friends, self-identity, or well-being, although it does *indirectly* encourage an older self-identity and discourage well-being through its effect on community activities. Lack of involvement in community activities was the strongest predictor of an older self-identity for both working *and* retired men, whereas involvement in community activities has the strongest effect on the well-being of both working men and retirees.

Mutran and Reitzes (1981, 739) suggest that "involvement in community activities emerges as a possible intervening variable between retirement and social psychological measures"—self-identity and well-being. Further, they point out that the impact of retirement on other roles, such as that of active community participant, may affect well-being but may go unnoticed if researchers are not careful about how retirement is operationalized in their analyses.

Preretirement programs have been around since early in the post–World War II period. In general, their appearance is evidence of the belief that the work role is central and an important source of self-identity and status. As we have already seen, some believe that the notion of work as central to self-identity has been given undue consideration in research on adjustment to retirement. Almost despite this ongoing discussion in the gerontological literature, there has been a substantial growth in the prevalence of preretirement programs. Two important questions are: Do workers participate in such programs? And, do preretirement programs work?

Campione (1988) has used data from the National Longitudinal Survey of Mature Men to estimate the probability of participation in a retirement preparation program. The final sample employed in the study included 294 retired men who reported having had the opportunity to participate in a preretirement program and for whom longitudinal data were available. Most workers who do participate in such programs do so within two years of their retirement. Campione finds that those individuals who prepare for retirement during their working lives are more likely to participate in retirement preparation programs. In addition, those who are married and have families to plan for, those who have minimal health problems, and those of higher occupational status are more likely to plan for retirement. She concludes that program sponsors are failing to attract a broad cross-section of employees into preretirement preparation programs. Apparently those most likely to succeed in retirement anyway are those most likely to be given an opportunity to participate in such programs (Beck 1974).

Recently, Glamser (1981) has reported on a longitudinal study to determine the longer term impact of two different preretirement programs. Two experimental groups and one control group were used to test the merits of a "comprehensive group discussion program" and an "individual briefing program." Those male industrial workers in the group discussion program met eight times during a one-month period with sessions lasting approximately ninety minutes each. Those assigned to the individual briefing program met with the plant personnel officer for thirty minutes and received four booklets to read dealing with retirement planning, income, health, and leisure activities.

Questionnaire data were collected prior to program initiation and again six years later. The results showed no significant effect on the retirement experience of individuals by either program. Further, no substantive differences with the control group were noted in the length of the adjustment period, accuracy of expectations, level of preparation, life satisfaction, attitude toward retirement, or job deprivation. Glamser suggests that the major impact of preretirement programs may be of considerably shorter duration than six years. Further, their primary value may actually be in the period immediately prior to the employees' departure from the work setting.

Retirement in Cross-Cultural Perspective

As already indicated, retirement is a modern industrial phenomenon, with the emphasis on "industrial." There are numerous examples of retirement patterns in contemporary preindustrial societies that are different than those in America. Holmes (1972) reports that in Samoa there is the concept of retiring from the position of household head, an influential position in the village council. Sometimes this is done to allow younger men to achieve status and power, but stepping down does not mean a complete withdrawal from village council activities. Often, the former chief will become an elder statesman and function in an advisory capacity with the council.

Among the !Kung San of the Kalahari Desert in southwestern Africa, the aged are held in high esteem. They act as the following: (1) stewards of rights to water and resources in the area; (2) storehouses of knowledge, skills, and lore; (3) teachers and minders of children; (4) spiritual specialists and healers; and (5) ritually privileged figures. In this subsistence economy, these roles are based on reciprocal obligations across the life cycle, not on the accumulation of economic power and resources (Biesele and Howell 1981). Adult men are hunters, and many are healers. They do not know retirement. Aging men carry out these roles as long as they can and then replace them with less strenuous activities such as trapping, gathering, making artifacts, telling stories, and visiting. Women are gatherers, and many of them are healers also. With age, they also continue these roles and gradually move to less physically arduous activities, including child care and handicrafts work (Biesele and Howell 1981).

Japan provides an interesting case study of retirement in an advanced industrial society such as our own (Palmore 1975). Older Japanese men are more likely to work than are older American men. According to the 1965 census, 60 percent of the employed older men in Japan were between the ages of sixty-five and sixty-nine, compared with 37 percent for the United States. Most older Japanese workers are self-employed or work in a family business; over 50 percent are farmers, lumbermen, or fishermen. One recent survey reports that 41 percent of workers over sixty gave "duty" as the reason for continuing to work at an advanced age; 36 percent of those surveyed cited financial necessity as a reason for working (Palmore 1975).

About 75 percent of Japan's industries have compulsory retirement, and the most frequent retirement age is fifty-five. Yet almost all Japanese firms maintain the pattern of "permanent employment," which motivates them to provide some kind of employment for older workers even after compulsory retirement. This may take the form of extending the old job, creating a new job not subject to compulsory retirement, or offering a step-down job at reduced pay. Workers who retire to another job in the same company usually show a smaller decline in earnings than if they had moved to another company.

Currently, there are arguments in Japan about raising the retirement age and doing away with mandatory retirement. These arguments center around the needs of older people to work and maintain an adequate standard of living and the needs of the nation to utilize the productive capacities of older Japanese. Management specialist Peter Drucker (1971) believes that the Japanese system of retirement—mandatory retirement at age fifty-five and "permanent employment"—is a important contributor to Japan's economic growth. He says that this system reduces labor costs at no decline in worker productivity.

Women and Retirement

Most research on retirement has emphasized the experience of men, who traditionally have dominated in the labor force. The employment experience of women is changing, however, especially among younger cohorts. As these women enter old age, an increasing proportion will have participated in the labor force and will have done so for a longer period of time. This will have a positive effect on the economic position of women in old age; they will have accumulated more primary Social Security credits and more private pension benefits (Uhlenberg 1979). Further, retirement is likely to become more salient as an experience of older women.

In the short run, employment in the labor force will not be a major activity for older women. As Table 12-1 showed, the proportion of women aged sixty-five years and over participating in the labor force has declined since 1960; in 1980, only 8.1 percent of these women were working. The table also shows a slight decline in labor force participation rates among women fifty-five and sixty-four since 1970.

In the past, data on the retirement experiences of female workers were culled from studies of male workers. Today, there is an emerging literature on women's retirement. There is some evidence that women have different attitudes toward retirement than men do, even when these men are their husbands (Campbell 1979). For example, based on their analysis of a national personal interview survey, Barfield and Morgan (1978) report that husbands are more likely to plan early retirement than their wives are. Wives plan to work longer and think about early retirement only when there is a high family income and no mortgage payments or commitments to children.

Campione (1987) has used data from the University of Michigan's Panel Study of Income Dynamics to study the retirement decisions of married women aged fifty-five to seventy. She found the married woman's decision to be influenced significantly by changes in financial status, including Social Security wealth, wage wealth, pension wealth, and age. In addition, the married woman's retirement decision was significantly influenced by her spouse's labor force status. Thus, the retirement of her husband does increase the likelihood of the wife's retirement.

Working women seem to be opposed to mandatory retirement. Many do not start working until age forty or forty-five and are not ready to retire by age sixty-two or sixty-five (as long as they remain healthy and capable of job performance). Concentrated in occupations and industries where pensions are inadequate or nonexistent, working women receive lower wages on the average than men do, and the gaps in their work histories translate into low Social Security payments (Campbell 1979). Add to these conditions the probability of an older woman being widowed, divorced, or married to a man with a low income, and it becomes understandable that older women workers are willing to struggle to delay the years of reduced income that accompany retirement. Campbell (1979) believes that raising the mandatory retirement age will have the dual effect of allowing a large and growing population of low-income older women to continue working, while reducing the strain on Social Security and pension funds by keeping this population contributing to these funds rather than withdrawing from them.

Finally, some recent research suggests that men and women do not differ substantially in their adjustment to retirement. Schnore and Kirkland (1981), in their study of retirement in London, Ontario, report no sex differences in life satisfaction, satisfaction with the decision to retire, happiness, and attitudes toward work and retirement.

Is a woman's satisfaction with retirement different if she is married as opposed to widowed? Dorfman and Moffett (1987) addressed this question in their study of older women in two rural Iowa counties. The sample included women who reported that they had retired from a paying job in the last ten years. Two factors, self-perceived health status and increases in social participation in voluntary associations, were predictors of retirement satisfaction for married *and* widowed rural women. Perceptions of financial status and the frequency and perceived certainty of receiving aid from friends were predictors of retirement satisfaction among married women, whereas maintenance of pre-retirement friendships and frequency of contacts with friends predicted retirement satisfaction for widowed women. Should we be surprised by the fact that retirement satisfaction among rural widows seemingly was not affected by concerns about financial status or whether aid from close friends could be counted on in a crisis? According to Dorfman and Moffett (1987), these findings may simply reflect rural values of independence and the acceptance of unfavorable conditions of life without complaint.

Kroeger (1981) has provided what she aptly describes as a "tantalizing piece of data" on the relationship between duration of work experience and women's adjustment to retirement. The data come from a survey of recent retirees of all occupational classifications from the merchandising industries (major department stores, small retail shops, buying offices, and the like) in New York City. Adjustment to retirement was measured with a fourteen-item scale including statements on job satisfaction, social relationships, personal identity, and changes in activities since retirement. The average scores for women who reported having worked all their lives and those who reported having worked for about two-thirds of their lives were virtually identical. The average score for women who reported working only about one-third of their adult lives—about fifteen years—was lower (though not at a statistically significant level), reflecting greater dissatisfaction with retirement.

How do we explain the greater satisfaction with retirement experienced by those women who have worked all their lives? Do they really relish a return to house and hearth? Perhaps they do, at least in comparison with the more traditional housewife who, having had her fill of "good housekeeping" but only a taste of work life, finds less satisfaction in returning home.

LEISURE

Older people spend more time in leisure activities, on the average, than do people in their middle years (Riley and Foner 1968). This is no surprise. In general, old age brings retirement for men and a reduction in obligatory pursuits for women. This leaves more time free for leisure pursuits. According to Riley and Foner (1968), the leisure activities most frequently reported by older people include watching television, gardening, visiting, and reading. It appears that solitary activity receives increased time in old age, whereas social activities receive decreased time.

There is considerable controversy in the gerontological literature concerning leisure time pursuits. One argument, with which we are already familiar, is that leisure roles are not adequate substitutes for the work role. This is because leisure roles are not supported by norms that would legitimate the replacement (Miller 1965). Basic to this argument is the notion that work (and not leisure) is of dominant value in the United States, thus individuals are unable to develop self-respect from leisure time pursuits.

An opposing position is that leisure can, in fact, replace the work role and provide personal satisfaction in later life (Atchley 1971). This may be the case especially in the presence of adequate income (Barfield and Morgan 1969) and good health.

Thompson (1973) has tested the relative merits of these two positions. Data from personal interviews with almost 1,600 older men were analyzed in this study. The results challenged the position that argues for the centrality of work as a value in the lives of older Americans. Those retirees in the sample who were found to have low self-respect (the actual variable employed in the study was labeled "morale") were also found to be older, to have negative evaluations of their health, and to have more disability and less income. The research suggests that low self-respect is related to these factors, not to their lack of work role. As Thompson (1973) writes, "[I]t appears that given relative youth, an optimistic view of health, a lack of functional disability, and an adequate income, the retirement years can be as pleasant as the years of employment for a great many men and that leisure roles can adequately substitute for that of worker."

One reason why many people may have difficulty occupying leisure roles is simply that they lack the practice. Television, gardening, visiting, and reading are so popular precisely because older people have had so much practice time with these activities. Atchley (1977) points out many people are reluctant to engage in leisure activities because they feel incompetent at such activities. Miller (1965) argues that the prospect of embarrassment keeps many older people from participating in new leisure pursuits.

Americans have not been educated for leisure. Efforts should be made to prepare people for the life of leisure. When people are already old, it is too late for such preparation, because older people tend to retain activity patterns and preferences developed earlier in life. Leisure competence should be learned early. Doing so may be the only way to assure leisure competence in later life. In recent years, preretirement planning programs have been used to help workers identify activities and roles that may be rewarding after retirement, but such programs do little to enhance a lifelong learning approach to leisure.

SUMMARY

Labor force participation rates of old people have declined throughout the twentieth century. Currently, fewer than one-quarter of aged males and about one-tenth of aged females are in the labor force. Factors that have contributed to this decline include the health status of older people, new pension systems, changes in the population age structure, changes in economy characteristics, and age discrimination in employment.

Retirement is a modern industrial creation. According to Atchley (1976), the emergence of retirement as a social institution in a society requires four factors: longevity, economic surplus, pension systems, and acceptance of the idea of retirement. Recently, early retirement has become more acceptable, thereby reflecting a changing attitude (increasingly positive) toward retirement on the part of industrial workers. Most current retirees did not wait to be forced out by mandatory retirement policies before retiring.

Nevertheless, adjusting to retirement is seldom easy. Adequate finances, good health, and social activities may positively affect adjustment to retirement. Some gerontologists believe that retirement necessarily brings an "identity crisis," whereas others argue that self-respect can be gained from leisure pursuits. In the future, retirement is likely to become an issue that is salient to the experiences of older women as well.

Finally, although solitary leisure activities seem to be preferred by older people, it may be that most older people simply have more practice with such activities. Americans need to be educated for leisure, and this should begin early in life. When people are already aged, it is generally too late to prepare them for leisure participation.

STUDY QUESTIONS

1. Discuss the social conditions necessary for the emergence of retirement as a social institution.

2. In what types of jobs are older workers likely to be employed? How has the occupational distribution of the elderly work force changed during the twentieth century?

3. Discuss the relationship between health status and retirement.

4. Discuss age discrimination in employment in the United States, with emphasis on the Age Discrimination Employment Act. Why are age discrimination cases sometimes more difficult to prove than race or sex discrimination?

5. Within a historical context describe changing attitudes toward retirement in the United States.

6. Discuss the many social and psychological factors that contribute to or detract from adjustment to retirement.

7. Compare and contrast the *identity crisis* and *identity continuity* theories of adjustment to retirement.

8. Explain why leisure time can actually create problems for older people. What can older people do to prepare for more effective use of their leisure time?

BIBLIOGRAPHY

Achenbaum, W.A. 1978. *Old age in the new land.* Baltimore, Md.: The John Hopkins University Press.

Ash, P. 1966. Pre-retirement counseling. *Gerontologist* 6:97–99, 127–128.

Atchley, R. 1971. Retirement and leisure participation: Continuity or crisis. *Gerontologist* 11:13–17.

———. 1974. The meaning of retirement. *Journal of Communication* 24:97–100.

———. 1976. *The sociology of retirement.* New York: Halsted Press.

———. 1977. *Social forces in later life* (2nd ed.). Belmont, Calif.: Wadsworth Publishing Co., Inc.

Barfield, R. 1970. *The automobile worker and retirement: A second look.* Ann Arbor: Institute for Social Research, University of Michigan.

Barfield, R., and Morgan, J. 1969. *Early retirement: The decision and the experience.* Ann Arbor: Institute for Social Research, University of Michigan.

———. 1978. Trends in planned early retirement. *Gerontologist* 18(1):13–18.

Beck, S.H. 1982. Adjustment to and satisfaction with retirement. *Journal of Gerontology* 37(5):616–624.

———. 1984. Retirement preparation programs: Differentials in opportunity and use. *Journal of Gerontology* 39:596–602.

Benet, S. 1971. Why they live to be 100, or even older, in Abkhasia. *New York Times Magazine,* December 26.

Biesele, M., and Howell, N. 1981. The old people give you life: Aging among !Kung hunter-gatherers. In P.T. Amoss and S. Harrell (eds.), *Other ways of growing old: Anthropological perspectives.* Stanford, Calif.: Stanford University Press.

Bixby, L. 1976. Retirement patterns in the United States: Research and policy interaction. *Social Security Bulletin* 39(8):3–19.

Boaz, R.F. 1987. Work as a response to low and decreasing real income during retirement. *Research on Aging* 9(3):428–440.

Bowen, W., and Finegan, T. 1969. *The economics of labor force participation.* Princeton, N.J.: Princeton University Press.

Butler, R. 1975. *Why survive? Being old in America.* New York: Harper and Row.

Calhoun, R. 1978. *In search of the new old.* New York: Elsevier Scientific Publishing Company, Inc.

Campbell, S. 1979. Delayed mandatory retirement and the working woman. *Gerontologist* 19(3):257–263.

Campione, W.A. 1987. The married woman's retirement decision: A methodological comparison. *Journal of Gerontology* 42(4):381–386.

———. 1988. Predicting participation in retirement preparation programs. *Journal of Gerontology* 43(3):S91–95.

Cohen, W. 1957. *Retirement policies under Social Security.* Berkeley: University of California Press.

Collins, G. 1987. Wanted: Child-care workers, age 55 and up. *The New York Times* December 15:1,8.

Donahue, W., Orbach, H., and Pollak, O. 1960. Retirement: The emerging pattern. In C. Tibbitts (ed.), *Handbook of social gerontology.* Chicago: University of Chicago Press.

Dorfman, L.T., and Moffett, M.M. 1987. Retirement satisfaction in married and widowed rural women. *Gerontologist* 27(2):215–221.

Drucker, P. 1971. What can we learn from Japanese management? *Harvard Business Review* 49:110–122.

Ekerdt, D.J., Vinick, B.H., and Bossé, R. 1989. Orderly endings: Do men know when they will retire? *Journal of Gerontology* 44(1):528–535.

Ellison, D. 1968. Work, retirement and the sick role. *Gerontologist* 8:189–192.

Evans, L., Ekerdt, D.J., and Bosse, R. 1985. Proximity to retirement and anticipatory involvement: Findings from the Normative Aging Study. *Journal of Gerontology* 40(3):368–374.

Fillenbaum, G.G., George. L.K., and Palmore, E.B. 1985. Determinants and consequences of retirement among men of different races and economic levels. *Journal of Gerontology* 40(1):85–94.

Friedmann, E., and Havighurst, R. 1954. *The meaning of work and retirement.* Chicago: University of Chicago Press.

Gibson, R.C. 1987. Reconceptualizing retirement for black Americans. *Gerontologist* 27(6):691–698.

Glamser, F.D. 1981. The impact of preretirement programs on the retirement experience. *Journal of Gerontology* 36(2):244–250.

Goldberg, D. 1978. Mandatory retirement and the older worker. *Aging and work* 1:264–267.

Holmes, L. 1972. The role and status of the aged in changing Samoa. In D. Cowgill and L. Holmes (eds.), *Aging and modernization.* Englewood Cliffs, N.J.: Prentice-Hall.

Israel, J. 1971. *Alienation: From Marx to modern sociology.* Boston: Allyn and Bacon, Inc.

Kart, C. 1981. Attribution (and misattribution) of symptoms among the elderly. In M. Haug (ed.), *Elderly patients and their doctors.* New York: Springer Publishing Co.

Kasschau, P. 1976. Perceived age discrimination in a sample of aerospace employees. *Gerontologist* 18:166–173.

Kingson, E. 1981. Involuntary early retirement. *Journal of the Institute for Socioeconomic Studies* 6(3):27–39.

Kroeger, N. 1981. Women in retirement: Good housekeeping revisited. Paper presented at annual meeting of the Gerontological Society of America, Toronto, Canada.

Long, C.D. 1958. *The labor force under changing conditions of income and employment.* Princeton, N.J.: Princeton University Press.

Mechanic, D. 1968. *Medical sociology.* Glencoe, Ill.: The Free Press.

Miller, S. 1965. The social dilemmas of the aging leisure participant. In A. Rose and W. Peterson (eds.), *Older people and their social world.* Philadelphia: F.A. Davis Company.

Mutran, E., and Reitzes, D.C. 1981. Retirement, identity and well-being: Realignment of role relationships. *Journal of Gerontology* 36(6):733–740.

Palmore, E. 1975. *The honorable elders.* Durham, N.C.: Duke University Press.

Parnes, H.S., Adams, A.V., Andrisani, P.J., Kohen, A.I., and Nestel, G. 1975. *The preretirement years, Vol. 4. A longitudinal study of the labor market experience of men.* U.S. Department of Labor, Manpower Research and Development Monograph No. 15. Washington, D.C.: U.S. Government Printing Office.

Patton, C. 1977. Early retirement in academia: Making the decision. *Gerontologist* 17(4):347–354.

Quinn, J. 1975. *The microeconomics of early retirement: A cross-sectional view.* Social Security Administration Report. Washington, D.C.: USGPO.

Reno, V. 1976. *Reaching retirement age.* Social Security Administration Report No. 47. Washington, D.C.: USGPO.

Riley, M.W., and Foner, A. 1968. *Aging and society. Vol. One: An inventory of research findings.* New York: Russell Sage Foundation.

Schnore, M.M., and Kirkland, J.B. 1981. Sex differences in adjustment to retirement. Paper presented at joint meetings of the Canadian Association of Gerontology and the Gerontological Society of America, Toronto, Canada.

Schulz, J. 1976. *The economics of aging.* Belmont, Calif.: Wadsworth Publishing Co., Inc.

Schwab, K. 1974. Early labor force withdrawal of men: Participants and nonparticipants aged 58–63. *Social Security Bulletin* 37(8):24–38.

Select Committee on Aging, U.S. Senate. 1981. *The early retirement myth: Why men retire before age 62.* Washington, D.C.: U.S. Government Printing Office.

Shanas, E. 1968. The meaning of work. In E. Shanas, P. Townsend, D. Wedderburn, H. Friis, P. Milhhøj, and J. Stehouver (eds.), *Old people in three industrial societies.* New York: Atherton Press.

Sheldon, H. 1958. *The older population of the United States.* New York: John Wiley and Sons, Inc.

Sherman, C. 1974. Labor force status of non-married women on the threshold of retirement. *Social Security Bulletin* 37(9):3–15.

Simpson, I., Back, K, and McKinney, J. 1966. Orientation toward work and retirement, and self-evaluation in retirement. In I. Simpson and J. McKinney (eds.), *Social aspects of aging.* Durham, N.C.: Duke University Press.

Slavick, F. 1966. *Compulsory and flexible retirement in the American economy.* Ithaca, N.Y.: Cornell University Press.

Snow, R., and Havighurst, R. 1977. Life-style types and patterns of retirement of educators. *Gerontologist* 17(6):545–552.

Streib, G., and Schneider, C.J. 1971. *Retirement in American society.* Ithaca, N.Y.: Cornell University Press.

Terkel, S. 1972. *Working: People talk about what they do all day and how they feel about what they do.* New York: Random House, Inc.

Thompson, G. 1973. Work versus leisure roles: An investigation of moral among employed and retired men. *Journal of Gerontology* 28:339–344.

Uhlenberg, P. 1979. Older women: The growing challenge to design constructive roles. *Gerontologist* 19(3):236–241.

U.S. National Center for Health Statistics. 1964. *Health survey procedure.* Washington, D.C.: U.S. Government Printing Office.

U.S. Senate Special Committee on Aging. 1985. *Aging America: Trends and projections, 1985–86 edition.* Washington, D.C.: U.S. Government Printing Office.

Williams, R., and Wirths, C. 1965. *Lives through the years.* New York: Atherton Press.

Yankelovich, D. 1974. The meaning of work. In J. Rosow (ed.). *The worker and job.* Englewood Cliffs, N.J.: Prentice-Hall.

CHAPTER 13

THE POLITICS OF AGING

This chapter takes the view that in recent years age issues have become a substantial element in U.S. politics. Demographic trends already in place suggest that many future political issues are likely to be centered on questions of age. Do old people stick together in their voting attitudes and behavior? Will long-standing bases of political conflict such as race and social class be superseded by questions of age? Have old people become a favored political constituency in the United States? What is the future of the political economy of aging? These important questions have only recently become substantive concerns for gerontologists. Some of these questions have fragmentary and incomplete answers; on others, a growing body of literature is emerging.

Before beginning a discussion of these questions, and the answers emerging in the gerontological literature, it seems useful to remind readers of our discussion in Chapter 2 of the age/period/cohort problem. Interpretation of the political attitudes and behavior of older people involves the ability to understand and elicit the effects of the distinct perspectives represented by these three concepts (Hudson and Binstock 1976). First, we must consider the possibility that the political attitudes and behavior of older persons can be explained by developmental patterns inherent in the processes of human aging. This consideration describes what we could call the *age effect*.

Second, we must look at the possibility that changes in the political attitudes and behaviors of older people simply mirror the impact of historical or period effects on an entire population. If older people have become more conservative over a period of time, perhaps this tendency can be explained by showing that *all* age groups have become more conservative over the time period examined (Hudson and Binstock 1976). This describes the *period effect*.

The third perspective takes into account the possibility that the political attitudes and behaviors of older people result from the shared experiences and perceptions of a particular older generation. This perspective describes the *cohort effect*.

Only recently has gerontological research used quantitative techniques to distinguish among these three analytical perspectives effectively. Much of the work discussed in this chapter overlooks this important methodological and conceptual problem. Nevertheless, we must not be insensitive to these issues as we begin with a discussion of the relationship between political participation and age.

POLITICAL PARTICIPATION AND AGE
Voting Behavior

A basic indicator of participation in the political process is voting behavior. A variety of factors affect an individual's voting participation (Cutler and Schmidhauser 1975). Historically, it seems that men were more likely to vote than were women at all ages and that those with more education voted more frequently than those with low levels of education did.

Table 13-1 presents data on voting behavior by age, race, sex, region, employment status, and education for the United States in the 1984 Presidential election. Race, employment status, education, and age seem the most important contributors to variation in voting behavior in 1984. Whites were only slightly more likely to vote than blacks (61.4 percent versus 55.8 percent), and twice as likely to vote as individuals of Spanish origin (32.6 percent). The employed were about 40 percent more likely to vote than the unemployed (61.6 percent versus 44.0 percent), although, interestingly, the proportion of those reporting they voted among the employed was only slightly greater than the proportion voting among those unemployed so long that they are considered to be out of the labor force. College graduates report voting at a higher rate in the 1984 Presidential election than any other group (79.1 percent).

The proportion of individuals reporting they voted in the 1984 election is lowest in the youngest age group. Voter participation increases with successive age levels until old age, when a slight decline from previous levels appears. This pattern seems consistent with generalizations about the relationship between chronological age and voting behavior made by Milbrath in the mid-1960s.

Milbrath (1965) identified three factors that may help explain the relationship between age and voting exhibited in Table 13-1. First, younger people are typically not as well integrated into the communities in which they reside as are mature and older adults. Those who own homes, have families, enroll children in the local schools, and pay local taxes may be more affected by

TABLE 13-1   Voting-Age Population, and Percentage Reporting Registered and Voted, 1984 Presidential Election

Characteristic	Voting-Age Population (Mil)	Percentage Reporting They Registered	Percentage Reporting They Voted
Total	170.0	68.3	59.9
White	146.8	69.6	61.4
Black	18.4	66.3	55.8
Spanish Origin	9.5	40.1	32.6
Male	80.3	67.3	59.0
Female	89.6	69.3	60.8
Northeast	36.9	66.6	59.7
Midwest	42.1	74.6	65.7
South	57.6	66.9	56.8
West	33.4	64.7	58.5
18–20 years	11.2	47.0	36.7
21–24 years	16.7	58.3	43.5
25–34 years	40.3	63.3	54.5
35–44 years	30.7	70.9	63.5
45–64 years	44.3	76.6	69.8
65 years and over	26.7	76.9	67.7
Employed	104.2	69.4	61.6
Unemployed	7.4	54.3	44.0
Not in labor force	58.4	68.1	58.9
8 years or less of school	20.6	53.4	42.9
1–3 years high school	22.1	54.9	44.4
4 years high school	67.8	66.4	58.7
1–3 years college	30.9	74.4	67.5
4 years or more of college	28.6	83.8	79.1

Source: U.S. Bureau of The Census, 1985. *Statistical Abstract of the U.S., 1986* (106th ed.), Table 434, p. 256. Washington, D.C.

political issues (both local and national) and thus are more likely to vote. Second, as children grow up, become more independent, and leave home, mature and older adults may have more available leisure time to become active in the political process. Finally, although most older people are in good health with little activity limitation, age does bring an increased risk of deterioration in mental and physical health. The greater likelihood of experiencing a health impairment later in the life cycle may be associated with reduced participation in a variety of forms of social behavior, including the political process.

Active Participation in Politics

Voting is a relatively passive form of political participation, occurring infrequently and requiring minimal effort on the part of an individual. It is a far cry from active involvement in the political process through community or campaign activity. Two often cited investigations of older people's political involvement have been carried out by Verba and Nie (1972) and Nie, Verba and Kim (1974). In general, these authors find (1) that the level of older people's participation in the political process is higher than the population average and (2) that when variation in socioeconomic status is controlled for, older people show even higher participation scores. In fact, when this variation is controlled for, these authors find the peak period of political activity to occur in the sixth decade of life.

Verba and Nie have created a political participation typology and looked to the distribution of those aged sixty-five and over across the six types in this categorization schema. The six types are as follows:

1. Inactives: no political activity
2. Voting specialists: regular voters
3. Parochial participants: those who make occasional contact with a public official
4. Communalists: those working actively in community organizations
5. Campaigners: those working actively around campaigns, including working for a party or a candidate and contributing money
6. Complete activists: those highly involved in each of the preceding activities

The aged are overrepresented among the inactives, the voting specialists, and parochial participants. They are moderately underrepresented among the communalists and the campaigners and highly underrepresented as complete activists. Data reported by Nie, Verba, and Kim (1974) provide some support in a cross-national context for the findings presented above.

Glenn and Grimes (1968) suggest that older people turn to political activity because they have few other absorbing interests or activities. From the point of view of these authors, older people's involvement in politics may have more to do with attempting to achieve personal fulfillment than with achieving some instrumental political end. Schmidhauser (1968) has provided support for such a hypothesis by showing that age brings an increase in interest in politics while at the same time bringing an increase in cynicism about the ability of individual political action to have impact on the broader political process.

Approximately 1,800 adult Americans aged eighteen years and older were interviewed by the National Opinion Research Center (NORC) for the 1982 General Social Survey. Respondents were asked to assess their level of interest in government and public affairs and how much confidence they had in the executive branch of the federal government. For purposes of presentation here, respondents were divided into three approximately equal-sized age groups: eighteen to thirty-two years; thirty-three to fifty-four years; and fifty-five years and older. In general, older people pay more attention to government and public affairs than do the young; 43.1 percent of those aged fifty-five and older compared with 23.5 percent of those aged eighteen to thirty-two answered that they followed what was going on in government most of the time. Only 22 percent of the older respondents reported having a great deal of confidence in the executive branch of the federal government; 13.4 percent of the younger adults and 18.7 percent of the middle-aged reported similarly. Among the older respondents, there is no support for Schmidhauser's hypothesis mentioned above. In fact, 24.2 percent of those with the most interest in government affairs had a great deal of confidence in the executive branch; only 14.8 percent of those with the least interest in government had a great deal of confidence in the executive branch.

Political Leadership

Perhaps the most intense form of political participation involves occupying an office or holding a position of political leadership. It is widely believed that persons in late middle and old age disproportionately occupy positions of leadership in the United States and other advanced industrial nations. The visibility of national political leaders such as former President Reagan and former House Majority Leader "Tip" O'Neill provides support for these beliefs. In addition, the work of Lehman (1953) and Schlesinger (1966) shows that in a wide variety of political contexts—U.S. presidential candidates, Presidents, senators, U.S. representatives, governors, Supreme Court justices, U.S. ambassadors, cabinet members—positions of political leadership are held by relatively old persons. In the ninety-fourth Congress (1975), 39 percent (39/100) of the senators and 21 percent of the representatives (91/435) were sixty years of age or over. Ten years later, the ninety-ninth Congress showed fewer aged members with thirty-one senators and seventy-eight representatives aged sixty years of age or older.

Recently, Lammers and Nyomarkay (1980) have shown a changing age pattern among the appointees to cabinet level positions in five advanced industrial nations, including the United States. These authors find a growing concentration of middle-aged cabinet members, with aging populations increasingly underrepresented in the political leadership in these five nations. Table 13-2 shows the representation of the sixty-five and over group in the cabinets of Canada, France, the United Kingdom, Germany, and the United States over the last one hundred years or so. Through the 1950s, the general pattern was clearly toward overrepresentation. Only in France and the United States were the aged slightly underrepresented in cabinet positions in the late nineteenth century. By the 1960s (and through the 1970s), a significant and

TABLE 13-2 Representation: Individuals 65 Years of Age or Older in Total Population and in Cabinets (in percentages)

Year	Canada Population 65+	Canada Cabinet Members	Canada Difference	France Population 65+	France Cabinet Members	France Difference
1870s	4	6	+2	7	19	+12
1880s	4	16	+12	8	5	−3
1890s	5	16	+11	8	5	−3
1900s	5	14	+9	8	9	+1
1910s	5	19	+14	9	14	+5
1920s	5	13	+8	9	11	+2
1930s	5	12	+7	10	13	+3
1940s	5	15	+10	11	7	−4
1950s	8	16	+8	11	7	−4
1960s	8	8	0	12	7	−5
1970s	8	1	−7	13	6	−7

Year	United Kingdom Population 65+	United Kingdom Cabinet Members	United Kingdom Difference	Germany Population 65+	Germany Cabinet Members	Germany Difference	United States Population 65+	United States Cabinet Members	United States Difference
1870s	5	17	+12				3	8	+5
1880s	5	19	+14				4	12	+8
1890s	5	25	+20				4	0	−4
1900s	5	18	+13				4	17	+13
1910s	5	13	+8				4	10	+6
1920s	7	17	+10	6	6	0	5	28	+23
1930s	8	17	+9	7	7	0	6	30	+24
1940s	10	21	+11				7	22	+15
1950s	11	13	+3	10	15	+5	8	9	+1
1960s	12	4	−8	12	12	0	9	4	−5
1970s	14	3	−11	14	1	−13	10	2	−8

Source: Lammers, W.W. and Nyomarkay, J.L., 1980. The disappearing senior leaders, *Research on Aging* 2(3):329–349. Copyright 1980. Reprinted by permission of Sage Publications, Inc.

uniform shift had taken place: The underrepresentation of the elderly in cabinet positions has been the case in every country.

How do Lammers and Nyomarkay (1980) explain the increasing underrepresentation of the aged in the leadership groups of these advanced industrial societies? One answer is found in greater bureaucratization, which has caused career patterns to become more routinized. This has brought a more focused age structure, resulting in the exclusion of older cabinet appointees and a greater uniformity of ages at time of appointment and departure.

Will the aged suffer as a function of this underrepresentation? As these authors point out, it is certainly possible that more youthful leaders will develop an identification with the problems of the old age, perhaps out of a belief that they constitute a significant voting block. On the other hand, if it is true that "the wearer is the best judge of the shoe," then there are fewer individuals who both directly experience the vagaries of aging and are directly responsible for making public policy that affects the aged.

POLITICAL ORIENTATIONS AND ATTITUDES OF OLDER PERSONS

One indicator of political orientation is party affiliation. Currently, more aged voters are identified with the Democratic party than the Republican party. Nevertheless, among those who identify with the Republican party, the elderly outnumber the young and middle-aged (Campbell and Strate 1981). Some have taken this and other cross-sectional data from past years and mistakenly assumed that aging brings with it a conversion to Republicanism (Crittenden 1962). Glenn and Hefner (1972) have provided definitive evidence on this issue from their longitudinal research. Using data spanning 1945 to 1969, they conclude there is no support for the assumption that Republicanism is a consequence of aging. Rather, their work shows that the positive association between affiliation with the Republican party and aging is a function of cohort or generational differences. Thus, it is possible that early socialization experiences have made many of today's aged cohort Republicans.

Although the disproportionate number of older people compared with the middle aged who say they support the Republican party is a legitimate indicator of conservatism, we still must ask: Are old people conservative? Campbell and Strate (1981) have addressed this question while analyzing data from fourteen American National Election Studies conducted by the Center for Political Studies at the University of Michigan from 1952 to 1980. After using a variety of measures of political attitudes available in these studies, these authors warn against facile generalizations:

> [I]f one takes these results as a whole a general conclusion does emerge. The political orientations of older people are not peculiar. Knowing that someone

is old will not help very much in predicting how conservative he or she is, in most important respects. The elderly are very much in the mainstream of American political opinions. (pp. 590–591)

Recently, Cutler and his colleagues (1980) have studied this issue by examining the relationship between age and attitudes about legalized abortion. They found that, if controls for cohort differences are employed, little variation exists among the different age groups. Looking at changes over time in specific cohorts, they found that people who are now old, when younger, had more conservative views than presently younger cohorts do, but that their attitudes have become more liberalized at the same rate as those of the younger group.

Are old people more conservative? Aging per se does not appear to bring with it a set of conservative positions on prominent political issues. Yet, a different set of self-interests may be associated with age than with youth. In this respect, the answer to the original question (Are old people more conservative?) would seem to be both yes and no!

ARE THE AGED A FAVORED CONSTITUENCY?

The aged have been a favored social welfare constituency in the United States; that is, older persons have done relatively well in the arena of public policy in comparison with other population groups whose needs can be argued to be equally pressing (Hudson 1978). A 1979 publication of the Select Committee on Aging of the U.S. House of Representatives lists forty-eight federal programs benefiting the elderly. These are shown in Table 13-3. The program categories represented include employment and volunteer, health care, housing, income maintenance, social service programs, training and research programs, and transportation. Virtually every agency in the executive branch and many independent agencies are represented.

Robert Hudson of Brandeis University distinguishes between "breakthrough" and "constituency-building" policy enactments that may bring favored status upon a special interest group. *Breakthrough* policies consist of those pieces of legislation that involve the federal government in providing or guaranteeing some fundamental benefit. *Constituency-building* policies are those that recognize that different groups have common interests and give these interest groups a voice in the making of public policy. The aged have been the principal beneficiaries and most functional constituency in the federal government's involvement in breakthrough legislation to ensure health-care financing for high-risk populations (Medicare and Medicaid) and to guarantee minimum income for the impoverished (for example, Supplemental Security Income; SSI) (Hudson 1978).

Still, several recent commentators have described the differential success of federal intervention on behalf of the elderly. Kutza (1981) points out that

---

TABLE 13-3   Federal Programs Benefiting the Elderly, by Category

---

Employment and Volunteer

    Age Discrimination in Employment
    Community Based Employment and Training Programs
    Community Service Employment for Older Americans
    Employment Programs for Special Groups
    Foster Grandparent Program
    Retired Senior Volunteer Program (RSVP)
    Senior Companion Program
    Service Corps of Retired Executives (SCORE)
    Volunteers in Service to America (VISTA)

Health Care

    Health Resources Development Construction and Modernization of Facilities (Hill Burton Program)
    Community Mental Health Centers
    Construction of Nursing Homes and Intermediate Care Facilities
    Grants to States for Medical Assistance Programs (Medicaid)
    Program of Health Insurance for the Aged and Disabled (Medicare)
    Veterans Domiciliary Care Program
    Veterans Nursing Home Care Program

Housing

    Housing for the Elderly (Sec. 202)
    Low and Moderate Income Housing (Sec. 8)
    Mortgage Insurance on Rental Housing for the Elderly (Sec. 231)
    Rural Rental Housing Loans (Sec. 515)
    Community Development
    Low Rent Public Housing
    Rural Home Repair Program (Sec. 504)
    Rural Rental Assistance (Sec. 521)

Income Maintenance

    Civil Service Retirement
    Food Stamp Program
    Old Age Survivors Insurance Program (Social Security)
    Railroad Retirement Program
    Supplemental Security Income Program
    Veterans Pension Program

Social Service Programs

    Crime Prevention (LEAA)
    Education Opportunities for Older People
    Legal Services Corporation
    Multipurpose Senior Center Facilities
    Nutrition Programs
    Revenue Sharing
    Senior Opportunities and Services
    Social Services for Low Income Persons and Public Assistance Recipients (Title XX)
    State and Community Social Service Programs (Title III)

TABLE 13-3 (continued)

Training and Research Programs

Model Projects
Multi-Disciplinary Centers of Gerontology
Personnel Training (Title IV—Older Americans Act)
Research and Demonstration Program (Title IV—Older Americans Act)
Research on Aging Process and Health Problems

Transportation

Capital Assistance Grants for Use by Public Agencies
Capital Assistance Grants for Use by Private Non-Profit Groups
Reduced Fares
Capital and Operating Assistance Grants

Source: Select Committee on Aging, U.S. House of Representatives, 1979. *Federal Responsibility to the Elderly.* Washington, D.C.: U.S. Government Printing Office.

minority older persons and older women have not shared in the gains experienced by other elderly in this recent period of concentrated assistance provided to older people. She describes this as follows:

> Since 1969, elderly white women have made remarkable gains; their poverty rate has dropped to 14.4 (compared to 8.3 for elderly white males). Elderly black women cut their rate nearly in half, moving from 77 percent in 1969 to 41.2 percent in 1977. Yet, that two out of every five elderly black women live below the poverty level today points up the serious differential impact our federal income-support programs have had in the past ten years. While great progress has been made in providing a more adequate income standard for most older retired persons, several subgroups within the population—most especially nonwhites and women—remain seriously disadvantaged. (E.A. Kutza, *The Benefits of Old Age,* p. 85. Chicago: University of Chicago Press, 1981. © 1981 by The University of Chicago Press.)

Beth Hess (1983) has identified what she describes as a gerontological "gender gap" in the application of federal programs to the elderly. Three areas where older women are especially disadvantaged are income, health, and housing. As she reports, because of their lower incomes, increasing frailty, and singlehood, old women are the prime market for subsidized rental housing. During the administration of President Reagan, the major federal programs for the construction of such facilities—sections 8 and 202—have lost funding. In addition, eligibility has been limited and the share paid by renters has been increased. Hess argues that "public programs have been shaped by assumptions based on the life experience of men. . . . Yet, not only are the real problems of old age disproportionately experienced by women, but it is women who are increasingly expected to bear the brunt of dealing with these problems."

Despite this growing recognition of the differential impact of public policy efforts for the elderly, there is currently considerable debate about the economic costs of this favored status for the elderly. This may be part of a resistance to social welfare expenditures in general. Some writers see the costs of programs for the elderly as the dominant factor shaping federal spending and taxing decisions, and one analyst characterizes the cost of an aging America as having the potential to "bust the U.S. budget" (Samuelson 1978). This characterization deserves careful scrutiny.

According to Robert Samuelson (1978), spending for the elderly amounted to about one-fifth of the federal budget in 1969; by 1979, this figure had increased to approximately one-third of the federal budget. Almost 80 percent of federal spending for the elderly in 1979 was through the Social Security and Medicare programs. Samuelson believes there will be continued pressure on the federal budget in coming years. By 1984, federal outlays for Social Security and Medicare alone had more than doubled from 1979 and accounted for more than the entire outlay of federal spending for the elderly in that year. As the size of the elderly population increases, the government must raise taxes and reduce funding for other programs or run increasingly larger deficits. With current federal deficits in the vicinity of $150 billion, a political scenario including sharply higher taxes and further federal deficit spending does not seem to be a likely one at this time. Fears about recurring economic recession, the continued fight against inflation, energy costs, and continued increases in defense spending suggest an upcoming age of scarcity for education, urban, and social welfare constituencies. The specter of these needy and powerful political interest groups battling for scarce federal dollars is not inviting, but it is a scenario that many policy analysts consider will become a reality.

Not everyone ascribes to the age of scarcity scenario, however. Jack Ossofsky (1978), Executive Director of the National Council on the Aging, takes exception to Samuelson's characterization of the federal budget as ready to bust and to his calculations of expenditures on the aging in the federal budget. For example, Ossofsky reminds us that the Social Security program provides income to many millions of younger men, women, and children as part of its dependents, survivors, and disability program. Seven million people alone received survivor benefits in 1986 under Social Security. Today, about 40 percent of Social Security benefits go to nonretirees (Hardy 1987). In addition, we must remember that workers "buy in" to Social Security (as do employers): To include employee contributions when computing government expenditures on behalf of the aged makes little sense. Beyond simply confusing matters, it creates the impression that Social Security is just another government welfare program, rather than a return of money put aside during the course of a person's working years. This holds true as well for the Federal Civil Service Retirement System; redistributed employee contributions should not be counted as government expenditures. Finally, as Ossofsky points out, playing hocus pocus with the federal budget figures creates the impression that the elderly are receiving lavish treatment from the federal government. This is clearly not the case; 12.4 percent of American aged have incomes below the poverty level (1986 figure), and the proportion in near poverty is substantial as well.

Robert Butler (1978) takes a different tack. He suggests that the discussion over expenditures in the federal budget for the elderly is misdirected—a case of blaming the victims. Butler makes three important points:

1. The need for all those dollars in retirement systems might be lessened somewhat if we did not pressure people to leave the work force while they are still able and willing to continue working. If people were free to continue working after age sixty-five or seventy—and by law, this is now the case— they could continue to contribute to retirement systems, and the budget would become less menacing.

2. A considerable proportion of the federal budget reflects the existence of illness and disability in the aged population. What if we could identify the biomedical and socioenvironmental factors that produce illness and disability and prompt people to retire? If these "illness factors" could be minimized in any way it would reduce expenditures made through the Medicare and Medicaid programs.

3. Government expenditures for health-care services have increased dramatically in recent years. Nevertheless, the elderly now pay as much out of pocket for health care as they did before Medicare. To what extent is the increasing cost of health care to be attributed to the elderly? To what extent should it be attributed to the providers of health-care services?

What are the political consequences of this debate over federal expenditures for the elderly? Will proposed funding for programs for the aged face opposition in the future? Can the aged mobilize political pressure to serve their interests?

ARE THE ELDERLY A POLITICAL FORCE?

One commonly held image of the aged is as a political force capable of playing interest group politics. Political scientist Robert Binstock, former president of the Gerontological Society of America, believes this image to be inaccurate, though nurtured by several aging-based membership organizations:

There is little reason to believe that a phenomenon termed "senior power" will significantly increase the proportion of the budget devoted to the aging, or redirect that portion of the budget toward solving the problems of the severely disadvantaged. Whatever senior power exists is held by organizations that cannot swing decisive voting blocs. (Binstock, R.H. 1978. Federal policy toward the aging—its inadequacies and its politics. *National Journal*, November 11, 1978.)

Evidence of this may have been present in the 1976 Carter campaign for the presidency. The "seniors desk" had the lowest budget and fewest paid personnel among the eleven desks established by the Democratic Presidential Campaign Committee (Binstock 1978).

One reason the image of senior power persists lies in the belief that the elderly are a homogeneous group and thus a homogeneous political constituency. This is just not the case. The elderly are as heterogeneous politically as they are socially or economically. Binstock argues most older voters do not primarily identify themselves, and hence their self-interest, in terms of aging. When a person reaches age sixty-five, retires, or is widowed, he or she does not suddenly lose all prior self-identities; self-interest is still derived from race, education, religion, community ties, and so on.

Not everyone sees senior power as illusory. Pratt (1976) notes the elderly have come to expect some degree of income security as well as adequate health care. Theirs may be a revolution of rising expectations. Pratt cites the 1971 White House Conference on Aging as the watershed for old-age political influence. Through the Conference, he argues, national groups such as the National Retired Teachers Association (NRTA), the American Association of Retired Persons (AARP), and the National Council of Senior Citizens (NCSC) developed the political acumen necessary for effecting legislation that benefits the aged. Pratt credits the NCSC with helping to formulate and pass the Social Security Amendments of 1972. These amendments pegged increases in Social Security benefits to the rate of inflation and replaced welfare programs for the aged, blind, and disabled with SSI.

As indicated above, Pratt has described the 1971 White House Conference on Aging as a watershed for old-age political influence. The 1981 conference, however, seems to have been less successful. The year prior to the conference brought a change in president and a different political party to power. Organizational aspects of the conference were changed at the last minute—the result, some argued, of Reagan administration concerns that the conference, organized under a Democratic administration, would produce recommendations unacceptable to the new President.

Ultimately, 600 or so recommendations from fourteen different issue committees were approved by the conference participants. Prioritizing these recommendations would seem an impossible task. Recently, the Leadership Council of Aging Organizations, made up of representatives from a variety of organizations working on behalf of the elderly, prepared an agenda prioritizing eight of these issues. These were as follows:

1. Safeguard current eligibility conditions, retirement ages, and benefit levels in Social Security.

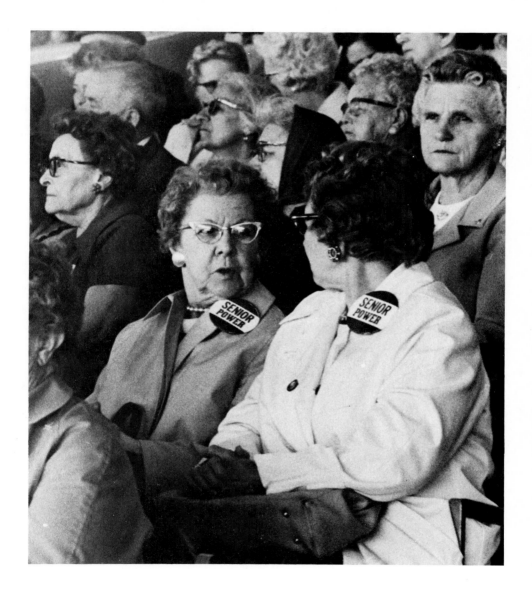

2. Broaden opportunities for older workers to remain active voluntarily in the labor force.

3. Assure older people an income sufficient to maintain a minimum level of dignity and comfort.

4. Enact a comprehensive national health plan for all Americans.

5. Take interim steps to improve health care for older persons.

6. Make available no fewer than 200,000 units of publicly financed housing for the elderly each year during the decade.

7. Set up comprehensive service delivery systems for older people at the community level in the 1980s.

8. Strengthen the federal commitment to gerontological research, education, and training.

Can an old-age political movement become institutionalized? According to Achenbaum (1983), such a "gray lobby" would differ from other interest groups in at least two important ways. First, there are ideological and political schisms within and among the organizations that purport to represent and work for the elderly. Second, the gray lobby is the only interest group to which every American can hope to aspire. Hence, it is especially important for leaders of these organizational entities to weigh the future ramifications of current policy decisions. What looks good in the short run may have devastating implications for the elderly of the next century.

Hudson (1987) sees great potential surrounding the organization of a political agenda "of and for the able elderly." Presumably, the *able elderly* are those not frail, in poverty or dependent; the concept captures a growing number of older people who are integrated, vigorous, affluent, and well. They constitute a political and economic generation "caught between the demands of a frailer generation ahead of it and the pressures of a command generation behind it" (p. 406). Still, as Hudson correctly notes, formalizing the concept of the able elderly and organizing a political agenda around this group creates potential problems for the less able old as well as for those who may properly be described as able. For example, in the area of employment, the concept of an able elderly highlights the contradiction between the desires to eliminate mandatory retirement rules (and thus allow older workers to continue in place) and to take early retirement. In areas such as income support and medical care, the improved education and economic status associated with being able is likely to bring new proposals for the self- and private-financing of pension and health benefits, as well as the imposition of more means-tested and needs-tested standards to better target services for the elderly.

How willing will current and future aged be to identify themselves as old? The development of a widespread *aging group consciousness* would bring recognition among the elderly of their common interests. Bengtson and Cutler (1976) present evidence that older people who identify themselves as "old" are more liberal, particularly on issues affecting the aged, such as government intervention in inflation and medical care. As Hudson notes, the development of an aging group consciousness may have important consequences beyond helping to create and sustain an old-age political movement. Not the least of these would be a lessening of the stigmatization and isolation of the aged, the maintenance of self-esteem, and a viewing of intergenerational policy proposals in a more favorable light (Wisensale 1988).

THE FUTURE OF OLD AGE POLITICS: AGE VERSUS NEED ENTITLEMENT

Much of the material contained in this text is aimed at describing a new set of realities regarding the aged and aging. In general, we have argued that many of the conditions prevalent in the early part of this century that led us to see old age as a social problem (for example, incapacity, isolation, and poverty) have changed dramatically. Such changes have resulted from collective political action that took the form of governmental legislation to create programs of income maintenance, housing, transportation, health services, social services, and tax benefits.

In creating these programs, which emanated from real concern about the welfare of older people, chronological age was used as a convenient indicator of need. Remember, older people in the United States were seen as a homogeneous population. Even through the 1950s and 1960s, they were described as poor and lacking in access to health services and the like. As Neugarten (1982) indicates, programs based on age eligibility did catch a large proportion of persons in need. The situation is different today, however. The elderly are currently described as a heterogeneous group, in many respects indistinguishable from the general population. For example, the proportion of those aged sixty-five years and over with incomes below the poverty line is approximately the same as the proportion of the total population with incomes below the poverty line. Further, as we have already indicated, there are subpopulations of the aged that have been differentially advantaged by governmental programs, and other groups such as minority elderly and older women who remain relatively disadvantaged despite these programs.

Rather than emphasizing the special disadvantages of minority elderly and older women, Nelson (1982) examines the relationship between social class and public policy for the elderly. Essentially, he argues that governmental programs for the aged act to perpetuate the existence of socioeconomic differences among the elderly that existed prior to old age. According to Nelson, three classes of elderly beneficiaries of governmental initiatives can be identified: (1) the marginal elderly; (2) the downwardly mobile elderly; and (3) the integrated elderly. Each class of elderly receives a different level of support that in total serves to sustain the social class inequalities that were present prior to the experience of old age. Let us briefly describe these three classes of elderly and exemplify how government provides different levels of support for the different classes.

Marginal Elderly. The marginal elderly are characterized by absolute need and poverty. For most of these individuals, poverty in old age is a continuation of a life of poverty. They are more likely to be living alone, female, minority, and old-old. Their work careers were in unskilled, semiskilled, or domestic labor that has been transient or interrupted during the adult years. Many such jobs were not covered by Social Security or other pension programs. These individuals represent the truly needy.

Downwardly Mobile Elderly. This class of elderly corresponds most closely to those who were considered middle-class or lower-middle class prior to old age. The downwardly mobile elderly experience need as a sense of relative deprivation. They are trying to maintain a preretirement life-style on more limited resources. Some are at risk of falling into poverty. They may prevent this by using available sources of public support.

Integrated Elderly. These are individuals who are presumed to be continuing a middle- and upper middle-class life-style. The integrated elderly are likely to be able to do this by marshalling personal and private resources and public support. Because these individuals are able to maintain their socioeconomic status, including social values, roles, and group and community memberships, we refer to them as the socially integrated elderly.

How does this three-tiered approach to the elderly affect government support for income-transfer programs? The central income-transfer program for the marginal elderly is SSI. As we have already noted, eligibility is determined by meeting certain income and assets standards. The program establishes a common minimum income benefit for the approximately 1.5 million marginal or poor elderly (May 1987 figure). Some states provide an additional supplement to the federal benefit. The average monthly amount (May 1987) of combined federal and state SSI payments for the aged was a high of $301.48 in California and a low of $99.40 in Maine. Still, many who are eligible for SSI do not receive it, and many who are receiving it are still living below the poverty level. It seems reasonable to conclude, as Nelson (1982) does, that the marginal elderly are guaranteed the most meager subsistence under the SSI income-transfer program.

The second tier of income support for the elderly is Social Security. Most of the work force is covered by this program, which is underwritten by the collected contributions of workers and their employers. Average monthly benefit amounts payable in May 1987 were $490.63 for retired workers and $487.65 for disabled workers. The downwardly mobile elderly includes most recipients of Social Security who were average wage earners. This group has a special reliance on the Social Security check plus accumulated private savings. For most of these individuals, the Social Security check is a guarantee against falling into near or absolute poverty.

The third tier of income support programs for the elderly includes those that are directed at the integrated elderly. Many of the integrated elderly receive Social Security; they are also recipients of governmentally supported public (railroad retirement, civil service, state and local governments) and private pensions and cash benefits from government-supported private savings plans (annuities, individual retirement accounts, and Keough plans) and favorable tax policies. The latter includes additional income tax exemptions for those sixty-five years and over and property tax reductions. These tax preferences, in conjunction with private and public pension supplements to Social Security, act to maintain the socioeconomic position of the higher income elderly.

The federal government's cost of maintaining the integrated elderly at a life-style consistent with that prior to retirement is staggering in comparison with the costs, for example, of maintaining the marginal elderly. In fiscal 1979, federal expenditures for all elderly on SSI amounted to less than $2.0 billion. Robert Ball (1978) estimates that in 1978 approved private pension plans were subsidized by the federal government at five times this figure, or $10 billion, the amount of taxes that would have been paid if tax exemptions had not been provided for private pension contributions. Comparable examples of higher governmental expenditures and subsidies for the elderly least in need are also available in the areas of health care and social services.

As Nelson's use of the term *integrated elderly* implies, the higher income elderly are more likely to be socially integrated into the broader society than other classes of elderly are. Yet, as we have already noted, age entitlement programs cause a considerable proportion of governmental resources to be directed at those elderly least in need. Is this fair? Shouldn't we redistribute public policy benefits on the basis of need?

The obvious answers seem *no*, it is not fair, and *yes*, we should redistribute benefits on the basis of need. Still, we have to decide who is needy. Careful readers of the analysis presented above might have us redistribute benefits to just the marginal elderly or some combination of the marginal and downwardly mobile elderly. One problem with such a reform is that it continues to employ age as a basic organizing principle in the development of policies and programs. After all, the elderly do not have a monopoly on need in the United States. As Elizabeth Kutza (1981) describes it, "No problem occurs in old age that does not occur also in other age groups, whether it be poverty, mental or physical disability, isolation, or malnutrition." Further, she quotes from a recent Administration on Aging study in which researchers were struck not by the differences among the young, the middle-aged, and the old but by the similarities: "[W]hen the picture is examined as a whole, the most striking aspect is how much alike were the values placed on quality of life factors regardless of age and how relatively little people's needs seem to change over time."

Reorganizing the distribution of federal policy benefits on the basis of need rather than age is an effort fraught with political liability. Benefits to the aged have been remarkably popular, especially those aimed at the downwardly mobile and integrated elderly. In part, this may result from the high value placed on independence by the elderly and their family members. It also may result from an understanding that the aged are a unique group—the one minority group to which we all anticipate belonging!

It seems likely that political support for the basic needs of the elderly will continue to be strong (Crystal 1982). In the current political environment, however, federal budgets are under constant pressure. As Crystal (1982) describes: "[I]f human services are to be cut, it is poor policy to slash benefits for the needy aged and spare those aiding mostly the middle-class and higher-income elderly."

Moving forward with entitlement programs based solely on need may reduce some pressure on the federal budget. Such a policy shift may also, in effect, "mainstream" the elderly. Continued insistence that the federal government underwrite the "special and unique needs" of the elderly tends to set up a tension between older persons and the rest of society (Etzioni 1976). Such tension may be extraordinarily dysfunctional for the elderly. Etzioni (1976) suggests that politically organized older Americans would be better served by supporting policies and social services needed by or favorable to the aged in the context of supporting more universalistic approaches. This may ultimately enhance how the rest of society views older people. More importantly, it may enhance how the elderly view themselves.

SUMMARY

Age-related issues have become a substantial element in U.S. politics, and the demographics of aging suggest that this trend will continue. Understanding the relevant questions and answers emerging from research into the politics of aging requires a sensitivity to the methodological and conceptual issues inherent in the age/period/cohort problem.

In recent elections the percentage of people reporting they voted has been lowest in the youngest age groups. With aging, there is an increase in voting until old age when a slight decline from previous levels appears. Factors contributing to this pattern include the (1) increased social integration of mature and older adults, (2) increased leisure time available to adults, and (3) the greater likelihood of the elderly experiencing a health impairment.

The aged are actively involved in partisan politics. They seem more likely than the young to make occasional contact with a public official. Many older people are also involved in working for community organizations and in political campaigns. Some suggest that older people's involvement in politics has more to do with their attempting to remain active and fulfilled than with a desire to achieve particular political goals.

The general impression many people have is that the elderly are overrepresented in positions of political leadership. Ronald Reagan notwithstanding, the trend in advanced industrial nations seems toward a significant underrepresentation of the aged in leadership positions. This is likely a result of a greater bureaucratization of government, which causes career patterns to become more routinized.

Are the elderly politically more conservative than the young? Probably, but not because aging brings with it a change to conservative positions on prominent political issues. Rather, today's older people, when younger, had more conservative views than currently younger cohorts do.

There is considerable debate about the impact of a growing aged population on the federal budget. Some analysts view the budget as being ready to bust as a result of increased outlays for the elderly. Others believe this characterization of the budget to be inaccurate. Unfortunately, it may create the impression that the federal government gives lavish treatment to the elderly. There is considerable debate about whether the aged constitute a political force that can mobilize to serve their own interests.

Several groups of aged, including the poor, minority elderly, and older women, have been especially disadvantaged by government initiatives on behalf of older people. Public policy appears to perpetuate the existence of social class differences among the elderly that existed prior to old age. Although there was a time when age entitlement programs seemed necessary to identify a large proportion of elderly persons in need, the current question is whether or not a change to need entitlement would more effectively target government programs for the truly needy elderly.

STUDY QUESTIONS

1. Explain how age, employment status, education, and race influence voting behavior in the United States.

2. Discuss how the three factors identified by Milbrath explain the relationship between age and voting.

3. List the six categories described by Verba and Nie in their typology of political participation. In which categories are the elderly overrepresented, and what could explain their overrepresentation?

4. Discuss the changing trend of political participation of the elderly in leadership positions in advanced industrialized nations.

5. Explain the difference between *breakthrough* and *constituency-building* policy enactments. Can you give examples?

6. Distinguish among the *marginal, downwardly mobile,* and *integrated* elderly. How does the distribution of policy benefits act to perpetuate social class differences among the elderly?

7. Discuss the concept of *senior power*. How does it relate to the presence or absence of *aging group consciousness*?

8. Discuss the relative merits of providing programmatic support to older people on the basis of age and need.

BIBLIOGRAPHY

Achenbaum, W.A. 1983. *Shades of gray: Old age, American values, and federal policies since 1920.* Boston: Little, Brown and Co.

Ball, R. 1978. *Social security today and tomorrow.* New York: Columbia University Press.

Bengtson, V., and Cutler, N. 1976. Generalizations and intergenerational relations: Perspectives on age groups and social change. In R. Binstock and E. Shanas (eds.), *Handbook of aging and the social sciences.* New York: Van Nostrand Reinhold Co.

Binstock, R. 1978. Federal policy toward the aging—its inadequacies and its politics. *National Journal* November 11:1838–1845.

Butler, R. 1978. The economics of aging: We are asking the wrong questions. *National Journal* November 4:1792–1797.

Campbell, J.C., and Strate, J. 1981. Are old people conservative? *Gerontologist* 21(6):580–591.

Crittenden, J.A. 1962. Aging and party affiliation. *Public Opinion Quarterly*. 26:648–657.

Crystal, S. 1982. *America's old age crisis: Public policy and the two worlds of aging.* New York: Basic Books.

Cutler, N.E., and Schmidhauser, J.R. 1975. Age and political behavior. In D.S. Woodruff and J.E. Birren (eds.), *Aging: Scientific perspectives and social issues.* New York: Van Nostrand Reinhold Co.

Cutler, S.J., Lentz, S.A., Muha, M.J., and Riter, R.N. 1980. Aging and conservatism: Cohort changes in attitudes about legalized abortion. *Journal of Gerontology* 35:115–123.

Etzioni, A. 1976. Old people and public policy. *Social Policy* November/December:21–29.

Glenn, N.D., and Grimes, M. 1968. Aging, voting and political interest. *American Sociological Review* 33:563–575.

Glenn, N.D., and Hefner, T. 1972. Further evidence on aging and party identification. *Public Opinion Quarterly* 36:31–47.

Hardy, D.R. 1987. The future of Social Security. *Social Security Bulletin* 50(8):5–8.

Hess, B. 1983. Aging policies and old women: The hidden agenda. Paper presented at the 78th Annual Meeting of the American Sociological Society, Detroit, August 31–September 4, 1983.

Hudson, R. 1978. The 'graying' of the federal budget and its consequences for old-age policy. *Gerontologist* 18(5):428–439.

———. 1987. Tomorrow's able elders: Implications for the state. *Gerontologist* 27(4):405–409.

Hudson, R., and Binstock, R.H. 1976. Political systems and aging. In R.H. Binstock and E. Shanas (eds.), *Handbook of aging and the social sciences.* New York: Van Nostrand Reinhold Co.

Kutza, E.A. 1981. *The benefits of old age: Social-welfare policy for the elderly.* Chicago: University of Chicago Press.

Lammers, W.W., and Nyomarkay, J.L. 1980. The disappearing senior leaders. *Research on Aging* 2(3):329–349.

Lehman, H.C. 1953. *Age and achievement.* Princeton: Princeton University Press.

Milbrath, L.W. 1965. *Political participation.* Chicago: Rand McNally.

Nelson, G. 1982. Social class and public policy for the elderly. *Social Service Review* March:85–107.

Neugarten, B.L. 1982. Policy for the 1980s: Age or need entitlement? In B.L. Neugarten (ed.), *Age or need? Public policies for older people.* Beverly Hills, Calif.: Sage Publications.

Nie, N., Verba, S., and Kim, J. 1974. Political participation and the life-cycle. *Comparative Politics* 6:319–340.

Ossofsky, J. 1978. Through the aging budget—one more time. *National Journal* March 11:408–409.

Pratt, H. 1976. *The gray lobby.* Chicago: University of Chicago Press.

Samuelson, R. 1978. Busting the U.S. budget—the costs of an aging America. *National Journal* February 18:256–260.

Schlesinger, J.A. 1966. *Ambition and politics: Political careers in the United States.* Chicago: Rand McNally.

Schmidhauser, J. 1968. The political influence of the aged. *Gerontologist* 8(1):44–49.

Verba, S., and Nie, N. 1972. *Participation in America: Political democracy and social equality.* New York: Harper and Row.

Wisensale, S.K. 1988. Generational equity and intergenerational policies. *Gerontologist* 28(6):773–778.

CHAPTER 14

RELIGION AND AGING

Writing in 1972, Heenan described the literature on religion and aging as "empirical lacunae." Have things changed since? Although the literature on death and dying (see Chapter 19) has grown dramatically in the last decade or so, empirical research on the religious attitudes and behavior of older people is still relatively scarce. One explanation for the scarcity of such research is that this aspect of older life is taken for granted. Elders are consistently portrayed as both more superstitious and more religious than younger people, and the assumption is that the role of older people in religious activities remains strong and enduring (Hess and Markson 1980; Orbach 1961).

Another explanation is that the relative scarcity of research on religion and aging may have roots in methodological concerns. First, most research in social gerontology is cross-sectional in design. Thus, it is difficult to disentangle age, cohort, and period effects on a wide variety of behaviors and attitudes, including religious behavior and attitudes (Maddox 1979). As Moberg (1965, 80) observes:

> Whether the differences in religious beliefs between the generations are a result of the aging process or of divergent experiences during the formative years of childhood and youth, which are linked with different social and historical circumstances, is unknown. Longitudinal research might reveal considerably different conclusions from the cross-sectional studies which provide the foundation for current generalizations about age variations in the ideological dimensions of religion.

Second, certain concepts are difficult to define in the area of religion. What constitutes a religious individual anyway? And how should religiosity be measured: church or synagogue attendance, or engagement in private devotional activities?

336

Third, though religious groups "differ in terms of the amount of participation and interest demanded of their adherents, the degree of organization
they possess and the opportunities they offer for the individual to achieve his
or her goals" (Atchley 1980, 331), there seems to be a general insensitivity
within the field of gerontology toward the need to distinguish among religious
groups. Thus, what few studies there are make no basic attempt to separate
Protestants, Catholics, and Jews, and further subdivision among these groups
is even more rare (Crandall 1980). A recent review of the measures used in
studies of age and religiosity indicates that most are Christian and church
oriented (Payne 1982). Insensitivity toward religious diversity among the aged
may simply be an extension of the development of the broader field of social
gerontology. Only recently has recognition of the ethnic and racial diversity
present in the aging experience begun to infiltrate the field.

Young and Dowling (1987) suggest that a period effect accounts for a
vacillating interest in religion on the part of researchers. Following World War
II and peaking in 1965, considerable work focused on religiosity and old age,
with particular emphasis on attendance at religious services. During the 1980s,
interest in religion has once again increased on college campuses and among
the U.S. population at large. One chronicler corroborating this perceived re-
surgence indicates that researchers in the field of aging have increasingly incorporated religion-related variables in their research designs (Fecher 1982).
Thus, Heenan's "empirical lacunae" appear to be closing.

Coloring the execution and any interpretation of this empirical research,
however, is a richness of history and myth. Many contemporary beliefs and
attitudes toward older people are built upon an orientation first recorded in
Scripture. This chapter uses such chronicles of life and humanity to assess the
relationship between religion and aging. Following Achenbaum's lead (1985),
we begin with a review of perceptions of age among the ancient Hebrews and
early Christians as these may be reflected in the Old and New Testaments.
Subsequently, the functions organized religion provides to society and to its
aged constituents are identified. Literature on the relationship between age
and religious commitment is reviewed, although, as already indicated, such
studies generally have not distinguished among individuals of different religious affiliation. Finally, the interactions among age, religion, and health are
examined.

IN THE BEGINNING . . .

As many commentators have pointed out, the images of old age presented in
the Old Testament are generally quite positive: "The hoary head is a crown of
glory, it is found in the way of righteousness" (Prov. 16:31). Longevity is
presented as the reward for service to the Lord. This is especially evident in

Moses' discourses on the religious foundations of the Covenant. For example, "Ye shall walk in all the way which the Lord your God hath commanded you, that ye may live, and that it may be well with you, and that ye may prolong your days in the land which ye shall possess" (Deut. 5:30).

In Genesis 5, the book of the generations of Adam, a list of individuals who lived abnormally long lives is provided. Adam is said to have lived 930 years, Seth 912 years, Enosh 905 years, and so on. Most biblical scholars doubt the accuracy of this chronology, however. Maimonides holds that only the distinguished individuals named in this chapter lived these long years, whereas others lived a more or less normal span (Hertz 1981).

The general respect and favorable position of the elderly in ancient Hebraic culture was a function of three vital roles they played (Achenbaum 1985). First, the aged were often instruments of the Lord's will. Noah exemplifies this function. In the face of God's decision to cleanse the earth of corruption and violence, Noah is instructed to "Make thee an ark of gopher wood" (Gen. 6:14) and bring "all thy house into the ark" (Gen. 7:1). Noah was 600 years old when "the flood of waters was upon the earth" (Gen. 7:6) and 601 years when instructed to "Be fruitful, and multiply, and replenish the earth" (Gen. 9:1); he died at the age of 950 (Gen. 9:29).

The second function fulfilled by the elderly was that of wielder of political influence and power. The Book of Numbers describes the wanderings of the Israelites after their departure from Egypt. In Chapter 11, Moses complains to the Lord that he is unable to bear alone the burden of all these people. The Lord instructs Moses as follows:

> Gather unto Me seventy men of the elders of Israel, whom thou knowest to be the elders of the people, and officers over them; and bring them unto the tent of meeting, that they may stand there with thee. And I will come down and speak with thee there: and I will take of the spirit which is upon thee, and will put it upon them; and they shall bear the burden of the people with thee. (Num. 11:16–17)

Finally, the elderly are viewed as custodians of the collective wisdom of the years. Job, who had his family and material possessions stripped from him and his body covered with boils, asks, "Is wisdom with aged men, And understanding in length of days?" (Job 12:12) One answer he receives is as follows: "Days should speak, And multitude of years should teach wisdom" (Job 32:7).

It is difficult, if not impossible, to discuss the positive themes attached to old age and aging in ancient Hebraic culture without speaking to the conception of parent–child relations presented in the Old Testament. The Fifth Commandment provides the basic guideline: "Honor thy father and thy mother, as the Lord thy God commanded thee; that thy days may be long, and that it may go well with thee, upon the land which the Lord thy God giveth thee" (Deut. 5:16). As Achenbaum (1985) points out, however, the Old Testament may have been written in a time when ideals were not always realized. Thus,

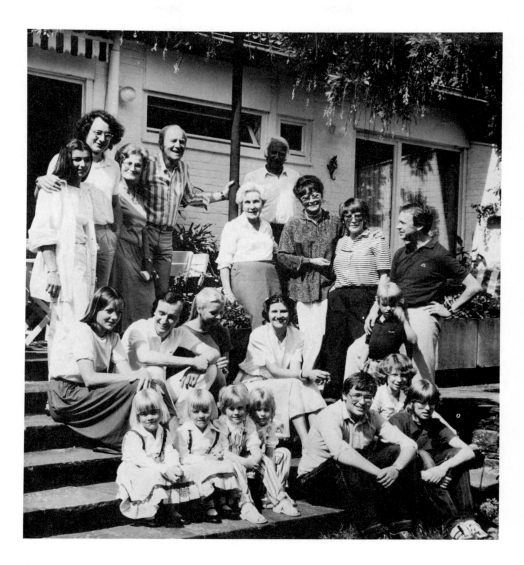

the Fifth Commandment can be juxtaposed with descriptions of the severe punishments assigned to children if a parental order was disobeyed or if a child cursed a parent. For example, an incorrigible son, whom milder measures failed to reclaim, might be tried by the elders at the gate of the city, and be liable to death by stoning (Deut. 21:18–21).

New Testament perspectives on old age and aging were built on Old Testament precedents. Honor to parents specifically and to the older generation generally is a device for expressing obedience toward God (Eph. 6:1–4). Yet distinctively Christian views of age and aging are put forth in the New Testament. For the most part these are intertwined with the conception of the personhood of Christ:

> But grace was given to each of us according to the measure of Christ's gift . . . until we all attain to the unity of the faith and of the knowledge of the Son of God, to mature manhood, to the measure of the stature of the fulness of Christ; . . . speaking the truth in love, we are to grow up in every way into him who is the head, into Christ, from whom the whole body, joined with which it is supplied, when each part is working properly, makes bodily growth and upbuilds itself in love. (Eph. 4:7, 13–16)

This image of aging posits that the goal of human development is to grow into the "mature manhood" of Christ. The theme of growth and continuity stretching through the course of human life is accentuated in the New Testament (Achenbaum 1985). Still, no Christian, no matter how old, can attain full maturity in this world. Presumably this results when one becomes fully incorporated into the Body of Christ. Achenbaum (1985) suggests that this may explain why no older person in the New Testament is portrayed as vividly or with the same stature as the patriarchs of the Old Testament; the central figure of the New Testament is a vigorous middle-aged Christ.

Another important difference between the Old and New Testaments is the portrayal of the relationship between death and aging. The Old Testament offers little comfort or consolation for the reality of death. Afterlife or immortal life are not substantive issues for the ancient Hebrews, or contemporary Jews for that matter. For Christians, Old Testament teaching has been transformed by the story of Christ's death, resurrection, and ascension. The New Testament proclaims victory over death, although, as Achenbaum notes, different Christian sects have come to visualize the afterlife in different ways.

FUNCTIONS OF RELIGION

As a social institution, religion fulfills several basic functions within human societies. For example, religion defines the spiritual world and provides explanation for events and occurrences that seem difficult to understand. On a more mundane level, religious institutional services provide a meeting ground for unattached and otherwise disaffiliated individuals. Three functions of religion worthy of our discussion here include integration, social control, and the provision of social support.

Social Integration. According to the French sociologist Emile Durkheim (1912/1965), ideas about the ultimate meaning of life and ritual ceremonies that express these ideas arise out of the collective experience of individuals. Beliefs, including religious beliefs, depend upon agreement among people for their meaning. The content of religious belief systems—ideas expressed, ritual ceremonies enacted, and values held sacred—all express the shared fate of the believers. For Durkheim, all systems of religious belief "have the same objective significance and fulfill the same function everywhere. . . . There are no religions that are false. All are true in their own fashion; all answer, though in different ways, to the given conditions of human existence."

The sharedness of religious bonds, the common adherence to a religious belief system, can overcome personal and divisive forces (Koenig, George and Siegler, 1988). It can act as a societal glue, holding together individuals and social groups with diverse interests and aspirations. It is exemplified in ritual ceremonies of passage such as confirmation, bar and bas mitzvahs, weddings, and funerals. The integrative function of religion is, perhaps, most apparent in traditional, preindustrial societies where agricultural events such as seeding and harvesting, kin relationships, and even the exercise of authority by leaders are governed by religious beliefs and rituals (Schaefer 1986).

Religion can be a powerful integrative force for older people in a society. Cowgill and Holmes (1972) in their analysis of aging and modernization in fourteen societies listed nine universals of human aging. *Universals* represent common denominators or constants of behavior that are found in the same form in most societies around the world. One of these universals is as follows: *Societies rich in ceremonialism and religious ritual tend to honor the aged and accord them prestige seldom found in less formalistic societies.* Old people can be the caretakers of ritual tradition. Not only can they teach the details of the ceremonies but they also represent a liaison between the affairs of earth and the realm of the supernatural (Holmes 1983). De Beauvoir (1972) adds:

> As the custodian of the traditions, the intercessor, and the protector against the supernatural powers, the aged man ensures the cohesion of the community throughout time and in the present. . . . Generally speaking, the services, taken as a whole, that the old are enabled to render because of their knowledge of the traditions, mean that they have not only respect but also material prosperity. They are rewarded with presents. The gifts that they receive from those whom they initiate into their secrets are of particular importance—they are the surest source of private wealth, a source that exists only in societies that are insufficiently well-to-do to have an advanced culture. (p. 83)

Many of the ceremonial and ritual roles performed by the elderly are described by Simmons (1945):

> They have served as guardians of temples, shrines, and sacred paraphernalia, as officers of the priesthood, and as leaders of the performance of rites associated with prayers, sacrifices, feast days, annual cycles, historic celebrations, and the initiation of important and hazardous enterprises. They also have been prominent in ceremonies with critical periods in the life cycle—such as birth, puberty, marriage, and death. (p. 164)

Amoss (1978, 1981) has described the Coast Salish Indians of Washington State and British Columbia as a society in which the aged have continued to be valued because of their knowledge of ritual and ceremonial detail. According to Amoss, contact with the white world in the late nineteenth century was initially devastating for the Coast Salish aged. With the shift to wage labor (away from hunting and gathering), old people's knowledge and skills became outdated and irrelevant. Religious leadership passed to younger men, and the supernatural powers of the old were challenged.

Since World War II, the Coast Salish have faced economic hardship, with jobs difficult to come by and many individuals on welfare. During the 1940s and 1950s, many sought relief in revivalistic Christianity. Christian churches were not able to offer the opportunity to feel dignity as Indians, however, and some ministers were even antagonistic toward Indian belief systems. Traditional religious ceremonies including the revival of traditional-type spirit dancing rituals began to reappear. These traditional rituals emphasized solidarity with past generations as well as among present-day Coast Salish. Old men and women became the focus of this new revivalism. The young wanted to be proud of their traditional culture, and it was the elderly who had preserved traditions from the past.

As Spencer and Jennings (1977) report, societies without a ceremonial tradition may provide little or no opportunity for the prestige or the participation of the elderly. Among the Chipewyn Indians of the western subarctic region of North America, elderly men no longer able to hunt command little respect. There is minimal interest in myth or legend about the past, and there are few, if any, remaining religious rituals. As a result, the elderly are left with almost no opportunities for participation in the society.

Social Control. Karl Marx agreed with Durkheim's view of the collective and socially shared nature of religious behavior. But Marx (1844/1963) was also concerned that religion produced an otherworldly focus that diverts attention from the circumstances and realities of life in this world. From this perspective, religion supports the status quo and helps to perpetuate patterns of social inequality. Long-held religious beliefs and practices enforce taken for granted beliefs that sometimes act as significant barriers to new or different ways of thinking and behaving. Traditional practices, handed down from previous generations, become defined as God-approved ways of doing things and are resistant to change. This is so even when the results of such traditional practices include inequalities and inequities. Racism, sexism, and, to some extent, ageism have been linked to religion, and when this occurs the social control functions of religion may be enhanced. For example, Vander Zanden (1988) quotes Louisiana State Senator W. M. Rainach in defending racial segregation in 1954: "Segregation is a natural order—created by God, in His wisdom, who made black men black and white men white."

Marx portrayed religion as a painkiller for the suffering experienced by all oppressed peoples, including the poor and indigent of all ages. Like other painkillers, it may suppress the symptoms for a while but the underlying condition remains.

> Religious suffering is at the same time an expression of real suffering and a protest against real suffering. Religion is the sigh of the oppressed creature, the sentiment of a heartless world, and the soul of soulless conditions. It is the opium of the people.

From a Marxist perspective, religion keeps people from understanding their living conditions in political terms. Marxists argue that religion induces a "false consciousness" among the disadvantaged that lessens the possibility of collective political action to change the material conditions of people's lives. Have the elderly experienced a false consciousness that hides from them the possibility of changing the material conditions of their lives? Or have they, in fact, enjoyed political and legislative successes far beyond their relative proportion in the U.S. population? These remain much-debated questions among students of aging (see Chapter 13, "The Politics of Aging").

Social Support. Religious institutions bring together people of all ages and help reduce the isolation of the elderly. For many elderly, especially those in smaller communities, religious pursuits help instigate and provide nurturance for social relationships (Twente 1970). Friendships, opportunities for reciprocal exchanges, sympathy, empathy, encouragement, and reassurance all represent supportive aspects of religious organizational environments and may contribute to well-being in later life (Koenig, Kvale, and Ferrel 1988). Even when capacities for firsthand participation in religious services and activities diminish, as Field (1968) describes below, the importance of continued interaction with representatives of the religious institution cannot be underestimated:

> An eighty-one-year-old woman, Mrs. Lang was suffering from a crippling form of arthritis which made her homebound. She had always been a warm, vital, outgoing person who, until three years earlier, was active in her church and contributed her handiwork to the Ladies' Circle. Now, she says, she understands what it means to 'cast one's bread upon the waters.' She does not know what she would have done were it not for the visits from her minister, who is a source of spiritual comfort, and from the members of the Ladies' Circle. Through these visits, she is kept informed as to what is happening in her church, and they make her feel that she still "belongs," that it does not matter that she can no longer help her church—now it is their turn to help her.

In the 1980s, women like Mrs. Lang have another option—that of the electronic church. Almost one in three U.S. viewers say they watch religous programming on television. These viewers are disproportionately older, female, southern, and from small towns and are less well educated than are people who do not watch religious programs (Clymer 1987). Although most use television as a supplement to participation in local religious activities, many elderly shut-ins use it as a substitute for attendance at religious services. Television allows viewers to "privatize" religious worship, to gain a feeling of immediate and personal help in coping with their troubles, and to enjoy the illusion of a face-to-face relationship with a dynamic religious leader (Hadden and Swann 1981).

AGE AND RELIGIOUS COMMITMENT

Data from the 1987 General Social Survey (GSS) show a strong relationship between age and religious commitment. Carried out by the National Opinion Research Center at the University of Chicago, the GSS is a survey taken annually of the attitudes and opinions of a representative sample of noninstitutionalized adults eighteen years of age and older in the United States. Some results are reported in Tables 14-1 through 14-3.

According to Table 14-1, older people are more likely than younger people to characterize themselves as being strongly religious. Almost six in ten (59.8 percent) GSS respondents aged sixty-five years and over described themselves as being strongly religious. This compares with 38.4 percent of those aged eighteen to forty-four years and 48.7 percent of those aged forty-five to sixty-four years of age who make the same claim.

Does this relationship between age and strength of religious affiliation hold up in a review of patterns of attendance at religious services? A decline in attendance at religious services and participation in organized religious activities is sometimes associated with physical limitations or disability as well as the lack of transportation. According to Moberg (1965):

> Persons who have commuted to church for as much as half a century blame their declining participation on poor eyesight, 'old age,' or failing health. Driv-

---

TABLE 14-1   Strength of Religious Affiliation, by Age, 1987

	Age		
	18–44 (%)	**45–64 (%)**	**65+ (%)**
Strongly religious	38.4	48.7	59.8
Not very strong	50.9	39.5	28.3
Somewhat strong	10.7	11.9	11.8

Data from the 1987 General Social Survey by the National Opinion Research Center at the University of Chicago.

ing to church, especially at night, has become an arduous task, and they do not wish to be a 'bother' or to become a burden upon someone else by 'begging' rides to all of the church's meetings.

Table 14-2 provides data on the variation by age in attendance at religious services among GSS respondents in 1987. Although those aged sixty-five years and over are almost twice as likely as those eighteen to forty-four years to attend religious services once a week or more frequently (39.9 percent versus 20.3 percent), there is virtually no difference in patterns of attendance at religious services between the old and middle aged; 62.4 percent of those forty-four to sixty-four years of age and 63.5 percent of those sixty-five years and over report attending religious services more frequently than once a month.

Table 14-3 shows that compared with young and middle-aged adults, the old pray more often. More than three-fourths (78.3 percent) of the GSS respondents aged sixty-five and over reported engaging in prayer more frequently than once a day. It is interesting to note, however, that more than one-half of respondents in each age category reported praying at least once a day.

General Social Survey data for 1987 provide a single snapshot of the relationship between age and religious commitment. Just what do we really know about how age affects religious behavior and commitment? Bahr (1970) analyzed prior research in this area and suggested that the relationship between aging and church attendance be interpreted with reference to four distinct models: traditional; lifetime stability; family life cycle; and progressive disengagement. According to the *traditional* model, there is a sharp decline in religious activity during young adulthood, with the lowest point in the life cycle being between ages thirty and thirty-five. Beyond age thirty-five, this model posits a steady increase in church activity until old age.

The *lifetime stability* model alleges that aging and church attendance or religious activity are not related. One interpretation of this model is made by Lazerwitz (1964, 433). He suggests that "perhaps church attendance is based upon patterns established fairly early in life and subject to little (if any) change with aging." Wilensky's (1961) review of studies of the variations in religious

TABLE 14-2   Attendance at Religious Services, by Age, 1987

	Age		
	18–44 (%)	45–64 (%)	65+ (%)
Once a week or more	20.3	38.8	39.9
Once a month or more	27.6	23.6	23.6
Once a year or more	33.6	23.5	19.6
Less than once a year/never	18.6	14.1	16.8

Data from the 1987 General Social Survey by the National Opinion Research Center at the University of Chicago.

TABLE 14-3   Frequency of Prayer, by Age, 1987

	Age		
	18–44 (%)	45–64 (%)	65 + (%)
Several times a day	18.4	31.7	46.4
Once a day	32.4	34.3	31.9
Once a week or more	26.1	19.8	10.2
Less than once a week/never	23.1	14.2	11.4

Data from the 1987 General Social Survey by the National Opinion Research Center at the University of Chicago.

participation by age supports this interpretation. He found that church membership and attendance was fairly stable in the middle years and did not drop off until after age seventy or seventy-five.

A third model derives from the view that religious participation is related to stage of *family life cycle*. In general, family life cycle seems to be a euphemism for presence or absence of children. According to this model, when children are young and tied to the home, parental involvement in religious services peaks; with children no longer in the home, regularity of religious participation falls off. Although this model speaks to the influence of the presence of children on parental involvement in organized religion, there is general agreement that parents' religious orientations are particularly important influences upon young people's development (Hoge and Petrillo 1978). Hunsberger (1985) reports that mothers have the strongest proreligious influence.

The *progressive disengagement* model is tied to the disengagement theory of aging. From the perspective of this theory, aging is seen as "an inevitable mutual withdrawal or disengagement," resulting in decreased interaction between the aging person and others in his or her social systems (Cumming and Henry 1961). Applied to participation in religious activities, the theory suggests a model of decline following middle age. Riley and Foner (1968) conclude that "the evidence, though slight, suggests that more individuals decrease than increase their attendance as they reach old age."

Bahr's own interviews with more than 600 men from three distinctive socioeconomic strata (skid row, urban lower class, and urban middle class) show substantial religious disaffiliation during adult life in all three groups; the progressive disengagement model is most congruent with the pattern of church attendance reported by his respondents. With advancing age, church attendance is increasingly less important as a source of voluntary affiliation among both well-to-do and poor men (Bahr 1970). As Bahr himself suggests, however, it may be that age brings a qualitative change in the nature of religiosity such that the decline in attendance is not matched by declines in religious belief or feeling.

Wingrove and Alston (1974) have argued that support for each of Bahr's four models varies by the type of sample and methodology used and by the year of data collection. Applying cohort analysis to data collected by the Gallup Poll between 1939 and 1969, these authors found that, although church attendance appears related to age, no consistent support for any one of the four models was provided. Each cohort was found to show its own church attendance pattern. Gender and social environment seemed to have greater impact on church attendance than did age.

Blazer and Palmore (1976) report the results of a longitudinal study of the religious attitudes and activities of 272 community residents over an eighteen-year period. Subjects were interviewed at two- to three-year intervals beginning in 1957. Measures included church attendance and Bible reading, among others. They found that positive religious attitudes remain fairly stable over time. If individuals were religious or nonreligious when young, chances are they will continue to have the same basic religious orientation when they become old. As Figure 14-1 shows, Blazer and Palmore's findings do show a gradual decline in religious activities in the later years.

Criticism of these and other studies of the relationship between age and religious behavior often centers on the fact that researchers have too narrowly conceptualized religiosity in terms of attendance or participation in formal organizations. As Mindel and Vaughn (1978) point out, the role of "religious person" encompasses more than simple participation in a religious organization and may include private or nonorganizational religious behavior. Some even suggest that, with aging, these more private and nonorganizational religious expressions increase in importance (Moberg 1972). Stark (1968) found that

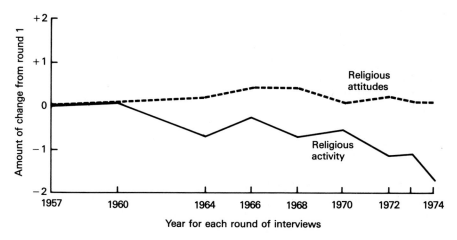

FIGURE 14-1   Religious attitudes and activities over time. *Source: Dan Blazer and Erdman Palmore, "Religion and Aging in a Longitudinal Panel," The Gerontologist, 16, No. 1 (1976), Pt. 1, 84. © The Gerontological Society of America.*

greater piety among the elderly compared with the young was manifested in the reported frequency of praying.

Employing a small sample of elderly from Central Missouri, Mindel and Vaughn (1978) observed that, although a majority did not attend religious services frequently, a majority of sample members maintained that they were nonorganizationally religious "very often." For the purposes of this study, examples of nonorganizational religious activity included engaging in individual or family prayer and listening to religious music or a religious service on the radio or television.

Young and Dowling (1987) have attempted to extend the work of Mindel and Vaughn by identifying factors that account for the variation in dimensions of religious participation. They sampled American Association of Retired Persons (AARP) members in El Paso, Texas, who were fairly evenly split between large "liberal" Protestant denominations (for example, Methodist, Presbyterian, or Episcopal) and "conservative/traditional" churches such as Baptist, Mormon, or Roman Catholic. Strength of religious conviction was the strongest predictor of organized religious activity and private religious behavior. These authors hypothesized that indicators of social or personal deprivation (including poor health, low income, reduced activity, and living alone) would predict higher levels of nonorganizational or private religious behavior. The assumption is that private religious behavior *compensates* for these deprivations. The researchers were forced to reject this hypothesis. Interestingly, they did find that strong kin and friend networks predict high levels of private devotion. Young and Dowling contend that frequent interaction in an informal social network contributes to the spiritual well-being of older persons through nonorganizational religious participation.

Kart, Palmer, and Flaschner (1987) studied the relationship between age and religiosity among Jews in Toledo, Ohio. Religiosity was measured in a variety of ways under two broad categories: organizational religious commitment and nonorganizational, or individual, religious commitment. Indicators of organizational religious commitment included synagogue attendance and the number of Jewish organizational memberships reported by each respondent. Indicators of individual religious commitment included whether the respondent follows religious dietary laws and keeps a kosher home, whether the respondent recites prayers of mourning for deceased parents and other family members, whether the respondent posts mezuzahs (parchment scrolls) on the doors of the household, whether female respondents light sabbath candles, and whether male respondents ritually pray over a cup of wine to consecrate the Sabbath. Respondents were also asked a question aimed at determining the strength of their religious beliefs.

For men in this sample, no statistically significant age differences could be observed on the array of organizational and individual measures of religious commitment. This is in contrast to Orbach's (1961) report made more than twenty-five years ago from the Detroit Area Study in which Jewish men showed increased synagogue attendance with age. In Toledo, only the number of Jewish organizational memberships showed age-related differences. Older men were much more likely to report holding multiple memberships in Jewish voluntary associations or organizations than were younger men.

Women in this study provide a different picture. Statistically significant age differences can be observed on a number of organizational and individual measures of religiosity, including synagogue attendance and the use of mezuzahs on the doorposts of the home. In all cases, older women evidence stronger religious commitment than do younger women. Only on a single scale made up of two items—observance of dietary laws and the lighting of Sabbath candles—did Kart and his colleagues find no apparent age differences.

Analyzing data from a large sample of Washington State residents, Finney and Lee (1976) found that age had a small, positive influence on private devotional practices but no effect on four other dimensions of religious commitment: belief, ritual, knowledge, and experience (Glock 1962; Glock and Stark 1965; Stark and Glock 1968). Finney and Lee suggest that older people may tend to employ religion as a means of reducing or alleviating anxieties, and the researchers point to the small effect of age on several dimensions of religious commitment as indicative of the need "to raise questions about recent thought in both social gerontology and the sociology of religion" (p. 17).

RELIGION, AGING, AND HEALTH

The general hypothesis that social ties may protect individuals from a variety of disease outcomes has received support from numerous researchers. The effect of marriage (for example, Gove 1973), contacts with relatives and friends (Zuckerman, Kasl, and Ostfeld 1984), and group membership (Berkman and Syme 1979) all have been reported as significantly associated with health status; those individuals most isolated (fewest contacts with others) have an increased risk to their health and greater mortality. Greater religiousness has been associated with lower levels of functional disability and symptoms of depression (Idler 1987). Researchers have reported an association between religious involvement and lower levels of hypertension (Graham et al. 1978) and myocardial infarction (Medalie et al. 1973) as well as lower risk of mortality (Berkman and Syme 1979; House, Robbins and Metzner, 1982; Schoenbach et al. 1986; Zuckerman et al. 1984). It is unclear, however, how or why health benefits may be derived from social ties.

Idler (1987) suggests focusing on the structure and support-giving characteristics of particular unique institutions, such as the church or synagogue, in order to discover the linking mechanisms between individual health status and involvement in the social environment. Presumably benefits from social ties are not only differentially distributed among social institutions in terms of frequency of occurrence; potential benefits may be qualitatively unique as well.

The question remains, as pointed out above, as to how and why social ties generate health benefits. Classical sociological theory holds at least four explanations for the influence of religiosity or participation in religious organizational activity over health status (Idler 1987; Norgard and Kart 1989).

1. Religious organizations comprise distinctively normative patterns from which individuals may structure their behaviors and attitudes. Religious guidelines may influence health status through restrictive behavioral habits associated with health risk such as smoking, drinking, or diet (*health behaviors hypothesis*).

   Mormons have been shown to have low cancer rates. This likely reflects adherence to their Church doctrines advocating abstention from the use of tobacco and alcohol. All Mormons do not adhere equally to the health practices of the Church, however. Gardner and Lyon (1982a) studied cancer in Utah Mormon men in relation to their adherence to Church doctrines. Cancer rates for 1966–1970 indicate that the most devout group had lung cancer rates 80 percent lower than those of the least devout group. The same was seen for all smoking- and alcohol-associated cancer sites combined. Cancer rates of the stomach and the leukemias and lymphomas also were lower in the most devout group. Mormon women classified as having the strongest adherence to Church doctrine had lung cancer rates during 1966–1970 much lower than did women with the weakest adherence (Gardner and Lyon 1982b).

2. Religious involvement may also influence health status by providing individuals with an opportunity to participate in a "moral community" (Durkheim 1897/1951), whereby religious involvement is seen as an affirmation of belonging to a group of like-minded people. Belonging may provide emotional as well as material support (*social cohesiveness hypothesis*).

   Graham and his colleagues (1978) examined the relationship between blood pressure levels and church attendance patterns in a group of white male heads of households in the 1967 to 1969 follow-up examination of the Evans County, Georgia, Cardiovascular Epidemiologic Study. A consistent pattern of lower systolic and diastolic blood pressures was found among frequent church attendees. The findings held up when controls for age, obesity, cigarette smoking, and socioeconomic status were employed.

3. Another functional aspect of religion, as a "unified system of beliefs and practices relative to sacred things" (Durkheim 1897/1951), is to define the spiritual and give meaning to the divine. A belief system that emphasizes people's relationships to a spiritual world provides an explanation for events that may otherwise seem unexplainable. Religious involvement may, therefore, provide a coherent framework for interpreting uncertainties associated

with day-to-day experiences and may provide support in stressful, out-of-the-ordinary situations (*cognitive coherence hypothesis*).

Zuckerman, Kasl, and Ostfeld (1984) reviewed mortality data during a two-year follow-up of some 400 elderly poor residents of three Connecticut cities between 1972 and 1974. Religiousness, measured by frequency of attendance at services and by two measures of religious strength and intensity, had an important protective effect among the elderly of both sexes in poorest health. And, this is the case when sociodemographic variables and health status measures are controlled. Among the religious, 19 percent of the males and 12 percent of the females who were ill died; the comparable mortality figures for the nonreligious in poor health were 42 percent of the males and 20 percent of females. Virtually no differences in death rates were apparent between the religious and nonreligious elderly in good health. Borrowing from Antonovsky, the authors suggest that religiosity may provide individuals with a *sense of coherence* that events "are predictable and that there is a high probability that things will work out as well as can reasonably be expected" (Antonovsky 1979, 123).

4. Finally, religious involvement may act to modify how individuals perceive particularly stressful situations including hospitalization, disability, or other traumatic events. Typically, religious belief systems provide a variety of contexts for understanding and interpreting individual human suffering. In part, this function of religion may be an extension of the social support and cognitive coherence functions mentioned above (*theodicy hypothesis*).

Norgard and Kart (1989) have investigated the relationship between religiosity and health status using older white respondents aged fifty-five years and older in the 1984 and 1987 General Social Surveys. Because of their insufficient numbers, nonwhites were excluded from the study. The four hypotheses identified above were tested in this work. The dependent variable, health status, was operationalized in two ways: a subjective evaluation of health status ("Would you say your health in general is excellent, good, fair, or poor?"); and subjective evaluation of psychological well-being ("Would you say that you are very happy, pretty happy, not too happy?"). Self-assessment of health status has been reported as correlating well with other measures of health status and in predicting general emotional states and behavior (Maddox and Douglas 1973). A number of researchers have identified a positive relationship between religiosity and happiness or life satisfaction (Blazer and Palmore 1976; Hunsberger 1985).

Religiosity was also measured in two ways: the frequency of attendance at religious services and an attitudinal measure of strength of religious belief. Demographic variables and measures relevant to each of the four hypotheses were also used. These included age, education, income, sex, and marital status.

In general, and as predicted, religiosity was positively associated with subjective health and happiness among the elderly GSS respondents. In addition, some empirical support was provided for each of the four hypotheses. These hypotheses are not mutually exclusive. There is nothing exclusive or inconsistent, for example, about encouraging people to be supportive of their family members and friends and at the same time encouraging them not to smoke. Religious institutions have multiple functions, and individuals, including elderly individuals, have a relationship to the social environment that is multifaceted. Certainly an older person may receive qualitatively different positive contributions to perceived health and happiness from their religious beliefs and attitudes.

SUMMARY

The relative scarcity of research on religion and aging may have roots in methodological concerns. Most research is cross-sectional in nature, making it difficult for researchers to disentangle age, cohort, and period effects. Religiosity is a difficult concept to operationalize: Are organizational affiliations and attendance of more importance than measures of private devotional activity? Finally, most research simply does not distinguish between and among religious groups.

Contemporary beliefs and attitudes toward older people have roots in Scripture. Images of aging presented in the Old Testament are quite positive. Longevity is often presented as a reward for service to the Lord. The elderly often played vital roles as instruments of God, wielders of political power and influence, and custodians of the collective wisdom of the years. The Fifth Commandment offers the basic guideline in parent–child relationships. New Testament perspectives on old age and aging built on the Old Testament precedents. Distinctively Christian views of age and aging are intertwined with the conception of the personhood of Christ. Another important difference between the Old and New Testament is the portrayal of the relationship between death and aging.

Major societal functions of religion include social integration, social control, and social support. Religion can be a powerful integrative force for older people in society. Societies rich in ceremonialism and religious ritual tend to honor the aged and accord them prestige seldom found in less formalistic societies. Religion can also be a powerful force for social control. It can provide barriers to new ways of thinking and behaving. And it can force people to focus on otherworldly issues rather than on the material conditions of their lives. Has religion induced a false consciousness among the elderly?

Data from the 1987 General Social Survey show a strong relationship between age and religious commitment. Older people are much more likely than young adults to describe themselves as being strongly religious. There is virtually no difference between the old and middle aged when it comes to attendance at religious services, but the old report praying more often than the young or middle aged do.

Early research on age and religious commitment provided four distinct models: traditional; lifetime stability; family life cycle; and progressive disengagement. Criticism of the early work centered on the narrow conceptualization of religiosity strictly in terms of attendance at religious services. The distinction between organizational religious commitment and private or individual religious commitment has become relevant. In addition, different researchers have identified different dimensions of organizational commitment.

Religiosity may influence the health status of older people in at least four ways: health behaviors hypothesis; social cohesiveness hypothesis; cognitive coherence hypothesis; and theodicy hypothesis. Some empirical support exists for each hypothesis.

STUDY QUESTIONS

1. What methodological issues help explain the relative scarcity of research on religion and aging?

2. What is the general position of the elderly in ancient Hebraic culture as reflected in the Old Testament? How do the Old and New Testaments differ in their conceptions of the aging process and the elderly?

3. Describe three major functions of religion. Give examples.

4. Distinguish the old from young and middle-aged adults with regard to strength of religiousness, attendance at religious services, and frequency of prayer.

5. Describe Bahr's four models of the relationship between aging and church attendance. Which model does Bahr's own data support?

6. List some measures or dimensions of religiosity that are alternatives to attendance at religious services. What is the importance of being able to identify these alternative measures?

7. How may religion affect the health status of older people?

BIBLIOGRAPHY

Achenbaum, W.A. 1985. Societal perceptions of the aging and the aged. In R.H. Binstock and E. Shanas (eds.), *Handbook of aging and the social sciences* (2nd ed.). New York: Van Nostrand Reinhold Co.

Amoss, P. 1978. *Coast Salish spirit dancing.* Seattle: University of Washington Press.

————. 1981. Coast Salish elders. In P. Amoss and S. Harrell (eds.), *Other ways of growing old.* Stanford, Calif.: Stanford University Press.

Antonovsky, A. 1979. *Health, stress, and coping.* San Francisco, Calif.: Jossey-Bass.

Atchley, R. 1980. *Social forces in later life* (3d ed.). Belmont, Calif.: Wadsworth Publishing.

Bahr, H. 1970. Aging and religious disaffiliation. *Social Forces* 49:59–71.

de Beauvoir, S. 1972. *Coming of age.* New York: G.P. Putnam's Sons.

Berkman, L.F., and Syme, S.L. 1979. Social networks, host resistance, and mortality: A nine-year follow-up study of Alameda County residents. *American Journal of Epidemiology* 109:186–204.

Blazer, D., and Palmore, E. 1976. Religion and aging in a longitudinal panel. *Gerontologist* 16(1):82–85.

Clymer, A. 1987. Survey finds many skeptics among evangelists' viewers. *New York Times* March 31:1, 14.

Cowgill, D., and Holmes, L. 1972. *Aging and modernization.* New York: Appleton-Century-Crofts.

Crandall, R.C. 1980. *Gerontology: A behavioral science approach.* Reading, Mass.: Addison-Wesley.

Cumming, E., and Henry, W. 1961. *Growing old: The process of disengagement.* New York: Basic Books.

Durkheim, E. 1897/1951. *Suicide.* New York: Free Press.

———. 1912/1965. *The elementary forms of religious life.* New York: Free Press.

Fecher, V. 1982. *Religion and aging: An annotated bibliography.* San Antonio, Tex.: Trinity University Press.

Field, M. 1968. *Aging with honor and dignity.* Springfield, Ill.: Charles C Thomas.

Finney, J.M., and Lee, G.R. 1976. Age differences on five dimensions of religious involvement. *Review of Religious Research* 18(2):173–179.

Gardner, J.W., and Lyon, J.L. 1982a. Cancer in Utah Mormon men by lay priesthood level. *American Journal of Epidemiology* 116:243–257.

———. 1982b. Cancer in Utah Mormon women by church activity level. *American Journal of Epidemiology* 116:258–265.

Glock, C.Y. 1962. On the study of religious commitment: Review of recent research bearing on religion and character education. *Religious Education* (July–August):98–110.

Glock, C.Y., and Stark, R. 1965. *Religion and society in tension.* Chicago: Rand McNally.

Gove, W. 1973. Sex, marital status and mortality. *American Journal of Sociology* 79:45–67.

Graham, T.W., Kaplan, B., Cornoni-Huntley, J., James, S., Becker, C., Harnes, C., and Heyden, S. 1978. Frequency of church attendance and blood pressure elevation. *Journal of Behavioral Medicine* 1:37–43.

Hadden, J.K., and Swann, C.E. 1981. *Prime time preachers: The rising power of televangelism.* Reading, Mass.: Addison-Wesley.

Hames, C., and Heyden, S. 1978. Frequency of church attendance and blood pressure elevation. *Journal of Behavioral Medicine* 1:37–43.

Heenan, E.F. 1972. Sociology of religion and aged. *Journal of Scientific Study of Religion* 11:171–176.

Hertz, J.H. (ed.) 1981. *Pentateuch and haftorahs: Hebrew text, English translation and commentary.* London: Soncino Press.

Hess, B. and Markson, E. 1980. *Aging and old age.* New York: Macmillan.

Hoge, D.R., and Petrillo, G.H. 1978. Development of religious thinking in adolescence: A test of Goldman's theories. *Journal for the Scientific Study of Religion* 17:359–379.

Holmes, L.D. 1983. *Other cultures, elder years: An introduction to cultural gerontology.* Minneapolis: Burgess Publishing Co.

House, J.S., Robbins, C., and Metzner, H.L. 1982. The association of social relationships and activities with mortality: Prospective evidence from the Tecumseh community health study. *American Journal of Epidemiology* 116:123–140.

Hunsberger, B. 1985. Religion, age, life satisfaction, and perceived sources of religiousness: A study of older persons. *Journal of Gerontology* 40(5):615–620.

Idler, E.L. 1987. Religious involvement and the health of the elderly: Some hypotheses and an initial test. *Social Forces* 66(1):226–238.

Kart, C.S., Palmer, N.P., and Flaschner, A.B. 1987. Aging and religious commitment in a midwestern Jewish community. *Journal of Religion and Aging* 3 (3/4):49–60.

Koenig, H.G., George, L.K., and Siegler, I.C. 1988. The use of religion and other emotion-regulating coping strategies among older adults. *Gerontologist* 28(3):303–310.

Koenig, H.G., Kvale, J.N., and Ferrel, C. 1988. Religion and well-being in later life. *Gerontologist* 28(1):18–28.

Lazerwitz, B. 1962. Membership in voluntary associations and frequency of church attendance. *Journal of Scientific Study of Religion* 2:74–84.

———. 1964. Religion and social structure in the United States. In L. Schneider (ed.), *Religion, culture, and society*. New York: Wiley.

Maddox, G. 1979. Sociology of later life. *Annual Review of Sociology* 5:113–135.

Maddox, G., and Douglas, E. 1973. Self-assessment of health: A longitudinal study of elderly subjects. *Journal of Health and Social Behavior* 14:87–92.

Marx, K. 1844/1963. Estranged labour—economic and philosophic manuscripts of 1844. In C.W. Mills (ed.), *Images of man*. New York: George Brazilier.

Medalie, J.H., Kahn, H.A., Neufeld, H.N., Riss, E., and Goldbourt, U. 1973. Five-year myocardial infarction incidence II: Association of single variables to age and birthplace. *Journal of Chronic Disease* 26:329–349.

Mindel, C.H., and Vaughn, C.V. 1978. A multidimensional approach to religiosity and disengagement. *Journal of Gerontology* 33:103–108.

Moberg, D.D. 1965. Religiosity in old age. *Gerontologist* 5(2):80–85.

———. 1972. Religion and the aging family. *The Family Coordinator* (January):47–60.

Norgard, T., and Kart, C.S. 1989. Religiosity and health status among the elderly: Replication with national samples. Paper presented at the annual meeting of the North Central Sociological Association, Akron, Ohio, April 1989.

Orbach, H. 1961. Aging and religion. *Geriatrics* 16:534–540.

Payne, B. 1982. Religiosity. In D.J. Mangen and W.A. Peterson (eds.), *Research instruments in social gerontology, Vol. 2. Social roles and social participation*. Minneapolis: University of Minnesota Press.

Riley, M., and Foner, A. 1968. *Aging and society, Vol. 1. An inventory of research findings*. New York: Russell Sage.

Schaefer, R.T. 1986. *Sociology* (2nd ed.). New York: McGraw-Hill.

Schoenbach, V., Kaplan, B., Fredman, L., and Kleinbaum, D.G. 1986. Social ties and mortality in Evans County, Georgia. *American Journal of Epidemiology* 123:329–349.

Simmons, L. 1945. *The role of the aged in primitive society*. New Haven, Conn.: Yale University Press.

Spencer, R., and Jennings, J.D. 1977. *The native Americans*. New York: Harper and Row.

Stark, R. 1968. Age and faith: A changing outlook as an old process. *Sociological Analysis* 29:1–10.

Stark, R., and Glock, C.Y. 1968. *American piety: The nation of religious commitment*. Berkeley, Calif.: University of California Press.

Twente, E. 1970. *Never too old*. San Francisco, Calif.: Jossey-Bass.

Vander Zanden, J.W. 1988. *The social experience: An introduction to sociology*. New York: Random House.

Wilensky, H.L. 1961. Life cycle, work situation, and participation in formal associations. In R.W. Kleemeier (ed.), *Aging and leisure*. New York: Oxford University Press.

Wingrove, C.R., and Alston, J. 1974. Age, aging and church attendance. *The Gerontologist* 11(4):356–358.

Young, G., and Dowling, W. 1987. Dimensions of religiosity in old age: Accounting for variation in types of participation. *Journal of Gerontology* 42(4):376–380.

Zuckerman, D., Kasl, S., and Ostfeld, A.M. 1984. Psychosocial predictors of mortality among the elderly poor: The role of religion, well-being, and social contacts. *American Journal of Epidemiology* 119:410–423.

PART V

SPECIAL ISSUES IN AGING

CHAPTER 15

RACIAL AND ETHNIC AGING

CHAPTER 16

**LIVING ENVIRONMENTS
OF THE ELDERLY**

CHAPTER 17

LONG-TERM CARE

CHAPTER 18

**HEALTH POLICY
AND AGING**

CHAPTER 19

DEATH AND DYING

CHAPTER 15

RACIAL AND ETHNIC AGING

The United States has been described as a "melting pot" in which ethnic minorities lose their distinctive character and become assimilated into the broader culture. Recently the ideology of the melting pot has been challenged by those who emphasize the pluralism of U.S. society. Cultural pluralism exists in a society when ethnic and racial groups are able to retain their unique character and when they are also able to participate equally in key roles in the society (Turner 1978). Unfortunately, U.S. society cannot be characterized as a place where opportunities to participate in key roles in society have been distributed equally. Still, whether the United States is a melting pot or a culturally pluralistic society may be an academic question. Clearly, as much as any society in the world, the United States has retained enormous ethnic and racial diversity.

Andrew Greeley (1974) uses the notion of ethnogenesis to explain this diversity. *Ethnogenesis* describes a model of ethnic relations in which pressures to assimilate exist alongside pressures to maintain ethnic identification. In this model, maintaining an ethnic identity becomes a device for expressing group interests and maintaining group identity. Glazer and Moynihan (1963), in their book *Beyond the Melting Pot*, anticipated the ethnogenesis perspective. They recognized, for example, that European immigrants often lost original customs and ways by the third generation yet still "voted differently, had different ideas about education and sex, and were still, in many essential ways, as different from one another as their grandfathers had been."

Recognition of the ethnic (and racial) diversity present in the U.S. experience has only recently begun to rub off on the field of social gerontology. Clearly, most of what we have come to learn of aging stems from studies of "middle-majority Anglos" (Moore 1971). As Robert Kastenbaum (1971) has remarked in characterizing the great majority of studies carried out on aged white samples, "any resemblance to the aging non-Caucasian is accidental and unintentional."

We must ask, however, whether there really is anything to learn from studying the aging experiences of U.S. minorities. After all, there are many commonalities among the elderly, which appear to cut across racial and ethnic lines. The greater number of older women, the higher remarriage rates of males, the relationships among living arrangements and income, isolation, and locale affect all elderly groups similarly, regardless of racial and ethnic identification (Moore 1971). The noted gerontologist Donald Kent (1971a, 1971b) believed that the study of minority patterns of aging was important for practical as well as theoretical reasons. According to Kent, from a practical point of view, it is important to remember that the aggregate number of minority aged is substantial, and these individuals are underrepresented among the prosperous and healthy. Thus, humanitarian considerations urge the study of minority aged. From a theoretical point of view, it is important that ideas about the aging process be generalizable across cultural groups. There is no way to accomplish this without studying a variety of aged groups. In addition, researchers often learn most about how their ideas work when they observe them in "extreme" situations. The position of minority aged in the United States makes it possible to test principles of aging in just such extreme situations.

MINORITY AGING—A CASE OF DOUBLE JEOPARDY?

Minority aging has been characterized by many as a case of *double jeopardy* (Jackson 1970, 1971; U.S. Senate, 1971).[1] This term is used to reflect the idea that the negative effects of aging are compounded among minority group members. The suggestion is that aged minority group members suffer both age *and* race discrimination. The U.S. Senate Special Committee on Aging (1971) notes that, compared with the white aged, minority aged "are less well educated, have less income, suffer more illnesses and earlier death, have poorer quality housing and less choice as to where they live and where they work, and, in general, have a less satisfying quality of life." The Senate Committee followed this up by suggesting that social policy be generated to reflect these differences.

Recently, Dowd and Bengtson (1978) empirically tested the hypothesis of minority aging as a double jeopardy. These authors analyzed data collected as part of a larger survey of adult (aged forty-five to seventy-four) black, Mexican

---

[1] Some social scientists have used the term *triple jeopardy* to represent the position of minority aged. The reference is to being old, poor, and a member of a minority group. Jackson (1971) has used the designation *quadruple jeopardy* to represent those who are black, female, old, and poor.

American, and Anglo residents of Los Angeles County. The researchers divided each group into three age strata—forty-five to fifty-four, fifty-five to sixty-four, and sixty-five to seventy-four years of age—and compared them on a series of variables that included (1) total family income, (2) self-assessed health, (3) a series of social interaction items, and (4) two measures of life satisfaction.

Income

The data showed that, although the incomes of all groups decline with age, the mean income reported by the oldest (sixty-five to seventy-four) black and Mexican American respondents is considerably lower than that of any other group. The relative decline in income from age forty-five to age seventy-four was also substantially greater for minority respondents than it is for whites. This decline was 36 percent for whites, 55 percent for blacks, and 62 percent for Mexican Americans.

Health

Older minority respondents reported poorer health than white respondents did when asked, "In general, would you say your health is very good, good, fair, poor, or very poor?" The average health scores of blacks and Mexican Americans declined 13 and 19 percent, respectively, across the age strata represented in the sample. The decline for whites was only 9 percent. This data on self-assessed health is quite consistent with observed differences on so-called "objective" measures of morbidity and mortality. Dowd and Bengtson attribute these health differences to past and present policies of racial discrimination, which have caused nonwhites to have lower incomes, inadequate nutrition, and poorer health than whites.

In general, the data on income and self-assessment of health from this study support the double-jeopardy hypothesis.

Life Satisfaction

Two measures of life satisfaction were analyzed in this study—*tranquility* and *optimism*. Both measures reflect different configurations of responses to eleven life-satisfaction items. A typical item related to optimism was "As you get older, do you feel less useful?" A negative response indicated life satisfaction. An item related to tranquility was "Do you worry so much that you can't sleep?" Presumably, a negative response here would indicate life satisfaction.

The tranquility scores of Mexican Americans aged sixty-five to seventy-four are significantly lower than those of whites and blacks. The decline in scores across the three age strata for Mexican Americans is so slight, however, it questions the impact of age on tranquility scores. This indicates that, at least with regard to this dimension, aging is not jeopardizing the life satisfaction of Mexican Americans. The pattern is different for the second measure of life satisfaction, optimism, and clearly supports the double-jeopardy hypothesis. Mexican Americans show a significant decline in optimism with age; their optimism scores are significantly lower than the scores of whites; and the differences in scores when compared with those of whites increase with age. Whites show a 2-percent decline in average optimism scores between those aged forty-five to fifty-four and those aged sixty-five to seventy-four, whereas the decline for Mexican Americans is 23 percent.

When blacks and whites are compared on the two life satisfaction measures, the differences present between younger respondents *narrow* and almost disappear entirely with age. This *leveling* phenomenon will be discussed in more detail below.

Social Interaction

One measure of social interaction involved asking respondents the frequency with which they had contact with children and grandchildren. This measure can be considered a quality-of-life variable. The reliable presence of family members can be an important social support for people making the transition into old age in U.S. society (Dowd and Bengtson 1978).

Mexican Americans at every age report the most frequent contact with their children and grandchildren. Relative to whites, blacks maintain an advantageous position on this measure in all but the oldest age stratum. A similar pattern exists on a second measure of social interaction, which asked respondents about their contacts with other relatives. Younger whites had fewer contacts with relatives than either blacks or Mexican-Americans did, although the differences become smaller in the older age groups. The result is a *leveling of differences* across the ethnic groups.

Finally, a third measure of interaction asked respondents about the frequency of their contacts with neighbors and friends. Whites report higher levels of contact with friends and neighbors than do blacks and Mexican Americans at all ages, and their contacts increase with age. The lower social interaction of blacks and Mexican Americans on this measure remains essentially stable across the age groups. Thus, although ethnic differences are present in frequency of contact with friends and neighbors, the absence of age as an influence on this variable for blacks and Mexican Americans creates a situation that does not constitute a double jeopardy.

In summary, this study finds the notion of double jeopardy to characterize accurately the situation of minority aged (blacks and Mexican Americans) on selected variables (especially income and self-assessment of health). Interestingly, the data also suggest that aging influences some variables in ways that *reduce* ethnic differences that existed in mid-life. Kent (1971a, 1971b; Kent and Hirsch 1969) has written of age as a *mediator* of racial and social differences. From this perspective, the problems faced by old people are seen as very similar regardless of ethnic or racial background. Kent goes on: "This is not to say that the same proportion of each age group faces these problems; obviously they do not. The point, however, is that if we concentrate on the group rather than on the problem, we shall be treating symptoms rather than causes."

There is another perspective on the concept of double jeopardy. Some believe that too much attention continues to be focused on the concept. They argue that, at best, the concept may be period-bound and unable to capture recent major social and political changes in the status of minority group members. At worst, investigators who have used the concept can be accused of providing very little useful information about age changes "in the statuses, roles, interpersonal relationships, attitudes, and values of adult minority individuals or populations as they age in their later years" (Jackson 1985, 284).

Schaie and his colleagues (1982) have used data on the life satisfaction of white and black respondents in the 1973 and 1977 General Social Surveys to show "the interacting effect of race not only with age, but also with cohort and period effects." They determined that there were significant cohort effects in life satisfaction favoring earlier born cohorts, regardless of race (even while controlling for health and income). Nevertheless, there were race differences across the period studied, with life satisfaction increasing for blacks while remaining stable for whites. The authors speculate that this finding may result from black respondents, on average, "beginning to perceive positive societal changes, which affect their overall levels of life satisfaction." This work may provide a model for moving beyond the double-jeopardy concept.

Manuel (1982) argues that we need to move beyond the assumption that application of a minority group label can be used as an indication that an individual has experienced the sociocultural events generally thought to be associated with the label. Given the complexity of racial and ethnic identity, the experience of some individuals may more closely resemble that of members of the majority than it will the experience of other members of what is only a nominal reference group. Clearly, there may be diversity within a minority group with regard to the extent and manner in which group members have been victimized by their minority group status. To paraphrase a question asked by Manuel, can we assume that black males of all ages, for example, have had significantly less opportunity than have their white counterparts to participate fully in U.S. institutions? To the contrary, he answers. It can be expected that there will be differential circumstances of aging within minority groups (Manuel 1982).

AGING AND THE
MINORITY EXPERIENCE

In this section we describe the situation of aged members of selected racial and ethnic minority groups. In each case, we begin by presenting demographic statistics and follow with discussion of some special aspects of the aging minority experience.

The Black Elderly

The diversity of experience represented in the population of older blacks cannot be overstated. Each cohort of blacks in the United States has been exposed to different cultural practices and social and political conditions (Greene and Siegler 1984). Wilson (1978) has identified three major stages that blacks in the United States have experienced historically. The first stage includes slavery and the post–Civil War period. Stage two is the period of industrial expansion beginning in the last quarter of the nineteenth century and continuing through World War II. The third stage comprises the contemporary era since the end of World War II.

During stages one and two, racial barriers were explicit and designed to systematically deny blacks access to economic, political, and social resources. Efforts to minimize, neutralize, and even negate the voting privileges of blacks exemplify these barriers (Simon and Eitzen 1982). According to Wilson 1978, very few blacks were employed in industrial plants prior to World War I. In the South, black labor was restricted largely to agricultural work and domestic services. The emergence of Jim Crow segregation effectively prevented the employment of blacks in industry. Mechanization reduced the need for farm labor during the 1920s and 1930s, and blacks suffered increased unemployment. Along with working-class members, the self-employed, and recent immigrants, blacks experienced particular hardship during the Great Depression.

The third stage brought change. World War II instigated a wave of black migrants to the industrial cities of the North. Following the war, this concentration of blacks in cities increased the likelihood of group actions in response to oppressive conditions in housing, employment, and the like. Increased educational opportunities allowed for the development of a cadre of black leaders, and the civil rights movement of the 1950s and 1960s helped reduce overt discrimination in employment, housing, education, and transportation, and provided blacks with access to economic and social resources (Eitzen 1986).

As Greene and Siegler (1984) point out, gains that occurred during the post–World War II period came too late to make appreciable impact on the educational level or economic condition of the oldest cohorts of black elderly. A black man who was eighty-five years of age in 1985 was already completing his work career by the time of the passage of the Civil Rights Act of 1964. Many in the younger cohorts of black aged have benefited, however, so that social and economic differentiation is greater among the young-old than the old-old.

By 1981 the black elderly made up about 8.2 percent of the total elderly population; about 11.8 percent of the total United States population is black. In general, the U.S. black population is younger than the population of whites. As Figure 15-1 shows, the proportion of the black population that is old (sixty-five years and over) is considerably smaller than that of the white population for both males and females. Most people attribute this to the lower life expectancy of blacks. Although the differential in life expectancy between the

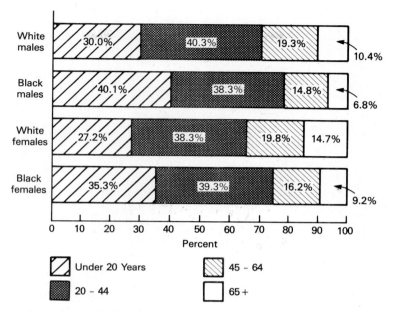

FIGURE 15-1   Age distribution of whites and blacks, 1984. *Source: U.S. Bureau of the Census (1986, Table 28).*

two races contributes moderately to the relative youthfulness of the black population, the key factor is the higher fertility among blacks. On the average, black women have 3.1 children, compared with the 2.2 recorded for white women. This disparity in fertility rates contributes to the fact that, whereas approximately 39 percent of all blacks are under the age of twenty-two, only about 30 percent of all whites are in this age grouping. The median age of blacks is roughly six years younger than that for whites; in 1981, black women had a median age of 26.5 years, white women, 32.5 years.

Readers should be reminded that the size and age composition of the black population show wide geographical variation. For example, in recent estimates of San Diego metropolitan residents over the age of sixty, only 4,500 or 2.2 percent of this total population were black (Stanford 1978). The proportion of aged blacks in Atlanta, Georgia, on the other hand, is 21 percent of the total aged population. These differences reflect the residential patterns of black Americans. Approximately 53 percent of all blacks live in the South; only 8.5 percent live in the West; furthermore, most aged blacks residing in the North and West have their roots in the South. As Dancy (1977) points out, these southern roots have greatly affected black cultural patterns, including religion, culinary habits, language, and life-style.

Despite the historical situation, black Americans have become urbanites.

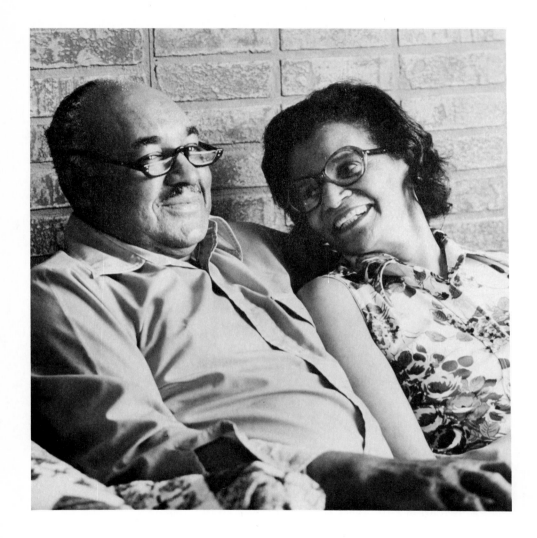

In 1980 about 85 percent of all blacks lived in metropolitan areas, and 75 percent of these resided in central cities. Black urbanization has come about at the same time as white suburbanization, leaving many central city areas without a sufficient tax base to support programs for the less affluent minority aged.

Aged blacks fare worse than aged whites across a variety of socioeconomic indicators. Elderly blacks have fewer years of education, lower incomes, and lower occupational status. Census data comparisons for the older population show that 38 percent of black men and 18 percent of black women had completed less than five years of formal education, as compared with 8 percent of white men and 7 percent of white women (Taylor and Taylor 1982).

The median income of older black couples and black singles was only 60 percent of the median income of white couples and 70 percent of white singles (Chen 1985). This disparity in income levels is reflected in the higher incidence of poverty among elderly blacks. As was reported earlier in Chapter 11 ("The Economics of Aging"), the poverty rate for aged blacks is about three times that for aged whites.

A study derived from the 1972 Social Security Survey of the Status of the Elderly (STATEL) shows the relationships between education and income for blacks (Abbott 1977). In general, the data indicate that education yields a lower economic return for blacks than for whites. At all education levels, white elderly were likely to have achieved a higher economic status than was the case for black elderly. Among those with a high school diploma or more, black elderly were twice as likely (20 percent versus 10 percent for whites) to be found in the lowest quintile of annual income and half as likely (19 percent to 36 percent for whites) to be located in the highest quintile. Many blacks achieved economic status despite less education. The proportion of blacks in the highest annual income quintile with less than eight years of schooling was 44 percent, while for whites, this figure was 8 percent.

Older blacks are found in the labor force in about the same proportion as are older whites; as with blacks at all other ages, however, their work brings them less income. The work histories of many blacks have clearly had impact on their retirement income. Black unemployment has been significantly higher than that of whites. Blacks have also been overrepresented in jobs (for example, domestic service) and industries (nonunionized) that do not afford protection from the whims of the marketplace. Interestingly, Belgrave (1988), using data gathered from black and white women aged sixty-two through sixty-six in Cleveland, Ohio, found that black women were more likely than whites to have worked steadily most of their adult lives, more likely to be eligible for pensions, but less likely to have retired.

Gender is probably the most widely studied predictor of socioeconomic status among aged blacks. In summarizing this body of work, Taylor and Chatters (1988, 436) report that "elderly black women tend to have more years of education than older black men." Despite this educational advantage, however, older black women have lower levels of occupational prestige, lower incomes, and a higher incidence of poverty.

The health status of older blacks is generally thought to be poorer than that of older whites (Ferraro 1987). Krause (1987) made a similar finding, although he identified different stress-related correlates of health status for whites and blacks. Chronic financial strain was found to be associated with ill health among older whites, while crisis events in the social support network were related to poor health among older blacks. Krause argues that older blacks may be more integrated into their communities than are older whites. As is indicated below, this social involvement often occurs within the context of family ties and church-related social networks. Still, as Krause points out, social support entails reciprocity, and greater involvement in the lives of others. Such involvement in the lives of others can be stressful and detrimental to health, especially when network members experience stressful events.

The disadvantaged health status of older blacks also is displayed in reduced life expectancy, particularly of black males. As a result, many blacks do not live long enough to collect the benefits of Social Security and other programs for the elderly—even those to which they have contributed through many years of taxation. Davis (1976) contends, for example, that for every dollar of Social Security taxes paid by the black community, only 28 cents comes back to it in the form of old-age benefits.

Income—or more accurately the lack of it—is probably the most serious problem faced by aged blacks in the United States. The high rate of poverty among aged blacks reduces their capacity to deal effectively with other major concerns, including health, crime, transportation, housing, and nutrition. Borrowing from Dancy (1977), we can put a human face on such dry assertions:

> Mrs. Mary C. was a widow. She eked out her existence on a tiny allotment from Social Security. Her husband's serious illness and subsequent death wiped out their lifelong savings in just a few months. Mrs. C. had suffered chronic health problems for ten years, a residual effect of a serious illness few friends had expected her to survive. Thus, regular check-ups by the doctor were important for maintaining reasonably stable health, and since Mrs. C. did not drive or have easy access to transportation, a friend agreed to take her for her medical check-up whenever this was needed. On one occasion, after Mrs. C. had left the doctor's office and returned to the car, she remarked that the doctor said she was coming along fine but needed medication, and he had written a prescription for her.
>
> Mrs. C.'s friend immediately turned her car in the direction of the drugstore. Seeing where her friend was headed, Mrs. C. said, "Oh, no, I'm not going to get the prescription filled now." Puzzled, the friend inquired whether someone would get it filled for her later that night. Mrs. C. replied that she was not going to get the prescription filled. As her friend continued to look puzzled, the older woman said, "I'm going to wait until the first of the month." (Dancy, J. 1977. *The Black Elderly: A Guide for Practitioners*, 12–13. Ann Arbor, Michigan: Institute of Gerontology, University of Michigan-Wayne State University. Reprinted by permission of the Institute of Gerontology.)

An unfilled prescription can do nothing to keep Mrs. C. healthy. Lacking resources, however, she must wait until the first of the month when the Social Security check arrives before filling the physician's prescription.

In a recent survey in Michigan, 65 percent of the white elderly expressed concern about health (Michigan Offices of Services to the Aging 1975). Income is not the only factor affecting the health status of elderly blacks. Elderly blacks in San Diego, when asked why they did not utilize available health services, offered several categories of response in addition to finances: fear of illness and consequences; mistrust of physicians and hospitals; language barriers; and transportation (Stanford 1978).

Fear of crime is a problem for elderly people of all races. Nevertheless, the Michigan survey referred to earlier reports 62 percent of elderly blacks worried about crime, compared with only 28 percent of whites. Many black elderly reside in poorer inner-city neighborhoods. Often the official crime statistics simply do not reflect all the victimization of the elderly in such neighborhoods. Old people fear attacks and robberies but also may feel that going to the police is useless. Many remember a time when they were accorded less than first-class citizenship by police and the courts. A similar feeling often arises in another context. One crime-prevention measure suggested by local police departments is direct-deposit mailing. This involves having Social Security and pension checks sent directly to a bank so they cannot be stolen from mailboxes at home. Many black elderly, however, do not have long experience dealing with banks and, in addition, mistrust bank personnel for sometimes failing to treat blacks with the same respect granted to whites.

Many elderly blacks are housing-poor. A M.I.T.–Harvard study on housing in America (Birch et al. 1973) found that in 1970 almost 13 million families (one-sixth of all American families) were in this condition. *Housing-poor* was defined as living in a housing unit with a deficiency in one or more of the following: (1) the ability of the household to afford the unit; (2) the location of the unit; (3) the physical condition of the unit; and (4) the degree of overcrowding.

Housing costs constitute a substantial portion of regular income. In 1970, 45 percent of the renting households headed by elderly individuals were paying 35 percent or more of their income for rent. Many elderly persons on fixed incomes are unable to keep up with the rising rents and maintenance costs.

Black aged are residentially concentrated in central cities and low-income areas; thus, they are somewhat more likely to reside in older housing. According to the 1970 Census, about 60 percent of homes owned by the elderly had been built before 1939. Many of these units are of high quality, but some are substandard. The slowed rate of housing construction in the past decade means that many of these physically substandard units that might otherwise have been removed from the housing inventory are necessary to provide some degree of shelter for individuals. This undersupply of housing, especially in the inner city, also means that the housing poor are often crowding two or three generations together in their homes or apartment units and are at great risk for homelessness.

Although, in general, the problems of aged blacks are related to income deprivation, two areas of strength emerge in which participation is not affected by income status: family and religion. These deserve special mention.

Black Family Ties. It has become part of the conventional wisdom that family ties are a source of strength among blacks. Interestingly, however, much evidence suggests that in the black experience (particularly the urban black experience) the notion of family extends beyond the immediate household. Stack has shown how family functions are carried out for urban blacks by clusters of kin who may or may not reside together. She offers the example of Viola Jackson's brother, who, after his wife died, "decided to raise his two sons himself. He kept the two boys and never remarried. His residence has been consistently close to one or another of his sisters who have fed and cared for his two sons" (Stack 1970).

Elderly blacks, especially black women, play an important role in this extended kin network, which so well characterizes the family life of many urban blacks. Hill (1971) reports that 48 percent of elderly black women have other related children living with them—in contrast to only 10 percent of similar white families. A more recent study shows 26 percent of black aged taking grandchildren into their homes, compared with 15 percent of the white aged (Jackson and Wood 1976).

One reason blacks may rely so heavily on family members is that they have minimal expectations for receiving effective service from social service agencies. This may especially be the case for older blacks, who have a painful history of inequality, rejection, and ejection when it comes to dealing with such agencies (Dancy 1977). Furthermore, as Dancy (1977) points out:

1. Elderly blacks often lack full knowledge or understanding of the service or benefits to which they are entitled.
2. They are cynical about promised services.
3. Most older blacks have no influence whatsoever on programs and services.
4. Few meaningful and needed services are located in their communities.

Family members often value their aged relations because they serve as important role models. Dancy (1977) lists four strengths of the black elderly, which may be useful to remember:

1. The accumulation of wisdom, knowledge, and common sense about life comes not only from age but from the experience of hardship and suffering.
2. A creative genius allows them to do much with little.
3. The ability to accept aging among the black elderly results from their belief that old age is a reward in itself. They are less likely to deny their age than those in the dominant society. Many elderly blacks voice this sentiment: "I thank the Lord that he spared me!"
4. They maintain a sense of hope and optimism for a better day.

The Black Church. In general, religion is a source of strength to the black elderly. Historically, the church has been a frame of reference for blacks for coping with racial discrimination and has played a role in their survival and advancement. The church is one institution that blacks control locally; it has remained relatively free from white authority.

The so-called black church is really many churches, including traditional black Protestant denominations such as the Baptists and Methodists as well as fundamentalist groups. Religious behavior within these churches often differs from that in comparable white churches. The black church is a place of expression, and worship frequently takes the form of celebration.

Religion is a main involvement of many black elderly. For most, this simply reflects the continuation of a lifelong trend. Church attendance and participation in church activities were important early in life and continue to be so in later life. Participation in church activities provides an opportunity for many to "be somebody." Black elderly receive high status and respectability in the community as a function of such participation.

> Mr. John Jordon worked as baggage handler for a large transportation company. He was in his late fifties and had worked for twenty-five years for the same company. Faithful to his job, he was never late and had seldom missed a day. Yet he had been passed over time and time again for a promotion to a job with more pay and responsibility. Each time he dared ask why he never advanced, he was told that he was "not ready" or lacked the skills or was given other excuses. Yet he saw whites with the same education as his—tenth grade—get better opportunities. What kept Mr. Jordon from becoming demoralized and bitter was his church. In those same twenty-five years he had moved from a pew member to a deacon. Now he was also treasurer of the church—a job of enormous responsibility which required banking a thousand dollars weekly. Mr. Jordon's church appreciated his talents, and Mr. Jordon was a faithful man and loved his church. There he was somebody. (Dancy, J. 1977. *The Black Elderly: A Guide for Practitioners,* pp. 22–23. Ann Arbor, Mich.: Institute of Gerontology, University of Michigan-Wayne State University. Reprinted by permission of the Institute of Gerontology.)

Finally, considering the influential position of the church in the black community, it is essential that service providers understand the roles the church plays in the lives of black elderly. The church is not only a place where large numbers of black elderly can be reached, but also a place where needs can be assessed and services delivered.

The Hispanic Aged

In 1980 Hispanic Americans constituted 6.4 percent of the U.S. population, or over 14 million people. Next to blacks, they make up the largest minority in the United States. The Hispanic population is fast growing, with birth rates and immigration rates relatively high. Officially, this population increased by 50 percent between 1970 and 1980, although there is little doubt that the actual rate of growth has been higher as a function of illegal immigration. Many experts believe that by some time in the 1990s, the Hispanic population will exceed the black population, making it the nation's largest minority group (Farley 1982).

The Spanish-American population is a heterogeneous group.[2] As Figure 15-2 shows, about 61 percent of all Americans of Spanish origin are Mexican, 15 percent are Puerto Rican, and 24 percent are of other Spanish heritage. The diversity of the population has created real problems for researchers and helps explain why so little systematic research is carried out on Spanish Americans. Spanish Americans are not easily categorized; attempts to make generalizations among Cubans in Florida, Puerto Ricans in New York, and Mexican Americans in California are likely to bear little fruit. In addition, Hispanics are one of the youngest ethnic groups in the United States; the elderly account for only about 5 percent of the total Hispanic population and, in light of the major problems faced by the population in general, the special concerns of the elderly have not emerged with a visibility in any way comparable to the situation among Anglos. Until this changes, gerontologists are forced to rely on widely varied sources for relevant materials. Because much of this available (although scarce) literature concerns itself with Mexican Americans, they dominate our presentation here.

The Spanish population is concentrated largely in the southwestern states of California and Texas, where 52 percent of all Spanish Americans were living in 1980. Most of these people are of Mexican descent. A majority of Puerto Ricans live in New York and New Jersey; Cubans have settled primarily in Florida. A majority of the Hispanic population resides in urban areas, with most living in central cities.

About half of the Hispanic elderly are foreign-born. Cubans and Puerto Ricans are more recent migrants than Mexican Americans, many of whom are descendants of original settlers of territories annexed by the United States in the Mexican-American War. The Spanish American population is an even younger population than blacks (43 percent under twenty years of age versus 39 percent for blacks). High fertility and large family size, in addition to immigration of the young and repatriation of the middle aged, contribute to the youthfulness of this group.

In terms of education, income, and occupational status, Spanish Americans lag behind other racial and ethnic minorities as well as behind whites (Lacayo 1977, cited in Barrow and Smith 1979). Although Hispanic elderly are literate in their native languages, only American Indian elderly have a higher rate of illiteracy. Median income for the group as a whole is about two-thirds of that for the white population. One in four Spanish-origin elderly persons lived below the poverty level in 1975. The proportion of Spanish Americans holding professional or technical jobs in less than half the proportion for whites. As

---

[2] We interchange the terms Hispanic and Spanish American for stylistic purpose only.

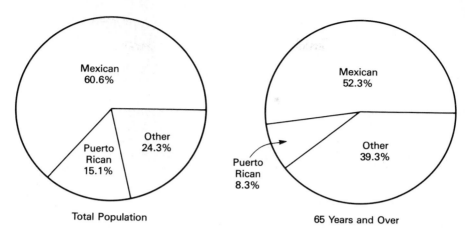

Mexican
60.6%

Puerto
Rican
15.1%

Other
24.3%

Total Population

Mexican
52.3%

Puerto
Rican
8.3%

Other
39.3%

65 Years and Over

FIGURE 15-2   Composition of Spanish American population (by percent), total and 65 +. *Source: U.S. Bureau of the Census (1986, Table 38).*

Hendricks and Hendricks (1977) point out, however, there are marked differences between Cubans and other Spanish-origin people, who more frequently hold high-paying jobs, and Mexican Americans and Puerto Ricans found in lower income manual labor occupations. Many elderly Hispanics work in unskilled labor or as farm workers. According to Barrow and Smith (1979), they stay in the labor force longer than white elderly. Few have had lengthy work careers in settings that provide retirement preparation. Others either entered the country illegally or have failed to maintain certification of their residential status as aliens. In either case, they forfeit benefits and services for which they might otherwise be eligible.

It would make sense that, as with the black elderly, the problem of Hispanic elderly emanates from their deprived income status. Yet one of the few available studies of the expressed needs of a Hispanic elderly population showed income to be fourth on the list (Valle and Mendoza 1978). For these elderly Hispanics in San Diego, health, transportation, and concerns about children preceded income as a "present cause of greatest concern." Steglich, Cartwright, and Crouch (1968) also found health to be a priority need among elderly Mexican Americans in Lubbock, Texas. Torres-Gil (1976) indicated lack of money, inadequate transportation, and health as major areas of concern among elderly Mexican Americans in San Jose.

Often the special needs of Hispanic elderly are understated because of the popular assumption that they are properly cared for within the context of the extended family. Aged Hispanics are seen as receiving positive emotional and social support because of their unique position as older family members. Historically, this popular view of Mexican Americans may have been correct; today, however, it is incomplete and misleading.

The traditional Mexican-American family has been described as a supportive and flexible structure that assumes a variety of functions in dealing with the environment and with the emotional and psychological aspects of the family unit and individuals (Sotomayor 1971). Such a family pattern maintains the elderly within the physical and social life of the family, thus reducing the likelihood of isolation. In general, the aged person holds high status and has considerable influence in the family's social life.

Recognition of the concept of *machismo* has led many to characterize the Mexican American family as a patriarchal structure. The most emphasized aspect of *machismo* has to do with sexual prowess (Alvirez and Bean 1976). From early childhood, males are given more freedom than females and are socialized into "manliness." This includes playing the dominant role in the family. Women are expected to be submissive and to subordinate their needs to those of the husband and other family members (Alvirez and Bean 1976).

Maldonado (1975) argues that this division of labor in the Mexican American family often changes as family members grow older. Close observation, he says, reveals that the woman plays an increasingly more active role as she grows older, to the point that the grandmother may be dominant in the extended family. In part, this family hierarchy may reflect the higher early death rate among Mexican American males.

To a great extent, the foregoing describes a picture of the Mexican American family that *does not* take into account the rapidly changing situation in the Mexican American community (Maldonado 1975). These changes, which may have a negative impact on the elderly, include the increased urbanization of Mexican Americans ("barrioization") and the gradual movement toward a stronger nuclear family. Many elderly now find themselves either in a small town or rural community isolated from their children, or in a barrio where, because of the social and educational mobility of the young, their status and influence have declined significantly. This generation gap leaves elderly Chicanos misunderstood by the society at large and by younger members of their own families. In addition, the general society, with its obsolete understanding of Chicano culture, believes that the Chicano family will provide for its older members, which the younger Chicano generation is having an increasingly difficult time doing (Maldonado 1975).

Despite the tension between the generations instigated by social changes in the Mexican American community, there is still some evidence that Chicano families are maintaining respect for the elderly. One example of this is reflected in the underutilization of nursing home facilities by Mexican American elderly. Eribes and Bradley-Rawls (1978) attribute this underutilization to the fact that nursing homes are not as yet viewed as a culturally viable alternative to the Mexican American family handling the housing and medical care of their elderly.

Nursing home placement may truly be the choice of last resort for Hispanics (Eribes and Bradley-Rawls 1978). Reviewing the records of admission to one nursing home in New York City, Espino and his colleagues (1988) found Puerto Rican/Hispanic patients to be younger and more impaired than their non-Hispanic counterparts. These researchers argue "that Puerto Rican/Hispanics are cared for in the community longer in that higher degrees of disability are reached and that these levels are reached at a younger age. At that point they or their families are forced to choose institutionalization" (pp. 823–824).

The Native American Aged

The aged American Indian population is small and relatively invisible. Despite the enormous diversity among Indian cultures, they suffer deprivation by any social or economic indicator employed. To a great extent, this reflects the special history of American Indians and their relationship with the U.S. government. Certainly, no other minority group has been as physically and socially isolated from the mainstream of American life as has the American Indian.

The total population of American Indians in 1980 (including Alaskan Natives) was approximately 1.4 million. A century or so ago, anthropologists estimated that the aboriginal population of North America before contact with the Europeans (circa 1600) was between 500,000 and 1.5 million persons. Some critics have suggested that these figures are too low and were generated for the purpose of legitimating European conquest of an allegedly unoccupied land (Feagin 1984). A considered estimate by Dobyns (1966) puts the number of Native Americans in North America at near 10 million at the time of the initial European contact. European diseases and firepower sharply reduced the number of Native Americans to a low point of about 200,000 in 1850.

Benedict (1972) considers this decrease to be a unique occurrence in American history. He has written, "Although other minority groups have experienced involuntary relocation and social and economic discrimination, none seems to have been subjected to a similar assault on life itself." Despite general agreement that high fertility and reduced mortality have contributed to an increase in the Indian population, current estimates should be regarded as crude. The Bureau of Indian Affairs (BIA) and the U.S. Census Bureau often disagree on their respective estimates. As an additional problem, the 1970 census initiated self-designation as an enumeration technique for the category "Native American."

About 51 percent of the American Indian population resides in the western United States, although the largest concentrations are found in Oklahoma, Arizona, California, and New Mexico. North Carolina, Washington, South Dakota, New York, and Montana all had in excess of 25,000 American Indians in 1970. Almost two-thirds of the native population resides on or near a reservation; the remainder are urbanized. Indians are the only minority group who are less urbanized than the U.S. population as a whole. Los Angeles has the most American Indians of any urban area, approximately 45,000. San Francisco, Tulsa, Oklahoma City, Minneapolis, Chicago, and Phoenix each have over 10,000 American Indians (Price 1976). The urbanization of this population is a relatively recent phenomenon. Bahr (1972) suggests this migration was triggered by the push factors of poverty and unemployment on reservations and the pull factor of expanding economic opportunities located in the cities.

The American Indian population is quite young. The median age in 1980 was twenty-three. The fertility rate is still considerably higher than that of either white or black Americans. Life expectancy among American Indians is approximately sixty-four years, with women living longer than men. About 5 percent of the Native American population is sixty-five years or older, and only one in three American Indians can expect to reach the age of sixty-five (Barrow and Smith 1979).

The contemporary American Indian experience is characterized by poverty. Unemployment is considerably higher than the national average. Typically, Native Americans are concentrated in unskilled, semi-skilled, and low-wage service jobs that are often seasonal. In 1980 the unemployment rate among American Indians was more than double that of whites, and these rates do not include the large numbers of Native Americans who have given up looking for work. According to Feagin (1984), one-third of all Indian families were classified as poor in 1970, including almost 50 percent of those in rural areas. Median income for Indian families in 1970 was far below the median for all U.S. families. The income level of Native American male earners was about 42 percent of that of all males in the United States in 1970. Retirement is both a luxury and a hardship for American Indians. For many, there has been no work to retire from; as Benedict (1972) points out, old age is simply a continuation of a state of economic distribution to which American Indians have had ample time to accustom themselves.

Formal educational attainment levels for Indians of all ages remain far behind those of whites. Let us remember, however, that aged American Indians were of school age at a time when only a small percentage of Native American children attended any type of formal school. Schooling took place within informal tribal circles. The few boarding schools (run by the BIA) and mission schools were often oppressive environments that attempted to enforce acculturation. Students were punished for speaking native languages, and Native American values were denigrated. Until very recently this remained an accurate characterization of the educational environments in which Native Americans found themselves.

Although the diversity of American Indian tribal culture makes generalization difficult, it is fair to say that the status of elderly American Indians has undergone enormous change in the last hundred years or so. According to Simmons (1945), most North American Indian societies ensured respect for the aged—at least until they were obviously powerless and incompetent. Close inspection, however, shows that respect was given not simply as a function of age but rather on the basis of some particular asset that an older person possessed. The range of avenues that afforded access to homage was great.

An individual might be respected for extensive knowledge, seasoned experience, expert skill, power to work magic, control of property rights, or skill in games, dances, songs, and storytelling. The Iroquois associated long life with wisdom. A common prayer began, "Preserve our old men among us. . . ." Among the Chippewa the elderly men held the central positions in council gatherings where the young were expected to sit in silence. Aged Navaho women were custodians of much property and highly regarded in both family and public life.

Much has changed. Today, elderly American Indians are for the most part ministered to by government bureaucracies. Social and financial services are provided by the Bureau of Indian Affairs, health needs by the Public Health Service (and into the 1980s, Native American health conditions are among the worst in the United States). The way these programs are operated often denies the old their traditional position in tribal society. For example, elderly Indians are required to transfer property rights to their heirs *before* they can receive financial assistance.

No program can immunize the Native American elderly from a lifetime of inadequate nutrition, housing, and health services. These deprivations usually take their toll long before old age. Clearly, many changes must be made in the situation of American Indians before future generations of elderly Native Americans can expect a better day.

The Asian American Aged

The median family income of Asian Americans was $22,075 in 1980—higher than for all other racial groups, including whites. No wonder, then, that Asian Americans are characterized as being a successful "model minority." This concept of *model minority* describes the general belief that Asian American families—and communities, for that matter—are stable and in full command of their social and economic concerns.

Kim (1973) argues that this view of Asian Americans as a model minority supports a myth and is a convenient device for excluding them from programs related to education, health, housing, and employment. He suspects that behind the prosperous shops of the Chinatowns and Little Tokyos are thousands of disaffiliated old people waiting out their remaining years in poverty and ill health. This view is supported by a White House Conference on Aging report (1972):

> The Asian American elderly are severely handicapped by the myth that pervades society at large and permeates the policy decisions of agencies and governmental entities . . . that Asian American aged do not have any problems, that Asian Americans are able to take care of their own, and that Asian American aged do not need or desire aid in any form.

This report characterizes older Asian Americans as

1. Having problems which are, in many respects, more intensive and complex than the problems of the general senior citizen population
2. Being excluded by cultural barriers from receiving their rightful benefits
3. Committing suicide at a rate three times the national average
4. Being among the people most neglected by programs presumably serving all elderly

Kalish and Moriwaki (1973) believe that the situation of older Asian Americans cannot be grasped without an understanding of four factors: (1) their cultural origins and the effects of early socialization; (2) their life history in the United States; (3) those age-related changes that occur regardless of early learning and ethnicity; and (4) their expectations concerning what it means to be old. We attempt to integrate these factors into brief discussions of two of the largest elderly Asian-American populations, the Japanese and the Chinese. First, however, let us describe the general characteristics of the older Asian American population.

Over 3 million Asian Americans were recorded in the 1980 census; this is equivalent to 1.4 percent of the total population and about 9 percent of the nonwhite population in the United States. Among the largest Asian American groups in the United States are the Chinese, Filipinos, Japanese, and Koreans. Most Asian Americans are urbanites, residing in ethnic enclaves in cities such as San Francisco, Honolulu, Los Angeles, Seattle, and New York.

Although the sex ratio among Japanese American elderly is comparable to that for whites, a majority of Chinese elderly and Filipino elderly are males. This reflects historically restrictive immigration laws, especially for Chinese and Filipinos, which often denied entry to women and children. Like earlier immigrants, without language and labor skills, Asian men were exploited. They were used as cheap labor in mining, canning, farming, and railroad work. Even now, this experience has an impact on elderly men who survived the exploitation. One study of the Chinese carried out under the auspices of the Community Service Society (CSS) of New York reported that nearly one-third of the older unattached men in the CSS caseload had no contact with a public or voluntary agency. Many were eligible for public support and needed it but refused to apply when they discovered the sort of personal information they were required to provide (Cattell 1962, cited in Fujii 1976).

Despite earlier comments about the exalted income status of Asian Americans in general, the income status of older Asian Americans is quite low. The median annual income in 1970 was $2,542 for Japanese men aged sixty-five years and older and $1,348 for Japanese women in this age group. Figures were lower for the other Asian American ethnic groups. Most elderly Asians have spent considerable employment time in low-paying jobs or in jobs not covered by Social Security or other pension programs. In a recent study of Chinese elderly in San Diego (Cheng 1978), median monthly income was reported to be $214. Many elderly Asians are still employed; 52 percent of a Japanese American group between the ages of fifty-five and ninety-four were currently working (Ishizuka 1978). Occupations most frequently cited by the men were gardener, farmer, fisherman, and nurseryman. Occupations commonly held by the women included garment factory or cannery work, assistant to their husbands in a family business, semi-skilled labor, and office or clerical worker.

Elderly Japanese Americans. The significant migration of Japanese to the United States occurred after 1890. Many came to this country as sojourners with an intent to stay a while, establish themselves financially, and then return home (Montero 1979). Migrants were young, uneducated, and unskilled. Hostility against the Japanese was great. Racist attitudes were prevalent: The Japanese were said to be wily, immoral, and unassimilable. Discriminatory laws and local nuisance ordinances were used to limit the activities of Japanese. Unions were successful in excluding Japanese, and city governments were pressured into refusing permits to Japanese businesses. In 1913 California passed an Alien Land Law, which disallowed land purchase or lease on the part of Japanese Americans. The Immigration Act of 1924 placed severe restrictions on Japanese immigration to this country. This hostility culminated during World War II when all people of Japanese ancestry were evacuated from their homes along the West Coast and placed in "relocation camps." No Italians or German Americans were similarly evacuated.

After the war, the camps were closed, and treatment of Japanese Americans improved. In general, the group has made enormous progress since 1950; they are upwardly mobile. This success has been attributed to Japanese American family life (Kitano and Kikumura 1976).

In traditional Japan, families occupied a central position. The extended family was an associational and supportive institution and most important for early socialization and upbringing. Marriage was often arranged by a father intent on maintaining family solidarity. The father–son relationship was preeminent in the family; women were dutiful and deferred to men. Caring for aged parents was the responsibility of the eldest son in particular, although clearly all adult children were expected to bear some responsibility in this area.

Among the first Japanese American families (called *Issei*), this traditional family picture survived in some modified form. As Kitano and Kikumura (1976) point out, there were no grandparents to serve as reminders of old traditions, and many immigrants felt free to Americanize. One powerful constraint on assimilation was the norm of *enryo* brought from Japan and still in existence in the United States. This norm is related to power and regulates how those who have power are to behave toward those without it (and vice versa). In the Japanese family and community, power and privilege were associated with the father. In the U.S. context, the norm *enryo* helped reinforce this association even when the Japanese father was subject to the humiliation and abuse of whites outside the family (Kitano and Kikumura 1976). Montero (1979) has described the continued importance of the family to Issei elderly. He points to data showing the disengagement of elderly Japanese Americans from many social and organizational ties, but the continued existence of a strong family support system. It is the adult children with whom Issei visit regularly and frequently who form the foundation of this family support system (Montero 1979).

Pressures to assimilate increased for subsequent generations of Japanese (*Nisei* and *Sansei*). Data presented earlier on the income status of Japanese Americans reflect their successful economic assimilation. Cultural assimilation, particularly in regard to language and religion, also advanced among Nisei and Sansei. Feagin and Fujitaki (1972), in a study from 1969 to 1970, found Nisei and Sansei showed significant acculturation with respect to speaking English at home, not reading Japanese literature, and not feeling it was essential to maintain Japanese traditions.

Kalish and Moriwaki (1973) have written of the problems created as different generations of Japanese come to reflect different degrees of assimilation to the U.S. context. As an example, they use the theme of filial piety—"honor thy father and thy mother"—which is common in Western as well as East Asian literature. Kalish and Moriwaki argue that the theme of filial piety is undermined by other themes in U.S. culture—independence, self-reliance, and mastery over one's own fate. This creates a situation whereby first-generation elderly retain expectations consistent with the theme of filial piety, whereas the second- and third-generation members become assimilated into a society "where future potential is more important than past accomplishments in evaluating the worth of a person, [and] the wisdom and the accomplishments of the elderly were often perceived as irrelevant or were forgotten and ignored." As Nisei and Sansei move into old age, these intergenerational incongruities should lessen. Increased interracial marriage and upward social mobility are also likely to reduce the relevance of traditional values among Japanese Americans. The Japanese American elderly in the future are likely to be more diversified in terms of social class and geographical distribution (Osako and Liu 1986).

Elderly Chinese Americans. Chinese began to arrive in California during the middle of the nineteenth century. Railroad and mining agents often went to China to recruit laborers with promises of work, higher wages, and free passage. Racism was rampant against the highly identifiable Chinese. Violence and murder were not uncommon and rarely punished by the authorities. Efforts to expel Chinese from California and other western states began almost with their arrival. California passed exclusion laws in 1852, 1855, and 1858; each was declared unconstitutional by the U.S. Supreme Court. Taxes and other discriminatory devices were used against the Chinese. Article XIX of the California State Constitution, initiated in 1879, prohibited corporations from directly or indirectly employing Chinese (Burkey 1978). Chinese were considered sinister and unassimilable, with vices bred into them over generations (Burkey 1978). Federal laws eventually passed in 1882, 1888, 1902, and 1904 severely limited Chinese immigration into this country until World War II. During this period the Chinese retreated into invisibility. Chinese Americans benefited somewhat from the war, however, because China was an ally of the United States. They were granted citizenship, exempted from land restriction, and permitted to enter professional and commercial activities that previously had been denied to them (Lyman 1974).

Many Chinese who arrived in the United States had no intention of staying. They came in order to provide for a family left behind with the expectation of returning in order to enjoy the fruits of their labors (Huang 1976). This may explain why they were able to withstand the racism and hostility encountered in the United States.

According to Huang (1976), before 1949, when the People's Republic of China assumed control of the mainland, it was the practice of many older immigrants to return to China after they retired. One of the traditional values of the Chinese family is filial piety. Thus, retired immigrants could enjoy a period of old age filled with respect and obedience and surrounded by children and grandchildren they may have never seen. Since 1949 the luxury of returning to the homeland has been taken away from the elderly Chinese immigrant (Huang 1976).

Like the Japanese, older Chinese Americans may have difficulty adjusting to the American values of children and grandchildren. Huang reports an anecdote in this respect:

> Recently a mother confided in this writer that she and her husband were shocked to receive a letter from their son and Caucasian daughter-in-law. They were happy to hear from them, but not to be addressed as "Dear Jeanie and Jack." "At least she could address us as Father Wong and Mother Wong," she stated, meaning that undoubtedly it was the American daughter-in-law who instigated such a big dose of democracy in their new relationship. [Huang, L.J. 1976. The Chinese American family, in C. Mindel and R.W. Habenstein (eds.), *Ethnic Families in America*, p. 141. New York: Elsevier Scientific Publishing Co., Inc.]

More serious problems beset aged Chinese Americans as a result of the changing values of the young. For example, drug abuse is apparently high among older men, especially those isolated from family and community.

Another problem for older Chinese Americans may involve a new sense of relative deprivation. These feelings result from the recognition that a new glory period for the aged has begun in China where, unlike their U.S. counterparts, the elderly are better off than other segments of the population. A recent *New York Times* report suggests that elderly in China are the beneficiaries of both the traditional Chinese chivalry toward old age and a munificent Communist retirement policy (Butterfield 1979). According to this report, a retiring worker may bring in one of his or her children as a job replacement. This is a very important consideration under conditions of high unemployment among the young and serves to support the position of aged persons in the family. In addition, early retirees (at age sixty) may find a second job, particularly if they are skilled or technical workers in much demand. Between pensions and a second income, earnings can exceed preretirement income. Women may retire at age fifty, and many remain at home to care for grandchildren. As another benefit, if retired people agree to move to the countryside, whence many of them came, they receive a stipend from the state to build a new house. In general, it appears that policy decisions in areas such as employment, retirement, and housing have had the consequence of underscoring rather than undermining the position of the aged in the Chinese family and community.

China is no utopia for the old, however, and disparities do exist among the elderly. For example, the oldest segment of the aged, who have not worked in state enterprises, are disadvantaged because they are generally not covered by retirement benefits. In addition, large numbers of older people are left with little to do, because no formally organized recreation programs exist for those elderly not in old age homes. As one Chinese social researcher interested in the problems of old age commented, "Many are just waiting to die" (Goldstein and Goldstein 1986).

Assimilation of Elderly Asian American Immigrants. Immigration of Asian American elderly to the United States has continued through the 1970s into the 1980s. How do these elderly immigrants who have grown old in a traditional Asian culture adjust to life in the contemporary United States? Kim and Schwartz-Barcott (1983) did periodic participant observation over seven years with fourteen Korean elderly women ranging in age from fifty-five to sixty-eight at the time of initial contact. Their results suggest that this small group of women did unexpectedly, though exceptionally, well. All these women arrived in the United States in the early 1970s. They were all from urban areas; seven were widows, two were separated from their husbands, and five were married and had come to the United States with their husbands. They all initially lived with either their son's or daughter's families in Providence, Boston, Los Angeles, and Toronto.

Most of these women experienced a typical progression of adjustment from an initial period of high involvement in family life to a series of steps involving employment in nontraditional roles, movement into a single or shared apartment, and finally development of social ties based on friendship rather than on family networks. All the women expressed satisfaction at residing with their children's families, although this may have represented the socially acceptable response. Traditionally, it is assumed that women (especially widows) prefer to live with their children rather than alone. Yet within a year or two of their arrival, many of these women began talking about living independently of the family.

The results of this study suggest (at least in this group of women) that having a living arrangement that allowed a peer-group social network to develop along with financial independence provided a greater degree of satisfaction with life than when only either one of these conditions was possible. Interestingly, it appears that after a short period of adjustment to life in the United States, elderly Korean women in this study began to realize that there might be a wide array of options available for independence and social ties outside of family life and traditional roles for elderly women. For these women, achieving independence was an attraction that provided a high level of self-esteem and satisfaction with life.

SUMMARY

Most studies of aging are carried out on samples of whites. Recognition of the ethnic and social diversity present in the U.S. experience has only recently begun to be presented in social gerontology.

Many have characterized minority aging as a case of double jeopardy. This term is used to reflect the idea that the negative effects of aging are compounded among minority group members. Although, in general, research supports the notion of double jeopardy among black and Mexican American aged, some data suggest that aging may reduce ethnic differences that existed in middle life. Recently, some have contested the importance of a double-jeopardy concept of minority aging.

Lack of income is probably the most serious problem faced by aged blacks in the United States. Approximately one-half of aged blacks live in poverty, which has major impact on the health status of elderly blacks and underscores problems related to transportation and housing. Two areas of strength that have emerged for black elderly that are not related to income deprivation are family and religion.

Next to blacks, Hispanic Americans make up the largest minority in the United States. This population is quite heterogeneous, although about 61 percent of all Hispanic Americans are of Mexican heritage. As with black elderly, the problems of Hispanic elderly emanate primarily from their deprived income status. In addition, a growing generation gap between old and young leave many elderly Hispanics misunderstood by the society at large and by the young in their own families.

The aged American Indian population is quite small and relatively invisible. Their special history has clearly contributed to the deprived situation of aged American Indians. No simple social program can immunize the Native American elderly from a lifetime of inadequate nutrition, housing, and health service.

Asian Americans have been described as a model minority. This may be myth. Despite the successful economic assimilation of Japanese and Chinese Americans, the accommodation of younger generations to U.S. values has left many aged Asian Americans isolated from family and community. If this pattern continues, we can expect future generations of elderly Asian Americans to have expectations and experiences more like those of elderly whites than is currently the case.

STUDY QUESTIONS

1. Define *double jeopardy* as it relates to the minority aged. According to the study by Dowd and Bengtson, how accurately does this term describe the social situation of the minority aged in the United States? Can you offer a critique of the double-jeopardy concept?

2. Explain the term *housing-poor*. Why is it so central to any discussion of the black elderly in the United States?

3. Despite the economic problems that still confront elderly blacks, two major strengths of black culture should not be ignored. Identify and discuss the importance of these strengths.

4. The special needs of the Hispanic elderly are often understated because of the belief that Hispanics take care of their own. Give a more realistic picture of the modern Hispanic family.

5. How has the status of elderly American Indians changed over the last one hundred years?

6. Explain what is meant by the concept of *model minority* in referring to Asian Americans. In what way has this view of Asian Americans been detrimental to the social conditions of their elderly?

BIBLIOGRAPHY

Abbott, J. 1977. Socioeconomic characteristics of the elderly: Some black-white differences. *Social Security Bulletin* (July):16–42.

Alvirez, D., and Bean, F. 1976. The Mexican-American family. In C. Mindel and R. Habenstein (eds.), *Ethnic families in America*. New York: Elsevier Scientific Publishing Co., Inc.

Bahr, H. 1972. An end to invisibility. In H. Bahr, B. Chadwick, and R.C. Day (eds.), *Native Americans today*. New York: Harper and Row.

Barrow, G., and Smith, P. 1979. *Aging, ageism and society*. St. Paul, Minn.: West Publishing Company.

Belgrave, L.L. 1988. The effects of race differences in work history, work attitudes, economic resources, and health on women's retirement. *Research on Aging* 10(3):383–398.

Benedict, R. 1972. A profile of Indian aged. In *Minority aged in America*. Ann Arbor: University of Michigan.

Birch, D., et al. 1973. *America's housing needs: 1970 to 1980*. Cambridge, Mass.: Joint Center for Urban Studies, M.I.T. and Harvard University.

Burkey, R. 1978. *Ethnic and racial groups: The dynamics of dominance*. Menlo Park, Calif.: Cummings Publishing Co., Inc.

Butterfield, F. 1979. China's elderly find good life in retirement. *New York Times* July 29:1, 13.

Cattell, S. 1962. *Health, welfare and social organization in Chinatown.* New York: Community Service Society of New York.

Chen, Y.P. 1985. The economic status of the aging. In R.H. Binstock and E. Shanas (eds.), *Handbook of aging and the social sciences (2nd ed.).* New York: Van Nostrand Reinhold Co.

Cheng, E. 1978. *The elder Chinese.* San Diego: Campanile Press, San Diego State University.

Dancy, J. 1977. *The black elderly: A guide for practitioners.* Ann Arbor: Institute of Gerontology, The University of Michigan-Wayne State University.

Davis, F. 1976. The impact of Social Security taxes upon the poor: The case of black community. In *Economics of aging.* Ann Arbor: Institute of Gerontology, The University of Michigan-Wayne State University.

Dobyns, H. 1966. Estimating aboriginal American populations. *Current Anthropology* 7:395–416.

Dowd, J., and Bengtson, V. 1978. Aging in minority populations: An examination of the double jeopardy hypothesis. *Journal of Gerontology* 33:427–436.

Eitzen, D.S. 1986. *Social problems* (3d ed.). Boston: Allyn and Bacon, Inc.

Eribes, R.A., and Bradley-Rawls, M. 1978. The underutilization of nursing home facilities by Mexican-American elderly in the southwest. *Gerontologist* 18:363–371.

Espino, D.V., Neufeld, R.R., Mulvihill, M., and Libow, L.S. 1988. Hispanic and non-Hispanic elderly on admission to the nursing home: A pilot study. *Gerontologist* 28(6):821–824.

Farley, J.E. 1982. *Majority-minority relations.* Englewood Cliffs, N.J.: Prentice-Hall.

Feagin, J. 1984. *Racial and ethnic relations* (2nd ed.). Englewood Cliffs, N.J.: Prentice-Hall.

Feagin, J., and Fujitaki, N. 1972. On the assimilation of Japanese Americans. *American Journal 1 (February):15–17.*

Ferraro, K.F. 1987. Double jeopardy to health for black older adults? *Journal of Gerontology* 42(5):528–533.

Fujii, S. 1976. Elderly Asian Americans and use of public services. *Social Casework* (March):202–206.

Glazer, N., and Moynihan, D.P. 1963. *Beyond the melting pot.* Cambridge, Mass.: Harvard University Press and The M.I.T. Press.

Goldstein, A., and Goldstein, S. 1986. The challenge of an aging population: The case of the People's Republic of China. *Research on Aging* 8(2):179–199.

Greeley, A. 1974. *Ethnicity in the United States.* New York: John Wiley and Sons, Inc.

Greene, R.L., and Siegler, I.C. 1984. Blacks. In E.B. Palmore (ed.), *Handbook on the aged in the United States.* Westport, Conn.: Greenwood Press.

Hendricks, J., and Hendricks, C. 1977. *Aging in mass society.* Cambridge, Mass.: Winthrop Publishers, Inc.

Hill, R. 1971. A profile of the black aged. *Los Angeles Sentinel* October 7.

Huang, L.J. 1976. The Chinese American family. In C. Mindel and R. Habenstein (eds.), *Ethnic families in America.* New York: Elsevier Scientific Publishing Company, Inc.

Ishizuka, K. 1978. *The elder Japanese.* San Diego: The Campanile Press, San Diego State University.

Jackson, J. 1970. Aged negroes: Their cultural departures from statistical stereotypes and rural-urban differences. *Gerontologist* 10:140–145.

———. 1971. Negro aged: Toward needed research in social gerontology. *Gerontologist* 11:52–57.

———. 1985. Race, national, origin, ethnicity, and aging. In R.H. Binstock and E. Shanas (eds.), *Handbook of aging and the social sciences* (2nd ed.). New York: Van Nostrand Reinhold Co.

Jackson, M., and Wood, J. 1976. *Aging in America, No. 5: Implications for the black aged.* Washington, D.C.: National Council on the Aging.

Kalish, R., and Moriwaki, S. 1973. The world of the elderly Asian American. *Journal of Social Issues* 29(2):187–209.

Kastenbaum, R. 1971. The missing footnote. *Aging and Human Development* 2:155.

Kent, D. 1971a. Changing welfare to serve minority. In *Minority aged in America.* Ann Arbor: Institute of Gerontology.

———. 1971b. The elderly in minority groups: Variant patterns of aging. *Gerontologist* 11:26–29.

Kent, D., and Hirsch, C. 1969. Differentials in need and problem solving techniques among low income Negro and White elderly. Paper presented at the International Congress on Gerontology, Washington, D.C., June 1969.

Kim, B. 1973. Asian Americans: No model minority. *Social Work* 18(May):44–53.

Kim, H.S., and Schwartz-Barcott, D. 1983. Social network and adjustment process of Korean elderly women in America: Some unexpected findings. *Pacific/Asian American Mental Health Center Research Review* 2(3):1–2.

Kitano, H., and Kikumura, A. 1976. The Japanese American family. In C. Mindel and R. Habenstein (eds.), *Ethnic families in America.* New York: Scientific Publishing Company, Inc.

Krause, N. 1987. Stress in racial differences in self-reported health among the elderly. *Gerontologist* 27(1):72–76.

Lacayo, C. 1977. Research and the Hispanic elderly. Paper presented at the Texas State Department of Public Welfare Conference, January 14, McAllen, Texas.

Lyman, S. 1974. *Chinese Americans.* New York: Random House, Inc.

Maldonado, D. 1975. The Chicano aged. *Social Work* (May):213–216.

Manuel, R.C. 1982. The dimensions of ethnic minority identification: An exploratory analysis among elderly black Americans. In R.C. Manuel (ed.), *Minority aging: Sociological and social psychological issues.* Westport, Conn.: Greenwood Press.

Michigan Offices of Services to the Aging. 1975. *The Michigan comprehensive plan on aging.* Lansing, Mich.: Offices of Services to the Aging.

Montero, D. 1979. Disengagement and aging among the Issei. In D.E. Gelfand and A.J. Kutzik (eds.), *Ethnicity and aging: Theory, research, and policy.* New York: Springer Publishing Co.

Moore, J. 1971. Situational factors affecting minority aged. *Gerontologist* 11:88–93.

Osako, M.M., and Liu, W.T. 1986. Intergenerational relations and the aged among Japanese Americans. *Research on Aging* 8(1):128–155.

Price, J. 1976. North American Indian families. In C. Mindel and R. Habenstein (eds.), *Ethnic families in America*. New York: Elsevier Scientific Publishing Company, Inc.

Schaie, K.W., Drchowsky, S., and Parham, I.A. 1982. Measuring age and sociocultural change: The case of race and life satisfaction. In R.C. Manuel (ed.), *Minority aging: Sociological and social psychological issues*. Westport, Conn.: Greenwood Press.

Simmons, L. 1945. *The role of the aged in primitive society*. New Haven, Conn.: Yale University Press.

Simon, D.R., and Eitzen, D.S. 1982. *Elite deviance*. Boston: Allyn and Bacon, Inc.

Sotomayor, M. 1971. Mexican-American interaction with social systems. *Social Casework* 5(May):321.

Stack, C. 1970. The kindred of Viola Jackson: Residence and family organization of an urban black American family. In N. Whitten and J. Szwed (eds.), *Afro-American anthropology*. New York: The Free Press.

Stanford, E.P. 1978. *The elder black*. San Diego: Center on Aging, San Diego State University.

Steglich, W., Cartwright, W., and Crouch, B. 1968. *Study of needs and resources among aged Mexican-Americans*. Lubbock, Tex.: Texas Technological College.

Taylor, R.J., and Taylor, W.H. 1982. The social and economic status of the black elderly. *Phylon* 43:295–306.

Taylor, R.J., and Chatters, L.M. 1988. Correlates of education, income, and poverty among aged blacks. *Gerontologist* 28(4):435–441.

Torres-Gil, F. 1976. Political behavior: A study of political attitudes and political participation among older Mexican Americans. Unpublished doctoral dissertation. Brandeis University, Waltham, Mass.

Turner, J. 1978. *Sociology: Studying the human system*. Santa Monica, Calif.: Goodyear Publishing Co., Inc.

U.S. Senate Special Committee on Aging. 1971. *The multiple hazards of age and race*. Washington, D.C.: U.S. Government Printing Office.

Valle, R., and Mendoza, L. 1978. *The elder Latino*. San Diego: Center on Aging, San Diego State University.

White House Conference on Aging. 1972. *The Asian American elderly*. Washington, D.C.: U.S. Government Printing Office.

Wilson, W.J. 1978. *The declining significance of race: Blacks and changing American institutions*. Chicago: University of Chicago Press.

CHAPTER 16

LIVING ENVIRONMENTS OF THE ELDERLY

Elderly Americans, like those of all ages, reside in a variety of settings—from single-room occupancy hotels to Palm Springs condominiums, urban homes and apartments, and isolated rural farmhouses. Although the first public housing units designated explicitly for the elderly were mandated in the 1959 Housing Act, not until about 1966 did attention and discussion among gerontologists begin to be directed toward the special problems of the elderly in securing physically adequate housing at a reasonable cost. Most recently, gerontologists have addressed the broader questions about the relationship between behavior and living environments. In particular, some have asked, "How and to what extent is the physical, social, and psychological functioning of an elderly individual influenced by the kind of environment in which he or she lives?" This chapter summarizes some of the growing body of literature that has appeared in response to this question. We begin by addressing some general issues important to understanding the impact of the environment on older people.

THE IMPACT OF ENVIRONMENT ON OLDER PEOPLE

According to the 1971 White House Conference on Aging, housing is probably the single most important element in the life of an older person, aside from his or her spouse. Still, as Carp (1976) points out, one sign of the growing maturity of this subfield of gerontology is recognition of the limited utility in considering housing out of context. Gerontologists have come to understand that, although number of rooms, square footage, or closet space are important, so is the broader living environment in which the housing unit is located.

The main elements of this living environment include characteristics of the neighborhood and community such as (1) the age and ownership of the dwelling unit, (2) the physical condition and availability of funds for maintenance and repair, (3) the location of the dwelling unit with regard to services needed by older people, (4) the proximity to commercial and recreational activities, (5) the proximity to relatives and age peers, (6) the accessibility and usability of transportation, and (7) the congeniality or threat in the surrounding environment—for example, poor street lighting or high crime rates (Carp 1966; Havighurst 1969).

What kind of neighborhood environment is most supportive for older persons? Chapman and Beaudet (1983) have explored the relationship between the neighborhood as a physical and social context and the well-being of a sample of relatively frail elderly persons living independently in a variety of community settings within Multnomah County (Portland), Oregon. Measures of the physical and social environments of the sample groups, the personal characteristics of the respondents, and their well-being were developed out of personal interviews. Environmental variables used in the analysis were house type, neighborhood quality, crime rate, age concentration of the neighborhood, distance to services, the social status of the neighborhood area, and distance to the city center.

The important part of this analysis involved determining whether, when personal characteristics are controlled for, environmental variables are useful predictors of the well-being of frail elderly people. Using a measure of life satisfaction as a global indicator of well-being, Chapman and Beaudet found that people living in higher quality neighborhoods were significantly more satisfied with their lives. How satisfied were people with their neighborhoods? Living in a higher quality neighborhood and living relatively far from downtown both significantly increased satisfaction with the neighborhood.

Three additional indicators of well-being were employed. Each provides a measure of social interaction with others. Interaction with neighbors was highest among those individuals residing in good-quality neighborhoods, relatively far from the center of the city, and with a low percentage of older people in the area. Frequent social contact with friends and relatives was associated with the environmental variables of good neighborhood quality, relatively low social status of the neighborhood, a low crime rate in the area, and relatively greater distance from the city center. No environmental variables were predictive of a general activity level measured by the frequency of visits to the bank, grocer, and other families.

The environmental variables most consistently associated with well-being were increased distance from the center of the city and the quality of the neighborhood. Quality of the neighborhood is a composite measure reflecting a residential area that is quiet, has little traffic, and is well maintained and landscaped. Such attributes suggest a neighborhood that is especially well suited to the competence levels of the frail elderly. One surprising finding is the failure of distance to services to show any value in predicting well-being. As Chapman and Beaudet point out, however, this may simply result from members of the study population having available social contacts and supports on whom they can rely to provide transportation.

Lawton and Nahemow (1973) have attempted to classify living environments on the basis of the demands they place on older people. Some living environments make greater physical, social, and psychological demands on people than others do. As a result, it is possible to place living environments on a hypothetical continuum from "very demanding" to "not demanding at all." Following the terminology of the noted psychologist Henry Murray (1938), Lawton and Nahemow use the term "environmental press" to describe this continuum. They posit that when a person of a given level of competence behaves in an environment of a given press level, the outcome can be placed on a scale from positive to negative (Lawton 1980a). Another way of describing this is to talk of the *fit* between an individual's competence and the environment in which that individual resides. When the fit is good, the competence of an individual will be consistent with the demands of the environment, and adaptation is positive. This may be the case for the great majority of older people. When environmental demands are too great, adaptation is poor and the outcome is negative.

An example may be useful. Mrs. L. is seventy years old and resides with her never-married brother. Mrs. L. has been a diabetic for thirty years and suffers from heart disease as well. She requires frequent medical care, including in-home personal care. When Mrs. L. began to show signs of mild confusion and forgetfulness, she was no longer able to meet the demands of the living environment. She was less able to participate in her own care and often found it difficult to navigate her way through the small house in which she and her brother resided. Her brother tried to find some home assistance, but this was scarce and expensive. Fearing for his sister's safety, the brother reluctantly sought a nursing home.

A small change in the environment, such as the presence of a homemaker, might have reduced the environmental press and made it compatible with Mrs. L.'s competence. She might have been able to defer entrance to the institution. Lawton and Simon (1968) stated this relationship between environmental press and individual competence in the form of a principle referred to as the *environmental docility hypothesis:* the less competent the individual, the greater the impact of environmental factors on that individual.

This principle is particularly relevant to older people because of the broad way in which Lawton (1980a) has chosen to view competence. Competence is reflected not only in terms of characteristics within the person—such as biological health, sensorimotor coordination, cognitive skills—it also reflects external processes, including age discrimination, social isolation, mandatory retirement, and reduced income. These social deprivations may be suffered by any of us as we age, although the elderly are particularly vulnerable to them.

The occurrence of one or more of these phenomena may tell us nothing about the competence of the individual who experiences them. Yet, the individual often experiences these occurrences as reductions in competence. Although the deprivation occurs outside the person, it may significantly affect his or her ability to deal with the environmental press (Lawton 1980a).

The environmental docility hypothesis has a positive side. If features of the broader living environment can deprive individuals of competence, then perhaps there are features of the living environment that can increase competence and elevate the quality of life. As Lawton (1980a) has stated, "[I]f we could design housing with fewer barriers, neighborhoods with more enriching resources, or institutions with higher stimulating qualities, we could improve the level of functioning of many older people more than proportionately."

Achieving the ideal fit between the individual and the living environment may be difficult in the real world. This is reflected in Lawton's (1980b) discussion of two contrasting developmental models of independent living environments: the constant model and the accommodating model. The *constant* model attempts to maintain the essential character of the environment and assumes that the needs of residents remain relatively stable over time. The *accommodating* model assumes that all aspects of the environment (including the resident) change over time.

According to Lawton (1980b), characteristics of the constant model are as follows:

1. Admission criteria for replacement tenants are the same as those for original tenants.
2. Criteria for continued residence are established so that administrators may initiate termination of residence when a tenant's physical or mental condition declines below a specific level.
3. Termination of residence because of reduced independence leads to transfer to either the home of a family member, congregate housing, or an institution. Some individuals will experience multiple transfers—to the home of a family member and then again to an institution—and much research (to be discussed) demonstrates that such late life relocations are undesirable.
4. The community continues to regard the housing environment as a place for independent living; thus, there is a continuation of the effort to recruit replacement tenants who are fully independent.

In some contrast, a typical accommodating environment might be characterized as follows:

1. Criteria for continued residence in the environment are considerably less stringent than those applied to the original applicants.
2. Changes in tenants' physical and mental condition require the addition of a variety of services, including on-site health services.

3. The provision of such services requires alteration in the physical environment to provide for the delivery of such services.

4. The needs of tenants do not change at an equal rate; thus, at first, new services provided are not cost-effective. Moreover, there will be a mix of independent and less-independent residents.

5. Admission criteria for replacement tenants may be relaxed as the service environment changes to be able to provide for less independent tenants.

6. The community image of the housing changes such that more marginally independent people apply in greater numbers. Over an extended period of time, such an accommodating environment could evolve into a long-term care institution.

As Lawton (1980b) points out, most housing environments are not as extreme as the two types characterized here. Still, housing that attempts to become accommodating certainly may face difficulty in remaining financially viable while attempting to provide services in physical settings not originally planned to function in this way. At the same time, those environments that attempt to remain constant and resist accommodation face the unpleasant task of terminating residence because of the lack of services or of maintaining marginal tenants without being able to provide them with needed services.

Ehrlich, Ehrlich, and Woehlke (1982) completed a needs assessment that examined the tenant population of the Delcrest Apartments for the Elderly in St. Louis, Missouri. Essentially, they asked, "Can a congregate housing program remain constant over a long period of time (thirteen years) without making some attempt to accommodate to an aging population?" Their findings failed to support an accommodating environment concept. Yet, the constant model embodied in the original program was not sufficient to take into account the diverse needs represented in a population of young-old and old-old residents.

The authors put forth what is described as a balanced environmental model that allowed for the maintenance of the traditional mobile-well independent environment while still guaranteeing some support for those with need. In many respects, this balanced model sits midway between the constant and the accommodating models described by Lawton. In particular, Ehrlich and her colleagues emphasized the importance of strengthening informal support networks, as evidence suggests the feasibility of elderly people assisting each other in all basic supportive tasks, such as crisis intervention, activities of daily living, and advice giving.

WHERE DO THE ELDERLY LIVE?

In Chapter 3, we discussed the geographical distribution of the elderly in the United States, including their residential mobility and concentration. This section describes the living arrangements of older people, the characteristics of

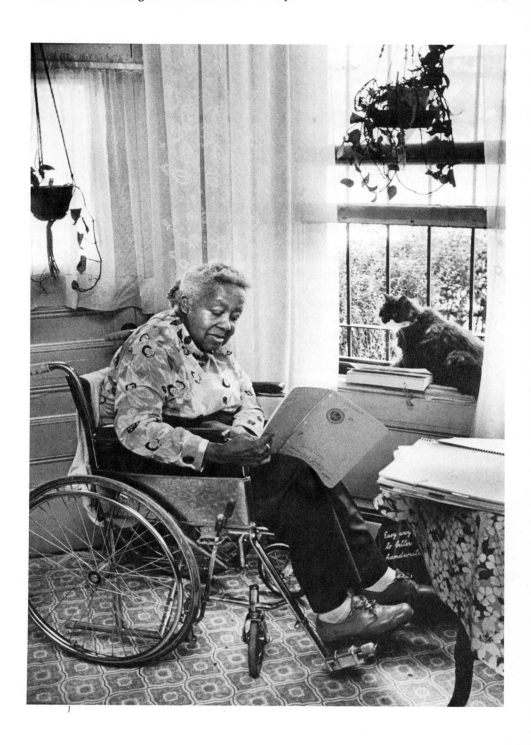

their housing, and the degree of satisfaction they have with their housing situations.

Living Arrangements

Nearly all elderly live in independent households. Approximately two-thirds of the elderly were living with family in 1980, with the great majority of these married and residing with spouse. Table 16-1 presents data on the living arrangements of the elderly, by sex and age, for 1980. In 1980 only about 5 percent of the elderly were in institutions on any given day. Chapter 17 discusses the elderly in old-age institutions.

The household composition of elderly men and women is strikingly different and reflects the differences in marital status between the sexes. In 1980, elderly women were about 2.5 times as likely to live alone as men (36.9 versus 14.1 percent), whereas almost three-quarters (71.8 percent) of all aged men are married and living with their wives.

The proportion of the elderly living alone is increasing. In 1965, for example, 29.9 percent of aged women lived alone as compared with 36.9 percent in 1980. In addition, the proportion of older men and women who live alone increases with age. This seems to be chiefly the result of the increasing number of widows among the elderly, and the fact that more elderly persons today can afford to live alone than in the past (Manard, Kart, and van Gils 1975). Among men, the percentage living alone increases from 10.9 at age sixty-five to sixty-nine to 21.7 among those eighty-five years and over. Among women, the percentage living alone increases from 29.5 at ages sixty-five to sixty-nine to 44.2 at ages seventy-five to seventy-nine but declines to 33.3 among women eighty-five and over. This decline is more than offset by the dramatic increase in the proportion of very old women living in group quarters. More than one-fourth (27.7 percent) of women aged eighty-five years and over live in homes for the elderly. This compares with 13.1 percent for women aged eighty to eighty-four.

Poverty and physical illness or disability are two reasons that may determine the choice of a shared household, even one with nonfamily members. Beth Soldo (1979) has analyzed 1970 census data and found that older people living with relatives are twice as likely to have low incomes as older people living independently. When the low income of the elderly person is pooled with that of the household in which he or she resides, a higher quality of living may be afforded all. Soldo found that 30 percent of elderly people living alone had incomes below the poverty level; among those living with younger relatives only 8 percent of the household incomes were below the poverty level.

Living in the household of a nonrelative or a relative other than spouse sometimes implies greater limitations in mobility and activity than does living with a spouse or alone. Although differences are not extraordinarily large, data from the National Health Interview Surveys do suggest that a shared household may act as protection when circumstances preclude maintaining an independent household.

TABLE 16-1 Living Arrangements of Persons 65 Years and Older By Age and Sex, 1980

Sex	65+	65–69	70–74	75–79	80–84	85+
				Age		
Male						
All males	10,262,568	3,880,624	2,859,530	1,842,694	1,011,742	667,978
In group quarters	4.0%	1.7%	2.6%	4.3%	7.9%	17.0%
In households	96.0%	98.3%	97.4%	95.7%	92.1%	83.0%
Householders or spouse	89.7%	93.6%	92.2%	89.1%	83.0%	67.9%
In families	74.8%	81.9%	78.4%	72.0%	62.1%	45.3%
Married, spouse present	71.8%	79.3%	75.6%	68.8%	58.2%	40.0%
In nonfamily households	14.9%	11.7%	13.8%	17.1%	20.8%	22.6%
Living alone	14.1%	10.9%	13.1%	16.4%	20.1%	21.7%
Other relatives of householder	5.0%	3.5%	4.0%	5.3%	7.8%	13.6%
Children or grandchildren	.2%	.4%	.2%	.1%	.0	.1%
Parent of householder	2.1%	1.0%	1.5%	2.3%	3.9%	7.7%
Males living with nonrelatives	1.3%	1.2%	1.2%	1.3%	1.3%	1.5%
Female						
All females	15,235,818	4,887,335	3,962,619	2,952,351	1,906,812	1,524,701
In group quarters	7.0%	1.7%	3.1%	6.3%	13.1%	27.7%
In households	93.0%	98.3%	96.9%	93.7%	86.9%	72.3%
Householders or spouse	80.7%	90.2%	86.9%	80.5%	69.4%	48.4%
In families	42.7%	59.7%	47.8%	35.1%	23.6%	13.9%
Married, spouse present	34.7%	51.8%	39.9%	26.8%	15.0%	5.9%
In nonfamily households	37.9%	30.5%	39.1%	45.4%	45.8%	34.5%
Living alone	36.9%	29.5%	38.1%	44.2%	44.7%	33.3%
Other relatives of householder	11.4%	7.1%	9.1%	12.2%	16.6%	22.8%
Children or grandchildren	.2%	.5%	.2%	.1%	.1%	.1%
Parent of householder	5.4%	2.8%	3.9%	5.8%	8.6%	13.1%
Females living with nonrelatives	1.0%	1.0%	1.0%	1.0%	1.0%	1.1%

Source: U.S. Bureau of the Census, 1980 Census of Population and Housing, Vol. 1, Chapter D, Table 265.

Housing Characteristics

Most Americans, including the elderly, live in single-family owner-occupied homes. Of the almost 18 million households headed by older persons in 1983, 75 percent were owner-occupied, and 25 percent were rental units. As Table 16-2 shows, patterns of home ownership vary widely by age, sex, and living arrangements. Among males up to age eighty and for all females, the elderly are more likely to own their own home than are householders aged twenty-five to sixty-four. Regardless of age, people who live alone are more likely to rent than are married persons. Generally, householders at advanced ages are more likely to be renters; 20 percent of males and 41.4 percent of females aged fifty-five to fifty-nine rent, whereas 35.4 percent of males and 49.2 percent of females aged eighty-five and over do similarly.

Homes owned by the elderly are older than those owned by younger people. In 1980 about 40 percent of elderly householders lived in structures built in 1939 or earlier; another 12 or 13 percent lived in structures built between 1940 and 1949. There is a difference in the age of the structures in which different cohorts live. For example, 62.2 percent of female householders aged eighty-five or older lived in structures built before 1940; 44.7 percent of female householders aged fifty-five to fifty-nine lived in such aged structures.

Despite the high visibility accorded elderly migrants to the South and West, most elderly people remain in the homes they have long lived in. Among persons sixty-five years and over, high percentages have been living in their houses for thirty or more years, and these percentages increase in each successive cohort. According to the 1980 census, about two-thirds of the elderly aged seventy-five years or older moved into their current homes before 1970.

Housing Quality. There has been poignant evidence of elderly persons living in dirty, unsafe, and thoroughly wretched conditions. In general, however, defining what constitutes adequate housing has been problematic. There is no consensus on what measures should be included in such a standard.

A commonly used indicator of inadequate housing is "incomplete plumbing." The U.S. Census category "with all plumbing facilities" is composed of housing units that have hot and cold piped water, a flush toilet, and a bath or shower—all within the structure and for the exclusive use of the occupants of the unit. Because of urban–rural differences and the fact, for example, that residents of an otherwise delightful lodging house may share shower facilities, "incomplete plumbing" does not always tell us much about housing quality.

A study completed by the Joint Center for Urban Studies and the Massachusetts Institute of Technology and Harvard University estimated that 31 percent of all homes with incomplete plumbing are also dilapidated, with such defects as "holes, open cracks, substantial sagging of floors and roof," and so on (Birch et al. 1973). The study provided no comparable estimate for the incidence of dilapidation among homes with complete plumbing.

According to the 1983 American Housing Survey, only 2.4 percent of elderly housing units had incomplete plumbing facilities. Viewed from a different perspective, however, elderly-headed housing units represented 21 percent of the units included in the 1983 survey, but they made up 25.7 percent of units lacking complete plumbing facilities. Elderly-headed households also made up 25.7 percent of units lacking complete kitchen facilities, and 22.9 percent with one or more bedrooms lacking privacy (U.S. Senate Special Committee on Aging 1985–86).

Struyk and Soldo (1980) used six indicators of deficiencies in their study of the quality of elderly housing. These indicators of housing inadequacy were related to plumbing, kitchen facilities, sewage, heat, maintenance, and public halls. For example, a housing unit must be declared deficient if either it lacks a complete kitchen or the household must share kitchen use or if the heating system was completely unusable for six or more hours at least three times during the past winter. The elderly were found to have a higher incidence than the nonelderly of incomplete plumbing and kitchen facilities. Elderly and nonelderly households had a similar proportion of heating system and sewage breakdowns, but elderly owners had slightly more maintenance deficiencies than did their nonelderly counterparts, and elderly renters had less.

What quality indicators do older people themselves identify as most salient in their housing? Lawton (1980c) lists two that appear stronger than the others. Having more bathrooms characterizes luxury dwelling units and is probably related to newness of housing. Central heating is also important and strongly related to housing satisfaction. In fact, Lawton suggests that if we are to choose a system whose improvement will add most to older occupants' perceived satisfaction with housing, it is the heating system that should be given highest priority.

High-quality living environments can show up in the most unlikely places. J. Kevin Eckert (1980) has studied the "unseen elderly" who reside in single-room occupancy (SRO) hotels in San Diego. A distinguishing feature of these living environments for older people is that men outnumber women. In virtually every other residential setting for older persons, older women predominate.

Ten women reside in one SRO, the Ballentine Hotel, on a permanent basis. Four of the women have lived in the hotel for more than ten years. They are old and retired. As a group, the women view the hotel as home and prefer it to other living arrangements they have experienced. Why would the SRO be preferable to an apartment? One woman answers:

> The advantages are that you have a lot of people. If you get tired of staying in your room, you can go to the lobby, then back to your room. I don't like apartments because here if you get sick or anything happens you get help right away. If you live in an apartment by yourself, you can drop dead and no one will know the difference. That's what I like about living here. I can get help right away if something happens, which is good health-wise. (p. 118)

The availability of social supports in the SRO is a theme expressed by both older men and women. As Eckert points out above, living in the hotel gives

TABLE 16-2   Housing Tenure for Specified Living Arrangements, by Age and Sex of Householder, 1980: Percentages

Age and Sex	Tenure	Number of Households	Living Arrangements						
			Living Alone	Living with Spouse	Living with Sibling	Living with Children	Living with Other Relatives	Living with Nonrelatives	Total
Male									
25–64	Own	26,100,960	28.2%	77.6%	44.9%	53.7%	54.5%	27.5%	70.0%
	Rent	11,169,480	71.8%	22.4%	55.1%	46.3%	45.5%	72.5%	30.0%
55–59	Own	3,193,120	36.2%	85.5%	66.7%	65.7%	62.7%	43.1%	80.0%
	Rent	799,840	63.8%	14.5%	33.3%	34.3%	37.3%	56.9%	20.0%
60–64	Own	2,656,760	40.3%	84.5%	69.4%	68.2%	65.3%	41.3%	79.1%
	Rent	700,760	59.7%	15.5%	30.6%	31.8%	34.7%	58.7%	20.9%
63–69	Own	2,094,940	43.9%	82.4%	67.0%	70.6%	60.0%	43.7%	76.8%
	Rent	632,140	56.1%	17.6%	33.0%	29.4%	40.0%	36.3%	23.2%
70–74	Own	1,460,260	46.2%	79.8%	65.9%	69.1%	63.1%	48.0%	74.0%
	Rent	512,740	53.8%	20.2%	34.1%	30.9%	36.9%	52.0%	26.0%
75–79	Own	860,980	48.8%	76.0%	66.9%	73.0%	66.1%	47.8%	70.2%
	Rent	365,860	51.2%	24.0%	33.1%	27.0%	33.9%	52.2%	29.8%
80–84	Own	422,320	51.0%	72.5%	66.9%	75.9%	69.4%	57.2%	66.8%
	Rent	209,540	49.0%	27.5%	33.1%	24.1%	30.6%	42.8%	33.2%
85 and over	Own	220,880	52.2%	70.2%	62.7%	78.9%	75.8%	65.5%	64.6%
	Rent	121,120	47.8%	29.8%	37.3%	21.1%	24.2%	34.5%	35.4%

							Female		
25–64	Own	4,879,700	36.9%	70.9%	47.7%	41.6%	56.1%	30.6%	42.8%
	Rent	6,534,400	63.1%	29.1%	52.3%	58.4%	43.9%	69.4%	57.2%
55–59	Own	804,180	51.6%	82.5%	66.2%	62.5%	59.7%	58.0%	58.6%
	Rent	568,500	48.4%	17.5%	33.8%	37.5%	40.3%	42.0%	41.4%
60–64	Own	864,980	53.1%	83.2%	65.6%	66.1%	63.2%	58.3%	58.7%
	Rent	609,800	46.9%	16.8%	34.4%	33.9%	36.8%	41.7%	41.3%
65–69	Own	949,520	53.0%	82.7%	65.0%	68.7%	63.0%	59.0%	57.4%
	Rent	704,860	47.0%	17.3%	35.0%	31.3%	37.0%	41.0%	42.6%
70–74	Own	896,180	51.7%	80.0%	65.8%	69.3%	62.8%	65.2%	55.5%
	Rent	719,580	48.3%	20.0%	34.2%	30.7%	37.2%	34.8%	44.5%
75–79	Own	717,980	49.3%	77.8%	62.1%	70.5%	63.4%	64.5%	52.9%
	Rent	640,120	50.7%	22.2%	37.9%	29.5%	36.6%	35.3%	47.1%
80–84	Own	452,260	47.2%	75.9%	63.5%	71.5%	63.1%	64.4%	51.0%
	Rent	434,040	52.8%	24.1%	36.5%	28.5%	36.9%	35.6%	49.0%
85 and over	Own	272,980	45.9%	71.2%	65.4%	71.6%	65.5%	65.9%	50.8%
	Rent	264,600	54.1%	28.8%	34.6%	28.4%	34.3%	34.1%	49.2%

Source: U.S. Bureau of the Census, 1980 Census of Population and Housing, Public Use Microdata Sample, special tabulations.

them instant access to a helping network. Women seem more likely than men to be involved in social networks and to have worked out supportive arrangements with others. Such arrangements are more likely worked out with other women, although, since the SRO is a predominantly male environment, the women do have a large pool of older men from which to choose relationships. For many of these older women, living in a hotel is an adaptive strategy that provides benefits over and above those of other living environments.

Cost of Housing. A principal problem for the elderly is that they have to pay too large a portion of their incomes to meet housing expenses. Struyk (1977) has suggested 30 percent or more of total income devoted to housing as a criterion for an excessive housing burden. Housing costs vary depending on homeownership status. Table 16-3 shows housing costs as a percentage of household income, by age and sex of the householder in 1980. Housing costs include gross rent or mortgage, basic utility costs—for all owners and renters if such fees are not included in rent—and real estate taxes and insurance for owners.

For males aged seventy to seventy-four in 1980, housing costs are 23.5 percent of income for renters and 24 percent for owners with a mortgage, but only 12.5 percent for owners without a mortgage. Housing costs as a percentage of income increase with age. The general pattern is the same for females, although percentage of household income spent on housing is higher for females. For females aged seventy to seventy-four in 1980, housing costs are 30.8 percent of income for renters and 36.5 percent for owners with a mortgage; housing costs for owners without a mortgage are 19.1 percent of household income.

Three important points on the housing costs of the elderly are evident from Table 16-3 and additional data (U.S. Senate Special Committee on Aging 1985):

TABLE 16-3   Housing Costs as a Percentage of Household Income, by Age and Sex of Householder

	Median Percentage by Age							
	25 to 64	55 to 59	60 to 64	65 to 69	70 to 74	75 to 79	80 to 84	85 plus
Male								
Rent	18.4	16.2	17.8	21.7	23.5	24.6	25.5	25.8
Own, with mortgage	18.1	13.9	15.6	20.5	24.0	27.6	30.5	33.4
Own, without mortgage	7.2	7.0	8.1	10.9	12.5	13.5	14.6	15.6
Female								
Rent	27.2	25.9	27.2	29.8	30.8	31.4	31.7	31.8
Own, with mortgage	24.7	22.8	26.1	33.1	36.5	37.4	38.4	39.3
Own, without mortgage	13.1	12.8	14.6	17.5	19.1	20.5	21.4	22.3

Source: U.S. Bureau of the Census, 1980 Census of Population and Housing, Public Use Microdata Sample, special tabulations.

1. Lower income households pay a higher proportion of their income for housing. This occurs regardless of age, sex, or homeownership status.

2. At more advanced ages people pay a higher proportion of their income for housing. This is consistent for males and females and homeownership category.

3. Female householders pay proportionately more for their housing than do male householders, at all ages and in all homeownership categories.

Satisfaction with Housing. There have been a number of efforts to assess the satisfaction older people have with their housing. In general, the elderly view their housing *and* their neighborhoods in much the same way younger people do. If anything, their assessments are likely to be somewhat more positive. In part, this may reflect a strong attachment of older people to their homes and neighborhood. As we have seen, a great proportion of the elderly have spent the better part of their adult lives in their present homes and neighborhoods.

Another explanation for the high satisfaction elderly have with their living environments reflects the options available. When an individual has no options, assessments of even highly deficient environments may be satisfactory. Several studies report favorable ratings by residents of housing that "objective" investigators rated as poor (Britton 1966; Hamovitch, Peterson, and Larson 1969). Their evaluations contain an element of psychological defense on the part of the elderly. This view is supported by Carp's (1976) report of changes in evaluations of housing that occurred when an option became available. In each of two situations of public housing, before anyone moved in, evaluations of current housing became more negative among applicants who were offered apartments and remained stable for those who were not.

This is not to say that there is no correlation between subjective assessments of housing by the elderly and more objective indicators of housing quality. Using data in the Annual Housing Survey, Lawton and Hoover (1979) found a modest correlation (.36) between older people's subjective ratings of housing quality and a summed index based on higher socioeconomic status households, owner-occupied structures, and newer housing.

O'Bryant (1982) investigated the housing satisfaction of elderly living in a large midwestern metropolitan area. She was particularly interested in whether the subjective or objective factors better explained satisfaction with housing. She found that subjective factors—including, for example, feelings of competence and emotional security that can be derived from a home—explained more of the variation in housing satisfaction than did demographic characteristics of residents or objective housing characteristics.

When controlling for individual differences, Golant (1985) identified six social and physical environmental experiences that helped explain life satisfaction among a sample of aged respondents in Evanston, Illinois. In the order of their contribution (from high to low), these measures were feeling bored in dwelling, thinking about memories of personal things, having a good time in the community or neighborhood, being satisfied with stores and shopping in the community, feeling lonely, and becoming annoyed because appliances have broken down. As Golant (1985) points out, these social and physical environmental experiences that influence life satisfaction emphasize the multidimensional content of the environment that impinges on the lives of older people.

In an overall assessment of the neighborhood, Struyk and Soldo (1980) report that the distinction between homeowners and renters appears to be more salient than that between elderly and nonelderly; 25 to 30 percent of renters rate their neighborhood as "fair" or "poor"; only 12 to 13 percent of homeowners give such ratings. Interestingly, the elderly and nonelderly both viewed the lack of adequate public transportation as the greatest service inadequacy in their neighborhoods. Table 16-4 summarizes the views of elderly and nonelderly toward neighborhood conditions and services. In general, the elderly found fewer bothersome conditions in their neighborhoods than did the nonelderly. Street noise and neighborhood crime lead the list of complaints for both groups.

Fear of Crime. Over the twenty years or so, any number of writers and researchers have reported on the reality and pervasiveness of fear among the elderly. Some have described the elderly as living under "house arrest." Many have pointed out, however, that such fear is out of proportion to the actual probability of an elderly person being a victim of crime. Generally, older people are victimized least often, but the rate for "larceny with contact" (for example, purse snatching and wallet stealing) is selectively high for older people (Yin 1980).

More recently, the relationship between age and fear of crime has been the subject of renewed scrutiny. This seems to be the result of two different motivations. On the one hand, researchers have sought to distinguish segments of the elderly population that are more or less fearful of crime. On the other hand, investigators have employed a variety of test factors, including residential location and income, to explain the relationship between age and fear of crime. For example, Braungart, Braungart, and Hoyer (1980), using a nationwide sample, found that the elderly were only somewhat more fearful of crime than were their younger and middle-aged counterparts. These researchers identified gender as more strongly related to fear of crime than either age or community size. Using Washington State residents, Lee (1982) reports that elderly urban dwellers showed more fear of walking alone in their own neighborhood than did elderly residents of rural areas, although they did not estimate their chances of being victimized much differently. Interestingly, when the actual incidence of recalled victimization was introduced into the analysis, the statistical significance of residential location disappeared.

Petee, Kart, and Palmer (1985) used 1982 General Social Survey data to test the effects of age, sex, income, and residential location on fear of crime. Several different analyses yielded the same final results. Sex and residence had direct effects on fear of crime. Females and big-city dwellers tended to show fear;

TABLE 16-4 Percentage Distribution of Resident Opinions of Neighborhood Conditions, by Age of Household Head, Type of Household Headed by the Elderly, and Tenure Status, 1976

Condition	Renters					Owner-Occupants				
			Elderly Household Type					Elderly Household Type		
	Nonelderly	Elderly	Husband–Wife	Single Persons	Other	Nonelderly	Elderly	Husband–Wife	Single Persons	Other
Neighborhood conditions viewed as bothersome										
Street noise	15	12	13	12	11	12	12	12	9	13
Heavy traffic	12	9	10	9	7	10	9	9	8	11
Roads in poor condition	10	4	5	4	8	13	8	8	6	9
Roads impassable due to rain, snow	6	3	4	2	4	7	4	4	3	4
Inadequate street lighting	10	4	4	4	6	10	5	5	5	4
Neighborhood crime	16	13	15	13	12	13	12	9	7	10
Trash, litter, and junk	13	7	8	7	8	9	10	8	9	10
Abandoned buildings	4	2	2	2	2	2	2	1	3	2
Occupied housing in poor condition	7	3	4	2	4	6	3	3	4	3
Commercial or industrial activities	3	2	1	2	1	3	2	2	3	2
Odors, smoke, or gas	7	4	5	4	4	6	5	5	5	4
Noise from airplane traffic	6	6	7	6	6	6	6	6	5	5
Inadequate services										
Public transport	23	20	22	14	23	41	37	38	36	34
Stores	12	16	12	13	10	14	17	14	19	20
Police protection	9	8	10	7	7	10	8	9	8	9
Fire protection	3	2	3	2	2	6	5	5	5	5
Hospitals	10	8	9	9	8	14	13	12	15	12
Rating of neighborhood										
Excellent	20	28	27	29	22	41	41	43	40	34
Good	50	47	45	47	49	46	45	44	46	49
Fair	25	20	23	18	24	11	12	12	11	14
Poor	5	4	4	4	5	1	1	1	2	3

Source: Struyk, R. and Soldo, B. *Improving the Elderly's Housing.* Copyright 1980, Ballinger Publishing Co. Reprinted with permission of Ballinger Division, Harper & Row Publishers, Inc.

males and rural residents tended not to show fear. There were no effects of age.

FEDERAL SUPPORT OF HOUSING FOR THE ELDERLY

In 1908, a Presidential housing commission examined the problem of slums in America's cities. Appointed by President Theodore Roosevelt, the commission was particularly interested in those eastern seaboard cities that had become the entry point for masses of new immigrants (Jacobs, Harney, Edson, and Lane 1986). Federal intervention in housing in the country's major cities was recommended. Not until 1918, after World War I, however, did Congress intervene by authorizing a loan program for housing construction for shipyard workers. In 1918 Congress also created the U.S. Housing Commission and authorized the development of twenty-five community housing projects for defense workers.

The Great Depression of 1932 marked the beginning of large-scale federal intervention in housing. Between 1932 and 1937 several important government initiatives were begun. For example, direct funding of low-income housing and slum clearance was provided under the Emergency Relief and Construction Act of 1932, and The National Housing Act of 1934 created the Federal Housing Administration (FHA) to provide government insurance for mortgages made by private lenders.

Jacobs and his colleagues (1986) describe the Housing Act of 1949 as the beginning of the modern era in federal housing and development programs. This Act declared that the quality of life of the nation's people required "housing production and related community development sufficient to remedy the serious housing shortage, the elimination of substandard and other inadequate housing through the clearance of slums and blighted areas, and the realization as soon as feasible of the goal of a decent home and a suitable living environment for every American family."

The Housing Act of 1959 provided public housing specifically for the elderly, with the creation of two new programs. Section 231 of the National Housing Act provided Federal Housing Administration mortgage insurance for rental projects for the elderly, and Section 202 created a direct-loan program for elderly rental housing developed by private nonprofit corporations. Since that time, a considerable amount of construction has taken place. According to Carp (1976), under its various programs the U.S. Department of Housing and Urban Development (HUD) has rehoused approximately 750,000 older people; about 600,000 live in special housing for the elderly. To the uninformed, these numbers seem impressive. Yet the 1971 White House Conference on Aging called for the annual production of 120,000 units of new housing for the elderly. By

1983 one estimate was that a minimum of 136,000 replacement units (new and rehabilitated) would be needed annually to supply the elderly in the United States over the next twenty years (Handler 1983). The need certainly exists, but these goals may have been unrealistically high. One problem is that, as Lawton (1980a) points out, most federal housing programs lead a precarious existence. They may be initiated and terminated within the time of one or two national political administrations. The Reagan years (1981 to 1988) have been noteworthy by the absence of a federal housing policy with new initiatives for the low-income and elderly.

Another kind of barrier to the development of housing for the elderly can be called "community resistance" (Mangum 1985). Lawton and Hoffman (1984) have observed, "Community response to the announcement of plans to construct elderly housing in a neighborhood is frequently hostile, sometimes to the point of a local group's taking legal action to bar the construction" (p. 42). Community resistance may result from (1) threats associated with perceived change in the characteristics of people in the area, (2) concern about the development of stigmatizing service facilities, (3) concern that neighborhood may be disturbed by a secondary set of resource users, and (4) the fact that any increase in density is threatening (Winkel, cited in Lawton and Hoffman 1984).

Mangum (1985) makes four recommendations to help overcome possible community resistance to housing for the elderly: (1) If possible, build in a "nice," semi-commercial area; (2) if housing can only be built in a predominantly single family home residential area, obtain community input; (3) if there is opposition from the community, efforts should be made to reach a compromise with opposing residents; and, (4) if a compromise cannot be reached, sponsors should look for an alternative site.

Most public housing construction has involved low-cost, high-rise apartment buildings. To be eligible for public housing designed specifically for the elderly, a person must be aged sixty years or over, the spouse of a person aged sixty-two or over, or handicapped (without age restrictions). Restrictions on income and assets are usually set at the local level. Almost uniformly, tenants pay rent on a sliding scale to a maximum of 30 or 35 percent of total income.

The most popular federal housing programs for the elderly are Section 8, Section 202, Section 231, Section 232, and several programs of the Farmers Home Administration. Each deserves a brief description.

Section 8

This program is currently the principal federal means of providing housing assistance to the elderly. The Section 8 program, created by the Housing and Community Development Act of 1974, provides housing subsidies to lower-income families generally. These subsidies are designed to compensate a family for the difference between the cost of housing it can afford (some percentage of adjusted family income) and the cost of standard housing in the local area where it resides. To be eligible for Section 8 housing subsidies, families and single persons must have incomes below 80 percent of the area median (classified as lower income households). The federal government pays the difference between the contract rent and the rent paid by the tenant, usually 30 percent of adjusted family income. Federal expenditures per unit in fiscal 1983 averaged about $2,900 per year or $240 per month.

With the repeal of the statutory authority for new construction and substantial rehabilitation, moderate rehabilitation and existing housing are the major components of the Section 8 program (Jacobs et al. 1986):

1. In 1978 at the request of the Department of Housing and Urban Development, the Congress created a new moderate rehabilitation component of the Section 8 program for units needing some fixing up but not major repairs. Such activities included repair of leaky roofs, replacement and or repair of heating, electrical, or plumbing systems. Typically a local public housing agency (PHA) oversees the repair work.

2. The existing housing program, in which households find existing housing units in the private market, is the basic structure of the Section 8 program. A PHA determines the eligibility of applicants, based on their income. A Certificate of Family Participation is issued to eligible applicants. With this certificate, a family can look for housing on the private market, provided the housing meets standards of quality and is suitable for the family. The units are inspected by a PHA to make sure they are of standard quality. The PHA then makes rental payments to the owners on behalf of the households.

Section 202

This program, enacted as part of the Housing Act of 1959, was designed to provide "independent living" for elderly and handicapped persons. Suspended because of criticism in 1969, the program was revived in 1974 under an amendment to the Housing and Community Development Act of that year.

The program authorizes direct loans to nonprofit organizations so that they can develop and operate multifamily housing projects. These housing projects are expected to be small in scale (no more than 300 units) and aimed primarily at low- and moderate-income elderly persons. According to a recent HUD report (U.S. Department of Housing and Urban Development 1979), the program has produced approximately 45,000 housing units in 335 projects located throughout the nation, although an additional 46,000 units of the combined Section 202/Section 8 programs obtained fund reservations from HUD in the fiscal years from 1975 to 1977 (Struyk and Soldo 1980).

Most Section 202 projects are located within cities and in predominantly residential neighborhoods that offer little or no other public or subsidized housing. The residents of these neighborhoods tend to be white, middle to lower income, and nonelderly (USDHUD 1979). Aside from age, many of the status characteristics of neighborhood residents are quite similar to those of Section 202 project tenants. The program appears to be serving primarily white, elderly females who have middle-socioeconomic status backgrounds and current income that, although low in absolute terms, are in the moderate to middle range of elderly incomes. As a result, it seems dubious that the program has provided significant improvement in housing quality for its residents. Males, blacks, other minorities, the handicapped, and persons with very low incomes appear poorly served by the program (U.S. Department of Housing and Urban Development 1979).

Section 202 housing has been involved in a demonstration project since 1978 that attempts a marriage between housing and services to meet the needs of frail elderly in subsidized housing. It is a direct effort to put off premature institutionalization. In the Congregate Housing Services Program (CHSP), federal monies were given directly to the managers and administrators of public housing and Section 202 projects, who had to deal with the problem of "aging in place" (Nachison 1985). The demonstration covers sixty-two projects nationwide and served about 3,500 people from 1978 to 1983. The CHSP is generally thought to be a success. According to Nachison (1985), costs are less than the delivery of services through agencies in the general community, and there seems a real and measurable impact on unnecessary institutionalization.

Section 231

This section of the Housing Act of 1959 has been HUD's main program for unsubsidized rental housing for the elderly and handicapped. The Section 231 program is an FHA mortgage insurance plan designed to offer frail but mobile elderly an alternative to institutionalization. Different from Section 202, mortgagors under this program can be either profit or nonprofit groups. There are currently about 320 Section 231 projects in existence (45,000 units), although most of these projects were generated in the early 1960s. A large number of Section 231 projects failed because of overbuilding in particular regions of the country, high rents, inexperienced sponsors, and management and program design deficiencies (U.S. Department of Housing and Urban Development 1979). There has been very little activity under Section 231 in recent years. Nonprofit orgnizations seem to prefer the 202 program and, because loan limits are higher under other FHA programs, many private developers do not use the program.

Section 232

Section 232 of the National Housing Act provides insurance for loans for the construction or rehabilitation of nursing homes and related facilities. The homes may be for those who require skilled nursing care or a protective living environment. Section 232 nursing homes may be operated by private, proprietary, or nonprofit organizations. The mortgagor may lease the home to another operator with the approval of HUD (Jacobs et al. 1986).

Farmers Home Administration

Assistance to the elderly can be provided under both the Farmers Home Administration's (FmHA) programs: the Section 502 single family and Section 515 rural rental housing assistance programs. Section 502 provides subsidized and unsubsidized direct loans and unsubsidized guaranteed loans. An unsubsidized Section 502 loan can be used to finance the construction or acquisition of a new, substantially rehabilitated, or existing home. Homes are limited to those "modest in size, design, and cost." The maximum loan term is thirty-three years, and interest rates are adjusted periodically according to market changes (Jacobs et al. 1986).

In 1962 Congress added Section 515 in recognition of the need for rental housing in rural areas and small towns as well. This section authorizes loans to finance cooperative and rental housing projects. Nonprofit, limited-dividend, and profit-motivated sponsors may participate in the rental housing program. The 515 program is open to low- and moderate-income families and those sixty-two years or older (Jacobs et al. 1986).

RETIREMENT COMMUNITIES

Increasingly, gerontologists are giving attention to the phenomenon of retirement communities. When the term *retirement community* is used, many people immediately think of wealthy older people residing in a country club setting. This is one type of retirement community, although a retirement community may also look like an urban ethnic neighborhood, a suburban town, or a single apartment building. Hunt and Gunter-Hunt (1985) describe naturally occurring retirement communities (NORCs) as housing developments that are not planned or designed for older people, but which over time come to house largely older people.

Retirement communities may be defined more by their membership than by their geographic boundaries. Longino (1980) defines a retirement community as any living environment most of whose residents have relocated there since they retired. The essential elements of the definition are *retirement* and *relocation*. Although many residents of retirement communities still work, almost all who have worked have also retired from full-time employment at least once. In addition, the definition excludes communities of retirement-aged people who have aged in place; only the settings to which retired people move may be defined as retirement communities.

Retirement communities can be distinguished by the amount of conscious planning that goes into developing and operating them. Some are designed specifically for individuals of a certain chronological age. These *de jure* retirement communities are designed to take into account the more common needs of retirees. Planned communities may be separated into two types: subsidized and unsubsidized (Longino 1980). A housing project built under the auspices of many of the federal programs described in the previous section can be classified as a subsidized retirement community. Unsubsidized planned communities for retirees range along a continuum from planning limited to housing alone, to life-care communities which attempt to provide a full range of services.

Some retirement communities place no age restrictions on new residents, yet attract people who are retired. These *de facto* retirement communities are not designed as such but in them a series of organizations and services arise that cater to older people (Longino 1980). Why do people move to retirement communities? According to Longino (1981), there are positive (pulls) and negative (pushes) triggering mechanisms in the relocation decision process. Residents of three different retirement communities in the Ozark region connecting the states of Missouri, Arkansas, and Oklahoma were all asked for the single most important reason for their move. In general, Longino reports a congruence between personal needs and community selection.

Residents of the Ozark Lakes County, a *de jure* retirement community that attracts relatively younger couples who are in better physical and financial health than residents of the existing towns of the region, report the outstanding natural beauty of the region as primary justification for relocating there. Fifty-four percent of residents gave this as the single most important reason for their relocation. Another 21 percent reported social needs as the most important reason for their move.

Horizon Heights is a *de facto* subsidized retirement community, part of a public housing facilities network in a midwestern city with a population of almost 200,000. It is exclusively for less affluent people of retirement age who pay 25 percent of their adjusted income toward the rent. Almost one in four (23 percent) gave financial reasons as the most important for the move. Another 25 percent offered the push factor of wanting to leave an unhappy neighborhood situation.

Finally, over one-half (51 percent) of the residents of Carefree Village, a nonsubsidized life-care retirement community inhabited by upper middle class migrants, cite health needs as the major reason for selecting this community. Another 19 percent indicate the availability of other services as the primary reason for the move.

Planned communities specialize in providing services and meeting special needs of older people. They make their advantages known to prospective residents, and they attract people who, because of unhappy events in their lives or changing circumstances, feel they must move. Such people generally show a higher push level of explanation for their relocation. People who reside in unplanned or *de facto* communities generally have more positive or pull factors as explanation for their move (Longino 1981).

Although the literature on retirement communities is not large, several interesting ethnographic studies have been carried out. Ethnography is a branch of anthropology that studies and reports on everyday lives of particular cultural groups. Two of these studies are worth noting, for they help highlight a question of practical and theoretical importance to gerontologists today: Are older people better served by age-integrated or age-segregated environments?

Merrill Court

Merrill Court is an apartment building housing forty-three retired individuals. Most of the residents are women who are widowed, fundamentalist Christians, and of working-class background. Hochschild (1973) worked there in a variety of jobs including recreation director. When she began, Hochschild expected to find a disengaged, lonely group of individuals. Instead, she found an "unexpected community" of active and engaged older people who appeared to be quite satisfied with their lives. Residents have a great deal of interaction, much of which began with the installation of a coffee machine in the recreation room. Visitation among residents and between residents and their families occurs frequently. Having frequent contact with their neighbors provides these women with the gratification of friendship as well as an opportunity for relaying information about other people. Although the status equality among residents led Hochschild to characterize their relationships as a sibling bond, informal status distinctions are made among the residents.

According to Hochschild, within Merrill Court there is a status system based on a distribution of honor accumulated through holding offices in the service club. A parallel hierarchy existed based on the distribution of "luck": Being young-old, having good health, and living close to one's children were defined as having luck. Those who fall short on the criteria for luck are called "poor dears." This hierarchy ran in one direction. Someone who was a "poor dear" in the eyes of another seldom called that other person a "poor dear" in return. Many residents applied the term to those in nursing homes they visited. Hochschild explained the "poor dear" hierarchy as follows:

> The way the old look for luck differences among themselves reflects the pattern found at the bottom of other social, racial, and gender hierarchies. To find oneself lucky within an ill-fated category is to gain the semblance of high status when society withholds it from others in the category. The way old people feel above and condescend to other old people may be linked to the fact that the young feel above and condescend to them. The luck hierarchy does not stop with the old. (Hochschild, A. 1973. *The Unexpected Community*. Englewood Cliffs, N.J.: Prentice-Hall, Inc.)

Despite these informal status differences among the residents of Merrill Court, no one is isolated. The widows of Merrill Court are independent. They do not use "poor dear" when referring to themselves. They take care of themselves, fix their own meals, pay their own rent, shop for their own food, and make their own beds. And, when it is necessary, they do these things for others.

Fun City

Jacobs (1974, 1975) has written of a different retirement community, Fun City (a pseudonym). This is a retirement community of about 6,000 residents located ninety miles from a large western metropolitan area. Fun City is a planned community of single-level ranch-style tract homes. A nearby shopping center caters to the needs of residents; an activity center houses ninety-two clubs and organizations available to residents. Fun City residents are predominantly white and middle to upper class; the average age is seventy-one years.

Fun City bills itself as promoting "an active way of life." From Jacobs' reports, however, it seems clear that Fun City is a "false paradise." The retirement community exhibits many of the negative aspects residents associate with life on the "outside." Fun City has no public transportation, no police department, and no adequate health-care facilities. It is geographically isolated. Despite all the scheduled activities, fewer than 10 percent of the residents participated in any activity on a given day, and generally the same individuals participated in different activities on different days. Thus, inactivity is the norm for Fun City residents.

Jacobs concludes that many residents were withdrawing from society when they moved to Fun City and simply continued this withdrawal after arrival. Despite the promise of Fun City ("an active way of life"), the environment was organized in a way that promoted disengagement. No transportation, geographical isolation, and a lack of ties among the residents led to dissatisfaction with life on the part of many in Fun City. Those in the retirement community expressing the highest degree of satisfaction with Fun City were those whose financial situation allowed for travel, vacations, and visits with family.

Age Integration Versus Age Segregation

Merrill Court and Fun City are both age-segregated living environments; nearly all the residents of both retirement communities are older people. Both are planned retirement communities. Merrill Court represents public housing for the elderly, whereas Fun City is an unsubsidized retirement community. In contrast, there are the Ozark lakes region retirement communities that developed on a *de facto* basis and remain age integrated.

Much discussion in the gerontological literature has evaluated the relative merits for older people of age-segregated and age-integrated housing. Very influential in this discussion has been the research of Irving Rosow (1967), who examined the social behavior of older people living in apartment buildings in

Cleveland (privately developed and public housing). In particular, he was interested in how social behavior was affected by the concentration of age peers in the buildings. Rosow classified apartment buildings into three categories of age density: those buildings in which the elderly represented 1 to 15 percent of the residents; those in which 33 to 49 percent were elderly; and those in which 50 percent or more of the residents were elderly. For both working class and middle class aged, Rosow found that the presence of more age peers was positively associated with social interaction with neighbors. In addition, he demonstrated that this relationship was even more advantageous for those with lower status.

Generalizing from Rosow's evidence is difficult. For example, both Merrill Court and Fun City have age densities that are higher (almost 100 percent) than Rosow's highest category (50 percent plus). Yet, Merrill Court shows high sociability among its residents, whereas social interaction among Fun City residents is minimal. Accounting for this difference is no easy task. Carp (1976) cities five reasons why she believes generalizing from Rosow's work is so difficult. These reasons point to differences between Merrill Court and Fun City and may help explain why social interaction among residents was high in one and low in the other.

1. Rosow's work was not conducted in new housing for the elderly, but in older apartment buildings.
2. In the most age dense of Rosow's apartment buildings, only about half of the residents were elderly. In public housing for the elderly and other planned retirement communities such as Fun City, the percentage of elderly in the environment approaches 100 percent.
3. Rosow studied long-time residents of apartment buildings, whereas tenants in newly constructed public housing or newly developed tract housing for the elderly are often the first in-movers.
4. Rosow studied people in old housing located in older established neighborhoods. In-movers to retirement communities have left accustomed living environments and have relocated, often in new housing in newer neighborhoods.
5. Rosow's respondents may have been a special population, and no one knows how it differs from the population of other age-segregated environments or from the general population of older people.

Certainly one important difference between Merrill Court and Fun City that affected the potential for social interaction is the physical layout. For example, it would be considerably easier for interaction to occur among the 43 residents of a five-story building at Merrill Court than among 6,000 residents distributed one or two to each home in the sprawling tract home community of Fun City (Jacobs 1975). Hochschild (1973, 4) makes this clear in her description of the design of the building:

> There was an elevator midway between the apartments, and a long porch
> extended the length of all the apartments. It was nearly impossible to walk
> from any apartment to the elevator without being watched from a series of
> living room windows that looked out into the porch. . . . A woman who was
> sewing or watching television in her apartment could easily glance up through
> the window or wave to the passerby.

No such arrangement existed at Fun City. Other factors that likely contributed to the generation of an "unexpected community" at Merrill Court
included the greater status similarity and "good health" that existed among
Merrill Court residents compared with residents of Fun City.

Fun City notwithstanding, the evidence from most studies of age-segregated living situations show them to be satisfactory environments for aging.
Generally, the studies show higher rates of activity and social interaction in
age-segregated housing. Research on morale or life satisfaction in age-segregated versus age-integrated housing is less clear. Messer (1967) measured morale and social interaction of elderly living in two public housing projects. One
was age-segregated, the other a mixture of older and younger families. In the
age-integrated setting, there was an association between the morale of older
tenants and the amount of social interaction they engaged in; no such association appeared in the age-segregated project. Messer believes morale was
linked to activity in the age-integrated environment because the norms of that
environment were based on standards of youth; the older person who did not
succeed in becoming active would feel deficient in light of these standards.
The age-segregated environment fostered social norms appropriate to the ages
of its residents; lack of activity did not reflect a deficiency, and it was commonly
recognized that some individuals preferred to be active whereas others did not.

Data from two large-scale research studies (reported in Lawton 1980a) show
that older people *themselves* approve of age-segregated living arrangements.
Still, there is great danger in concluding that achieving the ideal social situation
for older persons is contingent on their residing in age-segregated housing.
Although such environments do provide friendship and social needs for many
elderly, others' needs may not be filled by such arrangements. Apparently,
age segregation in Fun City did little to enhance the social relationships of
many residents there.

One special problem with much of the research on age-segregated versus
age-integrated housing for the elderly is that it is virtually impossible to isolate
the age composition of an environment from other variables that may be operating in that environment. As Carp (1976) points out, it is very difficult to
locate sites for research that are otherwise equivalent and whose tenants are
similar. Thus, it is possible (perhaps even likely) that reports of high satisfaction
on the part of the elderly tenants of age-segregated housing have more to do

with what we earlier in this chapter called the *fit* of the physical and social environment than with age-segregation in itself.

SUMMARY

Housing is an important element in the life of an older person. Yet, gerontologists have come to understand that the physical characteristics of housing represent only one part of the broader living environment in which an older person resides.

Lawton and his colleagues have been particularly interested in the relationship between an older person's competence and the demands the living environment places on that individual. This relationship is stated in the form of a hypothesis: The less competent the individual, the greater the impact of environmental factors on that individual. Lawton sees competence in the broadest possible terms. It may be affected not only by internal biological or physiological factors, but also by external social processes such as age discrimination and social isolation.

Nearly all elderly Americans live in independent households; the majority live with a spouse or other relatives, but women are more than twice as likely as men to live alone. Poverty and physical disability have an important impact on the choice of living arrangements.

Most elderly Americans live in single-family, owner-occupied homes. Homes owned by the elderly are older than those owned by younger people. Similarly, the elderly live in household units that are more modest than those of the nonelderly; they are more likely to have incomplete plumbing and kitchen facilities.

Determining how many elderly live in inadequate housing is problematic, primarily because there is no consensus on what measures should be included in a definition of inadequate housing. A principal problem for the elderly is that a large proportion of their incomes is used to meet housing expenses. Housing costs as a percentage of income increase with age. Lower income households pay a higher proportion of their income for housing. At all ages and in all home-ownership categories, females pay proportionately more for their housing than do male householders.

In general, the elderly are quite satisfied with their housing arrangements. They often give higher assessments of their housing *and* neighborhoods than do the non-elderly. This tendency reflects the strong attachment of older people to their homes and neighborhoods as well as the limited housing options that may be open to them.

Federal involvement in housing for the elderly has increased in the last two decades. Nevertheless, the 1971 White House Conference on Aging called for an annual production of 120,000 units of new housing for the elderly. By 1983 estimates were that 136,000 replacement units would be needed annually to supply the elderly in the United States over the next twenty years. The principal federal housing programs for the elderly have been Sections 8, 202, 231, and 232 of the National Housing Act and several programs of the Farmers Home Administration.

Gerontologists have given increasing attention to retirement communities—living environments defined by the retirement and relocation experiences of the residents. Retirement communities may be planned or not, and planned communities may be subsidized or unsubsidized. There is considerable discussion in the gerontological literature about whether age-segregated or age-integrated housing is more advantageous for older people. Although the evidence from most studies of age-segregated environments show them to be satisfactory for the aging, it is still too early to conclude that achieving the ideal social situation for older persons is contingent on their residing in age-segregated housing.

STUDY QUESTIONS

1. List the major neighborhood and community characteristics influencing the study of housing for the aged. How do these relate to the concept of *environmental press*?

2. Define and discuss the accommodative model of independent living environments. How does it differ from the constant model?

3. Discuss the living arrangements of the elderly in contemporary society. What is the impact of sex and marital status on those arrangements?

4. How does the housing of elderly homeowners differ from that of the nonelderly with regard to quality and cost?

5. Discuss the federal housing programs aimed at helping to provide for housing needs of the elderly.

6. Define *retirement community*. Distinguish between *de facto* and *de jure* communities. Describe the elderly who reside in this type of housing and reflect on the selection processes that operate to get them there.

7. In examining the relative merits of age-segregated and age-integrated housing for the elderly, why is it so difficult to generalize conclusively from current studies?

BIBLIOGRAPHY

Allen, C., and Brotman, H. 1981. *Chartbook on aging.* Washington, D.C.: Administration on Aging.

Birch, D., et al. 1973. *America's housing needs: 1970 to 1980.* Cambridge, Mass.: Joint Center for Urban Studies, M.I.T. and Harvard University.

Braungart, M., Braungart, R., and Hoyer, W. 1980. Age, sex, and social factors in fear of crime. *Sociological Focus* 13(1):55–66.

Britton, J. 1966. Living in a rural Pennsylvania community in old age. In F. Carp (ed.), *Patterns of living and housing of middle-aged and older people.* Washington, D.C.: U.S. Government Printing Office.

Carp, F. 1966. *A future for the aged.* Austin, Tex.: University of Texas Press.

———. 1976. Housing and living environments of older people. In R. Binstock and E. Shanas (eds.), *The handbook of aging and the social sciences.* New York: Van Nostrand Reinhold Co.

Chapman, N.J., and Beaudet, M. 1983. Environmental predictors of well-being for at-risk older adults in a mid-sized city. *Journal of Gerontology* 38(2):237–244.

Eckert, J.K. 1980. *The unseen elderly: A study of marginally subsistent hotel dwellers.* San Diego: Campanile Press.

Ehrlich, P., Ehrlich, I., and Woehlke, P. 1982. Congregate housing for the elderly: Thirteen years later. *Gerontologist* 22(4):399–403.

Golant, S.M. 1985. The influence of the experienced residential environment on old people's life satisfaction. *Journal of Housing for the Elderly* 3(3/4):23–49.

Hamovitch, M., Peterson, J., and Larson, A. 1969. Perceptions and fulfillment of housing needs of an aging population. Paper presented at the 8th International Congress of Gerontology, Washington, D.C., June 1969.

Handler, B. 1983. *Housing needs of the elderly: A quantitative analysis.* Ann Arbor: University of Michigan, National Policy Center on Housing and Living Arrangements for Older Americans.

Havighurst, R. 1969. Research and development goals in social gerontology. *Gerontologist* 9:1–90.

Hochschild, A. 1973. *The unexpected community.* Englewood Cliffs, N.J.: Prentice-Hall.

Hunt, M.E., and Gunter-Hunt, G. 1985. Naturally occurring retirement communities. *Journal of Housing for the Elderly* 3(3/4):3–21.

Jacobs, B.G., Harney, K.R., Edson, C.L., and Lane, B.S. 1986. *Guide to federal housing programs* (2nd ed.). Washington, D.C.: Bureau of National Affairs, Inc.

Jacobs, J. 1974. *Fun city: An ethnographic study of retirement community.* N.Y.: Holt, Rinehart and Winston, Inc.

———. 1975. *Older persons and retirement communities.* Springfield, Ill.: Charles C Thomas, Publisher.

Lawton, M.P. 1980a. *Environment and aging.* Monterey, Calif.: Brooks/Cole Publishing Company.

———. 1980b. *Social and medical services in housing for the aged.* Rockville, Md.: U.S. Department of Health and Human Services.

———. 1980c. Housing the elderly: Residential quality and residential satisfaction. *Research on Aging* 2(3):309–328.

Lawton, M.P., and Hoffman, C. 1984. Neighborhood reactions to elderly housing. *Journal of Housing for the Elderly* 2(2):41–53.

Lawton, M.P., and Hoover, S. 1979. *Housing and neighborhood: Objective and subjective quality.* Philadelphia: Philadelphia Geriatric Center.

Lawton, M.P., and Nahemow, L. 1973. Ecology and the aging process. In C. Eisdorfer and M.P. Lawton (eds.), *Psychology of adult development and aging.* Washington, D.C.: American Psychological Association.

Lawton, M.P., and Simon, B. 1968. The ecology of social relationships in housing for the elderly. *Gerontologist* 8:108–115.

Lee, G. 1982. Residential location and fear of crime among the elderly. *Rural Sociology* 47(4):655–669.

Longino, C. 1981. The retirement community. In C. Kart and B. Manard (eds.), *Aging in America: Readings in social gerontology* (2nd ed.). Sherman Oaks, Calif.: Alfred Publishing.

————. 1980. The retirement community. In F. Berghorn and D. Schafer (eds.), *Dimensions of aging*. Boulder, Colo.: Westview Press.

Manard, B., Kart, C., and van Gils, D. 1975. *Old age institutions*. Lexington, Mass.: D.C. Heath and Co.

Mangum, W.P. 1985. But not in my neighborhood: Community resistance to housing for the elderly. *Journal of Housing for the Elderly* 3(3/4):101–119.

Messer, M. 1967. The possibility of an age-concentrated environment becoming a normative system. *Gerontologist* 7:247–251.

Murray, H. 1938. *Explorations in personality*. New York: Oxford University Press, Inc.

Nachison, J.S. 1985. Congregate housing for the low and moderate income elderly—A needed federal state partnership. *Journal of Housing for the Elderly* 3(3/4):65–80.

O'Bryant, S.L. 1982. The value of home to older persons: Relationship to housing satisfaction. *Research on Aging* 4(3):349–363.

Petee, T., Kart, C., and Palmer, N. 1985. Fear of crime: Are there age effects? Paper presented at Annual Meeting of the Gerontological Society of America, New Orleans, La., November 1985.

Rosow, I. 1967. *Social integration of the aged*. New York: The Free Press.

Soldo, B. 1979. The housing characteristics of independent elderly: A demographic overview. *Occasional papers in housing and urban development*, No. 1. Washington, D.C.: U.S. Department of Housing and Urban Development.

Struyk, R. 1977. The housing expense burden of households headed by the elderly. *Gerontologist* 17:447–452.

Struyk, R., and Soldo, B. 1980. *Improving the elderly's housing*. Cambridge, Mass.: Ballinger Publishing Company.

U.S. Department of Health, Education and Welfare. 1974. *Limitations of activity due to chronic conditions—United States, 1972*. Series 10, No. 96. Washington, D.C.: U.S. Government Printing Office.

U.S. Department of Housing and Urban Development. 1979. *Housing for the elderly and handicapped*. Washington, D.C.: Office of Policy Development and Research, U.S. Department of Housing and Urban Development.

U.S. Senate Special Committee on Aging. 1985–86. *Aging America: Trends and predictions*. Washington, D.C.: U.S. Government Printing Office.

————. 1985. *How older Americans live: An analysis of census data*. Washington, D.C.: U.S. Government Printing Office.

Yin, P. 1980. Fear of crime among the elderly. *Social Problems* 27:492–504.

CHAPTER 17

LONG-TERM CARE

Ruth E. Dunkle and Cary S. Kart

In the minds of most Americans, the phrase long-term care has been synonymous with nursing home care because so few other options were available. With the aging of the U.S. population and the increasing number of chronically ill persons in need of some care, alternative noninstitutional arrangements have evolved. In this chapter, we use the concept of long-term care to describe a continuum of services, from those delivered at home or in community settings to those delivered within institutional facilities.

Long-term care involves the provision of "one or more services . . . on a sustained basis to enable individuals whose functional capacities are chronically impaired to be maintained at their maximum levels of psychological, physical and social well-being" (Brody 1984). Koff (1982) specifies long-term care services as designed to provide diagnostic, preventive, therapeutic, rehabilitative, supportive, and maintenance care. According to the United States Senate Special Committee on Aging (1982), the goals of long-term care involve a three-part strategy: (1) to delay the onset of preventable disease in healthy adults; (2) to lengthen the period of functional independence in those elderly with chronic disease; and (3) to improve the quality of one's later life.

We begin this chapter with a review of the long-term care needs and the patterns of service utilization in the elderly population. Selected types of noninstitutional services are then described. The actual risks of an older person being institutionalized are discussed, as are the logic of institutional care in the United States and the effects institutionalization may have on the aged individual. Policy issues related to long-term care are explored in Chapter 18.

LONG-TERM CARE NEEDS AND PATTERNS OF UTILIZATION

The National Nursing Home Survey of 1977 (NNHS77) estimates approximately 1.3 million elderly in nursing homes at any given time (Van Nostrand et al. 1979). This represents approximately 5 percent of the elderly population. It is generally believed that an additional 10 percent of elderly living in the community are homebound and as functionally impaired as those in institutions (U.S. General Accounting Office 1977; Shanas 1977). Although the help needed by older people living in the community varies greatly, Brody (1981) estimates that anywhere from 12 to 40 percent require some kind of supportive services.

Who are those most likely to be in need of long-term care assistance? Based on her analysis of a national probability sample of community-dwelling elderly, Soldo (1980) reports women, those over eighty-five years of age, widows, and those living with relatives other than a spouse as groups most likely to be in need of assistance. The typical nursing home resident is white, female, widowed, and over eighty years of age (Van Nostrand et al. 1979).

Not every individual who needs long-term care assistance receives it. Service delivery barriers for older persons are numerous. Sometimes the elderly are reluctant to admit need or accept help; many even deny using services. Generally, those services they do use are perceived by them as being earned (Moen 1978).

Simply creating services and making them available is not enough to ensure that they are utilized. As Ward indicates (1977, 66): "Making services objectively available to older people is not sufficient—they must perceive a need, know about the service, view it as appropriate, etc." According to Little (1982), who delivers the service, where and when the service is delivered, and who receives the service are also important dimensions of the service utilization issue.

How older people choose the long-term care services they will use is determined by a complex set of interacting personal and environmental factors (McAuley and Blieszner 1985). Personal factors include demographic, psychological, economic, and health-related characteristics. Environmental issues relate to the availability of informal support and community and institutional services (Branch and Jette 1982; Deimling and Poulshock 1985; Soldo 1981).

Although researchers have identified predictors of institutional versus home-based, long-term care (Branch and Jette 1982; Greenberg and Genn 1979), few have examined how older people might select among various types of long-term care services (McAuley and Blieszner 1985). Stoller (1982) asked elderly living in the community what they would do if they were ill and needed constant care. Most frequently mentioned was the nursing home; 30 percent offered no strategy for obtaining care. Dunkle and her colleagues (1982) found that a majority of hospitalized elderly with long-term care needs had no idea what services were available in their own communities. Lack of knowledge about resources and services reduces the search for information about what services exist (Silverstein 1984). In addition, knowledge about services does not mean that people are able to see the connection to their own needs. Older people may not know how to negotiate receiving services from agencies (Bild and Havighurst 1976; Cantor 1975; Comptroller General 1977).

McAuley and Blieszner surveyed over 1,200 elderly Virginians on their attitudes toward different long-term care arrangements. Respondents favored paid in-home care, care from a relative in their own home, and adult day care to the nursing home. When arrangements require a change of residence, people identify a nursing home as the residence of preference more often than a relative's home. In addition, the nursing home is the long-term care arrangement of choice for nonwhites, single persons, and those with higher incomes who felt they did not have anyone to care for them for an extended period (McAuley and Blieszner 1985). Adult day care was the choice of younger persons and nonwhites in better health as well as those who had more emotional problems. Paid home care seemed more appealing for whites and those with emotional problems.

The preference of nonwhites for nursing homes described in the above study is somewhat curious. Kart and Beckham (1976) have reported that nonwhites tend to be less likely than whites to be admitted to nursing homes. They suggest that this lower rate of utilization among nonwhites may result from whites being generally more able to pay for care in proprietary nursing homes and discrimination in the admission of black elderly to nursing homes. More recently, Kart and Palmer (1987) identified factors that may be useful in explaining differences in the level of care received by the elderly within nursing homes. These factors include marital status, source of payment, age, sex, and number of chronic illnesses. Race was not included as a variable in this analysis.

A body of research has developed suggesting that presence of family is an important factor in delaying, if not preventing, the institutionalization of a chronically ill elderly person (for example, Brody, Poulshock, and Masciocchi 1978; McAuley and Prohaska 1982). Still, we really do not know enough about the views toward various long-term care arrangements held by family members of elderly who are prospective consumers of such services. We do not know if the views of the elderly and their family members differ with regard to the perceived efficacy of these various arrangements (Neu 1982) or even if congruence of view is related in any way to successful outcomes for the elderly person.

THE QUALITY OF INFORMAL AND FORMAL SUPPORTS

Many gerontological researchers and practitioners recognize the duality of informal and formal supports to the elderly (for example, Cantor and Little 1985). Litwak (1965, 1978, 1985), among others, argues that the needs of the frail and vulnerable elderly are best met if there is a proper balance between formal and informal support, with each system performing the tasks for which it is best suited.

The main source of informal support for older persons is the family. Barbara Silverstone (1985, 156) describes this support system as "a rich fabric of informal relationships which envelops the majority of elders in our society along a number of dimensions. This fabric is bonded most strongly by marriage, and adjacent generational and peer relationships and for racial minorities, by expanded kin as well." Yet research findings indicate that residing with other relatives is not the living arrangement of choice for most elderly (Kobrin 1981; Troll, Miller, and Atchley 1979). Living with relatives is typically a result of impaired health or low income. Certain living arrangements are more satisfying than others. Johnson (1983) found that dissatisfaction with caregiving arrangements is more likely when the caregiver is a child rather than a spouse. She suggests that dissatisfaction may result from change in the relationship between child and parent when the parent becomes ill.

Various family members seem to be used for caregiving, depending on the type of help required. For instance, the main source of support for the bedfast and homebound is the husband or wife of the invalid. When children are available, they provide a second important source of help. Childless elders rely on other sources of informal support.

It is generally recognized that family and other informal supports frequently have difficulty providing help on a long-term basis to elders who are impaired and disabled (Shanas 1979; Litman 1971). Emotional, physical, and financial strains appear associated with personal and situational characteristics of the caregiver, with emotional strain seemingly the hardest to bear (Cantor 1981; Horowitz 1981). The isolation of a caregiver as well as a decrease in emotional resilience and morale (Archbold 1980) may provoke many elderly persons and their families to turn to formal service providers for help.

The array of services available to older people outside of institutions covers a broad range including health, housing, and nutrition. Services have been designed to aid the informal caregiving structure. How these services are organized and delivered are the result of complex policy and financial issues. Below, some existing formal services are identified in order to help define the range of services available. Many communities have a substantial number of these services; however, only a limited number of communities are able to provide a complete set of services. The listing is not all-inclusive. Services are presented in order of most to least restrictive.

Adult Day Care

The term *day care* applies to any service provided during the day. Such services range from social to health-related care, from home care to hospital care, and include rehabilitation as well as physical and mental health care (Harder et al.

1986). Weiler and Rathbone-McCuan (1978) define day care as a unique service modality because it meets the long-term care needs of people while allowing for individual differences. These tailor-made services can have a therapeutic objective of prevention, rehabilitation, or maintenance. Day care can be used to provide respite for care givers as well.

Table 17-1 depicts the services available under the rubric of day care. Four different service modalities are presented: day hospitals; social/health centers; psychosocial centers; and social centers. A wide range of services are offered to various types of clients in many different service settings. Geriatric day services help the older person placed in day care and can be used to provide respite care for caregivers as well.

Home Health Care

Home health care entails the provision of coordinated multidisciplinary services including skilled nursing and therapeutic services as well as social casework, mental health, legal, financial, and personal care, and household management assistance (Berg, Atlas, and Zeiger 1974; Bloom and Blenkner 1970; Wahl 1974). As Noelker and Harel (1978, 37) state: "Its purpose is to aid the elderly person in the performance of activities of daily living which are essential for continued independence yet are problematic for many aged given their health problems and functional impairments."

Home health services include the in-home services of a homemaker, home health aid, or home aide assistant. Eligibility requirements for Medicare coverage limit access to this type of service at the same time need is growing with shortened hospital stays resulting from the prospective payment plan (DRGs) under Medicare. About 80 percent of home care patients are post-hospital referrals; the others are referred by a physician after an outpatient episode of illness or by family or friends who need help in providing care. Home health services are available from proprietary and private service organizations, although use of such organizations may be limited by availability and cost.

Historically, home health services were only available under voluntary or public auspices. Usually, this involved a visiting nurse service, public health or welfare department and, on rare occasions, an extension of hospital services. A recent study on home health-care costs was conducted by the U.S. House of Representatives' Subcommittee on Health and Long-Term Care (Shannon 1985). Findings showed that home health agencies were doing well financially; from 1980 to 1982, the average home health care agency's revenue increased by 52 percent. With the increased profitability of this sector of the health care market, there has been increased development of profit-making agencies that function as local franchises of national organizations.

Research findings support the fact that home health care reduces the need for institutional care and is less costly (Rozelle 1980). Nielson and associates (1972) report a study conducted by the Benjamin Rose Institute in Cleveland

TABLE 17-1 Geriatric Day Services

Modality	Major Service Objective	Type of Client	Service Setting
Day hospital	To provide daily medical care and supervision to help the individual regain an optimal level of health following an acute illness	Individual is in active phase of recovery from an acute illness and no longer requires intense medical intervention on a periodic basis.	Extended-care facility or hospital
Social/health center	To provide health-care resources when needed by chronically impaired individuals	Individual has chronic physical illness or disabilities; condition does not require daily medical intervention but does require nursing and other health supports.	Long-term care institution of free-standing center
Psychosocial center	To provide a protective or transitional environment that assists the individual in dealing with multiple problems or daily coping	Individual has a history of psychiatric disorder; could reactivate or suffer from mental deterioration (organic or functional) that places him or her in danger if not closely supervised.	Psychiatric institution or free-standing center
Social center	To provide appropriate socialization services	Individual's social functioning has regressed to the point where overall capacity for independent functioning would not be possible without formal, organized social stimuli.	Specialized senior-citizen center

Source: Weiler, P. and Rathbone-McCuan, E. 1978. *Adult day care: Community work with the elderly*, p. 7. New York: Springer Publishing Co., Inc. Used by permission.

in which a group of elderly persons receiving home health services was compared with a group that did not receive these services. The group with home health services spent an average of eight days per person per year in institutional care; those without care spent an average of fifty-three days per person per year in institutional care.

Foster Care

Foster family care approximates the normal living environment, with the added dimension of supervision. It allows the older person an element of privacy as well as freedom not possible in the larger protected environment of the nursing home. Adult foster care is considered among the least restrictive housing options available to help older persons remain in the community. It utilizes private residences for the care of a nonrelated elderly person who is in need of supervision or assistance with the activities of daily living. Definitions of foster care vary from state to state. In Ohio, only homes that have Supplemental Security Income recipients are subject to licensing regulations that control foster care.

Certain problems are inherent in the provision of adult foster care. For example, unlike foster care for children, where the child moves toward independence and gains the capacity to contribute to the foster family, the elderly person is often viewed as only moving toward greater dependence. As a result, many potential care providers are reluctant to offer their foster homes to the elderly.

Hospice

Hospice is a concept of care for the terminally ill, which is gaining popularity in the United States. This model of care is more than a program of medical health care for the terminally ill. These services are often directed by a physician with an interdisciplinary team to provide psychological, social, and spiritual services when needed by the patient or family members on a twenty-four hour, seven days a week basis. These services can continue for family and friends after the patient's death. Additional material on hospices is located in Chapter 19.

Protective Services

Protective or *surrogate services* describe visits by a social worker with supplemental community services such as visiting nurses, homemakers, clinical services, meals, telephone checks and transportation (U.S. Senate 1977). A myriad of needs are addressed under protective services and include daily living, physical health, psychosocial problems, household management, housing, economic management, and legal protection (Hall and Mathiasen 1973). These services are similar to those delivered through the social service delivery system, although their effects may vary because of the potential for legal intervention in the form of guardianship, placement, and commitment and emergency services.

Every older person who is incapacitated is not necessarily a candidate for protective services (Ferguson 1978). The decisive factor appears to be the availability of a reliable person to help the needy individual. Thus, protective services encompass a wider range of considerations than just the condition of the individual alone.

There are three dimensions of protective services provided to older persons (Hall and Mathiasen 1968). These are prevention, support, and surrogate service. *Protective* services strive to maintain the well-being of the older person through reducing or remedying conditions that place the older person at risk, thus preventing unnecessary institutionalization. *Support* services provide the aid necessary for the impaired older person to maintain independence and self-direction to the maximum level possible. In providing *surrogate* services, the service provider is required to act on behalf of or assist someone to act on behalf of the impaired older person. The task is to provide the necessary supportive services *with or without* the client's approval.

Respite Care

Respite care offers support to family caregivers so that they can continue to provide care for the frail elderly (Archbold 1980; Blazer 1978; Crossman, London, and Barry 1981; Howells 1980). There is clear evidence that families express a need for respite care (Hagan 1980; Upshur 1978) and that it may prevent or delay institutionalization (Townsend and Flanagan 1976). Even with these noted advantages, respite care is not widely available to families caring for disabled elders.

There are four models of respite care (Hagan 1980; Upshur 1978): (1) home based; (2) group day care; (3) group residential care; and (4) residential programs providing respite care as an adjunct service (Upshur 1983). These models are described in some detail in Table 17-2.

Home-based respite care uses trained sitters who provide the service in the client's home and are matched with the appropriate family. Residential care involves a residential facility that is established to provide respite care to small groups of disabled persons (Upshur 1983). More intensive care can be given in this setting to medically and behaviorally difficult clients. These services, offered in a facility designed and staffed for short stays, can also be given on an adjunct basis.

TABLE 17-2   Summary of Major Approaches to Respite Care

Home-based care	
Respite placement agency:	Community providers are recruited and trained to provide day or overnight care in their own home or in the client's home.
Funding conduit:	Agency reimburses families for respite care, which they arrange on their own.
Respite home or apartment:	Agency provides a homelike space for client and community provider to "live-in" while respite care is provided.
Individual provider:	Persons unaffiliated with an agency take clients into their own home for respite care.
Group day care	Groups of clients are provided daytime activities so family members are free to run errands, go to meetings, etc., for a few hours weekly.
Group residential care	Groups of clients are provided overnight care from one night to several weeks in a facility that provides only respite care.
Respite care as an adjunct service	
Community residences:	One or two beds are reserved for planned or emergency respite care in a home that primarily services long-term clients.
Residential treatment facilities:	Some beds are reserved for respite care in a program that primarily provides educational or therapeutic services to longer-term clients.
Nursing homes:	On a reserved or as-available basis, respite care is provided to clients with medical needs.
State institutions:	Respite-care clients are taken into groups of longer-term clients, or special respite beds are designated.

Source: Upshur, C. 1983. Developing respite care: A support service for families with disabled members. *Family Relations* 32:16. Copyrighted 1983 by the National Council on Family Relations, 1910 West County Road B, Suite 147, St. Paul, Minnesota 55113. Reprinted by permission.

THE LOGIC OF INSTITUTIONAL CARE

Formal supports consist of open and closed care (Little 1979, 1982). *Open care* is care provided in the community and encompasses all the formal social services aimed at allowing the individual to maintain life at home and avoid premature or unnecessary institutionalization. *Closed care* describes formal care in institutions such as acute care hospitals. Hospitals service more elderly than any other community agency (Brody and Persily 1984). About 20 percent of all older people use inpatient facilities at least once a year. When the hospitalization is associated with physical or mental impairment, plans must often be made for some other type of long-term care. A sense of urgency typically accompanies discharge from the hospital, and this may interfere with usual patterns of problem solving. Moreover, the extent to which the elderly patient participates in arriving at a decision may be limited by the circumstances under which the plans are made (Brody 1984).

The Risks of Institutionalization

As indicated earlier, approximately 1.3 million elderly or 5 percent of those sixty-five years and older are found in nursing homes at any one time. Estimates are that 2 million elderly (6 percent of those aged sixty-five years and over) will be in nursing homes by the year 2000 (Fox and Clauser 1980; Hing 1981). Assessments of the present overuse of nursing homes vary widely (Congressional Budget Office 1977; Comptroller General of the United States 1972).

Kastenbaum and Candy (1973) were the first to point out the fallacy of assuming that the number or proportion of elderly in nursing homes could be used as an estimate of their cumulative chances for institutionalization. They reviewed 20,234 death certificates for those aged sixty-five and over filed in the metropolitan Detroit area during the 1971 calendar year. They found that 20 percent of all these deaths were reported in nursing homes, and approximately 24 percent were reported occurring in a larger category of institutions that included all identifiable extended-care facilities. Palmore (1976) and Lesnoff-Caravaglia (1978–79), among others, have substantiated these findings. The consensus seems to be that "the total chance of institutionalization before death among normal-aged persons living in the community would be about one in four" (Palmore 1976).

Presenting a picture that shows that one in four elderly Americans can expect to be institutionalized in a nursing home or rest home makes it easier to understand why a major fear of many older persons is that they will become dependent and have to face institutionalization. Such figures also make it easier to begin to understand the potentially high financial and human costs of institutionalization and the tremendous strain this phenomenon may place on public and private resources in our society.

Who Gets Institutionalized?

A number of factors seem to influence who among the elderly gets institutionalized. A U.S. Department of Health, Education and Welfare report (1977) describes the "typical" nursing home resident as white, female, widowed, aged seventy-nine and living in the facility for 2.6 years. Most of the residents lived in another institution prior to entering the nursing home. Almost 81 percent of nursing home residents were admitted primarily for physical reasons. The chronic conditions that are most prevalent in the elderly institutionalized population are stroke, heart disease, arthritis, and rheumatism.

More than 71 percent of elderly nursing home residents are female. The disproportionate number of elderly women in old-age institutions reflects their predominance in the elderly population and the fact that considerably more elderly women than men are older than seventy-five. Nonwhites constitute about 8 percent of the institutionalized elderly population.

More than four out of five (81.5 percent) elderly nursing home residents

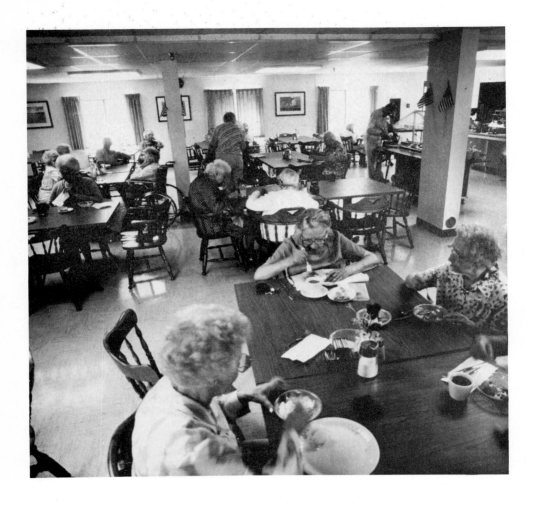

are seventy-five or older. One study found the age of an elderly population to be strongly associated with institutionalization. Manard and her colleagues (1975), using 1970 census data, found that those states with a high proportion of elderly who were seventy-five and above had a high rate of institutionalization. A factor that contributes to the relationship between age and institutionalization is that the chances of developing major health problems and of losing one's living companion (spouse, friend, or sibling) increase with age.

More than 60 percent (62.3) of aged nursing home residents are widowed; many of these people lived alone prior to institutionalization. Both widowhood and living alone appear to put some at risk for institutionalization. Generally speaking, people who grow old and sick will be less able to cope with the situation if they live alone. Still, almost 35 percent of nursing home residents between 1973 and 1974 moved there from a general or short-stay hospital. To some degree, this reflects Medicare regulations that allow coverage for extended care (up to one hundred days) only if the patient had recently been discharged from a hospital after a stay of three days or more.

Characteristics of Nursing Homes

The NNHS77 reports approximately 18,300 nursing homes in the United States. Using different criteria for inclusion in the Master Facilities Inventory, the National Center for Health Statistics reports 26,175 nursing homes in the United States in 1982 (Rabin and Stockton 1987). The great majority of these (74.3 percent) are run for profit (see Table 17-3). Although the nonprofit and government nursing homes comprised only about 26 percent of the facilities, their greater capacity (averaging ninety-seven beds versus sixty-eight beds for proprietary facilities) enable them to serve about one-third of all nursing home residents (NNHS77).

Nursing homes may also be classified according to their certification status. About 75 percent of all nursing homes in 1977 were certified either as skilled nursing facilities (SNFs), intermediate care facilities (ICFs), or both. ICFs constitute about 34 percent of all facilities and 45 percent of all certified facilities. Facilities certified as both a SNF and an ICF were larger (124 beds per facility) than the other facilities, and thus accommodate almost 36 percent of all nursing home residents.

Almost one-third of all nursing homes and more than one-third of all of their residents are located in the North Central region of the country. Facilities in the South are largest, averaging ninety-six beds in size (representing newer corporate-run facilities), whereas those in the West are smallest, averaging fifty-one beds in size.

Over the past three decades, medical care prices rose much faster than prices in general. Nursing home costs have been no exception. Through the 1980s to date, nursing home charges have continued to rise at a faster pace than the Consumer Price Index (CPI). According to a 1986 publication of the American Association of Retired Persons (AARP), nursing home costs range from a low of about $37 for custodial care to a high of about $140 a day for skilled nursing care.

THE DECISION TO INSTITUTIONALIZE
AN OLDER PERSON

Old-age institutions have been described as "dehumanizing" and "depersonalizing" (Townsend 1962). Nursing home critics describe many facilities as "human junkyards" and "warehouses" (Butler 1975). Studies of old persons

TABLE 17-3 Selected Characteristics of Nursing Homes, United States, 1977

Nursing Home Characteristics	Nursing Homes		Beds		Residents	
	Number	Distribution (%)	Number	Distribution (%)	Number	Distribution (%)
All Nursing Homes	18,300	100.0	1,383,600	100.0	1,287,400	100.0
Ownership						
Proprietary	13,600	74.3	926,100	66.9	851,700	66.2
Non-profit and government	4,700	25.7	457,600	33.1	435,700	33.8
Certification						
Skilled nursing facility	3,600	19.9	271,700	19.6	252,100	19.6
Skilled nursing and intermediate care facility	3,900	21.1	484,300	35.0	462,200	35.9
Intermediate care facility	6,200	33.7	455,700	32.9	414,300	32.2
Not certified	4,600	25.3	171,900	12.4	158,800	12.3
Number of Beds						
Fewer than 50	7,800	42.5	205,700	14.9	193,500	15.0
50–99	5,200	28.5	376,600	27.2	353,000	27.4
100–199	4,600	24.9	590,600	42.7	547,400	42.5
200 or more	[a]	[a]	210,800	15.2	193,500	15.0
Geographic Region:						
Northeast	4,300	23.4	302,100	21.8	274,600	21.3
North-central	5,800	31.8	472,300	34.1	446,700	34.7
South	4,200	22.9	404,000	29.2	377,800	29.3
West	4,000	21.9	205,300	14.8	188,300	14.6

Note: Figures may not add to totals due to rounding.

[a] Figure does not meet standards of reliability or precision.

Source: National Center for Health Statistics; An overview of nursing home characteristics: Provisional data from the 1977 National Nursing Home Survey, *Advance Data*, no. 35, DHEW Pub. No. (PHS) 78–1250. Hyattsville, Md.: Public Health Service, September 6, 1978.

residing in a variety of institutional settings have shown them to be more maladjusted, depressed, and unhappy; have a lower range of interests and activity; and be more likely to die sooner than aged persons living in the community (Lieberman 1969; Mendelson 1974; Townsend 1970).

Despite the unfavorable reputation of old-age institutions and the negative attitudes of elderly citizens toward them, many elderly individuals need and seek out institutional care. Usually, this need is apparent to family members or is based on a physician's recommendation. In fact, in cases involving physical illness or debility, the need may be apparent to the elderly patient as well.

As we have already indicated, the availability of adequate and applicable home-care and community services can prevent the institutionalization of many elderly patients. Family members are often very much involved in decisions concerning the institutionalization of an elderly person. When an aged family member is placed into a nursing home, many of the responsibilities for caring for that individual shift from the family to the institution. Still, many families continue to remain involved with that family member.

What is the most effective way for a family to remain involved with an institutionalized relative so as to promote higher quality nursing home care? What responsibilities do institutions have to provide support to families that want to stay involved? A first step in answering these questions and ultimately in providing optimal care is for both parties—families and nursing home staff— to understand and accept their respective responsibilities in providing services to the institutionalized individual.

Shuttlesworth and his colleagues (1982) have assessed the extent to which Texas nursing home administrators and relatives of institutional residents have congruous attitudes about whether the nursing home or the family is responsible for performing an inventory of tasks that are essential in nursing home care. Two findings are worthy of mention. First, both administrators and relatives assigned responsibility to the nursing home for the majority of tasks that they see as vital to care. These include technical tasks involving medical care, security, housekeeping, cooking, and the like.

Second, in most cases of discrepancies, relatives were more likely than administrators to assign responsibility to families. For the most part, these discrepancies involved nontechnical tasks such as room furnishings, leisure-time activities, clothing, and special foods.

This study suggests that a problem in engaging families in the care of institutionalized relatives is not with the willingness of families to claim responsibility for nontechnical aspects of care, but with administrators' insufficient recognition of family responsibility for nontechnical tasks. As a result, administrators may fail to offer sufficient support for family involvement in such tasks. They may overlook possible policy or procedural changes in institutional arrangements that could better facilitate family involvement in overseeing the nontechnical aspects of care.

INSTITUTIONAL EFFECTS:
REAL OR IMAGINARY

The gerontological literature is filled with descriptions of the institutionalized elderly as disorganized, disoriented, and depressed. Tobin and Lieberman (1976) review three explanations for this portrait: relocation and environmental change; preadmission effects; and the totality of institutions.

Relocation and Environmental Change

The relationship of environmental change to mortality and morbidity has been investigated in mental hospitals, nursing homes, and homes for the aged. And, much controversy exists regarding the effect of relocation on mortality and other health status outcomes (for example, Horowitz and Schulz 1983). Nevertheless, researchers generally agree that moving the older person from a familiar setting into an institution leads to psychologic disorganization and distress (Kasl 1972). This may be especially the case when the move is involuntary (Schulz and Brenner 1977).

Some investigators argue that the disruption of life caused by relocating an elderly individual into new surroundings may create many of the effects attributed to living in that new setting (Tobin and Lieberman 1976; Lieberman and Tobin 1983). Others argue that it is not simply the stress of relocation but rather *environmental discontinuity*, the degree of change between a new and old environment, that may explain the effects observed after institutionalization (Lawton 1974). Interestingly, some evidence suggests that environmental change can elicit desirable behavior and increase the competence of the older individual. Carp (1966) and Lipman (1968a) have both reported on favorable changes experienced by elderly individuals during the year after a move into an age-segregated housing situation. Important in such settings are the physical proximity of age peers and the development of behavioral expectations appropriate to the level of competence of the average resident (Lawton 1974).

Preadmission Effects

Anticipating and preparing for the actuality of moving into an institution can be very stressful. The effects of this stress on the older person before admission are often very similar to what is described as institutional effects. Tobin and Lieberman (1976) found old people who were awaiting institutionalization to be markedly different from those living in the community in cognitive functioning, affective response, emotional state, and self-perceptions. What is even more interesting is that the psychological status of the study sample awaiting institutionalization was not unlike the psychological status generally descriptive of aged persons in institutions: slight cognitive disorganization; constriction in affective response; less than optimal feelings of well-being; diminished self-esteem; and depression (Tobin and Lieberman 1976, 55–56). This evidence supports the existence of an anticipatory psychosocialization process in which forces are set into motion so that the individual comes to approximate the institutionalized elderly in frame of mind even before entering the institutionalized environment.

Another explanation that has been offered in the literature is that selection biases account for the usual portrait of the institutionalized elderly. In this context, the term *selection bias* refers to the fact that people who are admitted to institutions may have characteristics that sensitize them to respond negatively to living in those institutions. In this view, differences found between older persons living in the community and those living in institutions are not a function of institutional life but of population differences (Tobin and Lieberman 1976). If selection is playing a role, then, in Tobin and Lieberman's words, "[T]he institutionalized aged share some characteristics because of who they are and not where they are."

The Total Institution

The most compelling answer to the question, "What do institutions do to the old?" has been offered by Erving Goffman (1961) in his characterization of the total institution. According to Goffman, a basic social arrangement in contemporary society is that the individual tends to sleep, play, and work in different settings with different coparticipants. A central feature of total institutions is the breakdown of the barriers that ordinarily separate these activities so that all three activities take place in the same setting with the same people. One category of total institution includes those places that take care of persons who are perceived to be generally incapable of caring for themselves and harmless to themselves and others. Included in this category are nursing homes, homes for the aged, and homes for the poor and indigent.

Goffman argues that common to all total institutions is the fact that individuals in such institutions undergo a process of *self-mortification*. This process, which involves interacting with others in the institutional setting, strips the resident of his or her identity and reduces the control individuals perceive they have over events of daily life (Arling et al. 1986). Goffman (1961, 14–43) identifies the features of an institutional environment that he suggests contribute to the mortification process. These features are discussed here with particular emphasis on nursing home residents.

Admission Procedures. Admission procedures typically bring loss. The individual is often stripped of personal possessions, issued institutional clothing, and "shaped and coded" into an object that can be worked on smoothly by the institution. Such procedures are depersonalizing in that they serve to detach the individual from the social system at large. Jules Henry (1973) refers to this as "depersonalization through symbolic means" with a person losing his or her name, or being addressed as "you" instead of as "Mrs. Jones."

Barriers. The total institution places barriers between the resident and the outside world that result in a loss of the roles that are a part of the resident's self. Most institutionalized individuals are simply not able to play the roles of mother and father, grandmother and grandfather, aunt or uncle, and friend in the way these roles were played on the outside. All institutionalized persons face the loss of a familiar way of living. Most describe it simply in terms of losing others and leaving their families' possessions at home.

Deference Obligations. Because total institutions deal with almost all aspects of a resident's life, there is a special need to obtain the resident's cooperation. Thus, the resident may be required to show physical and verbal deference to the staff members or be subject to punishment. Such deference may be humiliating and result in loss of self-esteem. Often the individual is asked to engage in activity whose symbolic implications are incompatible with conceptions of self. Sharon Curtin (1972) describes the case of Miss Larson, at shower time in the Montcliffe Convalescent Hospital:

> I could hear Miss Larson. "No, no, I can bathe myself, just let me alone, I can do it." . . . Two aides, one on each side, would pick up the old carcasses, place them in a molded plastic shower chair, deftly remove the blanket, push them under the shower and rather haphazardly soap them down. . . . The aides were quick, efficient, not at all brutal; they kept up a running conversation between themselves about food prices, the new shoes one had bought, California divorce laws. They might have been two sisters doing dishes. Lift, scrub, rinse, dry, put away. And did you hear that one about. . . .

Verbal or Physical Humiliation. Residents may have to beg or humbly ask for little things such as a glass of water or permission to use the telephone. Staff or fellow residents may call the resident obscene names, curse him, publicly point out his negative attributes, or talk about him as if he were not there. At the extreme there may be loss of a sense of personal safety—beatings, shock therapies, or in some cases the understanding that one will be denied necessary treatment—which may lead residents to feel that they are in an environment that does not guarantee their physical integrity.

Contaminative Exposure. On the outside, the individual can hold his or her feelings about self, actions, thoughts, and some possessions clear from others. In the total institution these areas of self are violated. Facts about the residents' social statuses and past behaviors, including negative information, are collected upon admission and continually recorded and made available to staff. Physical contamination, such as unclean food, messy quarters, shoes and clothing soiled by previous users, and interpersonal contamination such as forced social relationships and denial of privacy may occur as well.

Admission procedures, barriers, deference obligations, verbal and physical humiliation, and contaminative exposure represent the mortifying processes that patients are subject to in old-age institutions (and other institutions). The patient must adapt to these processes. Goffman (1961) identifies four modes of adaptation to the processes of mortification that take place in an institution. The first, "situation withdrawal," occurs most frequently in old-age institutions and can be described in terms previously used to describe institutional effects. The patient withdraws attention from everything around him or her, and there is a drastic curtailment of involvement in interaction. "Regression" occurs and is often irreversible. A second mode of adaptation is what Goffman calls the "intransigent line": The inmate intentionally challenges the institution by flagrantly refusing to cooperate with staff members. This mode of adaptation can lead to patient abuse.

Two other modes of adaptation to the total institution, described by Goffman, are "colonization" and "conversion." Patients who take a colonization tack accept the sampling of the outside world provided by the institution and build a stable, contented existence by attempting to procure the maximum satisfaction available in the home. Such patients turn the institution into a home away from home and may find it difficult to leave. As Goffman (1961, 63) points out, the staff who try to make life in total institutions more bearable must face the possibility that doing so may increase the likelihood of colonization. Patients who convert take on the staff view of the patient and often attempt to act out the role of perfect patient. A patient employing this mode of adaptation might adopt the manner and dress of the attendants while helping them to manage other patients.

THE QUALITY OF INSTITUTIONAL CARE

Although Goffman implies that mortification of the self is characteristic of all total institutions (no matter how therapeutic the environment), it makes intuitive sense that some institutional settings are less mortifying than others and provide higher quality care. How such evaluations are made is often difficult to determine. Health-care practitioners and researchers find the issue of evaluating institutional care to be extraordinarily complex (Kart and Manard 1976; Lemke and Moos 1986). What is a good nursing home? Should quality be measured in terms of resident satisfaction or professional nursing care? Given limited resources, is it more important to spend money on gardeners, interior design, janitorial services, and food quality, or on an abundance of aides, orderlies, and health professionals?

A number of researchers have investigated the relationship between institutional characteristics and quality of care. Characteristics of institutions thought to be related to quality of care include ownership status (Lemke and Moos 1986; Levey et al. 1973), size (Greenwald and Linn 1971; Curry and Ratliff 1973), socioeconomic status (Anderson et al. 1969; Levey et al. 1973; Kosberg 1971, 1973), social integration (Jacobs 1969; Lipman 1968b; Gelfand 1968; Grant 1970), and staff professionalism (Holland et al. 1981; Levey et al. 1973).

Can high quality care be assured in nursing homes? Some cynics suggest that even the inspectors and regulators themselves admit regulation is a poor tool for assuring quality institutional care (U.S. Senate Special Committee on Aging 1974; Mendelson and Hapgood 1974). Approaches suggesting administrative change and accountability through greater community involvement have been offered in the past (Barney 1974; Gaynes 1973; Tobin 1974; Gottesman 1974). In recent years, government efforts to control abuse have been aimed primarily at reducing costs rather than improving quality of care. Still, cost containment efforts by the federal government could force better compatibility of patient needs and long-term care services. One approach involves some efficient substitution of long-term care services for acute services (Vladeck 1985). Another is the single or channeling agency, an organizational reform intended to provide opportunities for better matching resources in the community with needs of the area's elderly population (Brecher and Knickman 1985).

SUMMARY

Assessing the long-term care needs of the elderly and matching services to those needs can be difficult. There are many service delivery barriers for older people. Sometimes, the elderly are reluctant to admit that they have needs and many even deny using services. Just because services are created and made available to the elderly does not mean that those services will be utilized. How older people choose the long-term care services they will use is determined by a complex set of interacting personal and environmental factors.

The main source of support for older persons is the family. A body of research suggests that the presence of family is an important factor in delaying, if not preventing, the institutionalization of a chronically ill elderly person. Still, some argue that the needs of the frail and vulnerable elderly are best met if there is a proper balance between formal and informal support. A broad array of services is available to older people in the community, including health, housing, and nutrition. A limited number of these noninstitutional services are discussed in this chapter. These include adult day care, home care, foster care, hospice, protective services, and respite care.

Currently, more than 1.3 million elderly individuals (about 5 percent of the aged population) reside in nursing homes in the United States. The risks of an elderly person in the United States being institutionalized are about one in four. Typically, this population is white, female, widowed, over 75 and has lived in an institutional facility for more than two years. Over 80 percent of nursing-home residents were admitted primarily for physical reasons. There are more than 26,000 nursing homes in the United States today. The great majority of these are run for profit. Three-quarters of homes are certified to participate in Medicare or Medicaid or both.

Nursing homes have an unfavorable reputation and elderly individuals often have strong negative feelings toward being institutionalized even when institutional care is absolutely necessary. In part, this may result from the portrait the gerontological literature paints of the institutionalized elderly. This population is overwhelmingly characterized as disorganized, disoriented, and depressed. Three explanations for this negative portrait are discussed. These include problems of relocation, preadmission effects, and the totality of institutions.

A body of literature dealing with the quality of institutional care is reviewed. It was determined that the "best" institutions are nonprofit, small in size, wealthy in resources, sociable, and with staff that have positive attitudes toward the residents. Unfortunately, institutions with all these characteristics are scarce.

STUDY QUESTIONS

1. Identify the goals of long-term care.
2. Profile the long-term care service user. Does every individual who needs long-term care assistance receive it? What are the service delivery barriers?
3. What do we know about how older people select among long-term care alternatives?
4. What role does the family play in providing long-term care assistance?
5. Identify the following:
   a. Adult day care
   b. Home care
   c. Foster care
   d. Hospice
   e. Protective services
   f. Respite care
6. Why can't the institutionalization rate for the elderly be used as an estimation of their cumulative chances for institutionalization?
7. Describe the "typical" nursing home resident. Explain the disproportionate number of women and the underrepresentation of nonwhites in nursing homes.
8. List some major organizational dimensions along which nursing homes vary. How have nursing home costs increased in relation to prices in general? How and why do charges vary among different nursing homes?
9. What is the process of "self-mortification" as defined by Goffman? List and explain the features of institutional environment that he suggests contribute to the mortification process.

BIBLIOGRAPHY

American Association for Retired Persons. 1986. *Making wise decisions for long-term care.* Washington, D.C.: AARP (pamphlet).

Anderson, N., Holmberg, R., Schneider, R., and Stone, L. 1969. *Policy issues regarding nursing homes: Findings from a Minnesota study*. Minneapolis: Institute for Interdisciplinary Studies, American Rehabilitation Foundation.

Archbold, P.G. 1980. Impact of parent caring on middle-aged offspring. *Journal of Geriatric Nursing* 6(2):78–85.

Arling, G., Harkins, E.B., and Capitman, J.A. 1986. Institutionalization and personal control: A panel study of impaired older people. *Research on Aging* 8(1):38–56.

Barney, J. 1974. Community pressure as a key to quality of life in nursing homes. *American Journal of Public Health* 64:265–268.

Berg, W., Atlas, L., and Zeiger, J. 1974. Integrated homemaking services for the aged in urban neighborhoods. *The Gerontologist* 14:388–393.

Bild, B., and Havighurst, R. 1976. Senior citizens in great cities: The case of Chicago. *The Gerontologist* 16:4–88.

Blazer, D. 1978. Working with the elderly patient's family. *Geriatrics* 33:117–118, 123.

Bloom, M., and Blenkner, M. 1970. Assessing functioning of older persons living in the community. *The Gerontologist* 10:31–37.

Branch, L.G., and Jette, A.M. 1982. A prospective study of long-term care institutionalization among the aged. *American Journal of Public Health* 72:1373–1379.

Brecher, C., and Knickman, J. 1985. A reconsideration of long-term care. *Journal of Health Politics, Policy and Law* 10:245–273.

Brody, E. 1981. "Women in the middle" and family help to older people. *Gerontologist* 21(5):471–480.

Brody, S.J. 1984. Goals of geriatric care. In S. Brody and N. Persily (eds.), *Hospitals and the aged: The new old market*. Rockville, Md.: Aspen Publishing Co.

Brody, S.J., Poulshock, W., and Masciocchi, C. 1978. The family caring unit: A major consideration in the long-term support system. *Gerontologist* 18:556–561.

Brody, S.J., and Persily, N. (eds.). 1984. *Hospitals and the aged: The new old market*. Rockville, Md: Aspen Systems.

Butler, R.N. 1975. *Why survive? Being old in America*. New York: Harper and Row.

Cantor, M. 1975. Life space and the social support system of the inner city elderly of New York City. *The Gerontologist*. 15:23–27.

———. 1981. Factors associated with strain among family, friends and neighbors caring for the frail elderly. Paper presented at the Annual Scientific Meeting of the Gerontological Society of America, Toronto, Canada, November 1981.

Cantor, M., and Little, V. 1985. Aging and social care. In R. Binstock and E. Shanas (eds.), *Handbook of aging and the social sciences* (2nd ed.). New York: Van Nostrand Reinhold Co.

Carp, F.M. 1966. *A future for the aged*. Austin, Tex.: University of Texas Press.

Comptroller General of the United States. 1972. *Study of health facilities construction costs*. Washington, D.C.: General Accounting Office.

———. 1977. *The well-being of older people in Cleveland, Ohio*. Washington, D.C.: General Accounting Office.

Congressional Budget Office. 1977. *Long-term care for the elderly and disabled.* Washington, D.C.: CBO.

Crossman, L., London, C., and Barry, C. 1981. Older women caring for disabled spouses: A model for supportive services. *The Gerontologist.* 21(5):464–470.

Curry, T., and Ratliff, B.W. 1973. The effects of nursing home size on resident isolation and life satisfaction. *The Gerontologist* 13:296–298.

Curtin, S. 1972. *Nobody ever died of old age.* Boston: Little, Brown and Co.

Deimling, G.T., and Poulshock, S.W. 1985. The transition from family in-home care to institutional care. *Research on Aging* 7(4):563–576.

Dunkle, R., Coulton, C., Mackintosh, J., and Goode, R. 1982. The decision making process among the hospitalized elderly. *Journal of Gerontological Social Work* 4(3):95–106.

Ferguson, E. 1978. *Protecting the vulnerable adult.* Ann Arbor: The Institute of Gerontology, University of Michigan.

Fox, P.D., and Clauser, S.V. 1980. Trends in nursing home expenditures: Implications for aging policy. *Health Care Finance Review* 2 (Fall): 65–70.

Gaynes, N.L. 1973. A logic to long-term care. *Gerontologist* 13:277–281.

Gelfand, D.E. 1968. Visiting patterns and social adjustment in an old age home. *Gerontologist* 8:272–275.

Goffman, E. 1961. *Asylums.* New York: Doubleday.

Gottesman, L. 1974. Nursing home performance as related to resident traits, ownership, size, and source of payment. *American Journal of Public Health* 64:269–281.

Grant, D.P. 1970. Architect discovers the aged. *Gerontologist* 10:275–281.

Greenberg, J.N., and Genn, A. 1979. A multivariate analysis of the predictors of long-term care placement. *Home Health Care Services Quarterly* 1:75–99.

Greenwald, S.R., and Linn, M. W. 1971. Intercorrelations of data on nursing homes. *Gerontologist* 11:337–340.

Hagan, J. 1980. Report on respite care services in Indiana. South Bend: Northern Indiana Health Systems Agency, Inc.

Hall, G., and Mathiasen, G. 1968. *Overcoming barriers to protective services for the aged: Report of the National Institute on Protective Services.* New York: National Council on Aging.

———. 1973. *Guide to the development of protective services for older people.* Springfield, Ill.: Charles C Thomas.

Harder, W.P., Gornick, J.C., and Burt, M.R. 1986. Adult day care: substitute or supplement? *The Milbank Quarterly* 64(3):414–441.

Henry, J. 1973. Personality and aging—with special reference to hospitals for the aged poor. In J. Henry (ed.), *On shame, vulnerability and other forms of self-destruction.* New York: Random House.

Hing, E. 1981. *Characteristics of nursing home residents, health status and care received.* Vital and Health Statistics, Series 13, No. 51. Washington, D.C.: U.S. Government Printing Office.

Holland, T., Konick, A., Buffum, W., Smith, M.D., and Petchers, M. 1981. Institutional structure and resident outcomes. *Journal of Health and Social Behavior* 22:433–444.

Horowitz, A. 1981. Sons and daughters as caregivers to older parents: Differences in role performance and consequences. Paper presented at the 33rd Annual Scientific Meeting of the Gerontological Society of America, Toronto, Canada, November 1981.

Horowitz, M.J., and Schulz, R. 1983. The relocation controversy: Criticism and commentary in five recent studies. *Gerontologist* 23:229–234.

Howells, D. 1980. Reallocating institutional resources: Respite care as a supplement to family care of the elderly. Paper presented at the 32rd Annual Scientific Meeting of the Gerontological Society of America, San Diego, Calif., November 1980.

Jacobs, R. 1969. One-way street: An intimate view of adjustment. *Gerontologist* 9:268–275.

Johnson, C. 1983. Dyadic family relations and social supports. *Gerontologist* 23(4):377–383.

Kart, C., and Beckham, B. 1976. Black-white differences in the institutionalization of the elderly: A temporal analysis. *Social Forces* 54:901–910.

Kart, C., and Manard, B. 1976. Quality of care in old-age institutions. *Gerontologist* 16(3):250–256.

Kart, C., and Palmer, N. 1987. How do we explain differences in the level of care received by the institutionalized elderly? *Journal of Applied Gerontology* 6(1):53–66.

Kasl, S. 1972. Physical and mental health effect of involuntary relocation and institutionalization of the elderly: A review. *American Journal of Public Health* 62:377–384.

Kastenbaum, R., and Candy, S. 1973. The 4 percent fallacy: A methodological and empirical critique of extended care facility population statistics. *International Journal of Aging and Human Development* 4:15–21.

Kobrin, F. 1981. Family extension and the elderly: Economic, demographic and family cycle factors. *Journal of Gerontology* 36:370–377.

Koff, T.H. 1982. *Long-term care: An approach to serving the frail elderly*. Boston: Little, Brown and Co.

Kosberg, J. 1971. The relationship between organizational characteristics and treatment resources in nursing homes. Ph.D. dissertation, University of Chicago.

———. 1973. Differences in proprietary institutions care for affluent and nonaffluent elderly. *Gerontologist* 13:299–304.

Lawton, M.P. 1974. Social ecology and the health of older people. *American Journal of Public Health*. 64:257–260.

Lemke, S., and Moos, R.H. 1986. Quality of residential settings for elderly adults. *Journal of Gerontology* 41(2):268–276.

Lesnoff-Caravaglia, G. 1978–79. The five percent fallacy. *International Journal of Aging and Human Development* 9(2):187–192.

Levey, S., Ruchlin, H.S., Stotsky, B.A., Kinlock, D.R., and Oppenheim, W. 1973. An appraisal of nursing home care. *Journal of Gerontology*. 28:222–228.

Lieberman, M. 1969. Institutionalization of the aged: Effects of behavior. *Journal of Gerontology*. 24:330–340.

Lieberman, M., and Tobin, S.S. 1983. *The experience of old age: Stress, coping, and survival.* New York: Basic Books.

Lipman, A. 1968a. Public housing and attitudinal adjustment in old age: A comparative study. *Journal of Geriatric Psychiatry* 2:88–101.

———. 1968b. A socio-architectural view of life in three old peoples' homes. *Gerontologia Clinica* 10:88–101.

Litman, T.J. 1971. Health care and the family: A three-generational analysis. *Medical Care* 9:67–81.

Little, V. 1979. For the elderly: An overview of services in industrially developed and developing countries. In M. Teicher, D. Thursz, and J. Vigilante (eds.), *Reaching the aged: Social services in forty-four countries.* Vol. 4, Social service delivery systems: An international annual. Beverly Hills, Calif.: Sage Publications.

———. 1982. *Open care for the aging.* New York: Springer Publ. Co.

Litwak, E. 1965. Extended kin relations in an industrial democratic society. In E. Shanas and G. Streib (eds.), *Social structure and the family.* Englewood-Cliffs, N.J.: Prentice-Hall.

———. 1978. Agency and family linkages in providing services. In D. Thursz and J. Vigilante (eds.), *Reaching people: The structure of neighborhood, Vol. 3.* Social service delivery systems: An international annual. Beverly Hills, Calif.: Sage Publications, 59–95.

———. 1985. *Helping the elderly.* New York: Guilford Press.

Manard, B., Kart, C., and van Gils, D. 1975. *Old age institutions.* Lexington, Mass.: D.C. Heath.

McAuley, W., and Blieszner, R. 1985. Selection of long-term care arrangements by older community residents. *Gerontologist* 25(2):188–193.

McAuley, W., and Prohaska, T. 1982. Professional recommendations for long-term placement: A comparison of two groups of institutionally vulnerable elderly. *Home Health Care Services Quarterly* 2:44–57.

Mendelson, M.A. 1974. *Tender loving greed.* New York: Random House, Inc.

Mendelson, M.A., and Hapgood, D. 1974. The political economy of nursing homes. *Annals American Academy of Political and Social Sciences* 415:95–105.

Moen, E. 1978. The reluctance of the elderly to accept help. *Social Problems* 25:293–303.

Neu, C.R. 1982. Individual preferences for life and health: Misuses and possible uses. In R.L. Kane and R.A. Kane (eds.), *Values and long-term care.* Lexington, Mass.: D.C. Heath.

Nielson, M., Blenkner, M., Bloom, M., Downs, T., and Beggs, H. 1972. Older persons after hospitalization: A controlled study of home aide service. *American Journal of Public Health* 62:1094–1101.

Noelker, L., and Harel, Z. 1978. Aged excluded from home health care: An inter-organizational solution. *Gerontologist* 18:37–41.

Palmore, E. 1976. Total chance of institutionalization among the elderly. *Gerontologist* 16:504–507.

Rabin, D.L., and Stockton, P. 1987. *Long-term care for the elderly: A factbook.* New York: Oxford University Press.

Rozelle, G. 1980. If home care is effective, why is it underutilized? Ohio Home Health Observer.

Schulz, R., and Brenner, G. 1977. Relocation of the aged: A review and theoretical analysis. *Journal of Gerontology* 32:323–333.

Shanas, E. 1977. *The national survey of the aged.* Final report, ADA grant #90-A-369. Chicago: University of Illinois at Chicago Circle.

———. 1979. The family as a social support system in old age. *Gerontologist* 19:169–174.

Shannon, K. 1985. Home health care study paves way for fixed home care benefits. *Hospitals* 59(5):12.

Shuttlesworth, G.E., Rubin, A., and Duffy, M. 1982. Families versus institutions: Incongruent role expectations in the nursing home. *Gerontologist* 22(2):200–208.

Silverstein, N. 1984. Informing the elderly about public services: The relationship between sources of knowledge and service utilization. *Gerontologist* 24:37–40.

Silverstone, B. 1985. Informal social support systems for the frail elderly. In Institute of Medicine/National Research Council (ed.), *America's aging: Health in an older society.* Washington, D.C.: National Academy Press.

Soldo, B.J. 1980. *Family caregiving and the elderly: Prevalence and variations.* Final report, ADA grant #90-A-2124. Washington, D.C.: Kennedy Institute of Ethics, Georgetown University.

———. 1981. The living arrangements of the elderly in the near future. In S.B. Kiesler, J.N. Morgan, and V.K. Oppenheimer (eds.), *Aging: Social change.* New York: Academic Press.

Stoller, E.P. 1982. Sources of support for the elderly during illness. *Health and Social Work* 7:111–122.

Tobin, S. 1974. How nursing homes vary. *Gerontologist* 14:516–519.

Tobin, S., and Lieberman, M. 1976. *The last home for the aged.* San Francisco, Calif.: Jossey-Bass, Inc., Publishers.

Townsend, C. 1970. *Old age: The last segregation.* New York: Grossman Publishers.

Townsend, P. 1962. *The last refuge.* London: Routledge and Kegan Paul, Ltd.

Townsend, P.W., and Flanagan, J.J. 1976. Experimental preadmission program to encourage home care for severely and profoundly retarded children. *American Journal of Mental Deficiency* 180:562–569.

Troll, L., Miller, S., and Atchley, R. 1979. *Families in later life.* Belmont, Calif.: Wadsworth Publishers.

U.S. Bureau of the Census. 1985. *Statistical abstract of the United States: 1986.* Washington, D.C.: U.S. Government Printing Office.

U.S. Department of Health, Education and Welfare. 1977. *Characteristics, social contacts, and activities of nursing home residents, U.S. 1973 National Nursing Home Survey.* DHEW Pub. No. (HRA) 77-1778. Public Health Service. Hyattsville, Md.: U.S. Government Printing Office.

U.S. General Accounting Office. 1977. Report to the Congress on home health—The need for a national policy to better provide for the elderly. Washington, D.C.: U.S. Government Printing Office.

U.S. Senate. 1977. Protective services for the elderly: A working paper prepared for the Special Committee on Aging. Washington, D.C.: U.S. Government Printing Office.

U.S. Senate Special Committee on Aging. 1974. *Nursing home care in the U.S.: Failure in Public Policy.* Washington, D.C.: U.S. Government Printing Office.

———. 1982. *Developments in aging.* Vol. 1. Report 97-314, 97th Congress, Second session. Washington, D.C.: U.S. Government Printing Office.

Upshur, C. 1978. Final report on respite care policy development project. Boston: Providers' Management, Inc.

———. 1983. Developing respite care: A support service for families with disabled members. *Family Relations* 31:13–20.

Van Nostrand, J., Zappolo, A., Hing, E., Bloom, B., Hirsch, B., and Foley, D.J. 1979. *The national nursing home survey: 1977 summary for United States.* Vital and health statistics, series 13-1, no. 43. Washington, D.C.: U.S. Government Printing Office.

Vladeck, B. 1985. Reforming Medicare provider payment. *Journal of Health Politics, Policy and Law* 10:513-532.

Wahl, D. 1974. Model for protective-advisory-legal service project for the elderly: A multidisciplinary approach. Paper presented at the Gerontological Society meeting, Portland, OR.

Wahl, D., and Soifer, S. 1974. Determinants of physician utilization: A causal analysis. *Journal of Health and Social Behavior* 18:61–70.

Ward, R. 1977. Services for older people: An integrated framework for research. *Journal of Health and Social Behavior* 18:61–70.

Weiler, P., and Rathbone-McCuan, E. 1978. *Adult day care: Community work with the elderly.* New York: Springer Publishing Co.

CHAPTER 18

HEALTH POLICY AND AGING

We begin by identifying the patterns of health and medical service utilization among the elderly. Of particular interest are physician visits and the use of nonphysician professional and hospital inpatient services. In addition, policies, programs, and funding mechanisms available for the health and medical care of the elderly are assessed. The chapter concludes by placing health care in a broader political economy of aging perspective.

USE OF SERVICES

Table 18-1 presents data on physician visits per person per year by age for 1983. The average number of physician contacts by persons sixty-five years and over was 7.6 visits. This compared with 5.0 visits for persons of all ages and, as the data generally show, with the exception of children under six years of age, the average number of physician contacts per person increases with age. In 1983, the aged were more likely than the total population to receive care at the doctor's office (58.9 versus 55.9 percent) and less likely than the total population to be treated in a hospital outpatient department (12.3 versus 14.9 percent) or over the telephone (11.9 versus 15.5 percent). Physician visits are up only slightly over the last twenty years. In 1964 the average number of physician contacts among those aged sixty-five years and over was 6.7.

This lack of substantial change in the indicator for the entire elderly population may mask some changes that have taken place within the population. According to the U.S. Department of Health and Human Services, the number of physician contacts per person per year has *increased* for the elderly poor and

TABLE 18-1 Physician Visits, According to Source or Place of Care and Age; United States, 1982 and 1983 (data are based on household interviews of a sample of the civilian noninstitutionalized population)

| Age | Physician Visits (number per person) | | Source or Place of Care (percent of visits*) | | | | | |
| | | | Doctor's Office | | Hospital Outpatient Department† | | Telephone | |
	1982	1983	1982	1983	1982	1983	1982	1983
Total‡	5.1	5.0	56.9	55.9	14.5	14.9	14.9	15.5
Under 17	4.2	4.4	55.7	55.0	13.8	13.7	17.6	19.3
Under 6	6.0	6.5	54.3	54.3	12.7	12.8	20.4	20.6
6–16	3.2	3.2	57.0	55.8	14.9	14.7	14.8	17.9
17–44	4.6	4.5	56.0	54.4	15.2	16.4	13.7	14.6
45–64	6.1	5.8	58.2	58.7	15.5	15.2	13.5	12.5
65 and over	7.7	7.6	61.4	58.9	11.7	12.3	12.9	11.9

* Includes source or place unknown.

† Includes hospital outpatient clinic, emergency room and other hospital visits.

‡ Age-adjusted, includes all other races not shown separately.

Source: Division of Health Interview Statistics, National Center for Health Statistics; data from the National Health Interview Survey.

decreased for the nonpoor. This finding suggests that differences in the rate of physician utilization by the poor and nonpoor elderly have been narrowed or eliminated in recent years. One problem with this suggestion is that it fails to distinguish the differential need for health and medical services in various income groups. The inference here is that six or seven physician contacts a year may be sufficient given the need for services of an average elderly individual with income at or above the median for the total population. Nevertheless, six or seven office visits may not meet the needs of the average elderly individual with income at 125 percent or less of the poverty level. Aday (1975) has developed an index of use of services that takes into account need for care as measured by disability data. She reports that the poor continue to use fewer services relative to medical need than do those in higher socioeconomic circumstances.

Physician visits also vary by race and sex. Elderly whites report more physician visits per year than do elderly nonwhites; elderly women also report more physician visits than elderly men do. Differences in health and medical service use by race are generally explained by racial differences in socioeconomic status. The gender differential in utilization of physician services exists in all age groups except for those ages when a mother usually makes the health-care decisions. The largest differential occurs between the ages of fifteen and forty-four when women are most likely to be making use of obstetrical and gynecological services.

Explanations for these sex differences in utilization of medical services (and in morbidity rates) have focused primarily on the social situation of women. Nathanson (1975) groups these explanations into three categories: (1) Women report more illness than men and utilize medical services more frequently than men do because it is culturally more acceptable for them to be ill; (2) a woman's role is relatively undemanding, thus reporting illness and visiting the doctor are more compatible with her other role responsibilities than is the case for men; (3) women's assigned social roles are in fact more stressful than those of men—consequently, women have more real illness and need more care. As Nathanson points out, insufficient data are available to evaluate the merits of these explanations.

According to the National Center for Health Services Research, the elderly visit nurses, chiropractors, physical therapists, and other such health workers more than other Americans do. In 1977, 29.7 percent of the elderly had contacts with nonphysician providers; this compared with 23.2 percent of the total population (Berk and Schur 1985). "Nonphysician" providers is a category that also includes optometrists, podiatrists, and psychologists. Differences by age in the average number of nonphysician contacts for those with at least one contact were substantial. For example, on average, the aged had twice as many contacts per year (7.7 versus 3.9) as adults nineteen to twenty-four did (Berk and Schur 1985).

Table 18-2 presents data on one aspect of medical care service utilization

TABLE 18-2 Dental Visits and Interval since Last Visit, According to Age; United States, 1964, 1978 and 1983 (data are based on household interviews of a sample of the civilian non-institutionalized population)

| Age | Dental Visits (number per person) | | | Interval since Last Dental Visit (percent of population*) | | | | | | | | |
| | | | | Less Than 1 Year | | | 2 Years or More | | | Never Visited Dentist | | |
	1964	1978	1983	1964	1978	1983	1964	1978	1983	1964	1978	1983
Total†	1.6	1.6	1.8	42.0	49.9	51.8	28.1	25.1	23.7	15.6	10.5	10.8
Under 17	1.4	1.6	1.9	41.6	50.7	50.6	6.3	8.0	7.6	42.6	29.4	30.4
Under 6	0.5	0.6	0.5	16.5	21.2	23.1	0.6	0.9	1.0	80.4	74.3	70.5
6–16	2.0	2.1	2.6	56.9	64.2	66.1	9.8	11.2	11.3	19.6	9.1	7.8
17–44	1.9	1.6	1.8	50.0	54.3	56.6	27.8	25.1	24.9	3.2	1.9	1.6
45–64	1.7	1.7	2.0	38.4	48.8	51.9	45.5	37.0	34.3	1.3	0.6	0.6
65 and over	0.8	1.2	1.5	20.8	32.3	37.8	66.8	58.2	51.3	1.5	0.6	0.9

* Includes unknown interval since last dental visit.

† Age adjusted. Includes all other races not shown separately.

Source: Division of Health Interview Statistics, National Center for Health Statistics; data from the National Health Interview Survey.

that gets looked at all too infrequently—utilization of dental services. Dental problems increase with age. More than one-fourth of persons aged forty-five to sixty-four have lost all their teeth; almost 90 percent have diseases of the tissues supporting or surrounding remaining teeth (Shanas and Maddox 1977). Yet in 1983, elderly individuals averaged only 1.5 dental visits a year; this is up from 1.2 dental visits in 1978 and 0.8 visits in 1964. Unlike medical care, dental care is rarely financed by public programs or private health insurance. Thus, financial barriers to dental care are still substantial. Data from the National Health Interview Survey in 1975 reveal that an elderly individual with income of $15,000 or more makes almost three times as many dental visits a year as the elderly individual with income below $5,000 a year (2.0 versus 0.7).

The lack of dental care among the elderly is serious. Fully 50 percent of the elderly have no natural teeth. Of those, 10 percent have no false teeth or an incomplete set. Even those with false teeth do not use them all the time; many report that their dentures are improperly fitted. Increasing the availability of dental services could improve the quality of life of many older people. Fear and embarrassment about socializing because of oral health problems has led many old people to isolation. This could be overcome if dental care services were made available to more elderly. Nutritional status might also be improved by making it possible for those people who are edentulous or who have periodontal disease (and are thus restricted in diet) to eat a wider variety of foods.

Hospital utilization rates also vary according to age, gender, race, and family income. The elderly are the heaviest utilizers of hospital care; in 1977, each person aged sixty-five to seventy-nine years, on the average, spent almost 11.0 days in short-term, general nonfederal hospitals; this figure compares with 8.4 days for those aged forty to sixty-four years and 12.0 days for those aged eighty years and over (Granick and Short 1985). As data from the Hospital Cost and Utilization Project in Table 18-3 show, although more diagnoses are recorded for patients aged sixty-five and older, fewer surgical procedures are performed on this group.

Utilization of short-term hospitals has increased since Medicare was implemented in 1966. This increase was greatest among the elderly poor. According to Wilson and White (1977), discharge rates increased by 47 percent for the poor and by 18 percent for the nonpoor elderly between 1964 and 1975. Obviously, some financial barriers to inpatient hospital care for the poor have been lifted by Medicare and Medicaid, although in light of their greater need for care, the poor, relative to the nonpoor, are still undersubscribers to hospital care.

The elderly have lower rates of admission to inpatient psychiatric facilities than do all other age groups except those under eighteen years of age. Data for 1980 from the Veterans Administration Patient Treatment File and biennial inventories of mental health organizations show lower rates of admission for the aged for all diagnoses in an array of inpatient psychiatric organizations. In general, only for organic disorders do those aged sixty-five years and older

TABLE 18-3   Characteristics of Patients in Short-Term, General, Non-Federal Hospitals, by Age Group (HCUP Patient Sample, 1977*)

	40–64 years (n = 104,584)†	65–79 years (n = 64,603)†	80+ years (n = 23,773)†
Average length of stay (days)	8.4	10.8	12.0
Average number of diagnoses	2.5	3.1	3.5
Average number of surgical procedures	1.3	1.2	1.0
Percent operated upon	52.2	41.5	30.2
Percent discharged to another health facility	1.9	6.3	17.4
Percent Medicare	8.1	93.3	95.7
Percent female	54.2	53.5	62.3

* Hospitalizations for conditions that would not occur in the elderly are excluded; these include the entire range of conditions associated with childbirth, complications of pregnancy and abortions.

† Indicates differences between age groups significant at the .05 level using a standard two-tailed *t*-test.

Source: National Center for Health Services Research and Health Care Technology Assessment; Hospital Studies Program; Hospital Cost and Utilization Project.

have higher rates of admission to psychiatric facilities than is the case for the total population.

EXPLAINING USE OF HEALTH AND MEDICAL SERVICES

Although we have concentrated on the impact of age (and sometimes sex, gender, race, and income) on the utilization of medical services, other variables are included as well. Certainly, health beliefs or values and knowledge about health and the health-care system are related to use of health services (Andersen and Newman 1973). What Ward (1977) calls "community variables" also affect utilization. These include location of residence—central city, suburban, rural (Andersen, Greenley, Kravits and Anderson 1972), density of age peers, availability of local transportation, and availability of neighborhood-based services and social supports (Cantor 1975; Carp 1975; Lopata 1975).

Other writers and researchers have looked at how the health-care delivery system itself affects patterns of utilization. For example, Harris (1975) and Hammerman (1975) criticize the current system of service delivery as being too fragmented and disorganized. Such critics emphasize the extent to which financing programs are predisposed to fund inpatient care at the expense of community-based or home care and the way public funding mechanisms discourage preventive care and mental health services.

Determining the conditions under which people use health-care services is a difficult enterprise. The presence of an impairment or a self-assessment of poor health does not necessarily indicate a need for medical care. Even an objective indication of need for medical care may not be a foolproof predictor of whether an individual will use available health services.

A number of studies have implicated structural, social, and psychological factors in utilization behavior. The costs of medical care (Berki and Ashcraft 1979), gender (Verbrugge 1976), level of psychological distress (Tessler, Mechanic, and Dimond 1976) and the availability of social support (Schuval 1970) are among those variables that apparently have effects on the utilization of health services among the population at large.

Andersen (1968) and his colleagues (Andersen, Anderson, and Smedby 1968; Andersen and Newman 1973) have generated a conceptual framework within which to sort factors that contribute to the use of health services. Three groups of variables are identified in this conceptual framework: *Predisposing factors* are social structural variables (for example, race, religion, ethnicity) as well as family attitudes and health beliefs that may affect the recognition that health services are needed. *Enabling factors* include individual characteristics or circumstances, such as available family income and accessibility of service, that might hinder or accelerate use of a health service. *Need factors* include subjective perceptions and judgments about the seriousness of symptoms, the level of physical disability or psychological impairment, and an individual's response to illness. Using this categorization schema in a Swedish study, Andersen and his colleagues (1968) found that the social class (a predisposing factor) and income (an enabling factor) of an individual were important predictors of the use of health services.

Well-designed and executed studies focusing specifically on the use of medical care by the elderly are not well represented in the literature. Roos and Shapiro (1981), using data from a sample of Manitoba (Canada) elderly, suggest that a relatively few elderly account for a disproportionate share of health service utilization. The majority of older people in their study use services at approximately the same rate as younger people do. Having advanced age, low self-perceived health status, and several self-reported health problems seem to place individuals at a higher risk for the use of hospital services. Still, although the very old were at greater risk to be hospitalized, they used only marginally more physician services than did their younger counterparts. This finding is in opposition to a widely held belief that advancing age significantly increases the consumption of *all* types of health care (Roos and Shapiro 1981).

Several studies have recently tried to identify additional sociodemographic determinants of medical care use among the elderly. Haug (1981) has found older persons in general are more likely to get physical checkups and more likely to overutilize the health-care system for minor complaints than younger persons are. Yet, they are little different from the younger in underutilization for conditions that should receive a doctor's attention. Interestingly, currently married elderly are more likely than are younger marrieds to overutilize the health-care system. As Haug points out, this may be due to what Eliot Friedson (1961) has described as the *lay-referral system:* A spouse is turned to first for advice when a person is ill; it appears that spouses are more likely to recommend contacting a physician when an older husband or wife has a complaint.

Wan (1982) has studied the use of health services among almost 2,000 elderly individuals residing in low-income areas of cities such as Atlanta, Kansas City, and Boston, among selected others. He describes the regular user of neighborhood health centers as being black, with income under $5,000 per year, relatively uneducated, and on some form of public assistance. Persons using a hospital ambulatory clinic as a regular source of health care have a similar profile, though they seem more likely to be younger (aged sixty-five to sixty-nine years), male, and suffering from acute episodes of illness and a chronic disability.

In a multivariate analysis of his data, Wan (1982) found health status (as measured by number of acute illnesses experienced by an individual and level of chronic disability) to account for more variation in physician contacts than did access to a regular source of medical care. Access to medical care (as measured by the availability of a usual source of care and insurance coverage) did correlate with more frequent visits to physicians. Those with a regular source of care were three times as frequent users of ambulatory care as those with no regular source.

Interestingly, Wan's analysis showed Medicaid recipients and those with access to neighborhood health centers to be the most frequent users of physician care. Blacks also had a greater number of physician contacts than did whites. Previously, a number of studies had indicated that the poor have less accessibility to health-care services. At least in the United States this was the case prior to the implementation of Medicare and Medicaid when, for example, the lowest socioeconomic groups had fewer physician visits than those with more income (Mechanic 1978). According to Wan (1982, 104), poor elderly blacks appear to have significantly benefited from the advent of Medicaid and other forms of public assistance. They have also taken advantage of various services provided by the neighborhood health center. Wan concludes:

> One inference that can be drawn is that the removal of financial barriers, coupled with a concerted effort toward making health services readily available to the medically needy, has greatly facilitated the use of ambulatory physician care.

Recently, Coulton and Frost (1982) have reported on a study of health service utilization by the elderly, using the conceptual framework put forth by Andersen and his colleagues. The source of data was the *Study of Older People in Cleveland, Ohio, 1975, 1976,* conducted by the United States General Accounting Office. This data set includes over 1,800 noninstitutionalized elderly interviewed in 1975; approximately 1,500 were interviewed again a year later.

Variation in use of medical care services among the elderly was largely attributable to need factors, including perceived need as well as evaluated need. Enabling and predisposing factors offered little additional help in explaining why some older people use medical care services and others do not. Having an established pattern of utilization and a medical care provider with expectations for continued contact were additional determinants of health service utilization. This latter point is important. Some studies show that medical visits are often initiated by the medical care provider so that being affiliated with a source of care increases the likelihood of continued utilization. Finally, this study showed only weak effects of sex differences and psychological distress on utilization of health services among the elderly.

Wolinsky and his colleagues (1983) have studied the health services utilization patterns of the noninstitutionalized elderly in St. Louis, also using Andersen's (1968) model. They distinguish between the informal and formal use of health services among the elderly. Informal use of health services occurs when an individual gives provisional validation to being ill and initiates some form of self-treatment. In this study, informal use of health services is measured by self-reports of restricted-activity and bed-disability days. Formal health service utilization is measured in more typical fashion and includes measures of physician and dental contact, emergency room visits, and hospitalizations.

Four important trends are evident from this research. First, Andersen's model is more successful at explaining informal than formal utilization of health services. The level of dental contact evidenced by this population of elderly people is almost entirely explained by whether a regular source of dental care was available. Similarly, formal use of physician services was strongly influenced by the availability of a regular source of medical care.

Second, as is evident from previous studies (including Coulton and Frost, discussed above), the need characteristics are the most powerful predictors of the use of health services. Third, consistent with previous studies, predisposing factors show no significant effect on the use of health services after the effect of need. Fourth, there are no significant effects of any enabling factors aside from having a regular source of care. Also, the effect of having a regular source of care does not contribute to explaining informal utilization or the three most policy-relevant formal measures of utilization, that is, number of physician visits, number of emergency room visits, and hospitalizations.

PAYING FOR MEDICAL CARE

During the fiscal year 1974 the total cost of health care in the United States reached over 116 billion dollars, for an average of $522 per person. By 1984, these numbers had more than tripled. National health-care expenditures exceeded $387 billion with per capita expenditure reaching approximately $1,580. Health expenditures were projected at almost 10.6 percent of the gross national product (GNP) in 1984. For 1984, the annual percent increase in health-care costs was 9.1 percent, the lowest annual increase since the early 1970s. This is a radically different picture from 1965, the year Congress passed the Medicare and Medicaid legislation. Total health-care expenditures in 1965 amounted to $42 billion, 6.1 percent of the GNP, or $207 per person.

Health costs for the elderly have increased at a similar, if not a more rapid, pace. The amount of money expended on Medicare alone has increased more than eight times between 1970 and 1984 ($7.5 versus $64.6 billion). In 1981, the average medical care bill for the aged was three times that for those aged nineteen to sixty-four and seven times that for those younger than age nineteen. The source of funds to pay for health care of the elderly has also changed dramatically. During 1966, the year Medicare and Medicaid were implemented, only 30 percent of these funds were public; by fiscal 1981, 64 percent of the expenditures came from public funds.

The largest single item on the health-care bill of elderly individuals is hospital care. In 1981, this item cost $36.6 billion and accounted for 44 percent of all personal health-care expenditures for the aged. Public monies (including Medicare and Medicaid) paid for 85.5 percent of this bill. The 14.5 percent not covered by public funds must be paid by the individual or by some form of private health insurance.

Hospital care, nursing home care, and physicians' services together account for $71.6 billion or about 86 percent of the $83.2 billion spent on health care for the elderly in fiscal 1981. Items such as drugs, dental services, eyeglasses, and appliances constitute a very small part of the total bill as well as the privately funded bill. Still, expenditures for these items may be low because elderly people are going without them. As costs continue to rise (over the last decade medical care costs for the elderly have risen at an average annual rate of about 15 percent) and such services continue to remain outside the scope of most public funding mechanisms for health care of the elderly, we can expect continued low utilization. In 1981, private sources funded 82.3 percent of the costs of drugs and drug sundries for older people. How many older people go without needed drugs because public funding mechanisms do not generally underwrite the costs for drugs and personal funds are unavailable?

Payments for health care are made under a variety of public and private programs designed to provide care or access to care for specified population groups. The two largest programs are Medicare and Medicaid. They are the principal public funding mechanisms for health care of the elderly and deserve our special attention.

Medicare

In 1965, the *Social Security Act of 1935* was amended to provide health insurance for the elderly. This amendment, which became effective July 1, 1966, is known as Title XVIII or Medicare. It marked the inauguration in the United States of a national system of financing individual health services on a social insurance basis. It was not, however, the country's first attempt at establishing national health insurance. Such attempts and their failures date back to the beginning of the century. The historical record is worthy of a brief review.[1]

Between 1915 and 1918, a group of academics, lawyers, and other professionals who were organized under the American Association for Labor Legislation attempted to push a model medical care insurance bill through several state legislatures. They had no success. The American Medical Association (AMA) opposed the bills as did the American Federation of Labor (AFL). The AFL feared that any form of compulsory social insurance might lead to further government control of working people. It was not until the Great Depression that interest in governmental health insurance reappeared on a sustained basis.

In 1934 President Roosevelt created an advisory Committee on Economic Security. In the climate of destitution and poverty that accompanied the Great Depression, this committee was charged with drafting a social security bill providing a minimum income for the aged, the unemployed, the blind, and the widowed and their children. The result was the Social Security Act of 1935. The Social Security Act was originally intended to include health insurance provisions also. Nevertheless, as Feingold points out, the extent of this intention was little more than one line in the original bill that suggested that the Social Security Board study the problem and report to Congress. When opposition to this line became so strong that it appeared to jeopardize the Social Security bill itself, the line was dropped.

Although advocates of compulsory health insurance proposed congressional bills from 1939 on, it was not until Truman's "Fair Deal" that the possibility of passing such a bill became strong. In the interim (1939 to 1949), private health insurance (endorsed by the AMA) through Blue Cross, Blue Shield, and commercial insurance carriers became firmly established in the United States as a way of paying for medical expenses.

In 1949 President Truman requested congressional action on medical care insurance. In order to placate the AMA and its allies, it was specified that doctors and hospitals would not have to join the plan. In addition, doctors would retain the right to refuse to serve patients whom they did not want. This was not enough. The American Medical Association was adamantly opposed to "socialized medicine," and, despite Truman's characterization of the AMA as "the public's worst enemy in the efforts to redistribute medical care more equitably," efforts at passing a national health insurance bill were defeated.

What were the major objections to these early national health insurance proposals? According to Marmor, they were as follows: (1) Medical insurance was a "give-away" program that made no distinction between the deserving and undeserving poor; (2) too many well-off Americans who did not need

---

[1] Historical material on Medicare comes primarily from Marmor (1973) and Feingold (1966).

financial assistance in meeting their health needs would be helped; (3) utilization of health-care services would increase dramatically and beyond their capacity; and (4) there would be excessive control of physicians, constituting a precedent for socialism in the United States.

Clearly another strategy was necessary, and the one that developed shifted attention away from the health problems of the general population to those of the aged. There was great appeal in focusing on the aged, for as a group, they were needy yet deserving. Most had made a contribution to the United States. Still, through no fault of their own, many suffered reduced earning capacity and higher medical expenses. Proponents of this new strategy waged a public war of sympathy for the aged and a private war of pressure politics from 1952 until 1965. Not until then was the political climate ripe for amending the original Social Security Act to provide health insurance for America's aged (Medicare).

Medicare consists of two basic components. Part A is a compulsory hospital insurance (HI) plan that covers a bed patient in a hospital and, under certain conditions, in a skilled nursing facility or at home after discharge from the hospital. It is financed by employer–employee contributions and a tax on the self-employed. Most of the elderly are automatically eligible as a result of their own or a spouse's entitlement to Social Security. In 1983, almost 92 percent of those aged sixty-five years and over were covered by Medicare. If for any reason a person is not eligible for HI at age sixty-five, it can be purchased on a voluntary basis. The monthly premium became $248 on January 1, 1987.

Part B represents a voluntary program of supplemental medical insurance (SMI) that helps pay doctor bills, outpatient hospital benefits, home health services, and certain other medical services and supplies. Financing is achieved through monthly premiums paid by enrollees and matching funds by the federal government. As of January 1, 1987, the monthly premium is $17.90 or $214.80 for the year.

Hospital insurance (Part A) benefits are measured by periods of time known as *benefit periods*. Benefit periods begin when a patient enters the hospital and end when he or she has not been a hospital bed patient for sixty consecutive days. This concept is an important one to grasp since it determines how much care a Medicare beneficiary is entitled to at any particular point in time. Medicare will help to pay covered services for a patient for up to ninety days of in-hospital care, for up to one hundred days of extended care in a skilled nursing facility, and for posthospital home health care in each benefit period. If an individual runs out of covered days within a benefit period, he or she may draw upon a lifetime reserve of sixty additional hospital days. Use of these days within the lifetime reserve, however, permanently reduces the total number of reserve days left. For example, if a patient has been in the hospital for ninety days and needs ten more days of hospital care, he or she may draw ten days from the reserve of sixty, leaving a reserve of fifty days.

Part A Medicare benefits will pay for such services as a semi-private room, including meals and special diets, regular nursing services, lab tests, drugs furnished by the hospital, and medical supplies and appliances furnished by the hospital. It will not pay for convenience items, a private room, or private-duty nurses, for example.

A Medicare patient is financially responsible, through copayments and deductibles, for various components of his or her hospital insurance plan. As a bed patient in a participating hospital, he or she is responsible for the first $520 of costs in each benefit period (1987 figure). After this, Part A pays for covered services for the first sixty days of hospital care. From day sixty-one through day ninety-one in a benefit period, hospital insurance pays for all covered service except for $130 a day. If more than ninety days of inpatient care is required, reserve days may be used. The copayment after ninety days of care is $260 a day. Beyond 150 days in a hospital, Medicare pays nothing.

Extended-care benefits provide for covered services for the first twenty days in a benefit period. After the first twenty days, the recipient must pay $65 (1987 figure) a day for up to eighty days in a benefit period. Home health care, from a home health agency participating in Medicare, covers part-time nursing care by a registered nurse or under her or his supervision, physical or speech therapy, and medical supplies and appliances. It does not cover services of part-time health aides at home.

The medical insurance program (Part B) of Medicare is a voluntary one, and an individual must pay a monthly premium in order to be eligible for coverage. In addition, the subscriber pays a deductible each year and 20 percent of the remainder. Although Part B pays for a broad array of outpatient hospital services, doctors' services, home health care benefits, and other medical supplies, it does *not* cover such things as routine physical examinations, regular eye or hearing examinations, eyeglasses or hearing aids, prescription drugs, false teeth, or full-time nursing care.

Medicaid

Medicaid, or Title XIX of the Social Security Act, passed also in 1965, becoming effective July 1, 1966. According to Stevens and Stevens (1974), some observers of the time saw Title XIX as the "sleeper" of the 1965 legislation. After all, Medicare is limited in terms of who is covered (primarily the aged), the types of services covered (described above), and the presence of deductibles and copayments. Medicaid was intended as a catchall program to handle the medical expenses not covered by Medicare as well as to provide medical assistance to needy groups other than the aged. The program is jointly funded by federal and state governments with the federal government contributing in excess of 50 percent in poor states. Eligibility varies from one state to another, although one requirement seems to be almost universal. Wherever an individual qualifies for Medicaid, "pauperization" has preceded qualification. All persons, including the elderly, may find themselves eligible for Medicaid only after they have drained their resources and qualified as a member of the poor.

HEALTH POLICY: IS THERE A CRISIS
IN MEDICAL CARE FINANCING?

The Medicare program has made and continues to make various medical services available to many persons who would not receive them otherwise. Older people living on low, relatively fixed incomes might not be able to secure the services of a physician, a hospital, a skilled nursing home, or a home health-care program without Medicare. Nevertheless, the Medicare program is riddled with various out-of-pocket deductibles and copayments for its beneficiaries, not to mention limitations in services provided. Medicare now pays approximately 44 percent of the medical care expenditures of the elderly, leaving the rest to be paid for by Medicaid (17 percent) and by personal resources (39 percent).

A recent report by the Special Committee on Aging of the United States Senate (1978) indicates that many elderly Americans supplement their Medicare with some private health insurance plan. In 1975, almost 63 percent did so for hospital care, and up to 55 percent had some form of private insurance coverage for physician's services. Such plans have little impact and are not heavily drawn upon. Only about 5 percent of the health-care bill for older Americans is paid for by private health insurance coverage. Abuses are rampant. Senator Chiles of Florida reported on the case of an 87-year-old woman who had been sold nineteen separate policies from nine different companies by six agents in just over a year. The woman was committed to premium payments of almost $4,000 a year, most of which was worthless because of the duplication and overlap in coverage. May elderly Americans fear health-care costs beyond what Medicare will cover, but excessive insurance premiums are not a solution to limited coverage.

In the fall of 1986 President Reagan proposed an extension of Medicare to provide catastrophic health insurance coverage to older Americans. Under this proposal, a low monthly premium would protect an older person from being impoverished as a result of an acute illness; maximum out-of-pocket expenditures per year for the elderly ill would be about $2,000. By the end of 1987 both the House and Senate had passed different and expanded versions of the original Reagan proposal. Reconciliation brought added benefits for outpatient prescription drugs, increased benefits for outpatient and physician care, and some pegging of Medicare premiums to the income of elderly retirees. This latter fact has caused some outcry over the costs of the new plan (Tolchin 1988).

In addition to the problems of limited coverage, Medicare focuses too narrowly on providing acute care. The maintenance of chronic health conditions and quality of life issues do not receive appropriate attention. Eye examinations for eyeglasses, hearing examinations for hearing aids, orthopedic shoes, and false teeth are all excluded from coverage. Under this system, Medicare patients cannot take advantage of geriatric consultation clinics that are concerned with the prevention of illness and the maintenance of chronic conditions. Such clinics

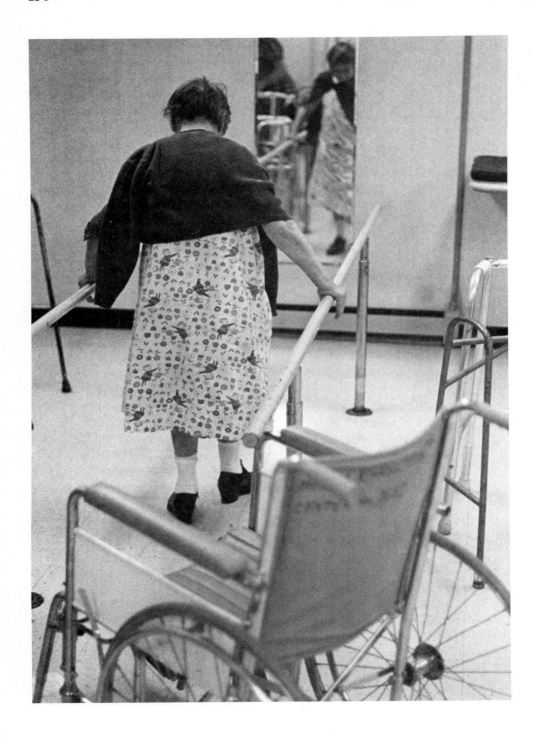

only exist for private, paying patients. The Reagan Administration proposal to offer catastrophic insurance coverage to older Americans continues the Medicare emphasis on acute care. This "extra" catastrophic insurance does not apply to long-term care needs of the elderly.

The language employed throughout the Medicare regulations refers to medical need, medical care, and medical necessity. Health teaching, health maintenance, prevention of illness, aspects of rehabilitation, and personal care are related to health care but not necessarily to medical care. The elderly are often in need of health-care services in far greater proportion than medical-care services (Schwab 1977). If the health needs of the elderly population are to be served and if suitable health maintenance programs are to be developed, then a financing system must be initiated that allows for funding of services that prevent illness and maintain health.

Because Medicare and Medicaid result from legal entitlements to services, there has been some concern that expenditures from these programs are uncontrollable. The costs of providing medical care under these programs have increased at a rate exceeding the growth of the federal economy and the consumer price index. Frustration over apparently uncontrollable costs has led to major reform in Medicare and Medicaid. Starting in October 1983 a new system began that fixed Medicare hospital-payment rates in advance. Under this *prospective payment system,* hospitals know in advance what Medicare will pay them for treating a patient with a particular ailment. A fee is set for the treatment of 467 illnesses and injuries categorized into *diagnosis-related groups* (DRGs). Fees vary by region, according to whether the hospital is in an urban or rural setting, and according to the prevailing wage rate in the area. Rates will likely be adjusted annually. Psychiatric care, long-term care, rehabilitation, and children's hospitals were initially excluded from this prospective payment system.

The fixed fee will have to be accepted as payment in full for treatment of a Medicare patient who has been hospitalized. Those hospitals that can provide the care for less than the fixed payment rate will be allowed to keep the extra money. If hospitals are unable to provide the care for the fixed payment rate, they may charge patients only for the deductibles and copayments that already are part of the Medicare payment system. Some argue that this prospective payment system provides incentives to hospitals to admit patients at a later stage in the progress of illness and discharge them at an earlier stage of illness recovery. Only analysis of hard data will determine if such incentives are at work.

An additional important reform of Medicare is the payment for *hospice* care for the dying. Under new hospice provisions, the federal government will purchase a comprehensive package of services for those terminally ill who no longer receive curative medical care (Rabin 1985). This package includes the cost of institutional as well as home care, drugs, counseling, and other medical and social services. The Congressional Budget Office estimates that the availability of reimbursement for hospice care will reduce the time patients would otherwise spend in hospitals and nursing homes, thus saving Medicare tens of millions of dollars annually.

Medicaid has also experienced reform. As Rabin (1985) reports, states have been given greater program autonomy over which services to provide. They may limit the freedom to select a medical care provider, develop new formulas for hospital reimbursement, and emphasize community-based alternatives to institutional care. Furthermore, states are now in a position to negotiate with providers about the organization and price of health- and medical-care delivery.

Despite these reforms, Medicare and Medicaid still represent legal entitlement to medical care. Although the price of medical care is more regulated than in the past, costs continue to rise. It was expected that combined spending for Medicare and Medicaid in 1985 would exceed $100 billion. The Medicare Board of Trustees has reviewed the actuarial status of the HI and supplementary medical insurance (SMI) trust funds (Klees and Warfield 1986). Using intermediate assumptions (somewhere between optimistic and pessimistic), the Board found the present financing schedule for the HI program barely sufficient to ensure the payment of benefits through the late 1990s. The SMI program is actuarially sound, but the Board recommended that Congress take action to curtail the rapid growth in this part of Medicare (Klees and Warfield 1986).

HEALTH POLICY: LONG-TERM CARE ISSUES

Services that are delivered across the continuum of long-term care (as described in Chapter 17) are fragmented. Community-based, long-term care programs comprise a heterogeneous collection of agencies, institutions, and programs of both a private and public nature (Somers 1985). Eligibility is frequently determined by a means test. This can eliminate persons in need from the service delivery system.

Recent amendments to Medicare have shown increased sensitivity to connecting acute care services to long-term care services. In particular, The Omnibus Reconciliation Act of 1980 liberalized Medicare home health-care benefits and made provisions for greater participation by proprietary home health agencies (Rabin and Stockton 1987). The limitation of one hundred home health visits was removed, as was the requirement of a prior hospitalization for Part A nursing home coverage (Somers 1983).

Medicaid benefits do attempt to meet the acute and long-term care needs of the elderly poor (Davis and Rowland 1986). Chore services, homemaker aid, and other types of social services are now covered by Medicaid under a waiver provision if a state can demonstrate that total expenditures are not increased by the use of this type of service. Unfortunately, a recent study by the General Accounting Office (1982) found that expanded home health services do not necessarily reduce nursing home or hospital use or total service costs. Even with these changes in Medicare and Medicaid, public spending has reinforced the use of institutions for providing long-term care (Davis and Rowland 1986).

Public expenditures for long-term care include nutritional and social services under the Older American's Act, Title XX of the Social Security Act, and various long-term care programs of the Veteran's Administration. Title XX of the Social Security Act provides federal block grants to the states for a broad range of social services to the poor. The Older American's Act of 1965 provides community health services.

Most people agree that reform is needed in the current system for financing health and long-term care services for the elderly. The conflict exists between the increasing need for acute and long-term health services and the budgetary constraints (Davis and Rowland 1986). Any change that the long-term care system will undergo will begin with those policies that shape and determine financing.

Cost seems to be the crux of any proposal to provide long-term care services. It has been recommended that Medicare simply be extended to include the types of services described above in this chapter. Some suggest a completely separate program with different funding methods, standards of eligibility, and administration. Somers (1983) has proposed a compromise between the two perspectives. She recommends that a schedule of benefits for institutional and home-based, long-term care be included in Medicare. These new benefits would be paid for by transferring funds now budgeted for long-term care of the elderly and disabled under Medicaid and Title XX. All Medicare providers should be paid on a prospective rate basis with no deterrent patient cost-sharing formulas developed by the federal government. Further, Somers proposes new federal and state community programs to coordinate long-term care for Medicare beneficiaries with administration at the community or county level.

Many policy proposals and initiatives contain latent functions that may be difficult to anticipate. One special concern involves the possibility that a new program or a program change might act as a disincentive to continuation of family care or that a newly developed service might simply act as a substitute to family care (Gibson 1984). Although there is no research to support this concern, no family policy for the aged has been developed in the United States (Kamerman 1976). The future trend in family support of older people is somewhat unpredictable as a result of uncertain fertility rates. Changes in family composition may cause changes in the quantity and type of care families can offer their elders.

Certain consumer incentives have been designed to aid with the payment for long-term care. Tapping home equity and employing private insurance are two approaches. Money accumulated in home equity can be released to the older person through reverse annuity mortgages and sale leaseback arrangements. Private insurance is being marketed to cover long-term care costs and to enable people who can afford to pay for services to have access to some sort of savings insurance mechanism (Brody and Magel 1986); only 1 percent of the $27 billion spent on nursing home care in the United States in 1982 was covered by private health insurance (Gibson, Waldo, and Levit 1983).

Is expansion of the long-term care component of the health-care market a necessity? Perhaps an alternative strategy can be devised. Health care, whether acute or long-term, reflects a continuum. Resources could be dispensed more effectively along that continuum. Further, the need for long-term care can be on two levels, permanent or extended care as well as temporary care. Many times the same client can require both.

"Short-term" long-term care is considered care that is offered for a period less than ninety days. "Stepdown" services can be used, which range from outpatient rehabilitation to community outreach services. Brody and Magel (1986) recommend the use of stepdown services to cross traditional service lines where service settings are organized to respond to a hierarchy of patient care needs. When "short-term" care is used, case management is frequently called into play: "It is a method of providing comprehensive, unified, coordinated, and timely services to people in need of them through the efforts of a primary agent who, together with the client (and the client's family), take responsibility for providing or procuring the services needed" (Kemp 1981).

Public policy initiatives should be expanded to include (1) elimination of homebound requirements for Medicare and provision of additional services such as homemakers; (2) expansion of Medicaid to a greater proportion of low-income elderly either by imposing federal standards of eligibility on states or by increasing the federal share of Medicaid payments; (3) tax incentives to family members who care for impaired elders; (4) payment under public programs to family caregivers for their services; (5) public funding for supportive services; and (6) changes in Supplemental Security Income and Food Stamp rules so that allocations under these programs would not be reduced if the elder moved in with a family member (Doty 1986).

Other suggestions for policy changes have been taken from the results of federally supported demonstration projects that have emphasized new approaches to the provision of community care (Benjamin 1985). Such suggestions include (1) coordinating and managing a mix of social services to meet clients' needs and reduce the rate of institutionalization; (2) providing Medicare and Medicaid coverage to pay for travel to medical services or changing the location of services to reduce costs; and (3) innovating with reimbursement methods that test whether costs are reduced without adversely affecting patient outcomes (Hamm, Kickham, and Cutler 1983). It should be noted, however, that not all students of long-term care view federal demonstration projects in positive terms (Trager 1981). Some argue that the money could better be put to use by funding additional services.

In some ways, fear has blocked legislation to expand noninstitutional long-term care benefits along the lines described in this chapter. These fears are related to predictions about the increasing numbers of older people, the difficulty in assessing need for long-term care, and the fear that with added services, families will abandon their elders.

TOWARD A POLITICAL ECONOMY OF HEALTH AND AGING

In attempting to understand the relationships among aging, health, and health services' utilization, students of aging in the United States have directed their analyses primarily at the individual older person. Resultant research has been concerned with biomedical, psychological, and social–psychological models of aging. Much of the material presented in this text can be located in one or more of these models. Thus, we ask, How do individuals adjust to the aging process? Why are certain aged persons healthier than others? Why do some elderly avail themselves of health services and others not?

As Estes and her colleagues point out, questions such as these make the economic and political structure of the society residual in explaining old age. These authors offer an alternative approach that "starts with the proposition that the status and resources of the elderly and even the trajectory of the aging process itself are conditioned by one's location in the social structure and the economic and social factors that affect it" (Estes, Swan, and Gerard 1984).

From this *political economy* perspective, the structure and operation of the major societal institutions (including the family, the work place, the medical and welfare institutions) shape both the subjective experience and objective condition of the individual's aging. In the area of health and aging, Estes and associates (1984) note that the political economy perspective emphasizes the following:

1. The social determinants of health and illness
2. The social creation of dependency and the management of that dependency status through public policy and health services
3. Medical care as an ideology and as an industry in the control and management of the aging
4. The consequences of public policies for the elderly as a group and as individuals
5. The role and function of the state in relation to aging and health
6. The social construction of reality about old age and health that both un-

dergirds and reinforces the institutional arrangements and public policies concerning health and aging in the society

Political economy provides a critical approach to the study of aging that does *not* attempt to psychologize the health problems of the aging. An analysis of health and aging from a political economy perspective emphasizes the broad implications of economic life for the aged and for society's treatment of the aged and their health. This view also examines the special circumstances of different classes and subgroups of older persons. It is a systematic view based on the assumption that old age cannot be understood in isolation from other problems or issues raised by the larger social order.

From this perspective, the future seems grim for positive health policy initiatives for the elderly. Minkler (1984), for example, sees a continuation of victim blaming and scapegoating of the elderly for economic problems and fiscal crises such as the federal budget deficit, although the character of victim blaming is changing. She describes how earlier efforts at victim blaming defined the elderly as a social problem, and consequently, solutions were devised for dealing with that problem. Medicare and Medicaid represent but two highly visible programs generated to deal with the problems of the aged. Victim blaming in the 1980s defines these solutions as part of the problem. Not only are the elderly themselves seen as a problem, but programmatic efforts to address their needs are characterized as "budget busting" and are targeted to be dismantled entirely or privatized.

Recently the terms of discussion have shifted to proposals for allocation of health care. For example, Longman (1987) argues that each new generation inherits valuable new medical technologies without the dedicated capital to pay for their use. The result is accumulating debt that can only be discharged by younger, coming generations. The pattern is exacerbated by efforts to prolong life to an advanced age. Implicit is the suggestion that those who benefit from such advances (the aged) are not those who will have to pay (the young).

Blank (1988) identifies three obstacles that stand in the way of traditional reform of our medical care system: (1) the belief that individuals have the right to unlimited medical care should they choose it; (2) the traditional acceptance of this maximalist approach by the medical community; and (3) the insulation of the individual from feeling the cost of treatment. He asks not whether we must ration health care, but how.

Callahan (1988) similarly argues that the "happy days" strategies are no longer working. We can no longer maintain the illusion of a health-care system that will be all things to all people. Presumably rationing will help restore the balance. And *age* may be the first standard we employ for the rationing or limiting of medical care.

The political economy perspective raises a whole new set of questions that need to be asked *and* answered as we proceed into the future. These questions and their answers will provide a significant opportunity for students of aging to rethink the relationship between society and its aged constituents.

SUMMARY

The average number of physician visits per person increases with age. Yet the number of physician contacts per aged person per year has not changed dramatically in the last twenty years. Although differences in the rate of physician utilization by the poor and nonpoor elderly have been narrowed or eliminated in recent years, the poor likely continue to use fewer services relative to their needs than do those in higher socio-economic circumstances.

There is a gender differential in the utilization of physician services in all adult age groups, but explanations have focused primarily on the social situation of women. In general, the utilization of dental services by older people is lower than among younger groups. This is despite the fact that dental problems increase with age. Few third-party reimbursement plans for health care include dental services. Hospitalization rates also vary according to age, sex, race, and family income.

Health-care expenditures have increased rapidly in recent years. The amount of money expended on Medicare alone has increased more than eightfold between 1970 and 1984. The source of funds to pay for health care for the elderly has also changed. By fiscal 1981, two out of three health-care dollars expended were public monies. The largest single item on the health-care bill of elderly people is hospital care. Public monies, including Medicare and Medicaid, pay for about 85 percent of this bill.

The Medicare program for the elderly contains many out-of-pocket deductibles and co-payments as well as limitations in services and focuses too narrowly on acute care problems. The language employed throughout the Medicare regulations refers to medical need, medical care, and medical necessity. The elderly are often in greater need of health promotion and illness prevention services than they are in need of medical-care services. Some reforms of Medicare have recently been made. The most notable among these are the institution of a prospective payment system for hospitals and the payment for hospice care for the dying. In the future, we may see catastrophic health insurance for the aged. Despite these reforms, Medicare and Medicaid still represent legal entitlement to medical care, and costs continue to rise.

The political economy perspective is a newer critical approach to understanding the relationships among aging, health, and health services' utilization. Rather than psychologizing the problems of health and aging, this perspective tries to place problems of health and aging in the broader context of the economic and political life of the society. Whereas earlier victim-blaming efforts identified the elderly as a social problem, current victim blaming defines programmatic efforts to address the health-care needs of the elderly as part of the problem. Consequently, suggestions to ration health care by age seem in some favor.

STUDY QUESTIONS

1. How does use of physician services vary by sex? What are some possible explanations for this difference in utilization of medical services between men and women?

2. What is the apparent relationship between age and dental problems? Dental visits? How do we explain the low rates of utilization of dental services among the aged?

3. Identify the three factors in Andersen's categorization schema that contribute to the use of health services. Give an example of each of these factors. How do the three factors rank in their ability to account for variation in health-care utilization by the elderly?

4. How have programs such as Medicare and Medicaid influenced the amount of physician contact among poor elderly blacks?

5. Distinguish between Medicare and Medicaid. What are the major gaps in these programs?

6. Is there a crisis in medical care financing? What reforms have been instituted to ensure the financial integrity of Medicare?

7. What reforms are needed in the current system of long-term care services for the elderly?

8. What is the value of the political economy perspective in understanding the relationships among aging, health, and health services' utilization? Why do you think that the allocation of health-care resources has become an issue in the 1980s?

BIBLIOGRAPHY

Aday, L. 1975. Economic and non-economic barriers to the use of needed medical services. *Medical Care* 13:447–456.

Andersen, R. 1968. *A behavioral model of families' use of health services.* Research Series 25. Chicago: Center for Health Administration Studies.

Andersen, R., Anderson, D., and Smedby, B. 1968. Perceptions of and response to symptoms of illness in Sweden and the U.S. *Medical Care* 6:18–30

Andersen, R., Greenley, R., Kravits, J., and Anderson, D. 1972. *Health service use: National trends and variations: 1953–71.* Chicago: Center for Health Administration Studies.

Andersen, R., and Newmen, J. 1973. Societal and individual determinants of medical care utilization in the U.S. *Milbank Memorial Fund Quarterly* 51:95–124.

Benjamin, A. 1985. Community based long-term care. In C. Harrington, R. Newcomer, C. Estes, et al. (eds.), *Long-term care of the elderly: Public policy issues.* Beverly Hills, Calif.: Sage Publications.

Berk, M.L., and Schur, C.L. 1985. *Non-physician health care providers: Use of ambulatory services, expenditures, and sources of payment.* DHHS Pub. No. (PHS) 86-3394. Rockville, Md.: National Center for Health Services Research.

Berki, S.E., and Ashcraft, M. 1979. On the analysis of ambulatory utilization. *Medical Care* 17:1163–79.

Blank, R.H. 1988. *Rationing medicine.* New York: Columbia University Press.

Brody, S.J., and Magel, J. 1986. Long term care: The long and short of it. In C. Eisdorfer (ed.), *Reforming health care for the elderly: Recommendations for national policy.* Baltimore, Md.: Johns Hopkins University Press.

Callahan, D. 1988. Allocating health resources. *Hasting Center Report* 18(2):14–20.

Cantor, M. 1975. Life space and the social support of the inner city elderly of New York. *Gerontologist* 14:286–288.

Carp, F. 1975. Life-style and location within the city. *Gerontologist* 15:27–34.

Coulton, C., and Frost, A.K. 1982. Use of social and health services by the elderly. *Journal of Health and Social Behavior* 23(40):330–339.

Davis, K., and Rowland, D. 1986. *Medicare policy.* Baltimore, Md.: Johns Hopkins University Press.

Doty, P. 1986. Family care of the elderly: The role of public policy. *The Milbank Quarterly* 64(1):34–75.

Estes, C.L., Gerard, L.E., Zones, J.S., and Swan, J.H. 1984. *Political economy, health, and aging.* Boston: Little, Brown and Co.

Estes, C.L., Swan, J.H., and Gerard, L.E. 1984. Dominant and competing paradigms in gerontology: Towards a political economy of aging. In M. Minkler and C.L. Estes (eds.), *Readings in the political economy of aging.* Farmingdale, N.Y.: Baywood Publishing Co., Inc.

Feingold, E. 1966. *Medicare: Policy and politics.* San Francisco: Chandler Publishing Company.

Freidson, E. 1961. *Patient views of medical practice.* New York: Russell Sage Foundation.

Gibson, M. 1984. Family support patterns, policies and programs. In C. Nusberg (ed.), *Innovative aging programs abroad.* Westport, Conn.: Greenwood Press.

Gibson, R., Waldo, D., and Levit, K. 1983. National health expenditures, 1982. *Health Care Financing Review* 5(1):1–31.

Granick, D.W., and Short, T. 1985. *Utilization of hospital inpatient services by elderly Americans.* DHHS Pub. No. (PHS) 85-3351. Rockville, Md.: National Center for Health Services Research.

Hamm, L.V., Kickham, T., and Cutler, D. 1983. Research, demonstrations and evaluations. In R. Vogel and H. Palmer (eds.), *Long term care: Perspectives from research and demonstrations.* Washington, D.C.: Health Care Financing Administration.

Hammerman, J. 1975. Health services: Their success and failure in reaching older adults. *American Journal of Public Health* 64:253–256.

Harris, R. 1975. Breaking the barriers to better health-care delivery for the aged. *Gerontologist* 15:52–56.

Haug, M. 1981. Age and medical care utilization patterns. *Journal of Gerontology* 33:103–111.

Kamerman, S. 1976. Community services for the aged. *Gerontologist* 16(6):13–18.

Kemp, B. 1981. The case management model of human service delivery. In E. Pan, T. Barker, and C. Vash (eds.), *Annual Review of Rehabilitation,* Vol. 2. New York: Springer Publishing.

Klees, B., and Warfield, C. 1986. Actuarial status of the HI and SMI Trust Funds. *Social Security Bulletin* 49(7):10–17.

Longman, P. 1987. *Born to pay: The new politics of aging in America.* Boston: Houghton Mifflin Co.

Lopata, H. 1975. Support system of elderly urbanites: Chicago of the 1970s. *Gerontologist* 15:35–41.

Marmor, T. 1973. *The politics of Medicare.* Chicago: Aldine Publishing Company.

Mechanic, D. 1978. *Medical sociology* (2nd ed.). New York: The Free Press.

Minkler, M. 1984. Blaming the aged victim: The politics of retrenchment in times of fiscal conservatism. In M. Minkler and C.L. Estes (eds.), *Readings in the political economy of aging.* Farmingdale, N.Y.: Baywood Publishing Co., Inc.

Nathanson, C. 1975. Illness and the feminine role: A theoretical review. *Social Science and Medicine* 9:57–62.

Rabin, D.L. 1985. Waxing of the gray, waning of the green. In Institute of Medicine/National Research Council (eds.), *America's aging: Health in an older society.* Washington, D.C.: National Academy Press.

Rabin, D.L., and Stockton, D. 1987. *Long-term care for the elderly: A factbook.* New York: Oxford University Press.

Roos, N., and Shapiro, E. 1981. The Manitoba longitudinal study on aging: Preliminary findings on health care utilization by the elderly. *Medical Care* 19:644–57.

Schwab, M. 1977. Implications for the aged of major national health care proposals. *Journal of Gerontological Nursing* 3:33–36.

Shanas, E., and Maddox, G. 1977. Aging, health, and the organization of health resources. In R. Binstock and E. Shanas (eds.), *Handbook of aging and the social sciences.* New York: Van Nostrand Reinhold Co.

Shuval, J. 1970. *The social functions of medical practice.* San Francisco: Jossey-Bass.

Somers, A.R. 1983. Medicare and long-term care. *Perspectives on Aging* (March/April): 5–8.

———. 1985. Financing long-term care for the elderly: Institutions, incentives, issues. In Committee on an Aging Society, Institute of Medicine, and the National Research Council (eds.), *America's aging: Health in an older society.* Washington, D.C.: National Academic Press.

Stevens, R., and Stevens R. 1974. *Welfare medicine in America: A case study of Medicaid.* New York: The Free Press.

Tessler, R., Mechanic, D., and Dimond, M. 1976. The effect of psychological distress on physician utilization: A prospective study. *Journal of Health and Social Behavior* 17:353–64.

Tolchin, M. 1988. New Health insurance plan provokes outcry over costs. *New York Times* November 2:1, 10.

Trager, B. 1981. In place of policy: Public adventures in non-institutional long-term care. Paper presented at the American Public Health Association Annual Meeting, Los Angeles, Calif. November 1981.

U.S. General Accounting Office. 1982. *The elderly should benefit from expanded home health care but increasing these services will not insure cost reductions.* Public No. GAD/IDE-83-1. Washington, D.C.: U.S. Government Printing Office.

U.S. Senate Special Committee on Aging. 1978. *Medi-gap: Private health insurance supplement to Medicare.* Washington, D.C.: U.S. Government Printing Office.

Verbrugge, L. 1976. Sex differences in morbidity and mortality in the United States. *Social Biology* 23:275–96.

Wan, T. 1982. Use of health service by the elderly in low income communities. *Milbank Memorial Fund Quarterly* 60:82–107.

Ward. R. 1977. Services for older people: An integrated framework for research. *Journal of Health and Social Behavior* 18:61–70.

Wilson, R., and White. 1977. Changes in morbidity, disability and utilization differentials between the poor and the non-poor, data from the Health Interview Survey, 1964 and 1973. *Medical Care* 15:636–646.

Wolinsky, F.D., Coe, R.M., Miller, D.K., Prendergast, J.M., Creel, M.J.M., and Chavez, M.N. 1983. Health services utilization among the noninstitutionalized elderly. *Journal of Health and Social Behavior* 24(4):325–336.

CHAPTER 19

DEATH AND DYING

Cary S. Kart and Eileen S. Metress

Age is an important variable in the study of a wide array of issues relating to death and dying. These issues include the relationship between age and the meaning of death, study of the grief and bereavement process, characterizations of the dying process, decisions about where death should take place and who should decide about the access of older people to life-sustaining medical treatments. This chapter presents an overview of a selection of such issues as they pertain to the older adult.

AGING AND THE
MEANING OF DEATH

The meanings that individuals give to death vary as a function of age. Nagy (1959) studied post-war Hungarian children and argued that the child's idea of death develops in three stages, each marked by a different view of death. She found that children under five did not recognize death as irreversible; they viewed it as a temporary departure or sleep, a type of separation. Between the ages of five and nine death was often personified and seen as a contingency. Although viewed as irreversible, it was not necessarily inevitable, at least as far as the child was concerned. Death existed but was remote. By nine or ten, the children understood death to be inevitable, final, and less remote, a part of the life cycle of all living organisms.

Some have questioned the universal application of Nagy's findings. McIntire and his colleagues (1972) found that unlike Hungarian children, American children are able to conceptualize "organic decomposition" as early as age five and in some cases as early as age three. The tendency to personify death noted by Nagy during stage two is not a common finding in more recent studies (Kastenbaum 1986). Kastenbaum considers that children since Nagy's research may have developed a fashionably scientific outlook in response to death. He notes one seven year old who likened death to "when the computer's down." Perhaps the children's tendency to personify is masked by contemporary images and terms. In addition, such work demonstrates the need to examine variations within cultural groups.

Bluebond-Langner (1977) summarizes research on the relationship between social class and children's views of death as follows: Children from lower socioeconomic groups are more likely to cite violence as the general and specific cause of death, whereas middle-class children are more likely to cite disease and old age as the general cause, and the arrest of vital functions as the specific cause of death. These variations seem to reflect differences in the life experiences of the children.

Two meanings of death with particular significance for the elderly are suggested by a large body of literature: death as an organizer of time and death as loss. To the elderly and the terminal patient, death is a clearly perceived constraint that limits the future (Kalish 1976). Anticipating the end of one's life may bring a reorganization of time and priorities. In work done over twenty years ago, Kastenbaum (1966) found that older persons projected themselves into a much more limited time frame than did younger persons when asked to report coming important events in their lives and the timing of these events.

Death also makes all possessions and experiences transient. For many elderly persons, the anticipation of death may generate feelings of meaninglessness. There is nothing meaningful to do because whatever is attempted will be short-lived or unfinished (Kalish 1976). Kurt Back (1965) asked residents of rural communities in the West what they would do if they knew they were to die in thirty days. The elderly were less likely than younger respondents to indicate that their activities would change at all. A more recent study by Kalish and Reynolds (1976) supported Back's findings. Using respondents in three age groups and extending the duration to the time of death to six months instead of thirty days, more of the older group were found unwilling to change their lifestyle. Nearly three times as many older persons as younger reported they would spend their remaining time in prayer, reading, contemplation, or other activities that reflected inner life, spiritual needs, or withdrawal.

Perception by the elderly of the finitude of life comes not only from within. Older persons receive many reminders of their impending death from other individuals and from social institutions. Society tends to perceive the older person as not having sufficient futurity to deserve a major investment of the resources of others.

GRIEF AND BEREAVEMENT

Bereavement refers to the state of having sustained a loss. For the elderly, losses accumulate and become very much a part of life. *Grief* is the reaction to loss. It is a painful yet necessary process that facilitates adjustment to the loss. Its course is quite variable; it may be short or long, taking months to a few years for the loss to be resolved and a normal life to resume. It may vary in its intensity. In addition to depression, reactions may include anger, guilt, anxiety, and preoccupation with thoughts of the deceased.

In his pioneering work, Lindemann (1944) described the physical symptoms of grief, which may include sensations of somatic distress lasting from twenty minutes to an hour. Stomach upset, shortness of breath, tightness in the throat, frequent sighing, an empty feeling in the abdomen, lack of muscular power, and "subjective distress" were found to be common among the grieving. Confusion, disorganization, absentmindedness, and insomnia were also expressed.

In part, the loss reaction is shaped by cultural norms and experiences. In less-developed societies with extended families, the trauma of death is only minimally disruptive. In preliterate families, the primary relationships involving parents, children, and spouses may be extended to other relatives. In this way, others may serve to "compensate" for a loss. For instance, among the Trobrianders the role of the father is assumed by the mother's brother. Such is *not* the case in the smaller nuclear family units that characterize industrialized societies. Nuclear family members are customarily left to their own resources to adjust to the psychological and social impact of loss.

In many societies, including our own, established rituals determine how life crises such as death are to be managed. Rituals have important social functions as well as utilitarian value to those who are grieving. They serve to channel and legitimize the normal expression of grief as well as to rally emotional support for the bereaved through the participation of friends and relatives. *Mourning,* the culturally patterned manner by which grief is managed, is quite variable from one society to another and among subcultures within our own society as well.

Many believe that, among blacks, funerals provide a number of psychological mechanisms that facilitate the grief process (Masamba and Kalish 1976). One factor that permits emotional expression at funerals in black churches is the visual confrontation with the deceased. This is carried out in at least two ways. First, the picture of the deceased uniformly appears on the program of the order of the service. According to a member of a deceased person's family, printing the picture in this fashion helped him accept the reality of the loss and generated a feeling of the spiritual presence of the deceased in the church (Masamba and Kalish 1976).

Second, the visual confrontation with the deceased is especially vivid when the remains are viewed by the living. In almost all the funerals attended by Masamba and Kalish (1976), caskets were closed at the beginning of the service

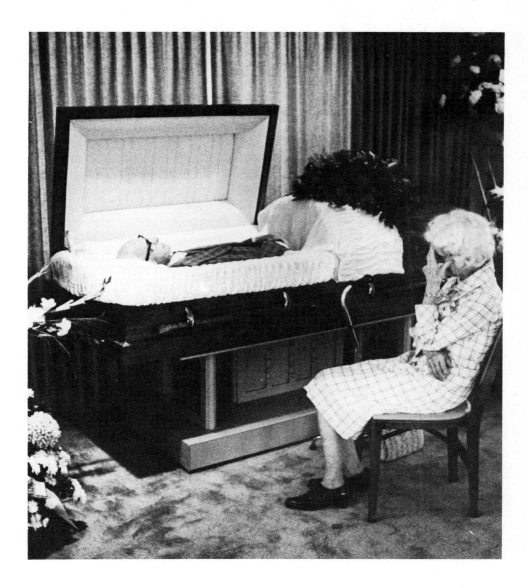

and opened at the end of the concluding sermon. Those present were asked to view the body. Responses varied: Some walked by silently, others touched and even talked to the deceased. Members of the family were always last to view the body, although this is usually done by bringing the body closer to where they are seated so that they can see the body without standing up. Overt expression can be quite strong, including vehement physical motion.

    According to Masamba and Kalish, emotion may not be expressed when

(1) there is a feeling that such expression may be seen as masculine inadequacy, (2) there is belief that such expressions should not be made in front of people who are not family members or friends of the family, and (3) the minister expresses a belief that such behavior implies a lack of acceptance of resurrection and hope in Christ.

The elderly in our society are not always provided an outlet for the expression of grief. Goodstein (1984) asserts that owing to their significant longevity, the elderly may be expected to grin and bear their losses rather than to grieve. Loss is expected with old age. When held by family, friends, and practitioners, such an attitude may compel older persons to act strong, fearing that doing otherwise might cause them to be labeled as weak.

Various types of losses accumulate with age, underscoring the possibility of severe grief reactions after the loss of a spouse, relative, friend, home, employment, financial security or health as well as the loss of personal belongings such as a domestic pet (Keddie 1977). Attachments to remaining people and objects may take on increasing value. Their loss may generate an intense response.

Symptoms of grief in the elderly may be mistaken for other conditions in what is referred to as a devious pattern of grief (Goodstein 1984). The clinician may attribute them to another physical illness or to dementia. As the grief remains ignored, episodic exacerbation of symptoms may result. Unresolved grief is one of the most frequently misdiagnosed illnesses in the elderly. Continued physical and emotional pain, if verbalized by the victim, may be dismissed as hypochondriasis.

Physical and emotional symptoms of grief usually subside in time, but some bereaved individuals are at increased risk for illness and possibly death (Osterweis 1985). Existing illness may worsen and new illnesses may be precipitated. Frederick (1976, 1982–1983) has suggested a pathway by which illnesses might be triggered. He has proposed that a chain of hormonal responses to the stress of loss leads to depression of the body's immune system; if the response pattern continues, the immune suppression can lead to the development of infection and cancer. Until approximately age seventy-five, widowed men are one and one-half times more likely to die than are married men (Helsing and Szklo 1981). Morbidity, hospitalization, and mortality exceed expected rates in the two-year period following a loss of spouse (Greenblatt 1978; Rowland 1977).

A number of factors appear to exert significant influence on the resolution of grief (Lieberman 1978; Osterweis 1985; Osterweis, Solomon, and Green 1984). The nature of the lost relationship is important. Loss of spouse has received considerable attention. More research needs to be directed at the loss of friends, siblings, and adult children. Gorer (1965) posits that the loss of a grown child would seem to be the most distressing and long-lasting of all griefs. Besides exerting emotional trauma, the death of an adult child might leave the older person without a caregiver. Yet research focusing on such a loss is extremely limited (Levav 1982). How the death occurred, the availability of a social support system, experiencing several deaths within a short period of time, the existence of illness prior to or at the time of loss, and life changes necessitated by the loss can all influence the intensity, duration, and consequences of the grieving process.

Although it is almost always best to allow the bereaved to experience the grieving process, problems may arise if the grieving appears interminable. In old age the depression involved in bereavement may not be self-limiting (Brocklehurst and Hanley 1976). Treatment may be necessary. Care may involve simple encouragement, personal warmth, understanding, and compassion, or it may require antidepressant drug therapy and psychiatric management. Life decisions related to finances, living arrangements, and personal care may have to be made. Counsel should be given carefully, lawfully, and together with the physician and family members. No irrevocable decisions involving such important matters should be made until the main period of grieving has passed.

Bereavement is a significant contributing factor to suicide. Suicide is more frequent among the widowed. The resolution of grief goes hand in hand with the resumption and development of interpersonal relationships. The psychosocial environment of the aged widow or widower may not furnish the opportunity for reestablishment or the building of important new links (Bromberg and Cassel 1983). Older persons who are married and who maintain contact with their children and other relatives are less likely to commit suicide (Robbins, West, and Murphy 1977).

The elderly are more likely than the young to complete a suicide effort (Maris 1981). Perhaps the older person who attempts suicide is less ambivalent about doing so and more likely to use a more lethal technique. Chapter 6 includes additional material on suicide and the mental health of the elderly.

THE DYING PROCESS

Death and the dying process itself are being looked upon more and more as the terminal phase of the life cycle. Professionals who work with the dying and those who study death and dying have made attempts to understand this final stage. It is hoped that such understanding will help health-care professionals to enrich the lives of the dying and their families and to provide personalized care for those who have been defined as terminal.

The Dying Trajectory

The Glaser-Strauss research team was the first to study and clarify the various sequences and distinctive characteristics of the terminal course. They observed the social process of dying in six medical facilities in the San Francisco area. The majority of their findings are published in two books: *Awareness of Dying* (1966) and *Time for Dying* (1968). Although their research was not limited to older patients, the results of their work are relevant to the elderly dying patient.

According to Glaser and Strauss (1968), staff members working with the ill must answer two questions for themselves about every patient: Will he or she die? If so, when? These questions are important because the staff generates expectations about a patient's death and takes its treatment and other attitudinal cues from the answers that are developed.

Perceptions about the course of dying are referred to as *dying trajectories*. The nature of staff interaction with the patient is closely related to the particular expectations they have formed about the patient's dying. This is the case regardless of whether or not the staff happens to be correct in its expectations. Patients' expectations about their own dying trajectories are greatly affected by staff expectations as well.

Two important cues that contribute to the perception of the dying trajectory are the patient's physical condition and the temporal references made by medical staff members. Physical cues are easiest to read and help establish some degree of certainty about the outcome. Temporal cues have many reference points. Doctors' expectations about the progression of a disease ("It's going fast," "He's lingering"), length of hospital stay, and even the work schedule—such as, can the patient continue to be bathed, turned, fed—are temporal cues that contribute to expectations about how much longer the patient will live (Glaser and Strauss 1968, 10).

In perceptions of a lingering trajectory, custodial care predominates. Aggressive treatment is rare. Health-care professionals tend not to find the support of such patients challenging or rewarding. Lower-paid staff may provide the majority of care for such patients (Friedman and DiMatteo 1982).

When staff perceives a patient as being in a lingering death trajectory, the patient may suffer a loss in his or her own perceived social worth and relinquish control over their care (Kastenbaum 1986). The staff members may feel that they have done everything that is possible to care for the patient, and they may view a downhill course as inevitable. Death of one who has been on a lingering trajectory may seem appropriate to the staff who rationalize that the patient's life held limited value. Intense emotional reactions at the death of such a patient may serve to confuse those who have made assumptions about the patient's present limited social worth. Or stress may result when the lingering patient does not die on schedule.

In contrast, the expected quick trajectory typically involves acute life-or-death crises. The patient's perceived social worth can influence the type of care delivered. The unexpected quick trajectory involves an unanticipated crisis that may challenge the professional caregiver's defenses regarding anxiety about death.

Dying: The Career Perspective

Julius Roth (1963, 93) has written that "when people go through the same series of events, we speak of this as a career and of the sequence and timing of events as their career timetable." Roth used the institutionalized tuberculosis patient as his career model. He argued that individuals involved in a career try to define when certain salient things will happen to them, developing time norms against which to measure their individual progress. The benchmarks on this timetable are the significant events that occur in the average career (Gustafson 1972).

Gustafson has applied Roth's notion of career timetables to the nursing home setting. She views the last phase of life as a career that moves in a series of related and regressive stages toward death. These stages, she argues, are defined by a series of benchmarks, which, for elderly patients, consist of the degree of deterioration indicated by their social activity, mobility, and physical and mental functioning. A successful career in this sense consists of the slowest possible regression from one stage to another.

Gustafson identifies bargaining as an important aspect of the career time-table, although she identifies it in a way that contrasts with Roth's original model. Roth depicts the tubercular patient as bargaining with medical and hospital authorities to move as quickly as possible toward the goal of restored health. Gustafson sees the elderly nursing home patient as bargaining with God, the disease, and the nursing home staff in an attempt to slow down the movement toward death.

By use of this perspective, the dying process is not conceptualized as an undifferentiated unbroken decline toward death. Rather, the dying career is viewed as comprising a social stage and a terminal stage. In the social stage the elderly patient is fighting against the tendency of society (as represented by relatives, staff, visitors, and peers) to impose a premature social death. Bargaining may involve holding onto status symbols that indicate the possibility of a future. An elderly woman may never read, but she indignantly demands a new pair of eyeglasses. An elderly man may not be able to walk yet demands a new walker or cane. In the terminal phase, when the signs of death are more dependable and its imminence cannot be avoided, the patient may begin bar-gaining directly with God or the disease in an effort to secure additional time.

According to Gustafson, a nursing home patient's dying career can be made less difficult if the staff adopts a view of the dying process as consisting of a social stage and a terminal stage. A nursing staff with this view might try to extend the social stage as long as possible and be supportive during the terminal stage. Later in this chapter we will discuss some ways in which health professionals, family members, and others can help ease the dying process for terminal patients.

The Stages of Dying

The best known conceptualization of the dying process is that proposed by Elizabeth Kubler-Ross (1969) in her landmark best seller *On Death and Dying*. In her view, various stages or emotional reactions mark an awareness of dying. The patient may experience denial, anger, bargaining, depression, and acceptance. The applicability and universality of these five stages are still empirical questions. Kubler-Ross (1974, 25–26) points out that patients may skip a stage, exhibit two or three simultaneously, or experience them out of order. Kalish (1976, 38) contends that Kubler-Ross's stages are in danger of becoming self-fulfilling prophecies: "Some health caretakers have been observed trying to encourage, or even manipulate, their dying patients through Kubler-Ross's stages; patients occasionally become concerned if they are not progressing adequately."

The first stage, denial, is most evident during the early period of awareness of impending death. It may be viewed as a coping mechanism to buffer the shock of such news; "No, not me, it cannot be true." Kubler-Ross (1969, 38) offers the case of a patient who went through a long and expensive ritual to support her denial.

> She was convinced that the x-rays were "mixed up." She asked for reassurance that her pathology report could not possibly be back so soon and that another patient's report must be marked with her name. When none of this could be confirmed, she quickly asked to leave the hospital, looking for another physician in the vain hope "to get a better explanation for my troubles. . . ." She asked for examination and re-examination, partially knowing that the original diagnosis was correct, but also seeking further evaluations in the hope that the first conclusion was indeed in error.

When the first stage of denial cannot be maintained any longer, it is often replaced by feelings of anger or rage. The patient finally realizes that denial is fruitless, "It is me, it was not a mistake." The next question becomes, "Why me?" This stage is perhaps the most difficult for staff and family members to deal with. Anger may be displaced and projected on anyone and everyone who comes into contact with the patient. Much of this anger is rational and should be expected. Place yourself in the terminal patient's position. You too would be angry if your life's activities had been interrupted and you could no longer enjoy life, especially if you had been kept too long in a hospital subject to unpleasant tests and treatments, and if you were constantly being reminded that you could no longer carry out your own affairs.

The third stage, bargaining, is really an attempt on the part of the patient to postpone the inevitable. As Kubler-Ross (1969, 82) indicates, the terminal patient in this stage uses the same maneuvers as a child; he or she asks to be rewarded "for good behavior." Most bargains are made with God and almost always include the wishes for removal of pain or discomfort and life extension.

Kubler-Ross (1969, 83) presents the case of a woman quite dependent on injections for painkillers. The woman had a son who was to be married, and she was sad at the prospect of being unable to attend the wedding. With great effort she was taught self-hypnosis and was able to be comfortable for several hours at a time.

> She had made all sorts of promises, if she could only live long enough to attend this marriage. The day preceding the wedding she left the hospital as an elegant lady. Nobody would have believed her real condition. She was "the happiest person in the whole world" and looked radiant.

Patients rarely hold up their end of the bargain. This same woman returned to the hospital and remarked, "Now don't forget, I have another son."

When the terminally ill person is unable to continue to deny the illness, when the rage and anger are dissipated, and when bargaining efforts are seen as hopeless, depression may begin. This fourth stage is characterized by feelings of loss, and two types of depression may be evident. *Reactive depression* is a result of the various other losses that accompany illness and dying. For instance, the patient may mourn the loss of a limb that has been amputated. The cancer patient may mourn the loss of her beautiful hair to radiation therapy. The second type of depression, *preparatory depression*, takes impending losses into account; that is, it prepares the individual for loss of all love objects. It facilitates the final stage of acceptance.

Acceptance should not be mistaken for happiness or capitulation. The dying patient can accept his imminent death without joy and without giving up the life that remains for him. According to Kubler-Ross (1969, 112–113), this is often a time when the dying individual will "contemplate his coming end with a certain degree of quiet expectation." This stage may represent "the final rest before the long journey."

Although many researchers and practitioners find Kubler-Ross's conceptualization of the dying process extremely valuable, others are critical (Feigenberg 1977; Metzger 1979; Schulz and Aderman 1974; Shneidman 1980). Weisman (1972), for example, rather than using the notion of "acceptance of death," encourages the concept of "appropriate death." Such a death means that the person has died in a fashion that resembles as much as possible the way that he or she wished to die. The totality of the person's life can be ignored in strict adherence to the stages of dying. The effects of age, gender, ethnic background, and one's life experience have not been studied as they apply to Kubler-Ross's stage theory (Kastenbaum 1986). Remember as well that the process of dying may be strongly influenced by the behavior and attitudes of those persons in the dying individual's social milieu.

Witness the inhabitants of the Etal Island in the Caroline Islands (Micronesia). They have no formal theory of dying, yet it is important to them that some resolution be achieved. "Dying is the last important social act an old person can perform. Past conflicts must be resolved. Also, this is the time for the old person to make a final decision about the disposition of property" (Nason 1981).

Islanders believe that the dying should pass on in an atmosphere of peace and solitude. A new ancestor, pleased with attention and respect provided by kin while he or she was alive, is likely to aid and protect islanders. On the other hand, a person who dies angry or dissatisfied with the inattention of relatives might take revenge on them. Actually, an older person might be driven to suicide to make a public protest against ill-treatment by relatives. To prevent this, relatives may stay constantly with the dying person. Such a suicide would bring public shame on the relatives and would cause trouble with the final settling of the estate, since suicides often make no final distribution of their property (Nason 1981). Just the threat of suicide by a dying person (or any elder, for that matter) can quickly bring about a change in relations with extended kin members.

Kubler-Ross's work has been of tremendous value in sensitizing us to the needs and rights of the dying. Shortcomings in the application of her work or its uncritical acceptance by some should not lead to a dismissal of her many useful insights or of the need for further research in this area (Kastenbaum 1986). Kubler-Ross argued that the physician can help the patient reach a calm acceptance of death. Schulz (1978) summarizes a body of literature that finds that physicians avoid patients once they begin to die. The nature and impact of the doctor–dying patient relationship on the dying process would seem an area ripe for additional research.

THE WHERE OF DYING

Today most people die in health-care institutions of one kind or another. In hospitals, rest homes, and nursing homes the dying process has become bureaucratized and, to a great extent, depersonalized. Such institutions, while treating the terminally ill, also isolate them from the rest of society. These institutions have routinized the handling of death for their own benefit. This may reduce disturbance and disruption for the institution. Standardized procedures render death nearly invisible. Bodies may not be removed during visiting hours to protect relatives and other visitors. When death appears imminent, the patient may be moved to a private room to protect other patients.

Many people, health professionals and laypersons alike, are aware of the depersonalized treatment provided the terminally ill in our health facilities. On the basis of their study of individuals in four ethno-racial communities in Los Angeles, Kalish and Reynolds (1976) report that most people of all ages would prefer to die at home, particularly those under forty and those over fifty-nine. Although many dying patients and their families wish for death in the home, the wish is not often realized. One recent study clearly indicates that, even when plans for home death have been made, they may be precluded by many factors, the most prominent of which appears to be the emotional and physical exhaustion of the family (Groth-Junker and McCusker 1983).

New options for caring for the dying are becoming available. One such option, called a *hospice,* combines the technical expertise for caring for the ill that is available in our health-care bureaucracies with the personalized attention of home care. The most widely known is St. Christopher's Hospice in London founded by Dr. Cicily Saunders.

A hospice is not a place, but rather a concept of care that combines various elements. It emphasizes *palliative care* rather than cure. Control of pain and distressing symptoms is viewed as a treatment goal in its own right. If a patient's preoccupation with suffering is of such intensity that everything else in life is excluded, then self-control, independence, human dignity, and interpersonal relations are sacrificed. Each patient is seen as a part of a family whose total well-being and life-style may be affected by the circumstance of having a terminally ill member. Caring does not stop when the patient dies but continues to help the family during bereavement. The hospice concept also views the home as a suitable domain for patient care. An interdisciplinary team involving physician, nursing, social work, counseling, and volunteer services provides hospice care.

The first hospice in the United States became operative in 1974. Known as the Connecticut Hospice (originally Hospice, Inc.), it provides both inpatient and home care services. Since its inception, hospice programs have developed in every state in the nation. They now take several forms in their organization. Home care programs have been preferred in the United States. Connecticut Hospice began as a home care program and later added an inpatient facility. Some hospitals are developing hospice units within their walls to deliver hospicelike care or other separate or free-standing facilities.

In the United States, hospice has evolved from a fringe alternative led by a group of idealistic professionals and volunteers to an accepted mainstream approach to terminal care (Tehan 1985). Much of this change has been precipitated by legislation that allows terminally ill patients over the age of sixty-five to receive Medicare reimbursable services from certified hospice programs.

The National Hospice Study conducted between 1980 and 1984 was spawned by a concern for the feasibility of a hospice Medicare benefit (Greer and Mor 1985). Its results presently represent the largest collection of carefully controlled data on hospice care in the nation. In general, results of the study demonstrate that hospice care tends to be less expensive than traditional hospital care and that hospice patients spend more time at home during the course of their terminal illness.

Medical anthropologist Robert Buckingham and his colleagues (1976) have, through participant observation, compared the relative merits of standard hospital versus hospice care for the dying. Using an elaborate and deceptive scheme that was aided by physicians, Buckingham played the role of a cancer patient. He prepared himself in a number of ways before entering the hospital. He went on a severe six-month diet and lost twenty-two pounds from his already spare frame. Exposure to ultraviolet rays made it appear that he had undergone cancer radiation therapy. Puncture marks from intravenous needles on his hands and arms indicated that he had also had chemotherapy cancer treatment. A cooperative surgeon performed minor surgery on him in order to produce biopsy scars, indicating that exploratory surgery had been performed. Buckingham reviewed medical charts and maintained close contact with patients dying of cancer of the pancreas. He was thus able to observe and imitate suitable behavior. A patchy beard and the results of several days of not washing or shaving completed the picture. He spent two days in the holding unit, four days on a surgical care ward, and four days on the hospice or palliative care ward of Royal Victoria Hospital in Montreal.

Buckingham's findings lend empirical support to the assumption that the hospice system of care for the terminally ill is effective. He lists certain hospital-staff practices that were observed in the surgical care ward that should be sources of concern in attempting to develop an optimal environment for the dying. These practices are as follows: (1) The tradition of physicians making their patient rounds in groups (this fostered social and medical discussion between the doctors but completely prevented doctor–patient communication on any but the most superficial level); (2) the lack of eye contact between staff members and patient (patients walked in the halls close to the walls, greetings were rare, and staff frequently crossed to the other side of the hall, walking by, heads averted); (3) reference to a patient by the name of his or her disease rather than by the name of the person; (4) the accentuation of negative aspects of a patient's condition; (5) the lack of affection given to the complacent patient; and (6) the discontinuity of communication among medical and nursing staff.

Staff–patient and staff–family relationships were qualitatively different on the hospice care ward. Buckingham and associates (1976) describe Buckingham's arrival on this ward as follows:

> The initial nursing interview was conducted by a nurse who introduced herself by name, sat down so that her eyes were on a level with [the patient's], and proceeded to listen. There was no hurry, her questions flowed from [the patient's] previous answers, and there was acceptance of the expression of his concerns. She asked questions such as "What do you like to eat?" and "Is there anything special you like to do?"
>
> In the hospice care unit Buckingham observed relatives enquiring for the doctor five times. On each occasion the doctor was reached and either came or spoke to the family on the phone . . . families also spent much time at the bedside participating in the care of the patient. They changed the bed linen, washed and fed the patient, brought the urinal and plumped the pillows frequently. The staff encouraged the family to experience the meaning of death by allowing them to help in the care of the dying.

A greater effort is necessary to accomplish total care of the terminally ill. Four observations made by Buckingham that are often overlooked by health-care professionals may facilitate consummating the total care effort:

1. The sharing and help provided by other patients form a powerful social support system for patients with terminal disease.

2. The need for the patient as a person to give and thus retain his or her individuality should be recognized.

3. The care given by families is a source of support for patients that must be recognized and emphasized.

4. The interest and care given by student nurses and volunteers are important, particularly in bringing the person out of the patient.

TERMINATION OF TREATMENT
Who Decides?

Central issues concerning who decides or exerts control in matters related to death and dying are exemplified in a series of recent court cases about the access of older people to life-prolonging medical treatments. One such case worthy of our attention here is that of Earle Spring (Kart 1981).

Earle Spring was born in 1901. In his working years, he was a chemist and metallurgist at a tool-and-die plant in Greenfield, Massachusetts. He was an avid outdoorsman who retired in 1966. In November 1977 Mr. Spring hurt his foot, developed an infection, and was hospitalized. He subsequently suffered pneumonia and then developed kidney failure and nearly died. Early in 1978 he was transferred to a hospital closer to his home, where hemodialysis treatments began. Within several weeks, Mr. Spring was returned to his home, where he received dialysis treatments three times a week, on an outpatient basis, at a private facility in the community.

According to the court record, Mr. Spring began showing signs of mental deterioration in conjunction with his progressive kidney failure. At home, he became destructive and was unable to care for himself. After being diagnosed as having chronic organic brain syndrome, he was admitted to a nursing home. By early 1979 his mental deterioration had continued to the point that he failed to recognize his wife and son. Yet he was ambulatory and, except for his kidney failure, in good physical condition.

On January 25, 1979, Mr. Spring's son and wife petitioned a local Probate Court for an order that hemodialysis treatments be terminated. The medical consensus was that Mr. Spring might live for four or five weeks following the termination of these treatments. The probate judge appointed a guardian for Spring in this case who opposed the petition. Yet in May 1979 the judge ordered the temporary guardian to "refrain from authorizing any further life-prolonging medical treatment." The guardian appealed; but after a stay of the order the judge ruled that the attending physician, together with the wife and son, was to make the decision to continue or terminate the dialysis treatments.

The guardian appealed this decision to the Appeals Court of Massachusetts, where it was affirmed. A further appeal was made to the Massachusetts Supreme Judicial Court, where, on May 13, 1980 (approximately one month after Earle Spring's death), it was reversed and remanded to the lower court. The Massachusetts Supreme Judicial Court acknowledged the substance of the lower court's decision yet opined that the ultimate decision-making responsibility should not have been shifted away from the probate court by delegating the decision to continue or terminate care to the physician and Mr. Spring's wife and son.

Who should decide in this matter? The court itself? The physicians? Spring's family members? What about Earle Spring himself? Let us look closely at some underlying issues in this case. A careful reading of the transcript of the probate court's hearing in the matter of Earle Spring shows that the court found that Mr. Spring would "if competent, choose not to receive the life-prolonging treatment." In so finding, the court followed a standard applied in another Massachusetts case, *Superintendent of Belchertown State School v. Saikewicz* (370 N.E. 2d 417, 1977), and invoked the principle of *substitute judgment.*

Joseph Saikewicz was sixty-seven years old, had a mental age of approximately three years, and had been a resident of the Belchertown State School for forty-eight years. He was well nourished and ambulatory, could make his wishes known through gestures and grunts, but was suffering from leukemia. In April 1976 the superintendent of the school filed a petition in local probate court asking for the appointment of a guardian for purposes of making a decision about Saikewicz's care and treatment for the leukemia. The judge did so, and the guardian filed a report with the court stating that the illness was incurable, that the indicated treatment would cause adverse side effects and discomfort, and that Saikewicz was incapable of understanding the treatment. In sum, it was the view of the guardian that the negative aspects of the treatment situation outweighed the uncertain and clearly limited extension of life the treatment could bring; in the guardian's opinion, treating Saikewicz would not be in his best interests.

In May 1976 the probate judge entered an order agreeing with the guardian; the Massachusetts Supreme Judicial Court concurred, and later that summer Joseph Saikewicz died without pain. It is noteworthy that in November of that year, the Supreme Judicial Court handed down a written decision in the Saikewicz case. In this written opinion the court argued that, like competent persons, incompetents must also have the right to refuse medical treatment. In making this argument, the court recognized what may currently be a widely held view—that medical treatment does not always further the best interests of the patient. The central problem the court faced, however, was in deciding how to determine what is in the best interest of an incompetent person (Glantz and Swazey 1979). The standard adopted was the substitute judgment test, which, according to the court, seeks "to determine with as much accuracy as possible the wants and needs of the individual involved."

In the case of Joseph Saikewicz, the use of the substitute judgment test would seem a "legal fiction" (Glantz and Swazey 1979). How is it possible to know the wishes of a sixty-seven year old who has been severely retarded all his life? In effect, the court substituted its own judgment for that of the incompetent person. Earle Spring's case is another matter, however. He was competent for the greater part of his adult life. Nevertheless, how did the Spring court ascertain that "if competent, Spring would choose not to receive the life-sustaining treatment"? Mr. Spring had never stated his preference regarding continuing or terminating life-sustaining medical treatment.

The probate court substituted the judgment of his wife, who indicated that, on the basis of their long years of marriage, she believed "he wouldn't want to live." In doing so, the court employed a variant of the substitute judgment standard used by the Supreme Court of New Jersey in *In re Quinlan* (355 A. 2d 647, 1976). Karen Quinlan was an adult woman in a persistent vegetative state from which her physicians felt she could not recover. Her father sought to be appointed her guardian so that he should have the power to authorize the discontinuance of all extraordinary medical procedures for sustaining his daughter's vital processes. The Quinlan court assumed that, if Karen were competent and perceptive of her irreversible condition, "she could effectively decide upon discontinuance of the life-sustaining apparatus, even if it meant the prospect of natural death." Since the patient was not competent, the court concluded that her father and other family members, with the concurrence of a hospital ethics committee, could assert this decision for her.

This variant of the substitute judgment test was applied by the probate court in the Spring case even though Spring's wife could offer no evidence in support of her conclusion about his wishes. No evidence was put forth that might provide a basis for believing that Earle Spring would reject life-sustaining medical treatment. Nothing was made of the fact that when Spring first began hemodialysis treatments, before he was believed to be incompetent, he cooperated in taking these treatments. In fact, the court took testimony from family members that Earle Spring's activity level had fallen off considerably before the diagnosis of organic brain syndrome. He was no longer able to hunt and fish as was the case in his younger years. This is precisely what some gerontologists argue is supposed to happen in old age. From this view, activity reduction in the later years is natural, expected, and even looked forward to by the aging.

The Massachusetts Supreme Judicial Court rejected the lower court's delegation of authority to withhold life-sustaining medical treatment to Earle Spring's wife, family, and physicians. In effect, the higher court rejected the approach employed in the Quinlan case and reasserted the standard employed in the Saikewicz case: "When a court is properly presented with the legal question, whether treatment may be withheld, it must decide the question and not delegate it to some private person or group" (Mass., 405 N.E. 2d 115, 122).

Is there basis in relevant literature for rejecting the substitute judgment of family members for that of an incompetent organic brain syndrome patient? Some would say yes. Several recent papers suggest that great stress is felt by family members of organic brain syndrome patients (Mace, Rabins, and Lucas 1980; Schneider and Garron 1980). Mace and her colleagues report that more than 90 percent of the families they studied showed anger—at the situation, the patient, other family members, or professionals—as a response to the presence of a dementia patient in the family. Other stress responses include depression, grief, conflict with family members, withdrawal from social activity, and the like. Such research suggests that family members may not be in the best position to substitute their judgment for that of an incompetent in the question of whether or not to continue life-sustaining medical treatment.

Some would argue that the decision about whether to continue medical treatment in cases like Spring, Saikewicz, and Quinlan should be based on quality-of-life issues. Defining the issue in these terms may serve to exclude physicians, since there is nothing inherently medical about a quality-of-life decision. Rather it seems, as some have indicated, that cases that raise quality-of-life questions are the ones that need to be resolved by a court of law.

Traditionally, decisions about how long to maintain a hopeless patient have been made by the physician, sometimes in concert with family members, and less frequently with input from the dying person. Many dying patients, particularly those who are very old and extremely deteriorated, have no input whatsoever into decisions about their own death. There have been several recent attempts to better represent the patient's wishes in such a decision. *Living wills* are being used by some to specify the conditions under which they would prefer not to be subjected to extraordinary measures to keep them alive. In September 1976 the state of California passed Assembly Bill 3060, the so-called Natural Death Act. The law authorizes the withholding or withdrawal of life-sustaining procedures from adults who have a terminal condition and who have executed such a directive. Several other states have passed similar legislation.

> Death is as much a reality as birth, maturity, and old age. It is the one certainty of life. If the time comes when I, _____, can no longer take part in decisions for my own future, let this statement stand as an expression of my wishes while I am of sound mind. . . .

These words begin the living will, a document first devised in 1969 by the Euthanasia Educational Council, now called Concern for Dying. In fifteen states and the District of Columbia, living wills have legal standing. With them, a competent person can instruct a physician not to use heroic measures to prolong life when "there is no reasonable expectation of recovery from physical or mental disability."

Still, controversy exists over the meaning and application of the document. In particular, some argue, difficulties may arise out of uncertainties of clinical prognosis that allow for misinterpretation of the living will. Two safeguards are in order. First, the details of the living will should be discussed with the personal physician at the time it is completed. This may lessen the chances of misinterpretation. If the physician refuses to carry out the wishes expressed in the will, the individual who wrote the will should consider finding another doctor. Second, the will should name someone who can interpret the exact wishes of the writer should he or she ever be unable to express them. This provision, known as a *durable power of attorney*, is especially important should the writer become incompetent. Such a person can then make decisions as to specific measures to be taken or not taken.

Removal of Food and Fluids

As Steinbock (1983) indicates, a substantial body of legal opinion views the disconnection of all life-support apparatus from irreversibly comatose patients as morally and legally permissible. Nevertheless, many fear that such permissiveness leads to the "slippery slope" whereby the lives of all terminally ill and handicapped individuals are endangered. Steinbock (1983) asks, for example, "[I]f it is permissible to remove a feeding tube from a permanently comatose patient, why not from a barely conscious, senile and terminal patient?"

In January 1985 the Supreme Court of New Jersey ruled that artificial feeding, like other life-sustaining treatment, may be withheld or withdrawn from an incompetent patient if it represents a disproportionate burden and would have been refused by the patient under the circumstances. This decision was made in the case of Claire Conroy, an eighty-four-year-old nursing home resident who suffered irreversible physical and mental impairments. She could move to a minor extent, groan, and sometimes smile in response to certain physical stimuli. She had no cognitive ability and was unaware of her surroundings.

She had been placed in a nursing home after having been declared incompetent. Eventually, she was transferred to a hospital for treatment of a gangrenous leg (a complication of her diabetes). Amputation was recommended, but Ms. Conroy's nephew and legal guardian refused consent. He maintained that she would have refused treatment. Surgery was not performed, but while in the hospital a nasogastric tube was inserted. Her nephew requested that its use be discontinued in the hospital and, likewise, in the nursing home where she eventually returned. On both requests, permission was denied by her attending physician.

Conroy's nephew filed suit to obtain court permission to remove her feeding tube. A lower court granted permission. The decision was appealed and reversed by the Appellate court in a declaration that termination of feeding constituted homicide. Ms. Conroy died during the appeal with the nasogastric tube still in place. Her guardian carried the case to the state Supreme Court.

The New Jersey Supreme Court ruling is consistent with that of the Barber case decided by the California Court of Appeals in 1983. In this case the cessation of intravenous feeding was equated with the removal of a respirator. The Conroy case represents the first time that a state Supreme Court has eliminated a distinction between artificial feeding and other artificial life supports (Nevins 1986).

While recognizing the legal rights of all patients to self-determination, the New Jersey court imposed very strict requirements in providing previously competent patients the right to exercise treatment refusal by proxy. Through the application of a "best-interest test" the court must ascertain the patient's known or suspected personal attitude toward life-sustaining treatment and the burden of pain.

The court feels a special duty to protect the rights of the now-incompetent nursing home patient. It maintains that the patient's guardian, next-of-kin, the attending physician, two consulting physicians (unaffiliated with the nursing home), and the state Office of the Ombudsman for the Institutionalized Elderly must all concur in the decision to remove life-sustaining treatment. The procedural portion of the court decision has received considerable criticism on the basis that it fosters a climate of distrust, is difficult to implement, and artificially distinguishes between nursing home and hospital patients (Annas 1985a, 1985b; Nevins 1985, 1986; Olins 1986).

The court does heavily involve the state *Ombudsman,* an office charged with guarding against and investigating allegations of elder abuse in conjunction with the state's Elder Abuse Statute. The Ombudsman must be notified before any such decision to terminate treatment is rendered and must consider every such decision as a possible case of abuse.

The court asserts that special precautions are necessary because elderly nursing home patients present special problems. Indeed, the court's holding is restricted to nursing home patients. Reasons cited are the patient's average age, their general lack of next-of-kin, the limited role of physicians in nursing homes; reports of inhuman treatment and understaffing in nursing homes; and, the less urgent decision-making that occurs within these facilities allowing for more time to review options.

It has been held by others that nursing home-based decisions can confound ethical considerations in a number of ways: (1) Personal autonomy may be lost because nursing home admission might result in a new physician's providing care rather than one who has previously treated the patient and is familiar with the patient's wishes; (2) the patient may view that life is diminished by virtue of entry into the nursing home; (3) the possibility of dementing illness does not allow for informed consent; and (4) the typically advanced age of the residents may influence decisions concerning treatment limitations (Besdine 1983).

Annas (1985b) charges that the court's strict differentiation between nursing home and hospital patients regarding life-sustaining treatment decisions is artificial. He states that almost all nursing home patients will be transferred to hospitals when invasive treatment is required. He adds that if Ombudsman intervention is appropriate, it should apply in both settings. More appropriately, the Ombudsman should be available to investigate cases of suspected abuse. Otherwise, the Conroy approach requires that time be wasted on cases that do not need investigation. Annas also posits that the court decision may create confusion in its applicability to nursing home residents who are temporarily hospitalized.

Changes in Medicare funding are moving patients from hospitals to nursing homes "sooner and sicker." Although differences exist, problems of the two patient populations promise to become more similar (Nevins 1986). Nevins concludes:

> So although their rhythms may differ, the two populations and their problems are becoming more homogeneous. No doubt differences exist, but to devise a totally new mechanism to resolve the same clinical issues depending on the locus of decision-making is unnecessary and unwise. (p. 143)

The court's ruling is binding only in New Jersey. Ultimately, how it influences decision making there rests largely with how the Ombudsman's office interprets and applies the court's rulings in Conroy. Although the mechanism set forth to allow incompetent patients to exercise the right to refuse treatment is cumbersome and restrictive, it stands as testimony to a sensitive concern for human dignity and patient autonomy for people of all ages.

SUMMARY

Although not an event that is unique to the elderly, death is something that must inevitably be faced. The deaths of friends, relatives, and others are more frequent occurrences for the older adult. Yet, death may have different meanings for people of different ages. Two meanings of death with particular significance for the elderly include death as an organizer of time and death as loss.

Bereavement refers to the state of having sustained a loss, while grief is a term that describes the reaction to loss. In part, the loss reaction is shaped by cultural norms and experiences. Mourning, the culturally prescribed manner in which grief is managed, varies from group to group within a society as well as between societies. And, a wide variety of factors appears to exert influence on the resolution of grief.

A number of conceptualizations of the dying process have been offered as attempts to understand this final stage of life. Dying has been described as a *trajectory*, a *career*, and a *five-stage process*. It is hoped that added understanding of the dying process will allow health-care professionals and family members to provide for personalized care to the dying.

Today most people die in health-care institutions. One response to this practice is the development of hospice—a new caring community that provides medical and psychosocial care to the dying and their bereaved family members. The Earle Spring case involves the question of whether the decision to continue life-prolonging medical treatments should be in the hands of the individual, the family, the physicians, or the courts. This is especially problematic in cases involving incompetent patients. The living will represents a possible solution to such dilemmas in the future.

Recently, the morality of withholding food and hydration in the case of severely demented or comatose elderly has emerged. Do such provisions constitute life-sustaining medical treatment? In the case of Clair Conroy, the Supreme Court of New Jersey ruled that artificial feeding, like other life-sustaining medical treatment, may be withheld from an incompetent patient if it represents a disproportionate burden.

STUDY QUESTIONS

1. Explain how the meanings individuals give to death vary as a function of age. Describe the two meanings of death found to have particular significance for the elderly.

2. Note some symptoms associated with the grieving process. Differentiate bereavement, grief, and mourning.

3. What factors might influence the expression of grief among the elderly? What is meant by a devious pattern of grief? Note various factors that might influence the resolution of grief.

4. Define the dying trajectory. What role does perception play in staff and patient definitions of the dying trajectory? What cues contribute to the perception of the dying trajectory?

5. Discuss Gustafson's concept of dying as a career timetable. How is bargaining used to manipulate the timetable?

6. List and explain the five stages of the dying process as conceptualized by Elisabeth Kubler-Ross. What has been the reaction to the stage theory of dying?

7. Define hospice, tracing its development in the United States. Explain how a hospice provides care for the terminally ill patient and his or her family.

8. Discuss the conflicting private and public interests involved in decisions about the continuance of life-prolonging medical treatments. Use the Spring and Saikewicz cases in your answer.

9. Explain the purpose of a living will. What are the arguments against the use of these instruments?

10. Present an overview of the Claire Conroy case. What has been the reaction to the Supreme Court of New Jersey's ruling in this case?

BIBLIOGRAPHY

Annas, G. 1985a. Fashion and freedom: When artificial feeding should be withdrawn. *American Journal of Public Health* 75:685.

――――. 1985b. When procedures limit rights: From Quinlan to Conroy. *Hastings Center Report* 15:24–26.

Back, K. 1965. Meaning of time in later life. *Journal of Genetic Psychology* 109:9–25.

Besdine, R. 1983. Decisions to withhold treatment from nursing home residents. *Journal of the American Geriatrics Society* 31:602.

Bluebond-Langner, M. 1977. Meanings of death to children. In H. Feifel (ed.), *New meanings of death*. New York: McGraw-Hill.

Brocklehurst, J., and Hanley, T. 1976. *Geriatric medicine for students*. Edinburgh: Churchill Livingston.

Bromberg, S., and Cassel, C. 1983. Suicide in the elderly: The limits of paternalism. *Journal of the American Geriatrics Society* 31:698–703.

Buckingham, R., Lack, S., Mount, B., MacLean, L., and Collins, J. 1976. Living with the dying. *Canadian Medical Association Journal* 115:1211–1215.

Feigenberg, L. 1977. *Terminalvard*. Lund: Liber Laromedel.

Frederick, J. 1976. Grief as a disease process. *Omega* 7:297–306.

――――. 1982–1983. The biochemistry of bereavement: Possible basis for chemotherapy. *Omega* 13:295–304.

Friedman, H., and DiMatteo, M. 1982. Interpersonal issues in health care: Healing as an interpersonal process. In H. Friedman and M. DiMatteo (eds.), *Interpersonal issues in health care*. New York: Academic Press, Inc.

Glantz, L., and Swazey, J. 1979. Decisions not to treat: The Saikewicz case and its aftermath. *Forum on Medicine* (January):22–32.

Glaser, B., and Strauss, A. 1966. *Awareness of dying*. Chicago: Aldine.

――――. 1968. *Time for dying*. Chicago: Aldine.

Goodstein, R. 1984. Grief reactions and the elderly. *Carrier Letter* 99:1–5.

Gorer, G. 1965. *Death, grief and mourning*. New York: Doubleday.

Greenblatt, J. 1978. The grieving spouse. *American Journal of Psychiatry* 135:43–47.

Greer, D., and Mor, V. 1985. How Medicare is altering the hospice movement. *Hastings Center Report* 15:5–9.

Groth-Junker, A., and McCusker, J. 1983. Where do elderly patients prefer to die? Place of death and patient characteristics of 100 elderly patients under the care of a home health care team. *Journal of the American Geriatrics Society* 31:457–461.

Gustafson, E. 1972. Dying: The career of the nursing home patient. *Journal Health Social Behavior* 13:226–235.

Helsing, G., and Szklo, M. 1981. Mortality after bereavement. *American Journal of Epidemiology* 114:41–52.

Kalish, R. 1976. Death and dying in a social context. In R. Binstock and E. Shanas (eds.), *Handbook of aging and the social sciences*. New York: Van Nostrand Reinhold Co.

Kalish, R., and Reynolds, D. 1976. *Death and ethnicity: A psychocultural study.* Los Angeles: University of Southern California Press.

Kart, C. 1981. In the matter of Earle Spring: Some thought on one court's approach to senility. *Gerontologist* 21:417–423.

Kastenbaum, R. 1966. *Death, society and human experience.* Columbus, Ohio: Charles E. Merrill.

Keddie, K. 1977. Pathological mourning after the death of a domestic pet. *British Journal of Psychiatry* 139:21–25.

Kubler-Ross, E. 1969. *On death and dying.* New York: Macmillan.

———. 1974. *Questions and answers on death and dying.* New York: Macmillan.

Levav, I. 1982. Mortality and psychopathology following the death of an adult child: An epidemiological review. *Israel Journal of Psychiatry and Related Sciences* 19:23–38.

Lieberman, S. 1978. Nineteen cases of morbid grief. *British Journal of Psychiatry* 132:159–163.

Lindemann, E. 1944. Symptomatology and management of acute grief. *American Journal of Psychiatry* 101:141–148.

Mace, N., Rabins, P., and Lucas, M. 1980. Areas of stress on families of dementia patients. Paper presented at the annual meeting of the Gerontological Society of America, San Diego.

Maris, R. 1981. *Pathways to suicide.* Baltimore, Md.: Johns Hopkins Press.

Masamba, J., and Kalish, R. 1976. Death and bereavement: The role of the Black church. *Omega* 7 (1):23–34.

McIntire, M., Angle, C., and Struempl, L. 1972. The concept of death in Midwestern children and youth. *American Journal of Diseases of Children* 123:527–532.

Metzger, A. 1979. A Q-methodological study of the Kubler-Ross stage theory. *Omega* 10:291–302.

Nagy, M. 1959. The child's theories concerning death. In H. Feifel (ed.), *The meaning of death.* New York: McGraw-Hill.

Nason, J.D. 1981. Respected elder or old person: Aging in a Micronesian community. In P.T. Amoss and S. Harrell (eds.), *Other ways of growing old: Anthropological perspectives.* Stanford, Calif.: Stanford University Press.

Nevins, M. 1985. Big brother at the bedside. *New Jersey Medicine* 82:950.

———. 1986. Analysis of the Supreme Court of New Jersey's decision in the Claire Conroy case. *Journal of the Amercian Geriatrics Society* 34:140–143.

Olins, N. 1986.. Feeding decisions for incompetent patients. *Journal of the American Geriatrics Society* 34:313–317.

Osterweis, M. 1985. Bereavement and the elderly. *Aging* 348:8–13.

Osterweis, M., Solomon, F., and Green, M. 1984. *Bereavement: Reactions, consequences and care: A report of the Institute of Medicine.* Washington, D.C.: National Academy Press.

Robbins, L., West, P., and Murphy, G. 1977. The high rate of suicide in older white men: A study testing ten hypotheses. *Social Psychiatry* 12:1–20.

Roth, J. 1963. *Timetables*. Indianapolis, Ind.: Robbs–Merrill.

Rowland, K. 1977. Environmental events predicting death for the elderly. *Psychological Bulletin* 84:349–372.

Schneider, A., and Garron, D. 1980. Problems of families in recognizing and coping with dementing disease. Paper presented at the annual meeting of the Gerontological Society of America, San Diego.

Schulz, R. 1978. *The psychology of death, dying and bereavement*. Reading, Mass.: Addison-Wesley.

Schulz, R., and Aderman, D. 1974. Clinical research and the stages of dying. *Omega* 5:137–144.

Shneidman, E. 1980. *Voices of death*. New York: Harper and Row.

Steinbock, B. 1983. The removal of Mr. Herbert's feeding tube. *Hastings Center Report* 13:13–16.

Tehan, C. 1985. Has success spoiled hospice? *Hastings Center Report* 15:10–13.

Weisman, A. 1972. *On dying and denying*. New York: Behavioral Publications.

EPILOGUE

CAREERS IN THE
AGING NETWORK

There is no clear consensus on what a degree or certificate in gerontology especially qualifies a person to do. Certainly, there are very few jobs titled "gerontologist." Does this mean that students in gerontology degree programs, or those interested in a career in aging, are being prepared for jobs that do not exist? Not at all! Hundreds of thousands of Americans earn their livelihood working with and for aged people.

Virtually every department in the executive branch of the federal government and a number of independent agencies are responsible for policies and programs meant to serve the elderly either directly or indirectly. These include the Departments of Health and Human Services (Medicare and Medicaid), Agriculture (food stamps), Housing and Urban Development (housing for the elderly and handicapped), and the Veterans Administration (pensions and medical care). The Departments of Transportation, Labor, Energy, Treasury, and Commerce also administer or monitor programs affecting the elderly. Moreover, state and local governments sponsor, monitor, and administer programs for older people.

The private sector also provides job opportunities in aging, including preretirement and retirement counseling, financial advising, and nursing home and health-care administration.

In a 1973 report, the U.S. Senate Special Committee on Aging estimated that by 1980 the need for new positions in the aging field would be significant. Estimates included 20,000 new managers of retirement housing, 25,000 new licensed practical nurses and 8,000 new registered nurses to handle the demand for nursing home care, and 17,000 recreation specialists to serve older people, to list a few. It is not clear that these needs were in fact met. Yet, we do know that the elderly population continues to grow, with expected dramatic increases in the population over seventy-five years of age.

Does this mean that finding a job in the aging field will be easy? Not necessarily. Recognition of the manpower needs in gerontology is widespread, and in recent years many students have sought training to prepare for entry into this job market. A recent survey found 1,155 college and university campuses on which at least one accredited course in gerontology was being taught annually (Peterson et al. 1987).

How can students best be prepared for the gerontological job market? First, they must obtain a clear picture of career alternatives in aging early enough in their academic lives so that they can obtain the best preparation for entry into the labor force. Part of this early preparation should involve contact with a general gerontological curriculum that contains information essential for all persons who will work with or for the elderly.

Finding a general gerontological curriculum, however, may not be as easy as it seems. A recent collaborative project of the Gerontological Society of America (GSA) and the Association for Gerontology in Higher Education (AGHE) (Johnson et al. 1980) found a consensus (defined by 90 percent agreement) to exist around the inclusion of only three topical areas in such a generalized curriculum: *psychology* of aging (with emphasis on normal changes), *health* and aging, and *biology* of (normal) aging.

In a survey of gerontology programs carried out by AGHE and the University of Southern California (USC), four courses were identified as most commonly offered and required in gerontological instruction programs in U.S. colleges and universities. An introductory course in social gerontology was the most frequently reported; 51 percent of gerontological instruction programs required it. A course on psychology of aging (50 percent) was second with biology/physiology of aging (42 percent), and sociology of aging (42 percent) courses following (Peterson et al. 1987).

Generally, content areas required by gerontology programs differ by a program's level of instruction. The core courses listed above were more likely to be required at the associate degree level than was the case at the bachelor's or master's level. For example, a social gerontology course was required by 75 percent of the associate degree programs, 67 percent of the bachelor's degree programs, and 39 percent of the master's degree programs. This suggests that students moving from an associate to a bachelor's level program, or from a bachelor's to a master's level, are likely to experience some repetition of course material.

Beyond the core courses, gerontological instruction programs show some variation in program level in substantive emphases. For example, associate degree programs are likely to include courses on death and dying (43 percent), nutrition (41 percent), and counseling (38 percent). On the other hand, master's degree programs provide more content in research methods (55 percent), public policy (36 percent), and statistics (26 percent).

Second, students must be made to understand the growing specialization in the field of gerontology and that different preparation may be necessary as careers in aging become further specialized. The collaborative project involving the Gerontological Society of America and AGHE (Johnson et al. 1980) has defined four different career clusters in gerontology. The *biomedical* career cluster involves direct contact with older people. The main foci of activity or inquiry include the biological aspects of aging and their effects on the health and physical functioning of the older person. Career examples include dieticians, nurses, physicians, and speech therapists. The *psychosocial* career cluster also involves direct contact with older people. Here the emphasis is on the psychological characteristics of the aged and the interplay among these characteristics and economic and familial situations and the effects of this interplay on the well-being of older people. Possible careers include clinical psychologist, social worker, retirement counselor, and legal advisor.

A third career cluster involves professional activities in the realm of the *socioeconomic environment*. Such professional activities may involve direct contact with the older person, but the emphasis is on the social, economic, and cultural aspects of the community and broader society and the effects of these on older people. Educators, program administrators, government officials, social workers, and sociologists exemplify professional groups concerned with the socioeconomic environment of older people.

A fourth career cluster involves the *physical environment* of older people. The main professional activity of careers in this cluster has to do with the natural and manufactured physical environment and the effects of this environment on older people. Architects, safety engineers, and transportation planners are professionals whose activities revolve around the relationship between people (including the elderly) and the physical environment.

Each career cluster demands different educational preparation, with some overlap. Table E-1 presents a comparison of areas of study considered essential for inclusion in a core curriculum and the curricula of three of the career clusters. Those topics included in the core curriculum (psychology of aging, health and aging, and the biology of aging) overlap somewhat with actual course offerings in U.S. gerontology programs referred to above and are also uniformly found in the curricula of the three career clusters. Only one additional topical area on the list, the demography of aging, is similarly included in the curricular content of all three career tracks. It is important to recognize that the consensus criterion used for inclusion in the curricular content of the career clusters is the same 90 percent agreement among experts used by GSA-AGHE in identifying topics to be included in a core gerontological curriculum. This standard is an arbitrary one. A number of additional topics were deemed essential for inclusion in the core curriculum (as well as in career clusters) by a relatively large proportion of experts in the GSA-AGHE project. Clearly, with a different standard (85 percent, for example), additional topics would have been included in the core curriculum. "Sensory change," "sociology of aging," and "mental health and illness" are examples of topical areas that would have been included

TABLE E-1 Comparison of Substantive Areas Deemed Essential for Inclusion in the Core Gerontological Curriculum and the Curricula of Three Career Clusters

Topics	Core	Biomedical	Psychosocial	Socioeconomic Environmental
Psychology of aging	yes	yes	yes	yes
Health and aging	yes	yes	yes	yes
Biology of aging	yes	yes	yes	yes
Demography of aging		yes	yes	yes
Mental health and illness		yes	yes	
Adaptive mechanism		yes	yes	
Sociology of aging		yes		yes
Environment and aging		yes		yes
Marital and family relationships			yes	yes
Sensory change		yes		
Health care and services		yes		
Nutrition and aging		yes		
Behavioral changes		yes		
Stress		yes		
Physiology of aging		yes		
Chronic conditions		yes		
Diseases of old age		yes		
Exercise physiology		yes		
Physical needs		yes		
Pathology		yes		
Pharmacology and aging		yes		
Cognition			yes	
Personality development			yes	
Economics of aging				yes
Attitudes toward aging and aged				yes
Public policy for aged				yes
Sociocultural context of aging				yes
Legislation concerning the aged				yes

Note: Inclusion is based on 90 percent agreement.

Source: Adapted from H.R. Johnson et al. 1980. Foundations for gerontological education. *Gerontologist* 20(3):25, Table III-9.

in the core curriculum if the arbitrary standard employed had been at 85 percent agreement.

Despite the emphasis on specialized training in gerontology, students should not lose sight of the value of a well-rounded, multidisciplinary undergraduate education. This undergraduate education should provide an appropriate grounding in the humanities and the social and natural sciences. Effective writing and communication skills, understanding of the research process and statistics, and familiarity with humanistic values should inform a student's gerontological expertise. In fact, given the availability and even the necessity of more specialized graduate training in gerontology for many positions in the field, the development of writing, communication, research and statistics skills—as well as broad contact with the humanities—should not be subordinate to specialized training in gerontology in the undergraduate curriculum.

A third component of proper preparation for entry into the gerontology job market includes job experience. Many college graduates, regardless of their field of study, often run into a barrier caused by their lack of experience when they seek their first professional-level job. Gerontology students are no exceptions. They may attempt to gain experience by taking a job below their level of training, or they may become discouraged and take a position unrelated to their field of study.

Field placements or job internships are frequently part of basic and specialized programs in gerontology. Such placements can give students a chance to sample work in the field of aging, while at the same time providing excellent job experience. Field placements and job internships that most effectively fulfill these functions are those that involve direct contact with older people while providing close supervision and allowing for continued evaluation of student progress. Table E-2 lists a variety of strategies for ensuring the most desirable characteristics in field placements and job internships. Obviously, careful planning is important, as well as "open and continuous communication between and among program faculty, staff of the placement institution and . . . students" (Johnson et al. 1980, 36).

A cautionary note about field placements is in order. Experience with the elderly may not be the most effective teacher. Placements in which students see older people only as dependent and sick may only serve to reinforce already held stereotypes. As described in Chapter 1, the consensus of third-year medical students was that 50 percent of the elderly are in ill health and as many as half of these were in institutional settings. Clearly this is not the case. Just as clearly, however, such an estimate was consistent with the nature of the contact these students had with older people in the hospital clinics where students received the bulk of their medical training. How many other students in job placements or internships associated with preparation for a career in the service of older people are similarly affected?

Field placements and job internships are likely to become more important components of gerontological education programs in the future. Effective use of such program components may be an appopriate strategy for dealing with the concerns expressed by groups in the gerontological community at the 1981 White House Conference on Aging. According to Harold Johnson (1982), a number of conference recommendations in the area of education were rooted in a general dissatisfaction with the quality of personnel serving the elderly. Unhappiness with health-care personnel in particular was expressed at committee meetings and in committee reports. Several recommendations call for expanding and strengthening the gerontological training of personnel serving the elderly. Moreover, as Johnson points out, more strident members of the

TABLE E-2 Ways Suggested to Ensure Desired Field Placement Characteristics

Communication

Install written "contract" between educational institution and placement institution regarding expectations, content, and supervision.

Have faculty present written objectives to agency and to students.

Require three-way agreement between student, school, and agency, plus ongoing communication.

Clearly define procedures between university and agency.

Arrange regular contact between agency staff and university.

Supervision

Use faculty as supervisor or as liaison.

Monitor continuously.

Put multidisciplinary program committee in charge.

Make field coordinator (liaison) a full-time position.

Make randomly timed visits.

Develop criteria for supervisors at setting.

Give adjunct university appointments to field work supervisors.

Hold periodic conferences between university and supervisor.

Have good people in charge—person with rank, pay, motivation, and intelligence.

Assess student's progress regularly.

Planning

Contract placements thoughtfully.

Establish accreditation procedures, criteria for placements.

Conduct on-site observation before assignment.

Match student and placement carefully.

Have people knowledgeable about agency do the planning.

Involve older persons in planning.

Commitment

Arrange performance contract between university and agency.

Reward faculty who are good teachers of practice.

Educational institution should assist agency, give time and effort to build mutuality.

Pay agency (dollars, consulting time, tuition breaks) for their cooperation.

Agency must be committed to student; they should assign responsibility for students to their own staff.

Obtain student stipends.

Other

Develop field manuals.

Use stable agencies, not ones in survival struggle.

Hold regular class periods to discuss topics of mutual interest.

Use students' abilities to fullest.

Require interview between student's adviser and agency.

Involve students in activities relevant to their goals.

Source: H.R. Johnson et al. 1980. Foundations for gerontological education. *Gerontologist* 20(3):37, Table III-18. Copyright The Gerontological Society of America, used with permission.

gerontological community proposed licensure requirements based on geron-
tological/geriatric training, especially for those in the health-care field, including
physicians and nurses.

I will briefly describe some careers in aging in one field, health care. Much
has been written about the inadequacy of health care for the elderly. One
crucial factor in the delivery of geriatric health care is the lack of availability
of adequately trained personnel. Further, a criticism of proposals for national
health policies in the United States is that they concentrate on the problem of
paying for health care and ignore the need to produce additional health services
for those populations, including some subpopulations of the elderly, who do
not have access to health-care services.

PHYSICIANS

Only a small number of physicians in this country practice geriatric medicine.
Further, a 1977 physician survey conducted by the American Medical Association found that fewer than 0.6 percent of the respondents indicated an
interest in geriatrics. Traditionally, the specialty of geriatrics has lacked prestige
and has been seen by prospective physicians as an unrewarding area in which
to work. Libow (1977) believes attitudes toward geriatrics may be changing.
He surveyed students in eight medical schools and found 75 percent of them
desirous of having a full course in geriatrics; 72 percent wanted to take an
elective course dealing with the elderly at some time in their clinical training.
Libow recommends a department of geriatrics in every medical school and
hospital.

Geriatrics seems to be a field that should grow if only to keep pace with
growing numbers of elderly. Kane and his colleagues (1981) have attempted
to make some manpower projections on the need for geriatricians in the United
States. Actually, they make four sets of projections based on four different
levels of geriatric activity in the United States, as follows:

1. A continuation of the current care-delivery pattern, with essentially no
   specially trained geriatricians
2. Geriatricians trained primarily for academic positions, but with some inevitable spillover into practice
3. Academic geriatricians plus a trained cohort of geriatric consultants, as are
   found in much of Western Europe
4. Geriatricians in academic roles and actively involved in practice as both
   consultants and providers of substantial amounts of primary care

Kane and his associates believe that about 1,500 geriatricians need to be trained
just to staff existing training programs in internal medicine and family practice,

as well as to provide a core group of geriatricians in each medical school. In addition, they project a need for 16,000 geriatricians today if we want geriatricians rendering some primary care to those in the population who are sixty-five years of age and older. A more intermediate estimate of need is for about 8,000 additional geriatricians by the year 1990, though even this intermediate estimate assumes that most specialized geriatric care will be directed at persons aged seventy-five and older; that there will be a moderate degree of delegation of care to nurse practitioners, clinical specialists, physician's assistants, and social workers; and, finally, that there be some increment of improved care for the elderly.

NURSES

In 1968 a geriatric nursing practice division was established by the American Nurses Association (ANA). In 1974 the *Guidelines for Geriatric Nursing Practices* were developed, and the ANA now certifies qualified nurses and nurse practitioners in geriatrics. Although geriatric courses are being added to nursing curricula, too few schools have a specialty in geriatrics. Three types of programs awarding different credentials prepare their graduates for licensure as registered nurses:

1. Hospital-based programs are usually three academic years in length and lead to a diploma.
2. Programs located at community colleges are two academic years and lead to an associate degree.
3. Programs located in colleges and universities most often lead to a four-year baccalaureate degree.

By 1981 there were about 1,400 nursing education programs preparing their graduates for licensure as registered nurses in the United States. The trend in nursing education is toward preparation in academic institutions. The number of baccalaureate programs has more than doubled in the past twenty years, to almost 400 by 1981. These programs differ from diploma and associate degree programs in two important ways: They prepare students to function as public health nurses in community settings as well as to provide service in institutional facilities, and they provide the base for advanced study in a clinical or functional area like geriatrics (U.S. Department of Health and Human Services 1982).

Qualified geriatric nurses are at a premium at all levels of training. This is especially the case at the baccalaureate, master's, and doctoral levels. A recent report on nurse supply, distribution, and requirements made by the U.S. Department of Health and Human Services (1982) to the Congress projected that the supply of baccalaureate nurses in 1990 (approximately 350,000) would be less than half of what would be required (747,000). For the master's and doctoral

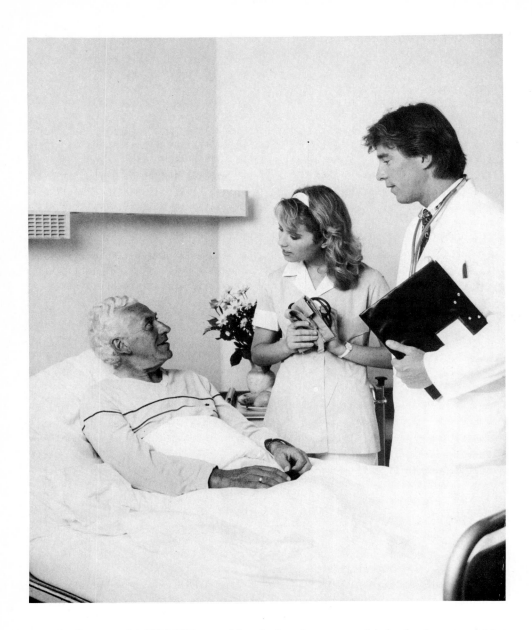

group, the supply (106,000) would only be about one-third of what would be required (270,000).

Geriatric nurses can form the backbone of care for the elderly in the community as well as in the institutionalized setting. The geriatric nurse is in a position to oversee primary nursing care of the institutionalized elderly and thus upgrade the care provided in nursing homes. Similar opportunities exist for visiting nurses for the homebound elderly.

Although they constitute a small fraction of the registered nurse work force, nurse practitioners also have significant potential for serving the elderly in a variety of settings. Nurse practitioners are registered nurses whose additional formal training prepares them for expanded nursing care functions, especially in the diagnosis and treatment of patients. In addition to delivering the traditional nursing services, they are qualified to perform some services more often delivered by physicians, such as managing self-limiting conditions and stabilized chronic illness. Their potential for serving the elderly is great because the scope of their practice is necessarily broad; they can facilitate movement into the health-care delivery system and provide continuity within the system as the patient moves from one part of the system to another (U.S. Department of Health and Human Services 1982).

There are approximately 200 nurse practitioner training programs in the United States. The majority of these programs lead to a certificate, though many do lead to a master's degree and the rate of growth in the latter type has been greater in recent years. It is noteworthy that programs established in the early years of the nurse practitioner movement focused primarily on pediatric practice. More recently, the specialty emphasis has shifted to family and adult health, which encompasses the geriatric population (U.S. Department of Health and Human Services 1982). This trend is likely to continue.

A very small proportion of currently employed nurses describe themselves as *nurse clinicians* or *clinical nurse specialists*. As the titles imply, these nurses are expected to be expert in a clinical practice area. Nurse clinicians and clinical nurse specialists provide patient care and, through teaching and by example, develop the competencies of less experienced nurses and students to meet the needs of patients whose nursing care management requires special knowledge and skills (U.S. Department of Health and Human Services 1982). This career title is likely to increase in importance within the nursing profession. Indeed, there is already some pressure to increase the supply of nurse clinicians with advanced training. One recommendation made by the Department of Health and Human Services (1982) in its 1982 report to the Congress, mandated by the Nurse Training Act of 1975, was as follows:

> The number of nurses with advanced nurse training should be augmented to assure sufficient numbers of expert clinicians, particularly in acute care settings, to direct the learning and clinical practice of students and to effect changes in the delivery of services both in institutions and community settings.

An important growth area here is likely to be the nursing home sector, where expertise in geriatric nursing is a critical element in maintaining patients at a maximum level of productive functioning.

GERIATRIC SOCIAL WORKERS

The vulnerability of many older people, the impact of their problems on family, community, and the broader society, and their relative lack of knowledge about how to secure the services they require make the aging population a prime concern of social work (Brody 1977). As Elaine Brody (1977, 73) has indicated, "On all levels, social work is an essential ingredient of health care and welfare systems and should have a major role in the identification of problems and in the delivery of preventive, supportive, and restorative services." Nevertheless, as recently as 1977, the National Association of Social Workers (NASW) issued a policy statement acknowledging that social work, along with some other disciplines, had "failed to recognize its unique contributions among the professions to the improvement of the quality of life for older Americans" (NASW 1977). In 1981 social work educators interested in gerontology and geriatric social work formed the National Committee for Gerontology in Social Work Education. The purpose of the committee was to promote the development of a gerontological focus in social work education (Nelson 1983).

In all its traditional forms—individual and group services, community organization, policy formulation, education and research—social work can participate in recognizing the potential of older people and in helping them overcome the prominent myths about the aged. The social worker who works with the elderly, sometimes referred to as a geriatric social worker, will likely require a Master of Social Work degree (MSW) and, no doubt, some positions will demand a specialization in geriatric or medical social work. Such specialization will be developed through course work and experience in the MSW curriculum or through a certificate program. This individual will be an expert on the variety of human resources available in the local community. These include nutrition programs, transportation services, home health services, homemaker services, and income sources. The social worker affiliated with a health-care institution assumes responsibility for all intake procedures, case work, and group work with patients and their families.

The geriatric social worker is often able to assume the role of an objective patient advocate. The aged (especially those who are ill) may be economically, socially, or psychologically vulnerable. They have little power or connections to power. One satisfaction of working in this field is that frequently the social worker can get the system that oppresses to work for the people who are most often oppressed. As Nelson (1983) has indicated, work force demands for gerontological and geriatric social workers will be a product of the growth of the aging population and governmental and private sector responses to the needs of the elderly. In 1980, the Administration on Aging provided $17 million to an estimated 14,000 individuals at fifty-eight institutions as part of the effort to encourage institutions and individuals to enter the field of gerontology. Social work majors led the list of those receiving these training monies and, according to one report (cited in Nelson 1983), approximately one-half of those who received gerontological training were working in the field of gerontology after graduation. The most frequently identified employment locations were human service agencies, hospitals and nursing homes, educational institutions and libraries, and government. Job activities included planning, evaluation and advocacy, direct service provision, counseling the elderly, supervision of direct services, provision of specialized service, research, and teaching (Nelson 1983).

What about the future? Recently, the Bureau of Labor Statistics published a list of the twelve fastest growing occupational titles. Geriatric social work was identified as one of the leading growth areas. The majority of jobs were in the high technology area, including industrial robot production; but geriatric social work was projected to account for 700,000 jobs by 1990. Unfortunately, cutbacks in the funding of social and health service programs by the Reagan administration should take some of the sheen off of these projections. Nevertheless, there definitely seems to be a place for gerontological and geriatric social work in the field of aging and the future job marketplace.

Many allied health specialists and others work with an elderly clientele. These include nurse practitioners, physician assistants, occupational therapists, speech therapists, geriatric aides, home health aides, physical therapists, recreation therapists, family and spiritual counselors, and a long list of other professions. These positions have wide and varying educational requirements and responsibilities on the health-care team. Although we cannot provide a detailed description of the career opportunities in each category, with patience, proper evaluation, and realistic goals, each can make an important contribution to geriatric health care.

BIBLIOGRAPHY

Brody, Elaine M. 1977. Aging. In J.B. Turner (ed.), *Encyclopedia of Social Work* (17th issue). Washington, D.C.: National Association of Social Workers.

Johnson, H.R. 1982. Perspectives on the 1981 White House Conference on Aging: Education. *Gerontologist* 22(2):125–126.

Johnson, H.R., Britton, J., Lang, C., Seltzer, M., Stanford, E., Yancik, R., Maklan, C., and Middleworth, A. 1980. Foundations for gerontological education. *Gerontologist* 20(3):1–61.

Kane, R.L., Solomon, D.H., Beck, J., Keeler, E., and Kane, R. 1981. *Geriatrics in the United States*. Lexington, Mass.: Lexington Books, D.C. Heath.

Libow, L. 1977. The issues in geriatric medical education and postgraduate training: Old problems in a new field. *Geriatrics* 32(2):99–102.

National Association of Social Workers. 1977. *NASW News* 22(3):17–18.

Nelson, G.M. 1983. Gerontological social work: A curriculum review. *Educational Gerontology* 9:307–322.

Peterson, D., Douglass, E., Bolton, C., Connelly, J., and Bergstone, D. 1987. *Gerontology instruction in American institutions of higher education: A national survey.* Washington, D.C.: Association for Gerontology in Higher Education and the University of Southern California.

U.S. Department of Health and Human Services. 1982. *Nurse supply, distribution and requirements: 3rd report to the Congress.* Hyattsville, Md.: Public Health Service, Division of Nursing.

GLOSSARY

Abkhasians The long-lived people of the Soviet state of Georgia; they attribute their longevity to practices in sex, work, and diet.

accommodating environment A model that assumes that all aspects of the environment (including the resident) will change over time.

activity limitation Limitations in activities of daily living, work outside the home, and housekeeping.

activity theory Often referred to as the implicit theory of aging, this theory states that there is a positive relationship between activity and life satisfaction. According to this theory, the individual who is able to maintain the activities of the middle years for as long as possible will be well adjusted and satisfied with life in the later years.

acute brain syndrome Reversible organic brain syndrome caused by the impairment of brain cell function. Specific cause may include alcoholism, drug abuse, and malnutrition.

acute illness A condition, disease, or disorder that is temporary.

Administration on Aging An administrative unit within the Department of Health and Human Services (formerly HEW) that oversees the operation of various services and programs provided in the Older Americans Act.

age composition Involves a quantitative description of the proportions of young and old people in a society. A population's age composition depends first on its level of fertility and only secondarily on mortality.

aged family Family in which the head of household is aged sixty-five or older.

Age Discrimination Employment Act A federal law passed in 1967 and amended several times since. The law prohibits discrimination in hiring, firing, and conditions of employment on the basis of age.

aged subculture Concept proposed by the sociologist Arnold Rose. It is based on the premise that, because of changes in the aged population and U.S. society, the aged have developed their own norms, system of stratification, and consciousness.

age-integrated environments Environments in which people of all ages live, work, and interact together.

ageism A term coined by Robert Butler to describe negative attitudes toward aging and the aged.

age-segregated environments Environments in which people of certain age groups live separated from individuals of other ages.

age-specific life expectancy The average duration of life expected for an individual of a given age.

age stratification A concept that perceives society as divided on the basis of age with each age stratum having its own set of rights, obligations, and opportunities.

aging group consciousness Arnold Rose believed that the development of an aged subculture would stimulate a group identification and consciousness among older people with the potential for social action.

Alzheimer's disease A progressively deteriorating form of senile dementia of unknown etiology. It involves a diminution of intellectual capabilities, memory loss, impaired judgment, and personality change.

ancestry group Defined by individuals in terms of the nation or nations of family origin.

antediluvian theme Involves the belief that people lived much longer in the past.

antioxidant A substance that prevents or retards cellular oxidation.

aphasia A term used to denote impaired ability to comprehend or express verbal language, and a clinical feature of stroke in many elderly victims.

appropriate death A concept developed by Avery Weisman. Such a death means that the person has died in a fashion that resembles as much as possible the way that he or she wished to die.

arteriosclerosis A generic term indicating a hardening of or loss of elasticity of the arteries.

arthritis Inflammation or degenerative joint change often characterized by stiffness, swelling, and joint pain. Some forms of arthritis are believed to be "autoimmune diseases."

atherosclerosis A condition whereby the inner wall of an artery becomes thickened by plaque formation.

autoimmune theory This theory maintains that, because of "copying errors" in repeated cell divisions, protein enzymes produced by newer cells are literally not recognized by the body. This brings the body's immunologic system into play, forcing it to work against itself.

baby boom A term often used to describe the higher fertility rates in the years immediately following World War II.

benefit periods Hospital insurance benefits under Part A of Medicare are measured by periods of time known as benefit periods. Benefit periods begin when a patient enters the hospital and end when he or she has not been a hospital patient for sixty days.

bereavement Refers to the experience of getting over another person's death. In part, the character that bereavement takes is shaped by society. Physical symptoms such as shortness of breath and psychological distress may accompany bereavement.

biological aging A term often used to describe the postmaturational changes in physical appearance and capability.

brain death A recently formulated conception of death that replaces the traditional heart death definition. Criteria include coma, apnea, cerebral unresponsivity, dilated pupils, absence of reflexes, and electrocerebral silence.

breakthrough policy A piece of governmental legislation that involves the federal government in providing or guaranteeing some fundamental benefit.

cataracts The most common disability of the aged eye. The normally transparent lens of the eye becomes opaque and interferes with the passage of rays of light to the retina.

centenarians Those who live one hundred years or more.

cerebrovascular disease A term used to describe impaired brain cell circulation. When a portion of the brain is completely denied blood, a cerebrovascular accident or stroke occurs.

chronic illness   A condition, disease, or disorder that is permanent or that will incapacitate an individual for a long period of time.

cohort   The term used for a group of persons born at approximately the same time. Although broadly defined, no two birth cohorts can be expected to age in the same way; each has a particular history and arrives at old age with unique experiences.

cohort-centric   Describes the fact that people in the same place on the life-course dimension experience historical events similarly and as a result may come to see the world in a like fashion.

collagen   A protein fiber distributed in and around the walls of blood vessels and in connective tissue, which has been implicated in age-related changes in physiological functions.

conductive hearing loss   Hearing loss resulting from the interrupted conduction of sound waves.

congestive heart failure   A state of circulatory congestion produced by the impaired pumping action of the heart.

constituency-building policy   A governmental policy that recognizes that different groups can have a common interest and allows "space" for these interest groups in the making of policy.

content analysis   A research technique that involves analyzing the content of records or documents.

constant environment   A model of the physical and social environment that assumes that the needs of residents remain relatively stable over time.

cross-cultural study   A method that involves gathering comparable data from different societies to test hypotheses, for example, about the status of the aged.

cross-sectional research   Studies based on observations representing a single point in time. Studies employing this research design are useful for emphasizing differences.

cultural pluralism   A situation in which ethnic groups may be able to retain their cultural uniqueness.

day care   Includes a wide range of services for older people who have some mental or physical impairments but who can remain in the community if supportive services are provided.

dementing illness   Any disease that produces a decline in intellectual abilities of sufficient severity to interfere with social or occupational functioning (memory disorder is usually prominent).

demographic transition   A three-stage conceptual model of population growth.

demography   The study of the size, territorial distribution, and composition of population and the changes therein.

dependency ratio   The ratio of the population of ages too young or too old to work to the population of working age.

depression   The most common functional psychiatric disorder among older people; it can vary in duration and degree and show psychological as well as physiological manifestations.

diagnostic-related groups (DRGs)   A categorization scheme for illnesses and injuries, which forms the basis for the prospective-payment system that fixes Medicare hospital payment rates in advance.

disengagement theory   Developed by Cumming and Henry, this theory postulates that aging involves a mutual withdrawal between the older person and society.

double jeopardy   A term used to reflect the idea that the negative effects of aging are compounded among minority group members.

the dying career   A concept used by Gustafson; she views the last phase of life as a career that moves in a series of related and regressive stages toward death.

dying trajectory   A term used by Glaser and Strauss to describe the dying process. All dying processes take time and can be visualized as having a certain shape through time. The combination of duration and shape can be charted as a trajectory.

early retirement   Retirement before that mandated by age or tenure.

ego integrity   Key concept in Erikson's eighth age that describes a basic acceptance of one's life as appropriate and meaningful.

empirical method   A broad category that includes quantitative and qualitative research techniques that can be replicated by many.

enabling factors   A term used by Andersen to describe individual characteristics and circumstances (for example, family income, accessibility of health service) that might hinder or accelerate use of a health service.

enculturation   The process by which new generations come to adopt traditional ways of thinking and behaving.

enryo   A norm brought from Japan and still in existence in the United States. It is related to power and regulates how those with it are to behave toward those without it. In the Japanese family and community, power and privileges are associated with the father.

environmental discontinuity   The degree of change between a new and an old environment that may explain the effects observed after institutionalization.

environmental docility hypothesis   "The less competent the individual, the greater the impact of environmental factors on the individual." (Lawton, M., and Simon, B. 1968. The ecology of social relationships in housing for the elderly. *Gerontologist* 8:108–115.)

ERISA   The Employee Retirement Income Security Act, passed by Congress in 1974, to establish minimum standards for private pension programs.

error catastrophe   Maintains that aging results from mutations.

exchange theory   A social–psychological theory recently applied to the situation of the aged. The basic assumption of the theory is that people will attempt to maximize benefits from an interaction while incurring the least costs.

extended care facility   Long-term care facility equipped to provide skilled nursing care around the clock.

extended family   Three or more generations living together in one household.

family dependency ratio   Defined in simple demographic terms (for example, population aged sixty-five to seventy-nine to population aged forty-five to forty-nine), this ratio crudely illustrates the shifts in the ratio of elderly parents to the children who would support them.

family life cycle   A concept used by family sociologists to characterize the changes that families undergo from their establishment through the postparental stage.

family of orientation   The family one is born into.

family of procreation   The family that adults form at the time of marriage.

fertility rate   The number of births that occur in a year per 1,000 women of childbearing age.

fibroblasts   Embryonic cells that give rise to connective tissue.

field research   A research strategy that is "observation-centered" and allows the researcher to establish close contact with subjects and their actions.

filial piety   Reflects the respect and deference owed to one's elders, perhaps especially to a father. Filial piety is most often present in traditional societies dominated by a patriarchal social order.

foster care   Use of private residences for the care of a nonrelated elderly person who needs supervision or assistance with daily living activities.

fountain theme   Based on the idea that there is some unusual substance that has the property of greatly increasing the length of life.

free radicals   Highly unstable molecules containing an unpaired electron. Their presence reduces cellular efficiency and causes an accumulation of cellular waste that may lead to cell aging.

fund of sociability hypothesis   According to this idea, there is a certain quantity of interaction with others that people require and that they may achieve in a variety of ways—either through one or two intense relationships or through a larger number of less intense relationships.

geriatric day center   An alternative to an extended care facility, such a center may provide care on an eight-hour-a-day, five-day-a-week basis.

geriatrics   A subfield of gerontological practice, the medical care of the aging.

gerontological gender gap   Term used by Hess to describe the differential application of federal programs to the elderly such that older women are disadvantaged in the areas of income, health, and housing.

Gerontological Society of America   The dominant professional society in the field of gerontology. Incorporated in 1945, it publishes the *Journal of Gerontology* and *The Gerontologist*.

gerontology   The systematic study of the aging process.

gerontophilia   Respect and reverence for the aged.

gerontophobia   A fear of and negative attitude toward the aged.

glaucoma   The most serious eye disease affecting the aged, it results from an increase in pressure within the eyeball.

gray lobby   A term used to describe all the groups and organizations that purport to represent the interests of the elderly.

health   Defined by the World Health Organization as "a state of complete physical, mental, and social well-being and not merely the absence of disease or infirmity."

heart failure   Condition where the heart fails to pump blood efficiently; fluid accumulates in peripheral tissues and lungs, producing edema and shortness of breath.

hemodialysis   The removal of waste products from the blood by mechanical means.

hidden poor   Those living in institutions or with relatives and not counted among the aged poor.

home health care   The provision of coordinated multidisciplinary services including skilled nursing and therapeutic services as well as social casework, mental health, legal, financial and personal care, and household management assistance.

hospice A facility that specializes in caring for and treating terminally ill patients and their families.

housing poor Defined as living in a housing unit with a deficiency in the physical condition of the unit, a high degree of overcrowding, or an inability of the household to afford the unit.

Hunza A group of allegedly long-lived people in the mountains of Kashmir, Pakistan.

hyperborean theme Involves the idea that in some remote part of the world there are people who enjoy a remarkably long life.

hypertension High blood pressure.

hypochondriasis Overconcern for one's health, usually accompanied by delusions about physical dysfunction or disease.

identity continuity theory Put forth by Robert Atchley, this theory argues that few people rest their entire self-identities on the work role. Most people have several roles on which identity is based; thus, they are able to adjust to retirement and gain self-respect and self-esteem from leisure pursuits.

identity crisis theory Because occupational identity is so much a part of a person's life, Stephen Miller argues, retirement necessarily brings an identity crisis. According to this theory, leisure roles cannot be expected to replace work as a source of self-respect and identity.

income replacement rate A term often used to describe the income position of a retiree relative to the income position of the individual before retirement. A replacement rate of 50 percent would indicate that a retiree received an income that was 50 percent of his or her preretirement earnings.

index of correlation A measure of the relationship between two interval level variables. The strength of a correlation ranges from .00, meaning no correlation, to 1.0, meaning a perfect correlation.

infant mortality Often used as a simple measure of the general welfare of a population, it usually reflects the number of infant deaths in a given year by the number of live births registered during that year.

in-kind income Income received indirectly or in the form of goods and services that are free or at reduced cost.

innate heat Believed by Hippocrates to be the essential factor in life. Individuals were believed to have a fixed quantity of this life force, and aging was equated with its continuous diminishment.

interiority of the personality Concept used by Neugarten to describe age-related increase in introspection, contemplation, reflection, and self-evaluation as characteristic forms of mental life.

intermediate nursing care Provision of health-related care and services (often in an institution) to those who need less than skilled nursing care but more than custodial care.

ischemic heart disease Another term for coronary artery disease. Tissue that is denied adequate blood supply is called ischemic.

laboratory experimentation A research technique that involves the systematic observation of phenomenon, under controlled conditions.

life expectancy Defined as the average number of years a person born today can expect to live under current mortality conditions.

life review Postulated by Robert Butler to describe an almost universal tendency of older persons toward self-reflection and reminiscence.

life span The extreme limit of human longevity, the age beyond which no one can expect to live.

life table Shows what the probability is of surviving from any age to any subsequent age based on the death rates at a particular time and place.

liquid assets Financial assets (for example, stocks or bonds) easily convertible to goods, services, or money.

living will A device used by some to attempt to specify the conditions under which they would prefer not to be subjected to extraordinary measures to keep them alive.

longitudinal research Studies designed to collect data at different points in time. This research design emphasizes the study of change.

lysosomes Saclike structures in the cell cytoplasm containing digestive enzymes that implement the breakdown of fats, proteins, and nucleic acids. Lysosomes have been implicated in cellular aging.

machismo An exaggerated manliness, with emphasis often placed on sexual prowess. From early childhood, Mexican American males, for example, are given more freedom than females receive and are expected to play a dominant role in the family.

maladjustment Behavior that does not completely satisfy the individual and social needs of the person.

malignant neoplasms Cancerous growth.

mandatory retirement Forced retirement, usually at age sixty-five or seventy.

Medicaid A public welfare program for indigent persons of all ages paid for with matching federal and state funds. Medicaid has become the principal public mechanism for funding nursing home care.

Medicare A federal insurance program financing a portion of the health-care costs of persons aged sixty-five and over.

melting pot A term often applied to the United States to describe a situation in which ethnic minorities lose their distinctive character and become assimilated into the broader culture.

menopause A term used to describe the conclusion of long-term changes in the female genital system. These changes usually progress at different rates in each individual. Menopause marks the end of childbearing potential.

migration Refers to the movement of populations from one geographical region to another.

minimum adequate diet Lowest cost food budget that could be devised to supply all essential nutrients using food readily purchasable in the U.S. market.

modernization theory Attempts to describe the relationship between societal modernization and the changes in role and status of older people. It holds that with increasing modernization the status of older people declines.

modified extended family A term used to describe several related nuclear families who do not share the same household but who do maintain strong kinship ties and have frequent social interaction and helping patterns.

morbidity The condition of being ill; often used to refer to the rate of illness per some unit of population in a society.

mortality crossover A concept used to describe the higher life expectancy and lower death rates of nonwhites of advanced ages relative to whites of similarly advanced ages.

mortality rate   The total number of deaths in society in a year per 1,000 individuals in the society.

mourning   Culturally patterned process by which grief is managed or resolved.

myth of desexualization   One stereotype of ageism: If you are old (or getting old), you are finished with sex.

National Institute of Aging   One of the institutes within the National Institutes of Health. Established in 1974, its mandate is to support research in the biomedical, social, and behavioral aspects of aging.

need factors   A term used by Andersen to describe subjective perceptions and judgments about the seriousness of illness symptoms and the need for health-care services.

nonliquid assets   Assets that are not easily convertible into cash.

normal distribution   An important theoretical model in statistics that assumes there is an average or central tendency around which are distributed higher and lower measurements. The normal distribution is often represented by the bell-shaped curve.

nuclear family   A family unit composed of husband, wife, and children.

nutrition   The science that deals with the effects of food on the body.

obesity   Excessive body fatness generally defined as a minimum of 15 to 20 percent overweight.

old age dependency ratio   Ratio of the population of those too old to work to the population of working age.

old age institution   A general term used to describe the entire array of rest homes and long-term care facilities for the aged.

old-old   Those seventy-five years of age and older.

organic brain syndrome (OBS)   A constellation of psychological or behavior signs and symptoms without reference to etiology.

organic mental disorder (OMD)   Designates a particular organic brain syndrome that has a known or presumed cause.

osteoarthritis   Degenerative joint change that takes place with aging. It is often referred to as "wear and tear arthritis."

osteomalacia   The adult equivalent of rickets or vitamin D deficiency.

osteoporosis   A demineralization of bone, often associated with aging.

palliative care   Care directed at symptom control rather than cure. Term is often used synonymously with hospice care.

paranoia   Form of psychopathology that involves delusions, usually of a persecutory nature.

Parkinson's disease   A common movement disorder among the elderly.

participant observation   A type of field research that includes observing and participating in events in a group.

pathological aging   As individuals grow older, they are more likely to become afflicted with diseases. Changes that occur as a result of disease processes may be categorized as relating to pathological aging.

period   The period of historical time through which a person lives influences how that person ages. Those who experience a historical point in time at different stages in the life cycle may be influenced differently.

periodontal disease   Pathology of the gum tissue.

peroxidation   Process of the transfer of oxidation out of the cell.

pneuma   A term used by Francis Bacon in place of the Greek notion of innate heat. Every body part was believed to contain a spirit; with use the spirits dissolved and, alas, old age ensued.

political economy   Critical approach that allows for broadly viewing old age and the aging process within the economic and political context of the society.

"poor dear" hierarchy   A status system based on the distribution of luck. Being relatively young, healthy, and close to one's children may be defined as having luck.

Poor Laws   Relief for the poor, passed during the reign of Elizabeth I.

population pyramid   A technique used to graphically depict the age and sex composition of a societal population.

portability   A term used to describe the rights of employees to transfer pension credits on a tax-free basis from one employer to another.

postparental family   That state of the family life cycle that occurs after the children have left home.

poverty index   An index developed by the Social Security Administration and based on the amount of money needed to purchase a minimum adequate diet as determined by the Department of Agriculture; it is the most frequently used measure of income adequacy.

predisposing factors   A term used by Andersen to describe social structural variables (for example, race, religion, ethnicity) as well as family attitudes and health beliefs that may predispose an individual to use health services even in the absence of symptoms of an illness episode.

preindustrial society   A premodern society characterized by a lack of technological sophistication.

preparatory depression   A type of depression, associated with the stages of dying, that takes impending losses into account. This depression prepares the individual for loss of all love objects.

presbycusis   Impaired hearing associated with aging.

presbyopia   Degenerative changes that occur in the aging eye.

prolongevity   A term used to describe attempts to significantly extend the length of the human life span.

proprietary nursing homes   Old-age institutions that are operated for profit.

prospective payment system   Medicare-based reimbursement system that fixes in advance how much payment a hospital will receive for care provided.

prostrate gland   A small gland that surrounds the base of the urethra in the male. It secretes a fluid that is discharged into the urethra at the time of emission of semen.

protective services   Visits by the social worker with supplemental community services such as visiting nurses, homemakers, clinical services, meals, telephone checks, and transportation.

psychological aging   A term often used to describe all the developmental processes, such as intellectual functioning and coping, that may be related to aging.

psychological autopsy   A method of inquiry in which researchers draw together medical, social, and psychiatric information about a patient in an attempt to understand the psychosocial context in which death occurs.

reaction time Measure of psychomotor performance affected by familiarity of task, practice at a task, task complexity, and other factors.

reactive depression A type of depression evident during the dying process that is a result of past losses. For example, the patient may have lost a job because of an inability to work.

respite care Temporary services that used trained sitters to provide relief for permanent caregivers of the frail elderly.

Retired Couple's Budget A measure of the adequacy of aged income used by the Bureau of Labor Statistics.

retirement community Any living environment to which most residents have relocated since retirement.

retirement test A "test" employed by the Social Security Administration to determine whether or not a person otherwise eligible for retirement benefits can be considered retired.

reverse annuity mortgage Mortgages under which a homeowner may sell some equity in his or her house and receive in return a fixed monthly sum based on a percentage of the current market value of the house.

rheumatoid arthritis A type of arthritis characterized by serious inflammation and joint destruction.

role loss Effect of life changes that involve loss of important social relationships and roles typical of adulthood.

role theory One of the earliest frameworks within which researchers in gerontology attempted to understand the adjustment of the aging individual. According to the theory, role loss (for example, retirement, widowhood) leads to maladjustment.

schizophrenia Chronic psychiatric disorder manifested by psychotic thinking, withdrawal, apathy, and impoverishment of human relationships.

secondary analysis A re-analysis of data produced by someone else.

selection bias Used in this context to describe those old people who may have characteristics that sensitize them to respond negatively to living in institutional settings.

self-mortification A process, associated by Erving Goffman with institutional settings, by which an individual is stripped of his or her identity.

senescence The term used by biological gerontologists to describe all the postmaturational changes in an individual.

senile macular degeneration Visual impairment as a result of damage to the macular area of the retina.

senile psychosis A common form of organic brain syndrome in the elderly, it is often characterized by progressive intellectual and cognitive impairments and by personality disorganization. The cause remains unknown. This condition is distinct from "senility," that all-too-frequently-used term that refers to mental incapacities believed to be associated with increased age.

senility A term often inappropriately used that describes all the age-related changes in intellectual functioning.

sensorineural hearing loss Hearing loss related to disorders of the inner ear where conducted sound vibrations are transformed into electrical impulses.

sex ratio The number of males for every one hundred females ($\times$ one hundred).

shared household   Two or more older persons (relatives or nonfamily members) who share a residence.

skilled nursing care   Typically offered in a specially qualified facility that has the staff and equipment necessary for providing high-level nursing care and rehabilitation services as well as other health services.

social gerontology   The study of the impact of social and sociocultural factors on the aging process.

social security   The colloquial term used to describe the Old Age Survivors, Disability, and Health Insurance (OASDHI) program administered by the federal government. The most well-known aspect of this program is the public retirement pension system, which provides income support to over 90 percent of U.S. elderly.

Social Security Act of 1935   The original piece of legislation, put forth by an advisory committee created by President Franklin D. Roosevelt, that created the so-called Social Security system. It has been amended and expanded numerous times. For example, Medicare and Medicaid represent Titles XVIII and XIX of the Social Security Act.

societal modernization   Perspective that looks to changes in the role and status of older people as society modernizes (in general, with increasing modernization the status of older people declines).

socio-environmental theory   A theory that is directed at understanding the effects of the immediate social and physical environment on the activity patterns of aged individuals.

sociological aging   A term often used to connote the role changes and adjustments associated with aging.

stages of dying   Prepared by Kubler-Ross, the most well-known conceptualization of the dying process. Dying is seen as a five-stage process through which most dying persons proceed.

status passage   Process of negotiating a passage from one age-based status to another, which may have both an objective and a subjective reality.

substitute judgment   A legal standard that allows for the substitution of another's judgment when a person is found to be incompetent.

Sun belt   Made up of those states in the southern and southwestern regions of the United States.

support system   System of relationships (friends, neighbors, and family) in which health and social services are provided to the aged.

Supplemental Security Income   A federal assistance program envisioned to supplement the existing incomes of eligible aged to bring them up to a minimal income level.

survey research   A currently popular form of social science research that involves collecting data directly from a representative sample of a relatively large population.

symbolic interactionism   A theoretical orientation based on the premise that people behave toward objects and others according to perceptions and meanings developed through social interaction.

total institution   An institutional setting within which the barriers that ordinarily separate the activities of work, play, and sleep are broken down so that all these activities take place in the same setting with the same people.

very-old Those aged eighty-five years and older.

vesting The nonforfeitable right of an individual to receive a future pension based on his or her earned credits, even if the individual leaves the job before retirement.

Vilacabamba A village in the Andean mountains of Ecuador where there is purported to be a high proportion of centenarians.

wear and tear theory of aging Theorists using this biological model of aging often employ machine analogies to exemplify the theory's underlying assumption that an organism wears out with use or stress.

widowhood Stage of life following the death of a spouse, which is experienced more by aged women than aged men.

young-old Those aged fifty-five to seventy-four years.

INDEX

Abkhasians, sexuality of, 86

Account of the State of the Body and Mind in Old Age, 25

Achenbaum, W.A., 204, 337–338, 340

Activity theory, 185–188, 209

Adams, John, 223

Adaptation: coping strategies for, 163; failure of, 178; life events model of, 178; to life stresses, 175–179; outcomes of, 176–178; styles of, 189

Adult day care, 421–422

Adult development stages, 141–142; theories of, 140–145

Age: change with, 38–39; changing attitudes toward, 4, 27; groupings by, 164; stratification, 204–208; veneration of, 4. *See also* Aging; Elderly

Age discrimination, 295–296, 309. *See also* Ageism

Age Discrimination Employment Act (ADEA), 295–296; amendments to, 299

Age mobility, 206–207

Aged population, 49–50; labor force participation of, 291–294, 309; negative attitudes toward, 3; number and proportion of, 46–49; trends in, 45–46. *See also* Elderly

Ageism, 3–4; late-life sexuality myths and, 86–87; perpetuation of, 4–5; subtlety of, 6–7; television viewing and, 6. *See also* Age discrimination

Age/period/cohort problem, 38–40

Agers, types of, 146

Age-vs.-need entitlement, 329–333

Aging: activity theory of, 185–188; age stratification and, 204–208; age/period/cohort problem in study of, 38–40; in ancient Greece and Rome, 23–24; antioxidants and, 97–98; biological, 27, 67–68, 94, 137–138; cellular theories of, 95–98; changing attitude toward, 4, 27; classic pattern of, 156; conferences on, 29; courses on, 29; demography of, 45–63; disengagement theory of, 187–190; due to accidental changes, 96–97; in early scientific era, 24–26; economics of, 208–209, 246–276; exaggerating effects of, 112–113; exchange theory of, 192–195; family life and, 217–240; fear of, 3; field research of, 31–33; free radicals and, 97; genetic programming for, 96; genital system changes with, 87–90; health policy and, 444–465; history of, 22–30; images of, 22–23; individual and, 184–197; laboratory experimentation in, 37–38; meaning of death and, 470–471; methodological issues in research of, 30–40;

Aging (continued):
modernization theory of, 200–204; myths of, 3–15; normal vs. pathological, 94; of older population, 49–50; personality types and, 146–148; physiological changes with, 77–86; physiological theories of, 98–101; political economy of, 208–209; politics of, 314–333; prolongevity theory of, 101–105; psychological changes with, 149–159; psychological study of, 26–27; psychology of, 137–159; questions about policy of, 209; in racial and ethnic groups, 359–383; religion and, 336–353; results of, 67–91; role theory of, 184–185; scientific study of, 40–41; senility and, 7–8; sexuality and, 86–90, 91; social aspects of, 163–179; society and, 197–210; socioenvironmental theory of, 190–192; sociological theories of, 183–210; study of, 5, 19–41; subculture of, 197–199, 210; survey research of, 35–37; symbolic interactionism and, 195–197; theories of, 94–105; in twentieth century, 26–30. *See also* Age; Elderly

Aging and Human Development, 28

Aging and Modernization, 200

Aging and Society, 28

Aging and the Professions, 28

Aging group consciousness, 328

Aging in Western Societies (Burgess), 28

Aging network, careers in, 494–505

Alcohol disorders, 124

Allied health specialists, 505

Alzheimer's dementia, 127–128, 131

American Association of Retired Persons (AARP), 29, 326

American family, old age and, 219–224. *See also* Family

American Geriatric Society, 28

American Medical Association, opposition of to Medicare, 454

American Society on Aging, 28

Ancestry groups, 59

Andersen, R., 452

Anderson, B., 228

Androgyny, 185

Angry agers, 146

Antediluvian theme, 19

Antioxidants, 97–98

Aphasia, 123–124

Archives, 33

Aristotle, 23